Important
Advances
in Oncology
1989

Edited by

Vincent T. DeVita, Jr., M.D.

Physician-in-Chief
Benno C. Schmidt Chair
  in Clinical Oncology
Memorial Sloan–Kettering Cancer Center
New York, New York

Samuel Hellman, M.D.

Dean and A.N. Pritzker Professor
Biological Sciences Division
  and Pritzker School of Medicine
Vice President for the Medical Center
The University of Chicago
Chicago, Illinois

Steven A. Rosenberg, M.D., Ph.D.

Chief of Surgery
National Cancer Institute
Professor of Surgery
Uniformed Services University of the Health
  Sciences School of Medicine
Bethesda, Maryland

35 Contributors

Important Advances in Oncology 1989

J. B. Lippincott Company

Philadelphia

Cambridge	London
New York	Singapore
St. Louis	Sydney
San Francisco	Tokyo

Sponsoring Editor: Richard Winters
Project Editors: Leslie E. Hoeltzel and Lynda Kenny
Manuscript Editor: Christy N. Wright
Indexer: Julia Schwager
Designer: Arlene Putterman
Production Manager: Carol A. Florence
Production Coordinator: Pamela Milcos
Compositor: TAPSCO, Inc.
Printer/Binder: Halliday Lithograph

6 5 4 3 2 1

ISSN 0883-5896
ISBN 0-397-51004-7

The authors and publisher have exerted every effort to ensure that
drug selection and dosage set forth in this text are in accord with
current recommendations and practice at the time of publication.
However, in view of ongoing research, changes in government
regulations, and the constant flow of information relating to drug
therapy and drug reactions, the reader is urged to check the
package insert for each drug for any change in indications and
dosage and for added warnings and precautions. This is
particularly important when the recommended agent is a new or
infrequently employed drug.

Contributors

Bruce N. Ames, Ph.D.
Professor and Chairman
Department of Biochemistry
University of California, Berkeley
Berkeley, California

John P. Bader, Ph.D.
Microbiologist, Laboratory of Molecular Oncology
National Cancer Institute
Bethesda, Maryland

Richard S. Bockman, M.D., Ph.D.
Associate Professor of Medicine
Cornell University Medical College
Head, Endocrine Service
The Hospital for Special Surgery
Associate Attending Physician
The New York Hospital
New York, New York

Paolo Boffetta, M.D., M.P.H.
Researcher, Unite of Cancer Epidemiology
University of Torino
Torino, Italy

Gianni Bonadonna, M.D.
Director, Division of Medical Oncology
Istituto Nazionale Tumori
Milano, Italy

Peter R. Carroll, M.D.
Assistant Professor of Urology
University of California, San Francisco
San Francisco, California

Jack S. Cohen, M.D.
Section Head, Biophysical Pharmacology Section
National Cancer Institute
Bethesda, Maryland

Graham A. Colditz, M.B., B.S., D.P.H.
Assistant Professor of Medicine
Harvard Medical School
Boston, Massachusetts

Neal G. Copeland, Ph.D.
Senior Scientist, Director–Mammalian Genetics
   Laboratory
BRI—Basic Research Program
NCI—Frederick Cancer Research Facility
Frederick, Maryland

Robert J. Fisher, Ph.D.
Biochemist, Laboratory of Molecular Oncology
National Cancer Institute
Bethesda, Maryland

Thomas W. Griffin, M.D.
Professor of Radiation Oncology
University of Washington School of Medicine
Seattle, Washington

Randall E. Harris, M.D., Ph.D.
Chief, Division of Epidemiology
American Health Foundation
New York, New York

Arnold M. Herskovic, M.D.
Associate Professor
Wayne State University
Detroit, Michigan

Amnon Hizi, Ph.D.
Department of Cell Biology and Histology
Sackler School of Medicine
Tel Aviv University
Ramat Aviv, Israel

Stephen H. Hughes, Ph.D.
Senior Scientist
National Cancer Institute
Frederick Cancer Research Facility
BRI—Basic Research Program
Frederick, Maryland

Nancy A. Jenkins, Ph.D.
Senior Scientist
Mammalian Genetics Laboratory
National Cancer Institute
Frederick Cancer Research Facility
BRI—Basic Research Faculty
Frederick, Maryland

V. Craig Jordan, Ph.D., D.Sc.
Professor of Human Oncology and Pharmacology
University of Wisconsin
Clinical Cancer Center
Madison, Wisconsin

Marc E. Lippman, M.D.
Director and Professor of Medicine
Lombardi Cancer Research Center
Georgetown University Medical Center
Washington, DC

Tom F. Lue, M.D.
Associate Professor of Urology
University of California, San Francisco
San Francisco, California

Connie Moore, M.D.
Assistant Professor of Psychiatry
Baylor College of Medicine
Houston, Texas

James J. Mulé, Ph.D.
Senior Staff Fellow
Surgery Branch, Division of Cancer Treatment
National Cancer Institute
Bethesda, Maryland

Norman D. Nigro, M.D.
Clinical Professor of Surgery
Wayne State University School of Medicine
Detroit, Michigan

Ian C. T. Nisbet, Ph.D.
President
I.C.T. Nisbet and Company, Inc.
Lincoln, Massachusetts

Takis S. Papas, Ph.D.
Chief, Laboratory of Molecular Oncology
National Cancer Institute
Bethesda, Maryland

Frederica P. Perera, D.P.H.
Associate Professor
Columbia University School of Public Health
New York, New York

Steven A. Rosenberg, M.D., Ph.D.
Chief of Surgery
National Cancer Institute
Professor of Surgery
Uniformed Services University of the Health
   Sciences School of Medicine
Bethesda, Maryland

Meir J. Stampfer, M.D., D.P.H.
Associate Professor of Epidemiology
Harvard School of Public Health
Assistant Professor of Medicine
Harvard Medical School
Boston, Massachusetts

C. A. Stein, M.D., Ph.D.
Senior Investigator, Medicine Branch
National Cancer Institute
Bethesda, Maryland

Sandra Meta Swain, M.D.
Director Comprehensive Breast Services
Assistant Professor of Medicine
Lombardi Cancer Research Center
Georgetown University Medical Center
Washington, D.C.

V. K. Vaitkeviceus, M.D.
Professor and Chairman
Department of Medicine
Wayne State University
Detroit, Michigan

Pinuccia Valagussa, B.S.
Chief, Operations Office
Istituto Nazional Tumori
Milano, Italy

Raymond P. Warrell, Jr., M.D.
Assistant Professor
Cornell University
School of Medicine
Associate Member
Memorial Sloan-Kettering Cancer Center
New York, New York

Walter C. Willett, M.D., D.P.H.
Professor of Epidemiology and Nutrition
Harvard Medical School
Boston, Massachusetts

Ernst L. Wynder, M.D.
President
American Health Foundation
New York, New York

Berton Zbar, M.D.
Chief, Cellular Immunity Section
Laboratory of Immunobiology
National Cancer Institute
Frederick Cancer Research Facility
Frederick, Maryland

Preface

Important Advances in Oncology 1989 is the fifth in a series of annual volumes, each of which contains the most significant changes in oncologic research and practice that have taken place during the preceding year. Each year the editors select approximately 15 areas of research and practice in which change has occurred, with each being described by one or more experts in that particular field. Topics are chosen for their currency and for their potential effect on the diagnosis, treatment, and prevention of cancer and on an understanding of its origins.

For the 1989 book, we have selected basic research that describes studies related to oncogenes and the mitogenic signal pathway; expression of the human immunodeficiency virus in *Escherichia coli;* chromosomal deletions in lung cancer and renal cancer; transgenic mice in cancer research; the potential therapeutic role of antisense compounds; and immunotherapy with lymphokine combinations.

The clinical progress section contains discussions of the treatment of patients with inflammatory breast cancer; the role of chemotherapy in stage I breast cancer; preservation of function in treatment of cancer of the anus; long-term tamoxifen therapy for breast cancer; treatment of impotence in cancer patients; gallium in the treatment of hypercalcemia and bone metastasis; and the status of clinical trials with neutron irradiation.

This year's volume marks the introduction of a new section that will address controversies in oncology. Chapters in this section will consider issues of particular scientific or clinical interest and will be structured to permit the presentation of differing points of view. Chapters in this year's book discuss the role of carcinogens in the etiology of human cancer, and whether alcohol consumption influences the risk of developing breast cancer.

One of the most important considerations in selecting topics for this 1989 book—as in the previous volumes—was timeliness, and timeliness will continue to be a major consideration in the choice of topics for the volumes to come. All topics will hold promise. The promise of some may not be fulfilled, whereas the promise of others will lead to major change in the way diseases are treated. It is our hope that these volumes will serve to speed such positive and beneficial changes.

VINCENT T. DeVITA, JR., M.D.
SAMUEL HELLMAN, M.D.
STEVEN A. ROSENBERG, M.D., Ph.D.

Contents

Part One   Basic Research

1. Robert J. Fisher
John P. Bader
Takis S. Papas
Oncogenes and the Mitogenic Signal Pathway   3

2. Amnon Hizi
Stephen H. Hughes
Expression of the Human Immunodeficiency Virus in *Escherichia coli:* Chemotherapy   29

3. Berton Zbar
Chromosomal Deletions in Lung Cancer and Renal Cancer   41

4. Nancy A. Jenkins
Neal G. Copeland
Transgenic Mice in Cancer Research   61

5. C. A. Stein
Jack S. Cohen
Antisense Compounds: Potential Role in Cancer Therapy   79

6. James J. Mulé
Steven A. Rosenberg
Immunotherapy With Lymphokine Combinations   99

xi

Part Two   Clinical Progress

7. Sandra Meta Swain **Treatment of Patients With**
Marc E. Lippman **Inflammatory Breast Cancer 129**

8. Gianni Bonadonna **Role of Chemotherapy in Stage I**
Pinuccia Valagussa **Breast Cancer 151**

9. Norman D. Nigro **Preservation of Function in the**
Vainutis K. Vaitkeviceus **Treatment of Cancer**
Arnold H. Herskovic **of the Anus 161**

10. V. Craig Jordan **Long-term Tamoxifen Therapy for**
Breast Cancer 179

11. Tom F. Lue **Treatment of Impotence in Cancer**
Peter R. Carroll **Patients 193**
Connie Moore

12. Raymond P. Warrell, Jr. **Gallium in the Treatment of**
Richard S. Bockman **Hypercalcemia and Bone**
Metastasis 205

13. Thomas W. Griffin **Status of Clinical Trials With**
Neutron Irradiation 221

Part Three

Controversies in Oncology

14.

What Are the Major Carcinogens in the Etiology of Human Cancer?

Bruce N. Ames

a. Environmental Pollution, Natural Carcinogens, and the Causes of Human Cancer: Six Errors   237

Frederica P. Perera

Paolo Boffetta

Ian C. T. Nisbet

b. Industrial Carcinogens   249

15.

Does Alcohol Consumption Influence the Risk of Developing Breast Cancer? Two Views

Walter C. Willett

Meir J. Stampfer

Graham A. Colditz

a.   267

Ernst L. Wynder

Randall E. Harris

b.   283

Index   295

Part One

Basic Research

Robert J. Fisher

John P. Bader

Takis S. Papas

Oncogenes and the Mitogenic Signal Pathway

1

Introduction ■

The exact process by which cancer cells arise and develop into malignant disease is an exceptionally perplexing medical question and an exciting scientific challenge. Discoveries made by molecular biologists over the past 10 years in areas of virology, cellular physiology, developmental biology, and molecular genetics have revolutionized the study of cancer biology. Researchers are now focusing on the specific areas of chromosomal translocations, mechanisms of molecular integration, control and regulation of gene activity, and the study of cellular growth factors and their role in the proliferation of cells. The concept that a single physiologic or morphologic aberration can define all cancer cells and distinguish them from their normal counterparts has been discarded, largely as a consequence of molecular biologic studies. We now know that several factors can perturb a cell's tightly controlled growth-regulatory properties, which often otherwise depend on the cell type or its state of differentiation. What can we learn by comparing these regulatory factors in malignant cells to those that operate in the normal cell?

The single obvious feature that defines a cancer cell is its ability to propagate under conditions that typically inhibit the growth of the normal cell. In normal cells with unaltered genetic constitution, restraints on growth are imposed by regulatory activities that take place at the cell surface. These activities, which may result from either cell contact or a decrease in the production or availability of growth factors, are communicated through the cytoplasm to the nucleus, thus regulating the synthesis of messenger RNAs (mRNAs) essential for the unique proteins needed to initiate subsequent DNA synthesis and mitosis. Cells can be relieved of this barrier to mitosis by cell dispersal or addition of growth factors; this molecular environmental change is recognized at the surface of the cell and transmitted through the cytoplasm to the nucleus. This signal transduction process activates the transcription and synthesis of specific proteins and other macromolecules that trigger the mitotic process. Any of a variety of genetic changes that hamper the regulation of mitosis may result in unrestrained growth and thus initiate malignancy. Similarly, factors involved in stimulation of mitosis may, when constitutively expressed, abrogate mitotic repression. Certain transforming retroviruses appear to play a role in the maintenance of an active mitotic state, and knowledge of the identity of their encoded proteins, and their interactions with various cellular signal transduction factors, is important to understanding carcinogenesis.

As a rule, a single genetic change is insufficient to drive a cell toward malignancy. The genetic change must be accompanied by either a temporary alleviation of the normal physiologic repression of control mechanisms or a second genetic disruption. Many chemical carcinogens are not sufficient alone to induce tumors in animals, but the addition of tumor promoters—which by themselves are noncarcinogenic—can effect tumor formation. Tumor promoters are known to induce mitogenic responses through signal transduction mechanisms—growth signals necessary to allow the expression of the genetic defect initiated by the carcinogen. It is generally thought that in humans (and in other animals) many potential cancer cells are initiated but remain latent until given the chance to respond to external mitotic stimuli. Only then do they develop into tumors.

The requirement for a second genetic change is established for functionally recessive mutations in growth-repressive genes (*e.g.,* retinoblastoma, Wilms' tumor), but even single dominant mutations may be inadequate to produce malignancy. There are several reasons for this, one of which involves an insufficient amount of altered gene product. Similarly, some retroviruses or retroviral genes are incapable of producing malignant transformation of cells without a second virus or another viral gene, or even a complementary cellular mutation. Transformation by a combination of retroviral genes is best exemplified experimentally by transfection using one gene that encodes a protein acting in the nucleus (*e.g., v-myc*) and another that encodes a protein acting in the cytoplasm (*e.g., v-ras*). Thus, it is perhaps not surprising that many of the most aggressive DNA- and RNA-containing transforming viruses encode at least two different proteins that act at different physiologic levels to render the cell malignant.

The retroviruses have been particularly useful in identifying and dissecting the metabolic pathways associated with mitosis, and in recognizing macromolecules that are potential determinants of the malignant process. These viruses have the unique capacity to acquire cellular genetic sequences, which they transfer to other cells by reverse transcription of viral RNA into DNA, integrating the proviral DNA into the host's chromosome. By transcription and processing of viral and cellular RNAs, retroviruses can form chimeric RNAs, which are then encapsidated into virions for subsequent rounds of infections.

The finding of endogenous retroviruses in mice and chickens led to the proposal that such viruses were components of all cells, and that the part of the virus that encodes transforming activity, the oncogene, was responsible for the genesis of tumor cells. Since that time, the term "oncogene" has been expanded to include *all* transforming genes in retroviruses that have nucleotide sequences homologous to cellular sequences, as well as all cellular genes that show transforming capability in DNA transfection assays. The complete cellular gene from which the transforming oncogene is derived is called the "proto-oncogene."

Although scores of oncogene-containing animal viruses have been identified, no human retrovirus has yet been found to contain an oncogene. However, the malignant transformation of cells by DNA extracted from human tumors or tumor cell lines led to the direct identification of human oncogenes, a discovery that provided the rationale for studying specific proto-oncogenes in certain types of malignancies.

Proteins encoded by oncogenes have been characterized by their cellular localization, enzymatic activity, and (poly)nucleotide binding affinities. The amino acid sequences predicted by the viral nucleotides of the viral oncogenes have been compared with homologous residues from a number of cellular proteins and examined for consensus sequences indicative of specific functional activities, such as adenosine triphosphatase (ATPase) and guanosine triphosphatase (GTPase) activity. The most exciting outcome of these comparative analyses is the finding that several oncogene proteins can be identified as altered variants of normal cellular proteins that are involved in signal transduction and growth-regulatory processes.

Molecular clones of oncogenes provide an excellent opportunity for detailed examination and comparison of the structural features of cellular proto-oncogenes. The general conclusion derived from such studies is that most viral oncogenes are truncated, mutated, or otherwise modified versions of normal cellular proto-oncogenes. Segments of coding sequences from proto-oncogenes are missing in homologous oncogenes. These oncogene-encoded proteins also lack specific peptides—a molecular alteration that would be expected to affect the localization or function of the encoded protein. The fusion of extraneous viral or cellular sequences to cellular proto-oncogenes would presumably produce a protein with altered activities. Also, specific point mutations could result in the replacement of crucial amino acids in active sites critical for function. It appears that some proto-oncogenes are transduced intact (albeit devoid of introns) into retrovirus genomes and thus seem relatively unaltered. However, the enhanced transcriptional activity afforded by the strong viral promoter would be expected to increase the level of the oncogene mRNA

FIG. 1–1 Schematic representation of responses to the signal transduction pathways in a typical cell. The pathway begins at the surface of the cell at its exterior (plasma) membrane, where a number of growth factors are symbolically represented interacting with their complementary receptors embedded in the membrane (*shaded area*). These shaded areas delineate the cellular barriers—the plasma membrane (*top*) and nuclear membrane (*bottom*)—along with various proteins and factors localized in these domains. The complex series of events illustrated is initiated by growth factors interacting with receptors and transducing their signals through the surface and into the interior of the cell to the nucleus, triggering mitogenesis. Oncogenes (*highlighted*) interface within this system, interacting at specific subcellular locations. Second messengers are highlighted to depict their intercession in the signal transduction processes. (DG = diacylglycerol; PKC = protein kinase C; IP_3 = inositol triphosphate; PIP_2 = phosphatidylinositol-4,5-biphosphate; PIP = phosphatidylinositol-4 phosphate; PI = phosphatidylinositol)

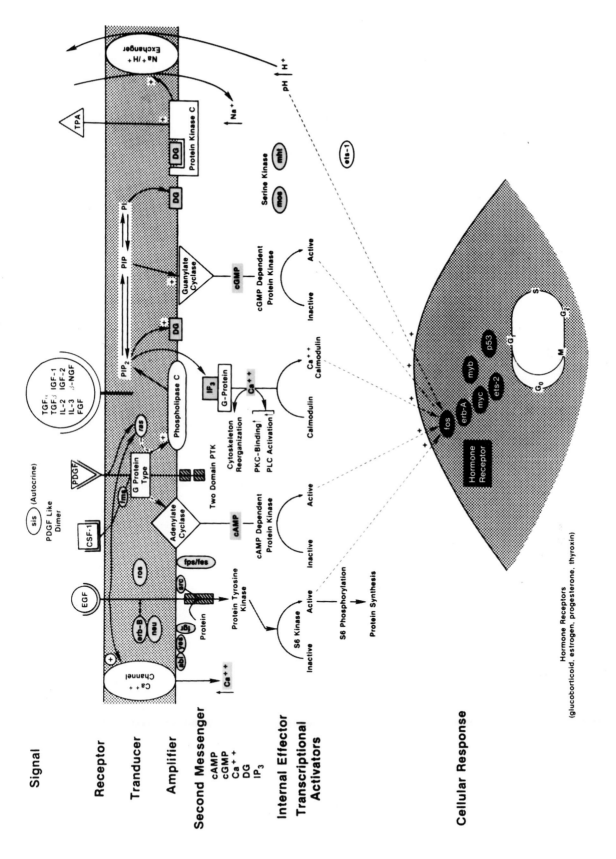

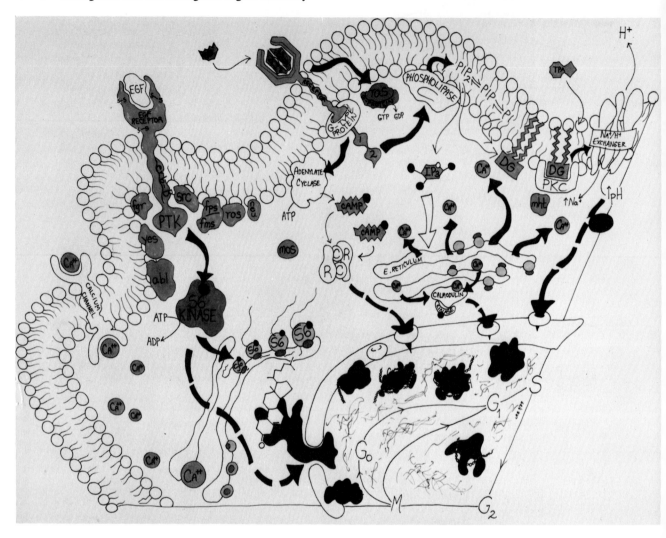

FIG. 1-2 Creative rendering of the signal transduction pathway presented in Figure 1-1. (Drawing prepared by Laura Bernstein, graduate student.)

and, hence, its protein product to an excessive and perhaps unregulated degree.

Identification of proto-oncogene products, and recognition of their relevance to components of the signal transduction pathways, has allowed researchers to create a cellular paradigm for the normal mitogenic pathway and has facilitated understanding of how disruption or amplification of the normal pathway can result in tumorigenesis. Alterations in the normal cellular transcriptional pattern are an essential feature of mitogenic stimulation and its regulation. Examination of the functional properties of the gene products involved promises to clarify much of this complex process. This review focuses on the relationships of oncogene and proto-oncogene products to the cellular structural features and metabolic events now

known to be crucial to mitogenic regulation and related growth processes.

The Cell Surface and the Mitogenic Response ■

The primary event in the induction or maintenance of the mitogenic process in vertebrate cells occurs at the cell surface. Growth factors present in serum interact as ligands with specific growth factor receptors associated with the cell surface membrane. At least one class of growth factor receptors, including those interacting with interleukins (IL-2, IL-3) and transforming growth factors (TGF-α, TGF-β), has a general structure that encompasses both an external growth factor binding site and a region that embeds the receptor in the plasma membrane. Little is known about how these receptors are activated or the consequent mitogenic stimulus, and no oncogene products have been identified that directly relate to this class of growth factor receptors or their ligands.

Another class of growth factor receptors contains large proteins (120–200 kDa) with an extracellular domain highly modified by glycosylation, a short transmembrane domain (22 or 23 uncharged amino acids), and an intracellular cytoplasmic domain. The binding of a peptide growth factor at the external domain induces enzymatic activity at the other (internal) end of the molecule. This binding initiates a cascade of events involving a variety of signals—cytoplasmic regulatory molecules that in turn effect transcription and, ultimately, mitosis.

The signal transduction pathway has been subdivided into several components (Figs. 1–1 and 1–2). Activation of a growth factor receptor results in the production of second messenger molecules by the enzymatic modification of cytoplasmic proteins. Second messengers, such as cyclic nucleotides or diacylglycerol, then act on internal effector sites, further elaborating cellular functions. It is important to understand that the signal transduction pathways are interconnected. Diverse agents acting through receptors alone, or in concert with other agents, can regulate events that allow continuation of the reproductive pattern of a cell, or that drive a cell out of G_0 into and through G_1 and S phases. Although much is now known about the components of the signal transduction apparatus, there is relatively little information on the sequence of events following receptor activation, especially the molecular events involved in transferring information to nuclear effectors.

Growth Factors and Growth Factor Receptors ■

Information on growth factors and growth factor receptors, as well as related oncogenes and their products, has accumulated rapidly over the last five or six years, and several general reviews are available.[1-3] Of particular interest are structural features of oncogene proteins that cause defective growth factor or abnormal receptor functions.

The prototype receptor, of which epidermal growth factor (EGF) receptor is one example, binds growth factor in its external domain. This region is typically located in the amino-terminal half of the protein molecule, a highly glycosylated region. Several receptors have abundant cysteine residues that are believed to stabilize the conformational structure of the mol-

ecule. Although receptors may be specific for individual growth factors, it is likely that certain receptors respond to more than one ligand. For example, the receptor for EGF can bind with equal affinity to at least three different peptides: EGF, TGF-α, and vaccinia virus growth factor.[4-6] These ligands appear to have little amino acid sequence homology, and presumably have substantial conformational similarities because they can bind equivalently to the same receptor.

The transmembrane domain of growth factor receptors contains a significant proportion of hydrophobic amino acids, a sequence characteristic of membrane associative capability. In addition to being a determinant in membrane localization, this hydrophobic region may be important to the receptor activation function: a single amino acid replacement in this region converts a normal receptor molecule into a transforming protein.

The cytoplasmic domain of the receptor appears to have the potential for enzymatic activity, which is a tyrosine kinase activity in at least several cases. This internal polypeptide portion of the receptor is phosphorylated at specific serine and threonine residues, as well as on its tyrosine residue. These phosphorylations may, in turn, affect and regulate the kinase activity of the receptor. It appears that ligand binding can activate kinase activity of receptors. Truncated receptor molecules, as represented by certain oncogene-encoded proteins, are devoid of the binding domain and are constitutively, enzymatically active and independent of growth factors.

Addition of EGF to purified EGF receptor is sufficient to activate tyrosine kinase, but concentration-dependence and other similar features of activation suggest that ligand-induced aggregation of receptor molecules may also be important in regulating enzyme activity. In support of this hypothesis is the finding that several growth factor proteins, including EGF[7] and colony-stimulating factor-1 (CSF-1), occur as bimolecular complexes that favor the association of receptors.[8] Also, platelet-derived growth factor (PDGF) consists of two peptide chains, A and B, which as heterodimers, or homodimers, are active in stimulating connective tissue-derived cell growth.[9]

Oncogenes, Growth Factors, and Receptors ■

The *sis* Oncogene and the PDGF Receptor ■

The most well-characterized oncogene known to encode a growth factor-like substance is v-*sis*. This oncogene encodes a protein (28 kDa) virtually identical to the 28 kDa precursor of the B chain of PDGF.[10,11] The precursor v-*sis* product is synthesized as a large protein, forms disulfide-linked dimers rapidly after synthesis, and then is processed at both amino and carboxy termini to form a molecule with structural and immunologic similarities to PDGF.[12] PDGF itself undergoes a similar transition from a larger to a smaller dimeric polypeptide protein.[13] The v-*sis* protein was shown to bind to PDGF receptors and to induce tyrosine phosphorylation of the receptor.[14] In that study, connective tissue cells exhibiting PDGF receptors were specifically stimulated to divide by the addition of v-*sis* protein, and the transforming activity of v-*sis* was found to be restricted to those cells possessing PDGF receptors.[14]

Characterization of the human c-*sis* proto-oncogene, located on chromosome 22, showed that it codes for the B chain of PDGF. When the human c-*sis* DNA was linked to a powerful promoter, it was able to transform cells *in vitro* following transfection.[15] These data, along with the fact that v-*sis* is the only transforming gene in simian sarcoma virus, suggest that excessive production of the B chain of PDGF can lead to cellular transformation.

Activation of PDGF receptors by v-*sis* protein appears to be an autocrine event. Chronic treatment with PDGF does not transform cells,[16] and antisera to PDGF has little effect on v-*sis*-mediated transformation.[17,18] Binding experiments with radioactive PDGF showed that few, if any, PDGF receptors are detectable in v-*sis*-transformed cells.[14,19] This finding was initially attributed to down-regulation of receptors caused by interaction of the v-*sis*-encoded protein with its receptors. Closer examination revealed that v-*sis*-infected cells synthesized PDGF receptors, but these PDGF receptors were not fully processed and never appeared on the cell's surface.[20] Because the intracellular form of the PDGF receptor was phosphorylated, the investigators concluded that v-*sis* protein activates PDGF receptors, but these receptors are unable to leave the cell.[20]

Although the immediate relevance of the proto-oncogene c-*sis* to human disease is not clear, increased mRNAs related to both c-*sis* and PDGF polypeptides have been found in human osteosarcomas, fibrosarcomas, and gliomas.[21] In chronic myelogenous leukemia (CML), the gene c-*sis*, located on the long arm of chromosome 22, is usually transposed to chromosome 9[22,23] (reciprocally with the c-*abl* gene). The c-*sis* gene was therefore an early suspected determinant in this disease. However, recent analysis has demonstrated that the c-*sis* gene is translocated intact, and this gene is considerably more distant from an important breakpoint cluster region (*bcr*) that occurs in CML and is associated with the so-called Philadelphia (Ph') chromosome. Thus, the importance of

c-*sis* in the development of CML appears to be diminished. In some Burkitt's lymphomas, the c-*sis* gene is also translocated to chromosome 8,[24] but it now appears that activation of the c-*myc* gene on chromosome 8 by a promoter for a lambda light chain gene, translocated from chromosome 22, is associated with this malignancy.[25]

A specific chromosomal translocation, t(11;22), has been reported to occur in Ewing's sarcoma, including both primary tumors and various established cell lines.[26-28] The c-*sis* gene is translocated to chromosome 11, and the recognized breakpoint is in a region where c-*sis* has been localized. Both the *bcr* and lambda light chain genes are unperturbed, suggesting that some other alteration, perhaps in the structural or regulatory region of the c-*sis* gene, may be responsible for tumorigenesis in Ewing's sarcoma. These observations suggest that such alterations result in the activation of the c-*sis* gene and lead to the constitutive synthesis and secretion of PDGF or related mitogens, and thus may be directly involved in certain specific malignant transformations.

The *fms* Oncogene and the CSF-1 Receptor ■

A variety of oncogenes encode proteins with receptor-like domains, or have tyrosine kinase activities similar to those associated with growth factor receptors. For example, a strain of feline sarcoma virus (FeSV) contains an oncogene, v-*fms,* whose product has been shown to be almost identical to a growth factor receptor. The protein, gp130[v-*fms*], is expressed in glycosylated form on the surface of cells transformed by FeSV. The gp130[v-*fms*] protein is oriented with its carboxy-terminal domain in the cytoplasm;[29] this protein undergoes endocytosis in coated pits.[30] Nucleotide sequence analysis[31] of the FeSV oncogene suggests a relationship to other tyrosine kinase-encoding oncogenes, and tyrosine kinase activity has been found in v-*fms* protein purified by the immunoaffinity method.[32] The analogous cellular product, encoded by the c-*fms* proto-oncogene, was found to have similar tyrosine kinase activity. Recently, the proto-oncogene product c-*fms* was found to be indistinguishable from the receptor specific for binding CSF-1, and CSF-1 also binds to the v-*fms* protein.[33]

The specific molecular defect in the v-*fms* product that confers transforming activity is not readily apparent. As with several other growth factor receptors, ligand binding activates the normal CSF-1 receptor-associated kinase, apparently providing a functional signal for cell growth. However, v-*fms* protein does exhibit tyrosine kinase activity, even in the absence of the growth factor CSF-1, and binding of CSF-1 to the v-*fms* protein has no obvious effects on this receptor-like activity.[34] Antibody to CSF-1, or an antibody that blocks CSF-1 binding to v-*fms* protein, failed to inhibit the growth of v-*fms*-transformed cells suspended in a semisolid medium.[34] In other experiments, myeloid cells that normally require IL-3 for growth lost this requirement after infection with a virus containing the v-*fms* gene.[35] Because these cells produced no IL-3 or CSF-1, either before or after infection, continuation of growth appeared to be directly related to the presence of the v-*fms* protein. Collectively, these data suggest that the tyrosine kinase of v-*fms* protein is constitutively activated and that the CSF-1 growth factor is irrelevant to this altered receptor's activity.

A number of observations indicate that the external domain of the v-*fms* receptor-like protein may be responsible for the transforming function of the protein. Interference with glycosylation by the use of antimetabolites[36] or site-directed mutagenesis[37] can attenuate the transforming ability of the v-*fms* protein without affecting tyrosine kinase activity. It is possible that such specific tampering with the external domain affects the localization of the v-*fms* protein or perhaps its orientation in the cell's membrane, which is critical to transforming activity. The human c-*fms* proto-oncogene was found to have coding sequences other than that of the 3' end of v-*fms*.[38] This deletion of amino acids could result in the loss of a regulating region at the carboxy end of the v-*fms* product, and thus may explain the tumorigenic activity of v-*fms*. Consistent with this possibility is the finding of a deletion in the 3' exon of the c-*fms* present in DNA derived from a patient with acute lymphocytic leukemia.[39]

The c-*fms* proto-oncogene has been localized to the long arm of chromosome 5,[38] and some patients with acute myelogenous leukemia or other hematologic disorders have cells with specific deletions in this region.[40] Cytogenetic evidence for the translocation of deleted segments of chromosome 5 to other chromosomes has not been reported. CSF-1 is a predominant growth factor known to stimulate growth and differentiation of precursor cells of the myelocyte lineage. Therefore, the possibility cannot be ignored that damage to the CSF-1 receptor, or an altered expression of c-*fms*, may be responsible for the manifestation of certain malignancies.

The *erb*B Oncogene and the EGF Receptor ∎

The *erb*B oncogene, one of two oncogenes originally described for the avian erythroblastosis virus (AEV), has an extremely high degree of sequence homology with the EGF receptor.[41,42] Both v-*erb*B and the EGF receptor map to the same region of human chromosome 7.[43] Despite the avian origin of v-*erb,* the cytoplasmic domain of the human EGF receptor, including the region containing the tyrosine kinase activity, is approximately 95% identical in amino acid residues to the v-*erb*B protein.[44] In contrast, only a small proportion of the sequences encoding the extracellular domain of EGF receptor is present in v-*erb*B. There is a small truncation of the cytoplasmic carboxy-terminal protein of the v-*erb*B oncogene that includes the primary sites of tyrosine autophosphorylation found in the normal EGF receptor. This latter region is thought to regulate the kinase activity of the normal receptor.

The c-*erb*B proto-oncogene of chickens is occasionally activated following infection by an avian leukosis virus (ALV) that possesses no oncogenes. Apparently, the leukosis virus genome is able to insert itself into the avian chromosome within the c-*erb*B (EGF receptor) gene locus,[45] eliminating upstream exons and enabling the strong viral promoter to activate the downstream transcription of c-*erb*B sequences. These virus-activated transcripts encode a protein that contains the entire carboxy-terminal region and transmembrane domain, which are similar to those of the EGF receptor, as well as a portion of the extracellular domain. Thus, the consequence ALV infection is an induction of erythroblastosis, similar to that induced by AEV. Other chickens infected with the leukosis virus develop lymphomas because of the viral integration and subsequent transcriptional activation of c-*myc* proto-oncogene sequences. It is easy to imagine how such retroviral infections could have diverse effects on mitotic regulation by integrating into various chromosomal sites that encode or control the expression of proto-oncogenes.

The observations made with v-*erb* suggest that the loss of the ligand-binding site of a receptor, in this case the EGF receptor, is sufficient to constitutively activate its tyrosine kinase and induce malignant transformation. Indeed, AEV—which encodes v-*erb*B that is deficient in both amino- and carboxy-terminal sequences—can easily transform fibroblasts and erythroid cells. AEV-related viruses that encode the entire carboxy terminus of the EGF receptor, however, are limited in transformation potential to cells of the erythroid lineage.[46] The other AEV oncogene, *erb*A, whose product is concentrated in the nucleus, may have a more direct role in preventing erythroid differentiation by altering transcriptional regulation. The development of erythroblastosis is complex, but the identification of *erb*B as an aberrant form of the gene for the EGF receptor provides a model for growth factor receptor-mediated malignancies, and is testable as such.

In addition to defective growth factor receptors, an overabundance of normal growth factor receptors may be a determinant in certain other malignancies. The EGF receptor was, in fact, first purified from cells derived from a human squamous cell carcinoma exhibiting excessive amounts of EGF receptor.[47] In addition, elevated expression of EGF receptors has been demonstrated in cells derived from other squamous cell carcinomas,[48] as well as pancreatic[49] and breast carcinomas.[50] Direct examination of tissue obtained from biopsies of squamous cell carcinomas of the lung and carcinomas of the brain has also revealed elevated EGF receptor levels.[51] The basis for this finding is unknown.

PDGF versus EGF Activation ■

There is an important biologic distinction between activation of the mitogenic response by PDGF and activation by EGF. PDGF alone can elicit DNA replication in mesenchymal cells, whereas agents such as EGF must work in concert with other growth factors present in serum, or with the PDGF growth factor, to be mitogenic.[52,53] When added to quiescent cells, both growth factors rapidly activate transcription of another nuclear oncogene, the *fos* gene. However, the enhancer element of the *fos* gene that responds to PDGF differs in sequence and locality from the enhancer element that responds to EGF.

In certain cell types, stimulation of the PDGF receptor leads to a large increase in cyclic adenosine monophosphate (cAMP). However, the cAMP elevation is an indirect result of a tortuous metabolic pathway, stemming from increased levels of arachidonate (a metabolite of diacylglycerol metabolism or of phospholipase A2), which leads to the formation of prostaglandins; these substances, in turn, stimulate cAMP synthesis through the prostaglandin receptor. Further, there is a significant structural difference between PDGF and EGF receptors. The tyrosine kinase domain of the PDGF receptor is divided into two parts that are separated by a non-kinase-related domain. This two-domain kinase is also found in the CSF-1 receptor and the receptor-related *fms* and v-*kit* oncogenes, implying that there is a subfamily of receptors with two-domain kinase.[54] In contrast, the tyrosine kinase domain of the EGF receptor is contiguous and similar to the kinase domains of receptor-related *neu* and *erb*B oncogenes, as well as the non-receptor-related *src, ros, abl, ves, fgr,* and *fps/ves* oncogene products. Therefore, it appears that the latter proteins may be functionally related and can be classed into another subfamily.

The *met* Oncogene ■

The c-*met* gene encodes a protein that is almost certainly related to a growth factor receptor. All three characteristic domains found in growth factors are present.[55] The cytoplasmic domain has the consensus sequences necessary for tyrosine kinase activity, and the expressed protein, p140^{met}, has tyrosine kinase activity.[56] However, the ligand for *met* binding to this receptor has not been identified.

The *met* oncogene from which c-*met* derives was isolated by transfection of DNA from human cells previously treated with a mutagenic carcinogen (N-methyl-N′-nitro-N-nytrosoguanidine [NMMG]). The oncogene was formed after chromosomal translocation that resulted in the fusion of a promoter locus from chromosome 1 to a portion of the c-*met* gene on chromosome 7.[57] This resulted in activation of sequences in the 3′ end of c-*met* and effected the translation of a severely truncated p65^{met} protein. This product not only has the receptor-binding domain removed, as with the v-*erb* protein, but the transmembrane portion is also removed. Thus, unlike the normal gene product, the *met* protein with intact tyrosine kinase activity is located exclusively in the soluble cytoplasmic portion of the cell. This severe molecular alteration may be directly involved in this cell's noted tumorigenic characteristics.[58]

The *neu* Oncogene ■

The oncogene *neu* was discovered after serial transformation of cells using rat neuroblastoma DNA.[59] The isolated oncogene hybridized with v-*erb*B and was subsequently observed to have about 50% sequence homology to the normal EGF receptor gene.[60] The *neu*-encoded glycoprotein reacts with antibody to EGF receptor, and has characteristic tyrosine kinase activity. The proto-oncogene for *neu,* designated c-*erb*-2, is localized to human chromosome 19;[61] obviously, it is different from the c-*erb*B gene located on chromosome 7. This receptor protein fails to bind to the ligand EGF and, presumably, is a receptor for some as yet undiscovered ligand. All three receptor domains of c-*erb*-2 appear to be intact in *neu*. However, the transforming activity of the *neu* protein appears to arise solely from a specific point mutation resulting in an amino acid replacement (valine to glutamic acid) in the transmembrane domain.[62]

Other Tyrosine Kinase-encoding Oncogenes ■

In addition to growth factor receptor-related oncogenes, a number of other oncogenes (*e.g., abl, fes/fps, fgr, kit, sea, src, yes*) encode *de facto* tyrosine kinases or at least contain sequences similar to those encoding tyrosine kinases. However, these oncogenes seem to have little else in common with other well-known growth factor receptors. Most contain neither the extracellular domain nor the transmembrane domain characteristic of membrane-associated receptors. Nevertheless, several of these oncogene-encoded products are membrane-associated, whereas others appear to be cytoplasmic but are often less definitively localized. Although the products of these oncogenes and their related proto-oncogenes have been identified, their general relevance to the mitogenic process remains obscure. For example, screening of normal and malignant tissue for the expression of c-src and its product revealed only negligible amounts, except in neural tissue,[63] whose cells are not known to actively proliferate. It is possible that these tyrosine kinase-encoding proto-oncogenes are involved in cellular differentiation or some other specialized aspect of cell responsiveness; for example, src may be related to neurologic functioning. These normal gene products may become mitogenic stimulants upon expansion of substrate specificity, unusual cellular localization, or some other aberration that may follow activation to an oncogene.

The p60^{src} protein encoded by Rous sarcoma virus has a potent tyrosine kinase activity; however, mutants that induce transformation at 37° but not at 41° produce a p60^{src} with tyrosine kinase activity at 37° but not at the higher temperature.[64,65] In fact, any deletions or mutations that alter the tyrosine kinase activity of p60^{src} coordinately affect the transforming potential of the oncogene.[66] As previously discussed, in the absence of growth factor, tyrosine kinase of the homologous receptor is inhibited. However, the continual presence of growth factor, the loss of a ligand-binding site, or an alteration in the transmembrane domain (as in neu) may result in a constitutive tyrosine kinase activity. Other factors are known to regulate the tyrosine kinase activity of receptor or oncogene proteins. Phosphorylation at specific sites in the cytoplasmic domain of receptor, or receptor-like, oncogene proteins can either activate or inhibit kinase activity. Autophosphorylation of a tyrosine residue is a common feature of many tyrosine kinases. For example, activation of EGF or insulin receptors results in autophosphorylation that further enhances protein kinase activity;[3] similarly, autophosphorylation in the N-terminal region of viral p60^{src} correlates with elevated tyrosine kinase activity.[67]

Phosphorylations other than autophosphorylations are often inhibitory. Protein kinase C, a serine-threonine kinase, phosphorylates the EGF receptor, attenuating tyrosine kinase activity.[3] It is interesting that exposure of cells to EGF itself induces protein kinase C activity, thereby autoregulating the cells' ability to respond to EGF.

The src Oncogene ■

In contrast to the protein encoded by v-src, p60^{c-src} has little tyrosine kinase activity and fails to transform cells. However, dephosphorylation of a tyrosine in the carboxy-terminal half of p60^{c-src}, or any exposure of a specific antibody directed against a peptide in this region, increases its kinase activity 5- to 10-fold. Replacement of the specific tyrosine in p60^{c-src} with phenylalanine (by site-directed mutagenesis) also results in activation of tyrosine kinase activity and increases the transformation potential. The carboxy-terminal region of p60^{c-src}, which contains the phosphorylated tyrosine, is absent in p60^{v-src}; thus, p60^{v-src} is not regulated by phosphorylation at this site. Therefore, the transforming activity of p60^{v-src} can be attributed to the constitutive activity of its tyrosine kinase.[66]

The abl Oncogene ■

Perhaps the most definitive proof of the involvement of an oncogene in human cancer is found in CML. This disease is characterized by the presence of the Ph' chromosome, which usually appears as a truncated chromosome 22 in leukemia cells[68] and progenitor cells. The distal portion of chromosome 9 is reciprocally translocated to the long arm of chromosome 22. The c-abl proto-oncogene, initially mapped to the end of chromosome 9,[69] was found to be in the translocated portion. Characterization of the breakpoints demonstrated that either one or both of two alternative first exons of c-abl remained on chromosome 9.[70] The downstream exons of c-abl became attached to chromosome 22 at any of a number of breakpoints, all located within the bcr.[71] The combined genes, using the bcr promoter, transcribe hybrid RNA containing bcr and abl elements,[72] and a 210 kDa bcr/abl fusion protein is synthesized.[73]

The v-abl protein encoded by a transforming mouse leukemia virus is also synthesized as a hybrid protein containing abl sequences attached to a viral structural polypeptide. This p160$^{gag-abl}$, with the amino-terminal sequences of c-abl replaced by gag sequences, has the same downstream elements of abl as the p40$^{bcr-abl}$. The normal c-abl protein (145 kDa), like p160$^{gag-abl}$ and p210$^{bcr-abl}$, exhibits tyrosine kinase activity.[74] Nevertheless, the hybrid fusion proteins differ in autophosphorylation properties from the normal proto-oncogene product, p145^{c-abl}. Also, the hybrid proteins are phosphorylated on tyrosine *in vivo,* whereas human and mouse c-*abl* proteins fail to become phosphorylated. This occurs despite the presence of the tyrosine phosphorylation acceptor amino acid at sites identical to those of p160$^{gag-abl}$.[75] Tyrosine phosphorylation of *gag-abl* and *bcr-abl* proteins in this common site may intensify the activities of the respective tyrosine kinase, as is also seen in the case of EGF receptor or p60^{v-src} kinase activation. However, the initial regulation of kinase activity is clearly determined in the amino-terminal portion of the protein, when a polypeptide encoded by a primary exon of c-*abl* is replaced by the *bcr* or *gag* polypeptide.

In addition to CML, other hematopoietic disorders such as acute myelocytic and lymphocytic leukemias (AML and ALL) occasionally exhibit the Ph' chromosome. Indeed, more than one-fourth of adult ALLs are Ph' positive,[76] with a high incidence of the t(9;22); the involvement of the *abl* gene is similar to that seen in CML. Some of these disorders develop following a chronic phase of CML and are manifestations of the same translocation. In several cases, however, novel p190^{abl} or p185^{abl} proteins were detected instead of the typical p210$^{bcr-abl}$ of CML.[77,78] Chromosome breakpoints were found upstream from the *bcr* region, but probably still lie within the larger gene encompassing *bcr*.[79,80]

To summarize, in these leukemia cells, a portion of the c-*abl* gene devoid of at least one primary exon is translocated in such a fashion that it interrupts the *bcr* gene. The *bcr* promoter produces transcripts that include a variable number of *bcr* exons and introns fused to *abl* exons and introns. Splicing removes introns and (if it is attached) the residual primary *abl* exon as well. Hybrid proteins are made that contain variable elements of *bcr* fused to all the major downstream elements of *abl*. Given the assumption that the *bcr-abl* proteins are, in fact, the direct cause of leukemogenesis in these CMLs and ALLs, it is curious that the presence or absence of coding sequences in the hybrid gene, and the corresponding changes of peptides in the proteins, can alter the specificity of cellular vulnerability.

Intermediate Steps in Signal Transduction ■

The immediate substrate responsible for initiating mitogenesis of the protein tyrosine kinases is as yet unknown. It is possible that several events essential to the cell's growth cycle must be changed to sustain the carcinogenic phenotype. In this light, we should recognize that a common substrate of both serine and tyrosine kinases, including the *src*-specific tyrosine kinase, is the ribosomal protein S6 kinase.[81–83] Phos-

phorylation of the abundant S6 protein, a 30S-ribosomal protein important in binding of the elongation factor TU, could lead to the overall stimulation of protein synthesis.[84] Alternatively, protein tyrosine kinase and possibly protein kinase C can phosphorylate lipocortin (p35/p36), an inhibitor of phospholipase A_2. Phospholipase A_2 is important in the metabolism of phospholipids, leading to formation of leukotrienes and prostaglandins[85]—agents with potent cellular activation effects.

Activation of the PDGF receptor rapidly [a] stimulates phosphoinositide turnover, [b] releases compartmentalized calcium, [c] increases production of inositol triphosphate and diacylglycerol (DG), [d] increases protein kinase C activity, and [e] raises cytoplasmic pH (see Fig. 1–1).[86] There is evidence to suggest an interrelated progression of these metabolic changes, which appear to be early events in mitogenic stimulation that are directly related to transcriptional activation.[87]

Metabolism of phosphatidylinositol (PI) involves progressive phosphorylation to PI-4-phosphate (PIP) and PI-4-5-biphosphate (PIP2). Activation of the growth factor receptor by the appropriate ligand results in hydrolysis of PIP2 by phospholipase C to DG and inositol triphosphate (IP3). These two products form two separate pathways for further activation, and metabolic products in each pathway may expand the initial signal. In the membrane, the released DG can activate protein kinase C, which in turn may be involved in a variety of regulatory events, including alkalinization of cytosolic pH and stimulation of cellular DNA synthesis. Also, DG can be hydrolyzed to release arachidonic acid, the precursor of other compounds (*e.g.,* prostaglandins and leukotrienes) that function as local hormones. Furthermore, phosphatidic acid (PA) results from the phosphorylation of DG, and PA is known to mimic growth factors in stimulating the hydrolysis of PIP2. The other metabolic product of PIP2, IP3 (see Fig. 1–1), stimulates the release of calcium sequestered in endoplasmic reticulum, and calcium availability is an important factor in mitogenic stimulation.

It is likely that not all of the steps outlined above are necessary to provoke a mitogenic stimulus. For example, phorbol esters and other tumor promoters with structural similarities to DG can activate protein kinase C directly, thereby circumventing a requirement for receptor activation.[88] Also, the mitogenic effect of EGF appears unrelated to PI turnover,[89] although calcium, sodium, and pH increases are found in EGF-stimulated cells.[90,91]

Although the tyrosine kinase activity of the *src* oncogene product is essential to transforming potential, the critical cellular substrate involved in initiating transformation has not been identified. Research attention therefore shifted to changes in PI and PI derivatives as the basis for malignant transformation. This direction was suggested by the possibility that the tyrosine kinase activity of the oncogene product could be a PI kinase that utilized PI or DG as alternative substrates.[92] However, subsequent experiments demonstrated that PI kinases are clearly separate from the v-*src* kinase.[93,94] Whether or not PI kinase activities increase in v-*scr* transformed cells remains a matter of contention. There is, however, a possibility that *src* may exert an effect directly through the PI pathway. This hypothesis is supported by the interaction between p60[c-*src*] and the middle T antigen of polyoma virus. Specific antibody against either protein coprecipitates both proteins in extracts of polyoma-transformed cells; yet in such complexes p60[c-*src*] that is normally attenuated in its kinase activity exhibits increased tyrosine kinase activity.[95] It seems that the interaction of the middle T antigen and p60[c-*src*] results in a form of p60[c-*src*] whose critical tyrosine cannot be phosphorylated, thus increasing its kinase activity.[96] It is significant that, in addition to the tyrosine kinase activity of p60[c-*src*] in the complex, a PI kinase activity was only found in immune complexes containing transforming middle T antigen.[97] Thus, the PI kinase activity has been attributed to a third component present in the immune complex.[98] These seemingly complex observations raise the possibility that an oncogene or proto-oncogene products may intervene in mitotic regulation by forming complexes with critical regulatory enzymes or signals, causing them to destabilize or augmenting their growth-influencing activities.

The gene for the Ca^{2+}-dependent and PI-specific phospholipase C has been cloned and its derived amino acid sequence determined.[99] The predicted amino acid sequence shows homology to the non-catalytic domains of tyrosine kinases (*src*). This regional homology suggests that phospholipase C and *src* may have similar regulatory domains. Recent findings show that the oncogene *crk* also has similar domains. The *crk* gene is part of the avian virus CT10, and cells transformed by this virus activate their cellular tyrosine kinases. It has been proposed that the gene product *crk* could act as a "sink" to bind negative regulatory factors, which, in turn, would activate the normally quiescent tyrosine kinases.[100]

GTP-Binding Regulatory Proteins ■

The GTP-binding proteins fall into three classes G-proteins, including G stimulatory (G_s) and G inhibitory (G_i); elongation factors, EF-TU, and related proteins involved in protein synthesis; and the *ras*-encoded proteins. The structure of the GTP-binding site characteristic for these proteins was first determined by x-ray crystallography of EF-TU.[101] Such studies showed that amino acid sequences on short segments surrounding the GTP-binding pocket are conserved in other G proteins and in the *ras*-encoded proteins.[102]

The G-proteins have been implicated in a variety of cellular process, including activation and inhibition of adenylate cyclase; stimulation of retinal cGMP phosphodiesterase; phosphoinositide hydrolysis by activation of phospholipase C; and regulation of ion channels.[103] All of these functions are part of the signal transduction processes (see Fig. 1–1). The G-proteins are heterotrimers composed of a GTP-binding protein (39–52 kDa α-chain) associated with two regulatory subunits (35 kDa β- and 8 kDa γ-chains). The α subunit binds GTP and determines the specificity, whereas the $\beta\gamma$ complex serves to anchor the α subunit to the cytoplasmic membrane. Stimulation of the receptor by growth factor results in the activation of the G-protein by releasing bound GDP and then binding to GTP. In the active conformation, the G-protein can regulate second messages (cAMP, cGMP, DG, IP3, and Ca^{3+}) by activating or inhibiting the enzymes responsible for their production. Hydrolysis of the bound GTP to GDP returns the activated G-protein to an inactive state, eliminating its regulatory effect.

The *ras* Oncogene ■

The fact that *ras* proteins bind guanine nucleotides suggests that they are related to G-proteins. Three *ras* genes (H-*ras*, K-*ras*, and N-*ras*) have been identified and their products localized to the cytoplasmic side of the plasma membrane, similar to the subcellular location of G-proteins.[104] Additionally, *ras* and G-proteins have highly conserved amino acid residues at their GTP-binding sites. However, there are no other amino acid homologies between these two classes of proteins. Therefore, although some functional similarities appear to exist for *ras* and the other G-proteins, these classes of protein remain clearly distinct.

The *ras* oncogene stimulates the PI signal transduction pathway. Rodent cells transformed by v-*ras* exhibit increased levels of both PIP2 and its second messages DG and IP3.[105] Consistent with this finding is the observation of rapid increases of PIP2, IP, IP2, and particularly DG following microinjection of a transforming p21[*ras*] protein into frog oocytes.[106] Microinjection of a monoclonal antibody to 21[*ras*] that effectively neutralizes intercellular p21[*ras*] activity will prevent the mitogenic activity of a phorbol ester or a calcium ionophore.[107] This suggests that *ras*-onco-gene-encoded proteins can function at more than one critical site in the signal transduction pathway.

The proto-oncogenes of *ras* have been highly con-served in evolution and are found over the entire eu-karyotic phylogenetic range.[104] In fact, p21[ras] from a mammalian source can functionally replace the ho-mologous genes in yeast. However, the function of p21[ras] in mammalian cells has not been reconciled to the finding that the p21[ras] of yeast functions in spor-ulation, an untenable process for mammalian cells. A further complication is the observation that all adult tissues contain p21[ras] proteins, and several terminally differentiated cells, including epithelial cells of en-docrine glands and neurons of the central nervous system, express high levels of p21[ras]. It is, in fact, the oncogenic variant—not the normal p21[ras]—that can induce the terminal differentiation of certain rat cells into neuron-like cells.

A role for the *ras* protein in mitogenesis of mam-malian cells was suggested by experiments using mi-croinjected monoclonal antibody, as mentioned above. This antibody prevented stimulation of DNA synthesis by serum (growth factors), phorbol ester, calcium ionophore, and prostaglandin and also re-versed the phenotype of cells transformed by tyrosine kinase-encoding oncogenes.[108] Specificity for the *ras* function was demonstrated by the inability of this antibody to reverse the phenotype of cells transformed by cytoplasmic oncogene-transforming proteins.[109] The *ras* proteins, although an apparently essential component in signal transduction, can be dispensable for transformation when similar factors farther along in the pathway are activated.

Purified *ras* proteins bind guanine nucleotides (GDP and GTP); the associated GTPase activity of these proteins is essential to normal biologic func-tion.[104] The *ras* oncogenes arise mainly by specific point mutations resulting in amino acid substitutions at critical points in p21[ras]. These mutated proteins retain nucleotide binding capability but have severely impaired GTPase activity. A reasonable model for *ras* function suggests that nonmutated p21[ras] is acti-vated to interact with an effector by binding GTP, and then reverts to the inactive state by hydrolysis of GTP to GDP. However, the inability to hydrolyze GTP stabilizes the mutated *ras* proteins in their active state.

Activated p21[ras] is actually a weak transformant compared to many other oncogene products. Cells apparently can acquire other growth-enhancing mu-tations or be transfected with a second oncogene that stimulates serial cell growth, thus permitting efficient transformation by p21[ras].[110] It is known that mor-phologic revertants of *ras*-transformed cells may still synthesize the full complement of active p21[ras] pro-tein, but these revertants contain elements that are able to overcome the transforming capability of this protein.[111] This feature of the *ras* transforming po-tential is particularly relevant to *ras*-related carci-nogenesis in humans, where at least two deleterious events are required for the generation of aggressive malignancies.

Transforming *ras* genes are found in a great variety of human tumor tissue studied by DNA transfection analysis; in fact, *ras* is the most frequent oncogene recovered from such tumors. Although a few of these tumors are related to the amplification of *ras* genes, there is no evidence that transcriptional activation of *ras* proto-oncogenes is a probable cause of tumori-genesis. Mutagenized *ras* oncogenes encoding an im-paired GTPase activity are the preponderant defect noted in these tumors.

Nuclear Oncogene Proteins ■

Stimulation of the mitogenic signal pathway induces transcription of a battery of genes without an inter-mediary requirement for protein synthesis.[112] Some of these induced transcripts have been cloned, and studies to identify and characterize their encoded products and their roles in mitogenic stimulation are in progress.[113] Interestingly, among these inducible genes are several proto-oncogenes that encode nuclear proteins. Expression of this family of nuclear proto-oncogenes is induced within a few minutes after growth factor stimulation, and proceeds in a sequen-tial manner beginning with c-*fos*, followed by c-*myc*, c-*myb*, and later c-*ets*-2.[114–116] Induction of these genes is independent of c-*fos*, and the protein synthesis in-hibitor cycloheximide does not interfere with induc-tion of any of these genes. The temporal differences in the responsiveness of these proto-oncogenes are probably due to their differential activities with respect to transcription-activating factors and the regulatory sequences with which they interact. This set of proto-oncogene-encoded nuclear proteins shares several properties: phosphorylation, rapid metabolic turn-over, and presumptive nucleic acid (DNA)-binding activity.[117–119] Characteristic of these nuclear proto-oncogenes is the ability to alter expression in response to modulators of cell proliferation and differentia-tion.[120–126] The *myc* and *fos* genes are the prototypes of this family of nuclear proto-oncogenes. Experi-mental evidence suggests that the products of these proto-oncogenes can stimulate the transcription of other cellular genes, implying that their normal func-tion is one of transcriptional regulation.[127–129] In this regard, newly characterized nuclear oncogene, *jun,* has been shown to code for a transcriptional activator protein, AP-1.[130]

The *fos* Oncogene ■

Both qualitative and quantitative differences have been reported for EGF and PDGF in mitogenic stimulation; these growth factors also exhibit differences in their stimulation of c-*fos* expression. An enhancer element (similar to sequences that enhance the promoters of polyoma, SV40, and the Moloney leukemia virus) is located about 300 bases upstream of the c-*fos* gene initiation site. This upstream enhancer region encompasses a sequence element with dyad symmetry (DSE)[131] that is required for the induction of c-*fos* by EGF, serum,[132] insulin,[133] or the phorbol ester TPA. A protein of about 65 kDa that has a strong affinity for the DSE sequence has been purified from extracts of human cells.[134,135] How this DSE-binding protein interacts with components of the mitogenic pathway is currently unknown.

Another element, located 30 to 40 bases upstream of DSE, responds to induction with conditioned medium from v-*sis*-transformed cells.[136] This upstream element may be the PDGF-inducible element, which binds to an inducible factor different from the DSE-binding protein. Moreover, EGF, TPA, and insulin fail to induce this DNA-binding factor.

A third region, located about 60 bases upstream from the initiation site, can be identified as a promoter element of the c-*fos* gene.[137,138] This region resembles the consensus sequence of cAMP-regulated promoters and binds to a nuclear factor, possibly a protein like the cAMP-binding protein. Thus, it may be responsible for the expression of mRNA induced by agonists of adenylate cyclase, such as dibutyryl cAMP, forskolin, or cholera toxin.[139,140] Depending on the initiating agonist, or the rate-limiting features of divergent pathways, transcription of c-*fos* is inducible by the action at least three different factors. A single agonist can induce transcription through divergent pathways, as is seen in the TPA activation of protein kinase C; this activation then leads to induction of the c-*fos* gene at the DSE site. The TPA-induced phosphorylation of adenylate cyclase[141] could also serve to activate the c-*fos* promoter. TPA induction, however, does not appear limited to the activation of the c-*fos* gene, since enhancer elements that respond to TPA have also been identified on human metallothionein and collagenase genes,[142] which obviously require different transcription factors from those mentioned above.[143]

The presence of distinct DNA sequence elements, and their responses to specific transcriptional activators (which are themselves activated by different components of the signal transduction pathway), probably explains the varied temporal appearance of different genes responding to the same initial stimulus. Thus, the regulation of c-*fos* gene expression is affected, both positively and negatively, by cell factors and their appropriate interaction with specific DNA sequences.

Inhibitors of protein synthesis characteristically superinduce the transcription of c-*fos* message and prevent repression of the gene,[144] and they may induce c-*fos* transcription in quiescent cells.[145] A labile protein apparently is present as an inhibitor of c-*fos* transcription. The presence of a protein synthesis inhibitor would rapidly reduce the level of this labile regulatory protein, as it requires replenishment. Also, it has been shown that transcription of c-*fos* can be induced by intracellular addition of large amounts of upstream regulatory sequences,[146] which apparently compete for the negative regulatory factors, releasing the cellular c-*fos* sequences from repression.

Although activation of the c-*fos* gene is the first transcriptional product noted upon mitogenic stimulation, the continued expression and availability of c-*fos* protein is probably not required for late events in the cell cycle or for the secondary generation of other mitogenic signals, as long as adequate levels of growth factors are present. The early expression of c-*fos,* however, may be essential to further progress through the cell cycle. Following its rapid induction, the c-*fos* gene is quickly repressed, and its mRNA is short-lived.[112,114] The c-*fos* protein disappears well before DNA synthesis begins, and c-*fos* apparently does not need to be induced until the next cycle begins.

Nuclear oncogene products are thought to be involved directly in the regulation of gene expression, mainly because of their ability to form binding complexes with DNA. The c-*fos* protein has been shown to be a component of such nucleoprotein complexes.[147,148] These complexes can regulate gene expression during adipocyte differentiation[149] and have also been shown to activate the α_1-collagen promoter.[150] Further, when specific DNA-interactive sequences are fused to c-*fos* or v-*fos* proteins, strong transcriptional activation occurs in yeast cells.[151] The *fos* protein complex recognizes DNA sequences homologous to the consensus binding sequence recognized by the transactivation factor AP-1,[152] similar to observations regarding the *jun* gene product (see below). Thus, there is accumulating evidence of a role for *fos* protein in transcriptional regulation.

The v-*fos* oncogene encodes a protein, p55$^{c\text{-}fos}$ (381 amino acids), which is similar in size to the c-*fos* product (380 amino acids).[153] Although these proteins differ in the last 50 amino acids of the carboxy-terminal region, it appears that this region has little obvious effect on function, given that both proteins become phosphorylated (mainly on their serine residues) and both can transform fibroblasts. However, transformation by the c-*fos* gene requires the removal of a 67 base pair AT-rich region from the 3' noncoding end. This region is known to transcribe sequences that render its mRNA unstable; its removal prolongs the half-life of c-*fos* mRNA. For whatever reason, it would seem that both extension of the longevity of the c-*fos* mRNA and constitutive expression of the oncogene are required for efficient tumorigenic potential. One could also anticipate that scissions in the c-*fos* gene deleting this 3' region from the *fos* mRNA might well contribute to malignant transformation, but such aberrations have not yet been reported in human tumors.

The *myc* Oncogene ■

Following mitogenic stimulation, c-*myc* is expressed more slowly than c-*fos,* but its expression is more sustained. In fact, once cells are growing, expression of c-*myc* RNA and protein remains constant throughout the cell cycle.[154] Continuous activation of the c-*myc* gene is thought to be responsible for the sustained levels, since the *myc* mRNA has a short half-life (about 30 minutes) and may be primarily determined, as in c-*fos* RNA, by the sequences in its 3' untranslated region.[155] The c-*myc* and v-*myc* proteins also have short half-lives;[156] most likely, these proteins are degraded by nonlysosomal proteases.[157] Expression of c-*myc* following mitogenic stimulation has been used to distinguish among signal pathways. Unlike the growth factor-stimulated pathways leading to the expression of c-*fos* (described above), stimulation of c-*myc* by PDGF, in some cells, appears to be independent of both phosphoinositol turnover and protein kinase C.[158] This observation suggests the possibility of other potential mitogenic intermediates.

Two promoter regions have been identified in molecularly characterized clones of the human[159] and mouse[160] c-*myc* genes, and the possibility of additional regulatory elements indicates a complex regulation for the expression of c-*myc.* In studies using human peripheral blood mononuclear cells, the two promoter regions are utilized differentially, depending on the mitotic stimulus. In fact, different c-*myc* transcripts are found after induction by IL-2, or following addition of the mitogen phytohemagglutinin.[161] This difference in expression is yet another demonstration that a single gene can be activated by different signal pathways. Attempts to understand the complex process of c-*myc* regulation are further complicated by the observation that elevated *myc* expression, presumably through excessive *myc* protein, can repress a c-*myc* promoter. For example, in Burkitt's lymphomas, the high level of c-*myc* expression noted after chromosomal translocation is thought to repress the expression of the normal allele.[162] Thus, much remains to be determined regarding the complex regulation of this proto-oncogene at the level of genomic expression, and the regulation of its product.

The c-*myc* gene is comprised of three exons, a presumptive noncoding first exon and two downstream exons, with a single large open reading frame spanning the last two coding downstream exons. This molecular organization is basically identical in several avian and mammalian species, including man.[163,164] Although the gene product is thought to be a single protein, based on the coding sequences, the immunoprecipitated c-*myc* proteins appear as two major bands. These data have been consistently obtained from a variety of species. Whereas the first AUG-initiating codon is known to occur in the second exon and encodes one of the *myc*-specific proteins, a second codon (non-AUG) near the 3' end of exon 1 can provide an alternative initiation site and is thought to be responsible for the larger species of protein.[165] Thus, it is possible that the different amino-terminal sequences found in the respective *myc* products may also be determinants for distinctive activities.

Several independent isolates of v-*myc* containing transforming viruses contain all or most of the c-*myc* coding sequences but are devoid of exon 1, as well as other regulatory sequences upstream of this exon. Although mutations resulting in amino acid substitutions have been recognized, and the v-*myc* proteins differ from those of c-*myc* in other aspects,[166] these features appear of little consequence with respect to the malignant potential of the oncogene. Rather, the transforming ability of v-*myc* can be attributed to the loss of transcriptional regulatory sequences, presumably occurring within and upstream from exon 1, as well as to the addition of a powerful promoter represented by the viral long terminal repeats (LTR).

Elimination of specific regulatory sequences of c-*myc* was noted in avian bursal lymphomas induced by ALV containing no cellular sequences (oncogenes). The insertion of the viral genome upstream from exon 2 was a consistent feature of these lymphoma cells,[167] suggesting that interposing viral sequences could interfere with the cellular regulation of the c-*myc* gene while, by way of the viral LTR, providing a strong promoter for c-*myc* transcription.[168]

The human c-*myc* proto-oncogene is normally located on chromosome 8; translocations with this chromosome to chromosomes 14, 22, or 2 are found in all Burkitt's lymphomas examined cytogenetically.[168] These translocations involve the human immunoglobulin loci, which are displaced in juxtaposition to c-*myc,* and which appear to affect the normal pattern of c-*myc* transcriptional regulation. Apparently, these specific translocations are caused by the enzyme involved normally in immunoglobulin gene recombination (V-D-J recombinase), which then mistakenly recognizes sequences in c-*myc* as immunoglobulin sequences and joins them to immunoglobulin sequences.[170] The recombinant translocation process produces a constitutive expression of the c-*myc* gene that ultimately results in an unrestricted proliferation of B-cells. Curiously, this effect of translocated immunoglobulin genes on c-*myc* deregulation is specific for B-cells and is not found in other lymphoid cell types.[171]

Another possible area of possible c-*myc* involvement in tumorigenesis is represented by the high frequency of c-*myc* rearrangements associated with hepatic carcinomas of woodchucks infected with hepatitis virus.[172] Investigations into the relevance of *myc* in hepatocellular carcinomas of man are therefore of prime interest, these tumors are rare in the United States, but very common in areas of endemic human hepatitis virus infections.

The *erb*A Oncogene ■

Avian erythroblastosis virus contains two oncogenes: v-*erb*B, which encodes a homologue of the EGF receptor described earlier; and v-*erb*A, whose product contains sequences homologous to the DNA-binding domains of steroid hormone receptors. The c-*erb*A proto-oncogene was recently shown to encode a high-affinity receptor for thyroid hormone;[173,174] at least two distinct *erb*A loci, located on chromosomes 3 and 17, have been identified in human cells.[175] These *erb*A genes code for products that have both a DNA-binding domain and a thyroid hormone-binding domain.

Like other oncogene homologues of growth factor receptors, the viral v-*erb*A product is damaged and has lost its ability to bind thyroid hormone,[173] apparently due to a mutation in the hormone-binding domain; the domain is otherwise intact, but the thyroid-induced regulatory property is lost. The v-*erb*A gene has no direct transforming effect,[176] but it does enhance the erythroid cell transforming potential of v-*erb*B; v-*erb*A can also cooperate with several other oncogenes (v-*src,* v-*fos,* v-*fms,* v-*sea,* and v-Ha-*ras*) in causing erythroid cell transformations.

This ability to specifically cause transformation in a semidifferentiated lineage has focused attention on erythroid-specific genes and how they are synergistically affected by v-*erb*A. It was found that v-*erb*A suppresses transcription of the erythrocyte anion transporter gene and, less efficiently, the δ-aminolevulinic acid synthetase gene, but does not affect other erythroid genes.[177] The anion transporter gene is not only important in anion transport in mature erythrocytes, but is the only protein known to anchor the erythrocyte cytoskeleton to the plasma membrane.[178] It is also part of the enzyme system that regulates intracellular pH in response to external CO_2, and thus could interconnect directly with a signal transduction pathway to sustain cell growth. Despite the interesting possibilities presented by the action of v-*erb*A on the transporter and synthetase genes, it is not yet known whether the v-*erb*A protein interacts with genes directly to effect transcription, or perhaps inhibits transcription by some as yet undiscovered process.

No specific human hematologic disorders have yet been attributed to alterations in the c-*erb*A genes. However, in small cell lung carcinoma (SCLC), deletions are often seen on the short arm of chromosome 3[179,180] in the region to which a particular c-*erb*A gene, c-*erb*A-β, has been localized. In all six cases of SCLC studied, at least one copy of *erb*A-β was deleted, suggesting that *erb*A-β may be a recessive gene required for the maintenance of normal lung cells.

The *jun* Oncogene ■

Cloning and sequencing of the v-*jun* gene present in avian sarcoma virus (ASV) 17 showed a high degree of homology with the yeast transcription factor GCN4 at the level of the predicted amino acid sequences. The homology was found mainly in the DNA-binding domain of GCN4, suggesting that v-*jun* might encode a sequence-specific DNA-binding protein.[181] A core consensus DNA sequence recognized by GCN4 is similar to the binding site of a human transactivating protein, AP-1,[182] and the possibility that human c-*jun* could be similar or identical to the gene encoding AP-1 was borne out. Expression of cloned c-*jun* in bacteria produced a protein with DNA-binding properties identical to AP-1,[183] and antibodies raised against c-*jun* peptides reacted specifically with purified AP-1. In addition, c-*jun* protein and AP-1 have tryptic peptides in common.

The relevance of *jun* and AP-1 to the mitogenic signal pathway becomes apparent when one considers that cells treated with TPA have elevated levels of AP-1 activity. Also, the genes whose expression is induced by phorbol ester promoters (*e.g.,* TPA) are identical to the genes responsive to AP-1.[184,185] Further, synthetic copies of the AP-1 consensus binding site act as intracellular enhancers in response to TPA. Because TPA directly activates protein kinase C, it would appear that experimental resolution of the intermediates between the mitogenic signal and transcriptional activation of *jun* is well within reach.

Analyses of both chicken and human c-*jun* protooncogenes revealed that an internal sequence corresponding to 27 amino acids had been deleted from v-*jun,* with two amino acid substitutions occurring in the DNA-binding region. It is possible therefore, that the oncogenic activity of the v-*jun* protein derives from the loss of these sequences in a regulatory domain, resulting from an inappropriate DNA sequence recognition.

The *ets-2* Oncogene ■

The human *ets-2* gene has a high degree of homology to the viral oncogene v-*ets.* This viral *ets* sequence was originally identified as a cell-derived sequence transduced into its genome by ALV E26. The genome of this transforming retrovirus codes for a single transforming fusion protein of 135 kDa that localizes in the nucleus. This oncogene-encoded protein, p135$^{gag-myb-ets}$, is capable of inducing erythroblastosis and myeloblastosis in infected birds. To better understand the conversion of the normal proto-*ets* gene to the malignantly transforming v-*ets* gene, our laboratory has cloned several proto-*ets* genes, including those from the original avian host and numerous other animal species, both vertebrate (*Xenopus,* mouse, and human) and invertebrate (*Drosophila* and sea urchin), and studied their molecular details[186–190] and their encoded products. The *ets-2* gene appears to be very highly conserved in all animal species, from *Drosophila* to human. In fact, at the level of amino acid residues, there is greater than 92% homology between the predicted D-*ets-2* product of *Drosophila* and the human predicted *ets-2* gene product.[191,192] This level of conservation for proto-oncogene-encoded products is the highest noted to date for species so widely separated on the evolutionary scale,[188] and implies that the *ets-2* gene products must have important, if not essential, functions in these species. Previous observations in our laboratory suggested that the *ets-2* gene has a role in cell proliferation.[193] The product of the *ets-2* gene was preferentially expressed in a variety of proliferative tissue; levels of *ets-2* expression were generally greater when tissue was obtained from various young organs compared to adult organs of the same type. This was most evident in testis tissue, where *ets-2* mRNA synthesis was maximal in 8-day-old samples, compared to 42-day-old preparations of the germinal tissue. In a model system of surgically induced regenerating hepatic murine tissue, *ets-2* gene expression peaked at 4 hours after partial hepatectomy, returning to basal levels within 24 hours. Densitometric scanning studies of the 4-hour samples of *ets-2* mRNA following partial hepatectomy showed a 10-fold increase above basal levels seen in sham-operated controls and in adult liver tissue. During the course of liver regeneration, DNA synthesis peaked at 48 hours after hepatectomy. Thus, the maximal *ets-2* peak at 4 hours occurs well before peak DNA synthesis, not unlike the kinetics observed with another proto-oncogene, c-*fos,* following partial hepatectomy in the rat.[193,194] Also, consistent with the proposed relationship of *ets-2* to proliferation is evidence that stimulation of quiescent fibroblasts by the addition of serum results in a marked increase in levels of *ets-2* mRNA. As is true of other known nuclear proto-oncogene (*fos* and *myc*) mRNAs, addition of cycloheximide superinduced levels of *ets-2* by more than 15-fold in hepatic tissue and even higher (20- to 40-fold) in cycloheximide-treated partially hepatectomized tissue. The temporal expression of *ets-2* was determined to be *fos* → *myc* → *ets-2*, and during hepatic regeneration, transcription of *ets-2* proto-oncogene, like *fos* or *myc,* does not require *de novo* synthesis. Thus, the product of the *ets-2* gene appears to be associated with the transition of cells from G_0 to G_1 (see Fig. 1–1). The human *ets-2* gene product has been identified by the use of specific antibodies directed against antigen obtained from the bacterially expressed partial cDNA clone of the *ets-2* gene,[195,196] as well as an oligopeptide antigen corresponding to a highly conserved hydrophilic region of *ets.* Using both types of sera, a 56 kDa protein has been identified as the human *ets-2* gene product; this protein, like the oncogene product p135$^{gag-myb-ets}$, locates in the nucleus. This localization supports the relationship of the human *ets-2* protein with other nuclear proto-oncogene products, (*e.g.,* those encoded by c-*fos* and c-*myc*) that are expressed in association with cellular proliferation.

We found that the *ets-2* protein is phosphorylated and has a rapid turnover—normally less than half an hour.[197,198] However, when cells are treated with a tumor promoter such as 12-0 tetra-decanuylphurbol 13-acetate (TPA), the level of *ets-2* protein is quickly and markedly elevated. This increase appears to result from stabilization of the protein, because the *ets-2* p56^{ets-2} product increases its half-life by more than 2 hours in the presence of TPA, whereas the *ets-2*-specific mRNA content does not increase. Because an inhibitor of protein kinase C also interferes with the stabilization of p56^{ets-2} and the effect of TPA can be mimicked by a synthetic DG, it appears that the protein kinase C signal pathway is probably involved in the induction of this nuclear proto-oncogene.

The ets-2 protein is, however, unique among nuclear oncogene products in its ability to respond to TPA posttranslationally. Other nuclear proto-oncogenes respond to TPA at the mRNA level and subsequently at the protein level, but thus far only the ets-2 protein level increases in the absence of any increase in net mRNA synthesis. In addition, the protein synthesis inhibitor cycloheximide enhances the effect of TPA on the level of ets-2 protein, further retarding its turnover, a finding consistent with a posttranslational mechanism. Taken together, these data suggest that expression of the proto-ets-2 gene and its encoded products is rapidly controlled by signal transduction, most probably involving, directly or indirectly, the protein kinase C pathway. This posttranslational response suggests that such a precisely controlled regulatory mechanism may be an essential feature of the function of the ets-2-encoded protein.[198] It can even be speculated that stabilization, and consequent transient elevation of this protein's level may be an intermediary step in the signaling process of the protein kinase C pathway, perhaps interconnecting this activation process with the regulation of other genes involved with proliferation. The deregulation of, or any subtle alteration in, these controlling mechanisms may then, through the signal transduction pathway, cause a profound change in intracellular physiology.

Activation of protein kinase C, as a result of receptor activation or action of TPA, alters the pattern of gene expression. Among the genes induced by this pathway are ornithine decarboxylase,[199] IL-2 and its receptor,[200,201] vimentin,[202] and the nuclear proto-oncogenes myc and fos.[121–124] This induction is not dependent on continuous protein synthesis, and occurs in the presence of protein synthesis inhibitors.[203,123] The pathways, as well as the mechanisms connecting protein kinase C activation at the cell membrane and the alteration of gene expression in the nucleus, are, however, largely unknown. One can assume that some modification is induced in the machinery for gene transcription or primary transcript processing, a modification that is assumed to be posttranslational. This assumption is reasonable because alteration in gene expression induced by the protein kinase C pathway is usually considered to be independent of continuous protein synthesis.

One of the more interesting examples of an intermediary process in signaling of the protein kinase C pathway, connecting enzyme activation with gene regulation, is the interaction of the immunoglobulin-enhancer-binding protein NF-κB[204] with the transcription activator proteins AP-1[1,30] and AP-2.[205,206] AP-1 and AP-2 are recently discovered examples of

nuclear transcription factors whose activities are also induced by TPA through posttranslational mechanisms. Like the ets-2 product, the level of NF-κB is superinduced in the presence of cycloheximide.[204] Moreover, a role for the nuclear transcription factors in proliferation has been demonstrated by the recent finding that the c-jun proto-oncogene codes for the AP-1 protein.[130] Given this linkage of a proto-oncogene product, with the example above of a TPA- and protein kinase C- activated transcription, one can not speculate that some of the properties of the normal c-ets-2 protein would be similarly related. Further, an analogous role can be suggested for the oncogene product of v-ets in usurping the normal ets function, based on the oncogene v-jun and its relationship to the cellular nuclear transcription factors as a potential factor in oncogenesis. In this regard, the human ets-2 gene may be of potential interest in oncology because this gene, normally located on human chromosome 21,[187] is translocated in certain leukemias that have been cytogenetically characterized.[207] Specifically, in certain nonrandom aberrations, the human ets-2 gene was transposed from chromosome 21 to 8 in t(8;21)(q22;q22)-associated translocations. This chromosomal event was also associated with altered expression of the ets-2 gene, although this gene was distal from the breakpoint and not visibly rearranged.[207–209] It is quite possible that such translocations could interfere with a regulatory region of the human ets-2 gene, an event with potentially profound biologic–oncogenetic ramifications, given the possible relationship of the ets-2 gene product to signal transduction. Further molecular details of this ets-2 interrelationship are required and will help expand not only our knowledge of cellular proliferation but possibly of the initiation of neoplasia.

Finally, it should be noted that the human ets-2 gene is located on the region of the chromosome 21 (21q22.3) implicated in Down's syndrome.[210–212] Trisomy of this small chromosomal domain results in the full manifestation of the Down's syndrome phenotype. Because the ets-2 protein level appears to be under precise control, the increase in the ets-2 gene dosage resulting from the trisomy may seriously affect control of the ets-2 protein. It is, thus conceivable that this deregulation is a contributing factor to the development of Down's syndrome.

Conclusion ■

We have limited this review to oncogenes or proto-oncogenes and their encoded proteins, many of which are similar or nearly identical to proteins involved in mitogenic regulation. Other oncogenes have been isolated, and their derived products can be placed in the categories of growth factor receptor, cytoplasmic tyrosine kinase, cytoplasmic (other than tyrosine) kinase, and nuclear binding proteins. Definitive characterization of these oncogenes is certain to expand our understanding of cellular division, and of the types of disruptions that occur in the normal proto-oncogenes to render oncogenes carcinogenic.

Identification of proto-oncogene products and specific components of the mitogenic signal transduction pathway allows us to follow the progression of cellular events, at least tentatively, from external stimulation to transcriptional activation. We can then reasonably assume that constitutive expression or independent, unregulated activity of an oncogene product can sustain continuous cell divisions and, hence, promote unremitting cellular proliferation. How transcriptional changes resulting from signal transduction, or alterations in DNA-binding proteins, affect the mitogenic program is not as obvious. At least 30 genes are activated by serum stimulation of quiescent cells, and transcriptional activating proteins, such as AP-1 (the c-*jun* product), may recognize sequences regulating only several of these genes. Thus, there remain numerous undiscovered regulatory factors and interactions within the nucleus alone that will help elucidate mitogenesis. At least some of these genes, if not their oncogenic variants, can relieve the restricted cell of growth factor requirements. Also, a major point to consider is that growing cells, especially malignant cells, excrete factors that can promote autologous growth and may also promote or repress the growth of heterologous cells.

Substantially less attention has been paid to genes that become repressed as a result of mitogenesis or oncogenesis then to those known to be inducible. For example, cells transformed by Rous sarcoma virus, and other dividing cells, synthesize less collagen,[213] fibronectin,[214] alkaline phosphatase,[215] and adenylate cyclase.[216] In the case of collagen at least, transcriptional repression is responsible for inhibition of synthesis. Thus, it would seem that signal transduction is not limited to the activation of enzymatic components or gene transcription and that specific repression is also an integral part of the mitogenic program. One could therefore consider recessive mutations as a basis for some oncogenesis, particularly when the elimination or depletion of an inhibitory regulator (or gene) may have dire consequences (*e.g.,* in retinoblastosis).

The recognition that oncogenes act through specific components of the mitogenic pathway has alerted researchers to the relevance of specific oncogene-encoded defects as significant factors intimately involved in certain types of malignancies. Thus, mechanisms by which oncogenes may induce malignancy can be proposed and experimentally tested. As we have seen for the oncogenes *myc, fos,* and *sis,* constitutive activation or synthesis of the altered proto-oncogene product is directly associated with the induction of malignancy. In some instances, the amplification of normal genes appears to be responsible for some *myc*-induced malignancies (perhaps by producing a genetic overload). This aspect of amplified expression should probably be a consideration for any gene product that can, in excessive amounts, enforce cell growth.

Chromosomal translocations, through rearrangements or disruption of regulation, can constitutively activate proto-oncogenes in appropriate cells and thus may be a significant basis for many human malignancies. In human Burkitt's lymphomas c-*myc* activation may be the sole initiating causative mechanism. The importance of cytogenetically correlating chromosomal constitution with a specific cancer and probing for consistent alterations in proto-oncogene expression is clear. Less obvious is the possibility that growth-promoting genes of human cells may be constitutively activated by insertion of proviral elements within the gene's regulatory program. This has been clearly demonstrated in avian bursal lymphomas and in some cases of avian erythroblastosis, where the promoter–enhancer elements of a nontransforming ALV activate c-*myc* or c-*erb*A genes, respectively. The prevalence (albeit restricted) of human T-lymphotropic viruses (HTLV-I and HTLV-II) and the rapid rise and spread of other infectious human immunodeficiency viruses, especially HIV-I, may prompt similar studies of the possible mechanisms of insertional activation by these human viruses in human oncogenesis. In addition to insertional activation, both the HTLV and HIV human retroviruses contain genes whose products are capable of transactivating their own (viral) or other cellular genes. Even if these transactivating (*tat*) genes are incapable of inducing malignancy on their own, they may contribute to neoplasia. For example, activation in an infected cell may lead to excretion of growth factors or other substances, which could affect heterologous cells in a fashion similar to transformed cells secreting growth factors. This type of activation is being considered as a plausible mechanism in the development of Kaposi's sarcoma, frequently observed in patients infected with HIV. Component cells of these sarcomas usually contain no evidence of viral infection; they are apparently mitogenically stimulated by factors secreted by other cells in these HIV-infected patients.

Proto-oncogenes, on the whole, seem to be converted to oncogenes by the truncation and loss of nucleotide sequences, which frequently changes the proto-oncogene's regulatory properties by deletion of a regulatory domain. A chromosomal translocation can easily produce this change, as exemplified in CML and ALL, where translocation of the c-*abl* gene results in loss of regulatory peptides from the normal protein. Chromosomal insertion of a provirus could not only result in transcriptional activation but also engender proto-oncogene mutations resulting in the deletion of key regulatory sites. This deletion mechanism has yet to be described in association with human cancers or human proto-oncogenes.

Point mutations that inactivate normal active regulatory sites are apparently the basis for at least one group of human oncogenes, the *ras* genes. Human tumors that frequently occur at sites most likely to be exposed to mutagens (*i.e.,* skin and alimentary tract) are those in which high incidences of activated *ras* oncogenes are detected.

The available information seems to suggest the possibility that every oncogene can, in some way, impinge on normal mitogenic signaling. One can anticipate that knowledge of factors that normally activate the mitogenic pathway (exemplified by growth factors and proto-oncogene products) will soon be complemented by the identification of components that keep the mitogenic program in check. Research on this aspect of mitogenic regulation encourages the notion that a real understanding of mitosis is possible and that carcinogenic growth may be arrested specifically. As the battery of proto-oncogenes and oncogenes enlarges and these genes become better characterized, the likelihood increases that we will achieve a comprehensive understanding of the complex cellular growth cycle. Extensive chromosomal analysis and correlation of specific aberrations and tumor types should continue to contribute important insights into the possible involvement of oncogenes in specific malignancies. Analyses of translocation breakpoints and characterization of adjacent genes may also reveal some specific genes important in mitotic regulation that would not be recognized otherwise. Each of the findings discussed here can be compared to a jigsaw puzzle piece; as the pieces are fitted together, a recognizable picture is emerging, one that should reveal a comprehensive molecular panorama of mitogenesis and cellular growth.

References ■

1. Goustin AS, Leof EB, Shipley GD, Moses HL: Growth factors and cancer. Cancer Res 46:1015–1029, 1986
2. Salomon DS, Perroteau I: Growth factors in cancer and their relationship to oncogenes. Cancer Invest 4:43–60, 1986
3. Carpenter G: Receptors for epidermal growth factor and other polypeptide mitogens. Annu Rev Biochem 56:881–914, 1987
4. Marguardt J, Hunkapillar WW, Hood LE, Todaro GT: Rat transforming growth factor type 1: Structure and relation to epidermal growth factor. Science 223:1079–1082, 1984
5. Stroobant P, Rice AP, Gullick WJ, Cheng DJ, Kerr IM, Waterfield MD: Purification and characterization of vaccinia virus growth factor. Cell 42:383–393, 1985
6. Brown JP, Twardzik DR, Marquardt H, Todaro GJ: Vaccinia virus encodes a polypeptide hemologous to epidermal growth factor and transforming growth factor. Nature 313:491–492, 1985
7. Carpenter G: Epidermal growth factor. In Baserga R (ed): Handbook of Experimental Pharmacology: Tissue Growth Factors, Vol 57, pp 89–132. New York, Springer Verlag, 1981
8. Das SK, Stanley ER: Structure function studies of a colony-stimulating factor (CSF-1). J Biol Chem 257:13679–13684, 1982
9. Stiles CD: The molecular biology of platelet derived growth factor. Cell 33:653–655, 1983
10. Doolittle RF, Hunkapiller MV, Hood LE, Devare SG, Robbins KC, Aaronson SA, Antoniades HN: Simian sarcoma virus *onc* gene, v-*sis,* is derived from the gene (or genes) encoding a platelet-derived growth factor. Science 221:275–277, 1983
11. Waterfield MD, Scrace GT, Whittle N, Stroobant P, Johnsson A, Wasteson A, Westermark B, Heldin C, Huang JS, Deuel TF: Platelet-derived growth factor is structurally related to the putative transforming protein p28^{sis} of simian sarcoma virus. Nature 304:35–39, 1983
12. Robbins KC, Antoniades HN, Devare SG, Hunkapiller MW, Aaronson SA: Structural and immunological similarities between simian sarcoma virus gene product(s) and human platelet-derived growth factor. Nature 305:605–608, 1983
13. Niman HL, Houghton RA, Bowen-Pope DF: Detection of high molecular weight forms of platelet-derived growth factor by sequence-specific antisera. Science 226:701–703, 1984
14. Leal F, Williams LT, Robbins KC, Aaronson SA: Evidence that the v-*sis* gene product transforms by interaction with the receptor for platelet-derived growth factor. Science 230:327–330, 1985
15. Igarashi H, Gazit A, Chiu I-M, Srinivasan A, Yaniv A, Tronick SR, Robbins KC, Aaronson SA: Normal human *sis*/PDGF-2 gene expression induces cellular transformation. In Cancer Cells 3: Growth Factors and Transformation, pp 159–166. Cold Spring Harbor, NY, Cold Spring Harbor Laboratory, 1985
16. Assoian RK, Grotendorst GR, Miller DM, Sporn MB: Cellular transformation by coordinated action of three peptide growth factors from human platelets. Nature 309:804–806, 1984
17. Huang JS, Huang SS, Deuel TF: Transforming protein of simian sarcoma virus stimulates autocrine growth of SSV-transformed cells through PDGF cell-surface receptors. Cell 39:79–87, 1984
18. Josephs ST, Guo C, Ratner C, Wong-Staal F: Human proto-oncogene nucleotide sequences corresponding to the transforming region of simian sarcoma virus. Science 223:487–491, 1984
19. Bowen-Pope DF, Vogel A, Ross R: Production of platelet-derived growth factor like molecules and reduced expression of platelet derived growth factor receptors accompany transformation by a wide spectrum of agents. Proc Natl Acad Sci USA 81:2396, 1984
20. Keating MT, Williams CT: Autocrine stimulation of intracellular PDGF receptors in v-*sis* transformed cells. Science 239:914–916, 1988

21. Eva A, Robbins KC, Andersen PR, Srinivasan A, Tronick SR, Reddy EP, Ellmore NW, Galen AT, Lautenberger JA, Papas TS, Westin EH, Wong-Staal F, Gallo RC, Aaronson SA: Cellular genes analogous to retroviral *onc* genes are transcribed in human tumor cells. Nature 295:116–119, 1982

22. Beutram CR, de Klein A, Hagemeijer A, Grosveld G, Hesterkamp N, Groffen J: Localization of the human c-*sis* oncogene in Ph¹-positive and Ph¹-negative chromic myelogenous leukemia by *in situ* hybridization. Blood 63:223–225, 1984

23. Groffen J, Heisterkamp N, Stephenson JR, Van Kessel AG, de Klein A, Grosveld G, Bootsma D: C-*sis* is translocated from chromosome 22 to chromosome 9 in chromic myelocytic leukemia. J Exp Med 158:9–15, 1983

24. De La Chapelle A, Lenoir G, Bove J, Bove A, Galamo P, Huerre C, Szijnert M-F, Jean Pierre N, Lalovel JM, Kaplan JC: Lambda I9 constant region genes are translocated to chromosome 8 in Burkitts lymphoma with t(8;22). Nucleic Acids Res 11:1133–1142, 1983

25. Erikson J, Martinis J, Croce CM: Assignment of the genes for human 1 immunoglobulin chains to chromosome 22. Nature 294:173–175, 1981

26. Avrias A, Rombautc C, Buffe D, Dubousset J, Mazbraud A: Chromosomal translocations in Ewing's sarcomas. N Engl J Med 309:496–497, 1983

27. Turc-Carel C, Philip I, Berger M-P, Philip T, Lenior GM: Chromosomal translocations in Ewing's sarcoma. N Engl J Med 309:497–498, 1983

28. van Kessel AG, Turc-Carel C, de Klein A, Grosveld G, Lenior G, Bootsma D: Translocation of oncogene c-sis from chromosome 22 to chromosome 11 in a Ewing sarcoma-derived cell line. Mol Cell Biol 5:427–429, 1985

29. Pettenheimer CW, Noussel MR, Quinn CO, Kitchingman GR, Look AT, and Sherr CJ: Transmembrane orientation of glycoproteins encoded by the v-*fms* oncogene. Cell 40:971–981, 1985

30. Manger R, Najita L, Nichols EJ, Hakemori S, Rohrschneider L: Cell surface expression at the McDonough strain of feline sarcoma virus *fms* gene product (9p140fms). Cell 39:327–337, 1984

31. Hampe A, Gobert M, Sherr CJ, Galibert F: Nucleotide sequence of the feline retroviral oncogene v-fms shows unexpected homology with oncogenes encoding tyrosine-specific protein kinase. Proc Natl Acad Sci USA 81:85–89, 1984

32. Barbacid M, Lauver AV: Gene products of McDonough feline sarcoma virus have an *in vitro* associated protein kinase that phosphorylates tyrosine residues; lack of this enzymatic activity *in vivo*. J Virol 40:812–821, 1981

33. Sherr CJ, Rettenmier CW, Sacca R, Roussel MF, Look AT, Stanley ER: The c-*fms* proto-oncogene product is related to the receptor for the mononuclear phagocyte growth factor, CSF-1. Cell 41:665–676, 1985

34. Sacca R, Stanley ER, Sherr CJ, Rettenmier CW: Specific binding of the mononuclear phagocyte colony-stimulating factor CSF-1 to the product of the v-*fms* oncogene. Proc Natl Acad Sci USA. 83:3331–3335, 1986

35. Wheeler EF, Askew D, May S, Ihle JN, Sherr CJ: The v-*fms* oncogene induces factor-independent growth and transformation of the interleukin-3-dependent myeloid cell line FDC-PI. Mol Cell Biol 7:1673–1680

36. Nichols EJ, Manger R, Hakomori S, Herscovics A, Rohrschneider CR: Transformation by the v-*fms* oncogene product: Role of glycosylational processing and cell surface expression. Mol Cell Biol 5:3467–3475, 1985

37. Lyman SD, Rohrschneider LR: Analysis of functional domains of the v-*fms* encoded protein of Susan McDonough strain feline sarcoma virus by linker insertion mutagenesis. Mol Cell Biol 7:3287–3296, 1987

38. Roussel MF, Sherr CJ, Barker PE, Ruddle FH: Molecular cloning of the c-fms locus and its assignment to human chromosome 5. J Virol 48:770–773, 1983

39. Verbeek JS, Roeroek AJM, van den Ovweland AMW, Bloemers HPJ, Van de Ven WJM: Human C-*fms* proto-oncogene: Comparative analysis with an abnormal allele. Mol Cell Biol 5:422–426, 1985

40. Sokal G, Michaux JC, van den Berghe H, Corbier A, Rodhain J, Ferrant A, Moriam M, de Bruyere M, Sonnet J: A new hamatopoietic syndrome with a distinct karyotype: The 5q--chromosome. Blood 46:519–533, 1975

41. Yamamoto T, Nishida T, Miyajima N, Kaeai S, Qoi T, Toyoshima K: The *erb*B gene of avian erythroblastosis virus is a member of the *src* gene family. Cell 35:71–78, 1983

42. Downward J, Yarden Y, Mayes E, Scarce G, Totty N, Stockwell P, Ullrich A, Schlessinger J, Waterfield MD: Close similarity of epidermal growth factor and v-*erb*B oncogene protein sequences. Nature 307:521–527, 1983

43. Spurr NK, Solomon E, Janson M, Sheer D, Goodfellow PN, Bodmer WF, Vennstrom B: Chromosomal localization of the human homologues to the oncogenes *erb*A and B. EMBO J 3:159–163, 1984

44. Ullrich A, Coussens L, Hayflick JS, Dull JJ, Gray A, Tam AW, Lee J, Yarden Y, Libermann TA, Schlessinger J, Downward J, Mayes ELV, Whittle N, Waterfield MD, Seeburg PH: Human epidermal growth factor receptor cDNA-sequence and aberrant expression of the amplified gene in A431 epidermal carcinoma cells. Nature 309:418–425, 1984

45. Nilsen TW, Maroney PA, Goodwin RG, Rottman FM, Crittenden CB, Raines MA, Kung H-J: c-*erb*B activation in ALV-induced erythroblastosis: Novel RNA processing and promoter insertion result in expression of an aminotruncated EGF receptor. Cell 41:719–726, 1985

46. Gannett DC, Tracy SE, Robinson HL: Differences in sequences encoding the carboxyl-terminal domain of the epidermal growth factor receptor correlate with differences in the disease potential of viral erb B genes. Proc Natl Acad Sci USA 83:6053–6058, 1986

47. Cohen S, Ushiro H, Stoscheck C, Chinkers M: A native 170,000 epidermal growth factor receptor-kinase complex from shed membrane vesicles. J Biol Chem 257:1523–1531, 1982

48. Conley GJ, Smith B, Gusterson B, Hendler F, Ozanne B: The amount of EGF receptor is elevated on squamous cell carcinomas. In Cancer Cells: The Transformed Phenotype, Vol 1, pp 5–10. Cold Spring Harbor, NY, Cold Spring Harbor Laboratory, 1984

49. Gamov S, Kim YS, Shimazu N: Different responses to EGF in two human carcinoma cell lines, A431 and NCVA-1, possessing high numbers of EGF receptors. Mol Cell Endocrinol 37:205–213, 1984

50. Fitzpatrick SL, LaChance MP, Schultz GS: Characterization of epidermal growth factor receptor and action on human breast cancer cells in culture. Cancer Res 44:3442–3447, 1984

51. Hendler FJ, Ozanne BW: Human squamous cell lung cancers express increased epidermal growth factor receptors. J Clin Invest 74:647–651, 1984

52. Pledger WJ, Stiles CD, Antoniades HN, Scher CD: An ordered sequence of events is required before BALB/c-3T3 cells become committed to DNA synthesis. Proc Natl Acad Sci USA 75:2839–2843, 1978

53. Stiles CD, Capone GT, Scher CD, Antoniades HN, Van Wyk JJ, Pledger WJ: Dual control of cell growth by somatomedins and platelet-derived growth factor. Proc Natl Acad Sci USA 76:1279–1283, 1979

54. Yarden Y, Escobedo JA, Kuang WJ, Yong-feng TL, Daniel TO, Tremble PM, Chen EY, Ando ME: Structure of the re-

ceptor for platelet-derived growth factor helps define a family of closely-related growth factor receptors. Nature 323:226–232, 1986

55. Park M, Dean M, Kaul K, Braun MJ, Gonda M, Vande Woude G: Sequence of MET proto-oncogene cDNA has features characteristic of the tyrosine kinase family of growth-factor receptors. Proc Natl Acad Sci USA 84:6379–6383, 1987

56. Gonzatti-Haces M, Seth A, Park M, Copeland T, Oroszlan S, Vande Woude GF: Characterization of the TPR-MET oncogene p65 and the MET protooncogene p140 protein-tyrosine kinases. Proc Natl Acad Sci USA 85:21–25, 1988

57. Dean M, Park M, Vande Woude GF: Characterization of the rearranged tpr-met oncogene breakpoint. Mol Cell Biol 7:921–924, 1987

58. Rhim JS, Park DK, Arnstein P, Heubner RJ, Weisburger EK: Transformation of human cells in culture by N-methyl-N'-nitro-nitrosoguanidine. Nature 256:751–753, 1975

59. Schechter AL, Stern DF, Vaidyanathan L, Decker SJ, Drebin JA, Greene MI, Weinberg RA: The neu oncogene: An erbB related gene encoding a 185,000 mr tumor antigen. Nature 312:513–516, 1984

60. Bargmann CI, Hung MC, Weinberg RA: The neu oncogene encodes an epidermal growth factor receptor related protein. Nature 319:226–230, 1986

61. Schecter AL, Hung ML, Vaidyanathan L, Weinberg RA, Yang-Feng T, Francke U, Ullrich A, Coussens L: The neu gene: An erb B homologous gene distinct from and unlinked to the gene encoding the EGF receptor. Science 229:976–978, 1985

62. Bargmann CI, Hung CH, Weinberg RA: Multiple independent activations of the neu oncogene by a point mutation altering the transmembrane domain of p185. Cell 45:649–657, 1986

63. Cotton PC, Brugger JS: Neural tissues express high levels of the cellular src gene product pp60c-src. Mol Cell Biol 3:1157–1162, 1983

64. Poirier F, Calothy R, Karess E, Erikson E, Hanfusa H: Role of p60src kinase activity in the induction of neuroretinae cell proliferation by Rous sarcoma virus. J Virol 42:780–789, 1982

65. Collett MS, Erikson RL: Protein kinase activity associated with the avian sarcoma virus src gene product. Proc Natl Acad Sci USA 75:2021–2024, 1978

66. Hunter T: A tail of two src's: Mutadis mutandis. Cell 49:1–4, 1987

67. Collett MS, Belzer SK, Purchio AF: Structurally and functionally modified forms of pp60v-src in Rous sarcoma virus transformed cell lysates. Mol Cell Biol 4:1213–1220, 1987

68. Rowley JD: A new consistant chromosomal abnormality in chronic myelogous leukemia identified by quinocrine fluorescence and Giemsa staining. Nature 243:290–293, 1973

69. Heisterkamp N, Groffen J, Stephenson JR, Spurr NK, Goodfellow PN, Solomon E, Carritt B, Bodmer WF: Chromosomal localization of human cellular homologues of two viral oncogenes. Nature 299:747–749, 1982

70. Ben-Neriah T, Bernards A, Paskin M, Daley GQ. Baltimore D: Alternative 5' exons in c-abl mRNA. Cell 44:577–586, 1986

71. Groffen J, Heisterkamp H, Stam K, de Klein A, Bartramm CR, Grosveld G: Philadelphia chromosomal breakpoints are clustered within a limited region, bcr on chromosome 22. Cell 36:93–99, 1984

72. Grosveld G, Verwoerd T, van Agthoven T, de Klein A, Ramachandran KL, Heisterkamp N, Stam K, Groffen J: The chronic myelocytic cell line K562 contains a breakpoint in bcr and produces a chimeric bcr/c-abl transcript. Mol Cell Biol 6:607–616, 1986

73. Ben Nariah T, Daley GQ, Mes-Masson A-M, Witte ON, Baltimore D: The chronic myelogenous leukemia-specific p210 protein is the product of the bcr/abl hybrid gene. Science 233:212–214, 1986

74. Konopka JB, Witte ON: Detection of c-abl tyrosine kinase activity in vitro permits direct comparison of normal and altered abl gene products. Mol Cell Biol 5:3116–3123, 1985

75. Groffen J, Heisterkamp N, Reynolds FH, Stephenson JR: Homology between phosphotyrosine acceptor site of human c-abl and viral oncogene products. Nature 304:167–169, 1983

76. Sandberg A, Kohna S, Wake N, Minowa: Chromosome and causation of human cancer and leukemia: XLII. Cancer Genet Cytogenet 2:145–174, 1980

77. Chan LC, Karhi KK, Rayter SI, Heisterkamp N, Eridami S, Powles R, Lawler SD, Groffen J, Foulkes JG, Greaves MF, Wiedemann LM: A novel abl protein expressed in Philadelphia chromosome positive acute lymphoblastic leukemia. Nature 325:635–637, 1987

78. Clark SS, Mclaughlin J, Crist WM, Champlin R, Witte ON: Unique forms of the abl tyrosine kinase distinguish Ph-positive cml from Ph-positive ALL. Science 235:85–88, 1987

79. Erikson J, Griffin CA, Ar-Rushdi A, Valtier M, Hoxie J, Finan J, Emanuel BS, Rovera G, Nowell PC, Croce CM: Heterogeneity of chromosome 22 breakpoints in Philadelphia positive (Ph+) acute lymphocytic leukemia. Proc Natl Acad Sci USA 83:1807–1811, 1986

80. Hermans A, Heisterkamp N, von Lindern M, van Baal S, Meijer D, van der Plas D, Wiedemann LM, Groffen J, Grosveld G: Unique fusion of bcr and c-abl genes in Philadelphia chromosome positive acute lymphoblastic leukemia. Cell 51:33–40, 1986

81. Blenis J, Erikson RL: Regulation of a ribosomal S6 kinase activity by the Rous sarcoma virus-transforming protein, serum or porbol ester. Proc Natl Acad Sci USA 82:7621–7625, 1985

82. Blackshear PJ, Witters LA, Girard PR, Kuo JF, Quamo SN: Growth factor stimulated protein phosphorylation in 3T3-L1 cells. Evidence for protein kinase C-dependent and -independent pathways. J Biol Chem 260:13304–13315, 1985

83. Stefanovic D., Erikson E, Pike LJ, Muller JL: Activation of a ribosomal protein S6 protein kinase in Xenopus oocytes by insulin and insulinreceptor kinase. EMBO J 5:157–160, 1986

84. Reddy P, Miller D, Peterkosky A: Stimulation of Escherichia coli adenylate clase activity by elongation factor TU, a GTP-binding protein essential for protein synthesis. J Biol Chem 261:11448–11451, 1986

85. Slivka SR, Insel PA: Alpha l-adrenergic receptor-mediated phosphoinositide hydrosis and prostaglandin E2 formation in Madin-Darby canine kidney cells. Possible parallel activation of phospholpase C and phospholipase A2. J Biol Chem 262:4200–4207, 1987

86. Whitman M, Fleischman L, Chahwala SB, Cantley L, Rosoff P: Phosphoinositides, mitogenesis and oncogenesis. In Putney JW (ed): Receptor Biochemistry and Methodology, pp 197–217. New York, Alan R Liss, 1986

87. Beridge MJ: Inositol triphosphate and diacylglycerol: Two interacting second messengers. Annu Rev Biochem 56:159–193, 1987

88. Edelman AM, Blumenthal DK, Krebs EG: Protein serine/threonine kinase. Annu Rev Biochem 56:567–613, 1987

89. Besterman JM, Watson SP, Cvatracacas P: Lack of association of epidermal growth factor, insulin and serum induced mitogenesis with stimulation of phospho-inositide degradation in BALB/c3T3 fibroblasts. J Biol Chem 261:723–727, 1986

90. Hesketh TR, Moore JP, Morris JDH, Taylor MV, Rogers J, Smith GA, Metcalfe JC: A common sequence of calcium and pH signals in the mitogenic stimulation of eukaryotic cells. Nature 313:481–484, 1985

91. Moolemaar WH, Yarden Y, Delaat SW, Schlessinger J: Epidermal growth factor induces electrically silent Na+ influx in human fibroblasts. J Biol Chem 257:8502–8506, 1982

92. Sugimoto Y, Whitman M, Cantly LC, Erikson RL: Evidence that the Rous sarcoma virus transforming gene product phosphorylates phosphotidylinositol and diacylglycerol. Proc Natl Acad Sci USA 81:2117–2121, 1984

93. Sugimoto Y, Erikson RL: Phosphatidylinosiol kinase activities in normal and Rous sarcoma virus-transformed cells. Mol Cell Biol 5:3194–3198, 1985

94. Sugano S, Hanfusa H: Phosphatidylinositol kinase activity in virus transformed and non-transformed cells. Mol Cell Biol 5:2399–2404, 1985

95. Bolen JB, Thiele JC, Israel MA, Yonemoto W, Lipsich LA, Brugge JS: Enhancement of cellular *src* gene product associated tyrosyl kinase activity following polyoma virus infection and transformation. Cell 38:767–777, 1985

96. Cartwright CA, Kaplan PL, Cooper JA, Hunter T, Eckhart W: Altered sites of tyrosine phosphorylation in pp60c-src associated with polyomavirus middle tumor antigen. Mol Cell Biol 6:1562–1570, 1986

97. Whitman M, Kaplan DR, Schaffhausen B, Cantley L, Roberts TM: Association of phosphotidylinositol kinase activity with polynoma middle T competent for transformation. Nature 315:239–242, 1985

98. Courtneidge SA, Heker A: A 81 Kd protein complexed with middle T antigen and pp60c-src: A possible phosphatidylinositol kinase. Cell 50:1031–1037, 198

99. Stahl M, Ferenz CR, Kelleher KL, Kriz RW, Knopf JL: Sequence similarity of phospholipase C with the non-catalytic region of *src*. Nature 332:269–272, 1988

100. Mayer BL, Hamaguchi M, Hanafusa H: A novel viral oncogene with structural similarity to phospholipase C. Nature 332:272–275, 1988

101. Jurnak F: Structure of the GDP domain of EF-T4 and location of the amino acids homologous to *ras* oncogene proteins. Science 230:32–36, 1985

102. Leberman R, and Egner U: Homologies in the primary structure of GTP-binding proteins the nucleotide-binding site of EF-T4 and p21. EMBO J 3:339–341, 1984

103. Gilamn AG: G Proteins: Transducers of receptor-generated signals. Annu Rev Biochem 56:615–649, 1987

104. Barbacid M: *ras* genes. Annu Rev Biochem 56:779–827, 1987

105. Fleischman LF, Chahwala SB, Cantly L: *ras*-transformed cells: altered levels of phosphatidylinositol 4,5 biphosphate and catabolitites. Science 231:407–410, 1986

106. Lacal JC, de la Pena P, Moscat J, Garcia-Barreno P, Anderson PS, and Aaronson SA: Rapid stimulation of diacylglycerol production in *Xenopus* oocytes by microinjection of H-*ras* p21. Science 238:533–536, 1987

107. Yu C-L, Tsai M-H, Stacey DW: Cellular *ras* activity and phospholipid metabolism. Cell 52:63–71, 1988

108. Mulcaly LS, Smith MR, Stacey DW: Requirement for *ras* proto-oncogene function during serum-stimulated growth of NIH3T3 cells. Nature 313:241–243, 1985

109. Smith MR, DeGudicibus SJ, Stacey DW: Requirement for c-*ras* proteins during viral oncogene transformation. Nature 320:540–543, 1986

110. Land H, Parada LF, Weinberg RA: Cellular oncogenes and multistep carcinogenesis. Science 222:771–778, 1983

111. Noda M, Selinger Z, Scolnick EM, Bassin RH: Flat revertants isolated from Kirsten sarcoma virus-transformed cells are resistant to the action of specific oncogenes. Proc Natl Acad Sci USA 80:5602–5606, 1983

112. Kruijer W, Cooper JA, Hunter T, Verma I: PDGF induces rapid but transient expression of the c-*fos* gene. Nature 312: 711–716, 1984

113. Cochran BH, Reffel AC, Stiles CD: Molecular cloning of gene sequences regulated by platelet-derived growth factor. Cell 33:939–947, 1983

114. Muller R, Bravo R, Burkhardt J, Curray T: Induction of c-*fos* gene and protein by growth factors proceeds activation of c-*myc*. Nature 312:716–720, 1984

115. Greenberg ME, Ziff EB: c-*fos* transcription is activated as an early response to 3T3 cell stimulation. In Cancer Cells 3: Growth Factors and Transformation, pp 307–314. Cold Spring Harbor, NY, Cold Spring Harbor Laboratory, 1984

116. Bhat NK, Fisher RJ, Fujiwara S, Ascione R, Papas TS: Temporal and tissue specific expression of mouse *ets* genes. Proc Natl Acad Sci USA 84:3161–3165, 1987

117. Curran T, Miller AD, Zokas L, Verma IM: Viral and cellular *fos* proteins: A comparative analysis. Cell 36:259–268, 1984

118. Hann SR, Eisenman RN: Proteins encoded by the human c-*myc* oncogene: Differential expression in neoplastic cells. Mol Cell Biol 4:2486–2497, 1984

119. Oren M, Maltzman W, Levine AJ: Post-translational regulation of the 54K cellular tumor antigen in normal and transformed cells. Mol Cell Biol 1:101–110, 1981

120. Curran T, Morgan JI: Superinduction of c-*fos* by nerve growth factor in the presence of peripherally active benzodiazepines. Science 229:1265–1268, 1985

121. Greenberg ME, Ziff EB: Stimulation of 3T3 cells induces transcription of the c-*fos* proto-oncogene. Nature 311:433–438, 1984

122. Kelly K, Cochran BH, Stiles CD, Leder P: Cell-specific regulation of the c-*myc* gene by lymphocyte mitogens and platelet-derived growth factor. Cell 35:603–610, 1983

123. Mitchell RL, Zokas L, Schreiber RD, Verma IM: Rapid induction of the expression of proto-oncogene *fos* during human monocytic differentiation. Cell 40:209–217, 1985

124. Muller RD, Muller D, Guilbert L: Differential expression of c-*fos* in hematopoietic cells: Correlation with differentiation of mono-myelocytic cells *in vitro*. EMBO J 3:1887–1890, 1984

125. Reich NC, Levine AJ: Growth regulation of a cellular tumor antigen, p53, in nontransformed cells. Nature 308:199–201, 1984

126. Torelli G, Selleri L, Donelli A, Ferrari S, Emilia G, Veenturelli D, Moretti L, Torelli U: Activation of c-*myc* expression by phytohemaglutinin stimulation in normal human T lymphocytes. Mol Cell Biol 5:2874–2877, 1985

127. Distel RJ, Ro H-S, Rosen BS, Groves DL, Spiegelman BM: Nucleoprotein complexes that regulate gene expression in adipocyte differentiation: Direct participation of c-*fos*. Cell 49:835–844, 1987

128. Kingston RE, Baldwin AS Jr., Sharp PA: Regulation of heat shock protein 70 gene expression by c-*myc*. Nature 312:280–282, 1984

129. Setoyama C, Frunzio R, Liau G, Mudryj M, de Crombrugghe B: Transcriptional activation encoded by the v-*fos* gene. Proc Natl Acad Sci USA 83:3213–3217

130. Bohman D, Bos TJ, Admon A, Nishimura T, Vogt PK, Tjian R: Human proto-oncogene c-*jun* encodes a DNA binding protein with structural and functional properties of transcription factor AP-1. Science 238:1386–1392, 1987

131. Greenberg ME, Siefried Z, Ziff EB: Mutation of the c-*fos* gene dyad symmetry element inhibits serum inducibility of transcription *in vivo* and the nuclear regulatory factor binding *in vitro*. Mol Cell Biol 7:1217–1225, 1987

132. Theisman R: Identification of a protein-binding site that mediates transcriptional response of the c-*fos* gene to serum factors. Cell 46:567–574, 1987

133. Stumpo DJ, Stewart TN, Gilman MZ, Blackshear PJ: Identification of c-*fos* sequences involved in induction by insulin and phorbol esters. J Biol Chem 263:1611–1614, 1988

134. Prywes R, Roeder RG: Inducible binding of a factor to the c-*fos* enhancer. Cell 47:777–784, 1986

135. Theisman R: Identification and purification of a polypeptide that binds to the c-*fos* serum response element. EMBO J 6: 2711–2717, 1987

136. Hayes TE, Kitchen AM, Cochran BH: Inducible binding of a factor to the c-*fos* regulatory region. Proc Natl Acad Sci USA 84:1272–1276, 1987

137. Fish TB, Prywes R, Roeder RG: c-*fos* sequences necessary for basal expression and induction by epidermal growth factor, 12-O-tetradecanoyl phorbol-13-acetate, and the calcium ionophore. Mol Cell Biol 7:3450–3502, 1987

138. Gilman MZ, Wilson RN, Weinberg RA: Multiple protein-binding sites in the 5'-flanking region regulate c-*fos* expression. Mol Cell Biol 6:4305–4316, 1986

139. Bravo R, Neuberg M, Burckhardt J, Almendral J, Wallich R, Muller R: Involvement of common and cell type specific pathways in c-*fos* gene control: Stable induction by cAMP TPA in macrophages. Cell 48:251–260, 1987

140. Kruijer W, Schubert D, Verma IM: Induction of the proto-oncogene *fos* by nerve growth factor. Proc Natl Acad Sci USA 82:7330–7334, 1985

141. Yoshimasa T, Sibley DR, Bouvier M, Lefkowitz RJ, Caron MG: Cross-talk between cellular signalling pathways suggested by phorbol-ester-induced adenylate cyclase phosphorylation. Nature 327:67–70, 1987

142. Angel P, Imagawa M, Chiu R, Stein B, Imbra RJ, Rahmsdorf HJ, Jonat C, Herrlich P, Karin M: Phorbol ester-inducible genes contain a common *cis* element recognized by a TPA-modulated *Trans*-acting factor. Cell 49:729–739, 1987

143. Lee W, Mitchell P, Tjian R: Purified transcription factor AP-1 interacts with TPA-inducible enhancer elements. Cell 49: 741–752, 1987

144. Greenberg, ME, Hermanowski AL, Ziff EB: Effect of protein synthesis inhibitors on growth factor activation of c-*fos*, c-*myc* and action gene transcription. Mol Cell Biol 6:1050–1057, 1986

145. Angel P, Rahmsdorf HJ, Poting A, Herrlich P: c-*fos* mRNA levels in primary human fibroblasts after arrest in various stages of the cell cycle. In Cancer Cells/Growth Factors and Transformation, pp 315–319. Cold Spring Harbor, NY, Cold Spring Harbor Laboratory, 1987

146. Sassone-Corsi P, Verma IM: Modulation of c-*fos* transcription by negative and positive cellular factors. Nature 326:507–510, 1987

147. Sambucetti CC, Curran T: The fos protein complex is associated with DNA in isolated muclei and binds to DNA cellulose. Science 234:1417–1419, 1986

148. Renz M, Verrier B, Kurz C, Muller R: Chromatin association and DNA binding properties of the c-*fos* proto-oncogene product. Nucleic Acids Res 15:277–292, 1987

149. Distel RJ, Ro H-S, Rosen BS, Groves DL, Spiegelman BM: Nucleoprotein complexes that regulate gene expression in adopocyte differentiation: Direct participation of c-*fos*. Cell 49:835–844, 1987

150. Setoyama C, Frunzio R, Liav G, Mudryj M, de Crombrugghe B: Transcriptional activation encoded by the v-*fos* gene. Proc Natl Acad Sci USA 83:3213–3217, 1986

151. Lech K, Anderson K, Brent R: DNA-bound *fos* proteins activate transcription in yeast. Cell 52:179–184, 1988

152. Franza BR, Rauscher FJ III, Josephs SF, Curran T: The *fos* complex and *fos*-related antigens recognize sequence elements that contain AP-1 binding sites. Science 239:1150–1153, 1988

153. Verma I, Sassone-Corsi P: Proto-oncogene *fos:* Complex but versatile regulation. Cell 51:513–514, 1987

154. Hann SR, Thompson CB, Eisenman RN: c-*myc* oncogene protein synthesis is independent of the cell cycle in human and avian cells. Nature 314:366–369, 1985

155. Jones TR, Cole MD: Rapid cytoplasmic turnover of c-*myc* RNA: Requirement of the 3' untranslated sequences. Mol Cell Biol 7:4513–4521, 1987

156. Hann SR, Eisenman RN: Proteins encoded by the human c-*myc* oncogene: Differential expression in neoplastic cells. Mol Cell Biol 4:2486–2497, 1984

157. Bader J, Hausman FA, Ray DA: Intranuclear degradation of the transformation inducing protein encoded by avian MC29 virus. J Biol Chem 261:8303–8308, 1986

158. Frick KK, Womer RB, Scher CD: Platelet-derived growth factor-induced c-*myc* RNA expression. J Biol Chem 263: 2948–2952, 1988

159. Broome HA, Reed JC, Godillot EP, Hoover RG: Differential promoter utilization by the c-*myc* gene in mitogen and interleukin-2-stimulated human lymphocytes. Mol Cell Biol 7: 2988–2993, 1987

160. Yang J, Bauer SR, Muchinski JF, Marcu KB: Chromosomal translocations clustered 5' of the murine c-*myc* gene quantitatively affect promoter usage: Implications for the site of normal c-*myc* regulation. EMBO J 4:1441–1447, 1985

161. Croce CM, Erikson J, Ar-Rushdi A, Aden D, Nishikura K: Translocated c-myc oncogene of Burkitts lymphoma is transcribed in plasma cells and repressed in lymphoblastoid cells. Proc Natl Acad Sci USA 81:3170–3174, 1984

162. Shih CK, Linial M, Goodenov MM, Hayward WS: Nucleotide sequence 5' of the chicken c-*myc* coding region: Localization of a noncoding exon that is absent from *myc* transcripts in most avian leukosis virus-induced lymphomas. Proc Natl Acad Sci USA 81:4697–4701, 1984

163. Stanton CW, Watt R, Marcu KB: Translocation, breakage and truncated transcripts of c-*myc* oncogene in murine plasmacytomas. Nature 303:401–406, 1983

164. Watson DK, Psallidopoulos EC, Samuel KP, Dalla-Fowern R, Papas TS: Nucleotide sequence analysis of human c-*myc* locus, chicken homologue and muelocytomatosis virus MC29 transforming gene reveals a highly conserved gene product. Proc Natl Acad Sci USA 80:3642–3645, 1983

165. Hann SR, King MW, Bentley DL, Anderson CW, Eisenman RN: A nonAUG translocational initiation in c-*myc* exon 1 generates an N-terminally distinct protein whose synthesis is disrupted in Burkitts lymphomas. Cell 52:185–195, 1988

166. Watson DK, Reddy EP, Duesberg PH, Papas TS: Nucleotide sequence analysis of the chicken c-*myc* gene reveals homologous and unique coding regions by comparison with the transforming gene of avian myelocytomatosis virus MC29 *gag-myc.* Proc Natl Acad Sci USA 80:2146–2150, 1983

167. Hayward WS, Neel BG, Astrin SM: Activation of a cellular *onc* gene by promoter insertion in ALV-induced lymphoid leukosis. Nature 290:475–480, 1981

168. Cory S: Activation of cellular oncogenes in hematopoietic cells by chromosome translocation. Adv Cancer Res 47:189–234, 1986

169. Croce CM, Nowell PC: Molecular basis of human B cell neoplasia. Blood 65:1–7, 1985

170. Tsujimoto Y, Jaffe B, Cossman J, Gorham J, Nowell PC, Croce CM: Clustering of breakpoints on chromosome 11 in human B-cell neoplasms with the t(11;14) chromosome translocation. Nature 315:340–343, 1985

171. Nishikura K, Ar-Rushdi A, Erikson J, Watt R, Rovera G, Croce CM: Differential expression of the normal and of the translocated human c-*myc* oncogene in B cells. Proc Natl Acad Sci USA 80:4822–4826, 1983

172. Moroy T, Marchio A, Biemble J, Trepo C, Tiollais P, Brendia MA: Rearrangement and enhanced expression of c-*myc* in

hepatocellular carcinoma of hepatitis virus infected woodchucks. Nature 324:276–279, 1986

173. Sap J, Munoz A, Damon K, Goldkey Y, Ghysdael J, Leutz A, Beug H, Vennstrom B: The c-*erb*A protein is a high-affinity receptor for thyroid hormone. Nature 324:635–640, 1986

174. Weinberger G, Thompson CC, Ong ES, Lebo R, Gruol DJ, Evans RM: The c-*erb*A gene encodes a thyroid hormone receptor. Nature 324:641–646, 1986

175. Benbrook D, Pfahl M: A novel thyroid hormone receptor encoded by a cDNA clone from a human testis library. Science 238:788–791, 1987

176. Graf T, Beug H: Role of the v-*erb*A and v-*erb*B oncogenes of avian erythroblastosis virus in erythroid cell transformation. Cell 34:7–9, 1983

177. Zenke M, Kahn P, Disela C, Vennstrom B, Leutz A, Keegan K, Hayman MJ, Cnoi H-R, Yew N, Engel JD, Beug H: v-*erb*A specifically suppresses transcription of the avian erythrocyte avian (Band 3) gene. Cell 52:107–119, 1988

178. Woods CM, Boyer B, Vogt PK, Lazarides E: Control of erythroid differentiation asunchionous expression of the avian transporter and the peripheral components of the membrane skeleton in AEV- and S13-transformed cells. J Cell Biol 103:1789–1798, 1986

179. Whang-Peng J, Bunn PA Jr, Kao-Shan CS, Lee EC, Carney DN, Gazdar A, Minna JD: A non-random chromosomal abnormality del 3p(14-23) in human small cell lung cancer (SCLC). Cancer Genet Cytogenet 6:119–134, 1982

180. Dobvovic A, Houle B, Belouchi A, Bradley WEC: *erb*A-related sequence coding for DNA-binding hormone receptor localized to chromosome 3p213p25 and deleted in small cell lung carcinoma. Cancer Res 48:682–685, 1988

181. Vogt PK, Bos TJ, Doolittle RF: Homology between the DNA-binding domian of the GCN4 regulatory protein of yeast and the carboxyl-terminal region of a protein coded for the oncogene *jun*. Proc Natl Acad Sci USA 84:3316–3319, 1987

182. Lee W, Haslinger A, Karin M, Tjian R: Activation of transcription by two factors that bind promoter and enhancer sequences of the human metallothionein gene and SV40. Nature 325:368–372, 1987

183. Bohman D, Bos TJ, Admon A, Nishimura T, Vogt P, Tjian R: Human proto-oncogene c-*jun* encodes a DNA binding protein with structural and functional properties of transcription factor AP-1. Science 238:1386–1392, 1987

184. Lee W, Mitchell P, Tjian R: Purified transcription factor AP-1 interacts with TPA-inducible enhancer elements. Cell 49:741–752, 1987

185. Angel P, Imagawa M, Chiv R, Stein B, Imbra RJ, Rahmsdorf HJ, Jonat C, Herrlich P, Karin M: Phorbol ester-inducible genes contain a common *cis* element recognized by a TPA-modulated trans-acting factor. Cell 49:729–739, 1987

186. Watson DK, Smith MJ, Kozak C, Reeves R, Gearhart J, Nunn MF, Nash W, Fowle JR III, Duesberg P, Papas TS, O'Brien SJ: Conserved chromosomal positions of dual domains of the *ets* proto-oncogene in cats, mice and man. Proc Natl Acad Sci USA 83:1792–1796, 1986

187. Watson DK, McWilliams-Smith MJ, Nunn MF, Duesberg PH, O'Brien SJ, Papas TS: The *ets* sequence from the transforming gene of avian erythroblastosis virus, E26, has unique domains on human chromosomes 11 and 21: Both loci are transcriptionally active. Proc Natl Acad Sci USA 82:7294–7298, 1985

188. Watson DK, McWilliams-Smith MJ, Lapis P, Lautenberger JA, Schweinfest CW, Papas TS: Human and mouse *ets*-2 genes: Members of a family of *ets* genes. Proc Natl Acad Sci USA (submitted)

189. Rao VN, Papas TS, Reddy ESP: *Erg*, a human *ets*-related gene on chromosome 21: Alternative splicing, polyadenylation, and translation. Science 237:635–639, 1987

190. Reddy ESP, Rao VN, Papas TS: The *erg* gene: A human gene related to the *ets* oncogene. Proc Natl Acad Sci USA 84:6131–6135, 1987

191. Pribyl LJ, Watson DK, McWilliams MJ, Ascione R, Papas TS: The *Drosophila ets*-2 gene: Molecular structure, chromosomal localization, and developmental expression. Dev Biol 127:45–53, 1988

192. Chen Z-Q, Kan NC, Pribyl L, Lautenberger JA, Moudrianakis E, Papas TS: Molecular cloning of the *ets* proto-oncogene of the sea urchin and analysis of its developmental expression. Dev Biol 125:432–440, 1988

193. Bhat NK, Fisher RJ, Fujiwara S, Ascione R, Papas TS: Differential regulation of *ets* loci during murine hepatic regeneration. In Voellmy RW, Ahmad F, Black S, Burgess DR, Rotundo R, Scott WA, Whelan WJ, (eds): Advances in Gene Technology: The Molecular Biology of Development, p 70. Cambridge, Cambridge University Press, 1987

194. Bhat NK, Fisher RJ, Fujiwara S, Ascione R, Papas TS: Temporal and tissue-specific expression of mouse *ets* genes. Proc Natl Acad Sci USA 84:3161–3165, 1987

195. Fujiwara S, Fisher RJ, Seth A, Bhat NK, Papas TS: Human *ets*-1 and *ets*-2 proteins: Identification and intracellular localization. In Voellmy RW, Ahmad F, Black S, Burgess DR, Rotundo R, Scott WA, Whelan WJ, (eds): Advances in Gene Technology: The Molecular Biology of Development, p 77. Cambridge, Cambridge University Press, 1987

196. Fujiwara S, Fisher RJ, Seth A, Bhat NK, Showalter SD, Zweig M, Papas TS: Characterization and localization of the products of the human homologs of the v-*ets* oncogene. Oncogene 2:99–103, 1988

197. Fujiwara S, Fisher RJ, Bhat NK, Papas TS: Human *ets*-2 protein: Nuclear location, phosphorylation, rapid turnover and induction by TPA. In Brew K, Ahmad F, Bialy H, Black S, Fenna RE, Puett D, Scott WA, Van Brunt J, Voellmy RW, Whelan WJ, Woessner JF (eds): Advances in Gene Technology: Protein Engineering and Production, p 107. Oxford/Washington, DC, IRL Press, 1988

198. Fujiwara S, Fisher RJ, Bhat NK, Diaz de la Espina SM, Papas TS: A short-lived nuclear phosphoprotein encoded by human *ets*-2 proto-oncogene is stabilized by protein kinase C activation. Mol Cell Biol (in press)

199. O'Brien TG, Simsiman RC, Boutwell RK: Induction of the polyamine-biosynthetic enzymes in mouse epidermis by tumor-promoting agents. Cancer Res 35:1662–1670, 1975

200. Clark SC, Arya SK, Wong-Staal F, Matsumoto-Kobayashi M, Kay RM, Kaufman RJ, Brown EL, Shoemaker C, Copeland T, Oroszlan S, Smith K, Sarngadharan MG, Lindner SG, Gallo RC: Human T-cell growth factor: Partial amino acid sequence, cDNA cloning, and organization and expression in normal and leukemic cells. Proc Natl Acad Sci USA 81:2543–2547, 1984

201. Shackelford DA, Trowbridge IS: Induction of expression and phosphorylation of the human Interleukin-2 receptor by a phorbol diester. J Biol Chem 259:11706–11712, 1984

202. Siebert PD, Fukuda M: Induction of cytoskeletal vimentin and actin gene expression by a tumor-promoting phorbol ester in the human leukemic cell line K562. J Biol Chem 260:3868–3874, 1985

203. Greenberg ME, Hermanowski AL, Ziff EB: Effect of protein synthesis inhibitors on growth factor activation of c-*fos*, c-*myc*, and actin gene transcription. Mol Cell Biol 6:1050–1057, 1986

204. Sen R, Baltimore D: Inducibility of κ immunoglobulin enhancer-binding protein NF-κB by a post-translational mechanism. Cell 47:921–928, 1986

205. Imagawa M, Chiu R, Karin M: Transcription factor AP-2 mediates induction by two different signal-transduction pathways: Protein kinase C and cAMP. Cell 51:251–260, 1987

206. Mitchell PJ, Wang C, Tjian R: Positive and negative regulation of transcription *in vitro:* Enhancer-binding protein AP-2 is inhibited by SV40 antigen. Cell 50:847–861, 1987

207. Sacchi N, Watson DK, Guerts van Kessel AHM, Hagemeijer A, Drabkin HD Patterson D, Papas TS: Hu-*ets*-1 and Hu-*ets*-2 genes are transposed in acute myeloid leukemias with (4;11) and (8;21) translocations. Science 231:379–382, 1986

208. Sacchi N, Cheng SV, Gusella JF, Drabkin HD, Patterson D, Tanzi RE, Haines JH, Papas TS: Genetic analysis of the chromosome 21 breakpoint of the acute myelogenous leukemia translocation (8;21). Proc Natl Acad Sci USA (submitted)

209. Sacchi N, de Klein A, Showalter SD, Papas TS: High expression of *ETS*1 gene in human thymocytes and immature T leukemic cells. Leukemia 2:12–18, 1988

210. Sacchi N, Gusella JF, Perroni L, Dagna Bricarelli F, Papas TS: Lack of evidence for association of meiotic nondisjunction with particular DNA haplotypes on chromosome 21. Proc Natl Acad Sci USA 85:4794–4798, 1988

211. Sacchi N, Nalbantoglu J, Sergovich FR, Papas TS: The *ETS*2 gene in Down syndrome genetic region is not rearranged in Alzheimer's disease. Proc Natl Acad Sci USA (in press)

212. Patterson D: The causes of Down syndrome. Sci Am 257:52–60, 1987

213. Auvedimento E, Yamada Y, Lovelace E, Vogeli G, de Crombrugghe B, Pastau I: Decrease in the levels of nuclear RNA precursors for alpha 2 collagen in Rous sarcoma virus transformed fibroblasts. Nucleic Acids Res 9:1123–1131, 1981

214. Marciani DJ, Bader JP: Polypeptide composition of cell membranes from chick embryo fibroblasts transformed by Rous sarcoma virus. Biochim Biophys Acta 401:386–398, 1975

215. Bader AV, Kondratick J, Bader JP: Decreased alkaline phosphatase in cells transformed by Rous sarcoma virus. Cancer Res 38:308–312, 1978

216. Otten J, Bader J, Johnson G, Pastan I: A mutation in Rous sarcoma gene that controls adenosine 3′:,5′-monophosphate levels and transformation. J Biol Chem 247:1632–1633, 1972

Amnon Hizi

Stephen H. Hughes

Expression of the Human Immunodeficiency Virus in *Escherichia coli:* Chemotherapy

2

Introduction ■

"Divide and Conquer" ■

The goal of cancer chemotherapy is the selective elimination of the malignant cells in a fashion analogous to the treatment of infectious pathogens with antibiotics. An ideal chemotherapeutic agent discriminates clearly between the host and the pathogen, selectively inhibiting the pathogen without harming the host. In evolutionary terms, bacteria and humans are quite distant, with substantial metabolic and biochemical differences. Thus, it is not surprising that one can find, using nonselective screening procedures, drugs that are substantially more toxic to pathogenic bacteria than to humans. In contrast to bacteria, which replicate autonomously, viruses rely to a greater or lesser extent on their host's cellular machinery for replication. Therefore, it is difficult to obtain effective antiviral drugs that are not toxic to the host. The problem is even more complex for viruses like human immunodeficiency virus (HIV), which encode only a small number of virus-specific functions and rely extensively on their hosts for replication.

Developing effective, nontoxic anticancer drugs is even more difficult. The fundamental differences between cancer cells and normal cells are so few that it is not yet possible to identify drugs that can selectively inhibit the replication of cancer cells without having substantial toxic effects on the host. However, we are now in a position to break down the replicative cycle of viral pathogens like HIV into individual steps and study the specific viral proteins associated with each step. Because the number of HIV viral proteins is small, it is possible to study each in detail and, through a better understanding of these proteins and the reactions in which they participate, to use a directed approach to drug screening. It may even be possible to design drugs to inhibit specific defined steps in viral replication.

Viral pathogens such as HIV present better targets for directed screens for chemotherapeutic agents than do cancer cells. Therefore, discussion of the current status of the work on HIV and HIV reverse transcriptase (RT) may provide a background for considering the application of similar technology to the more difficult problem of developing specific anticancer drugs.

The HIV life cycle can be conceptually divided into three stages. First, the virus must adhere to, and penetrate, a susceptible target cell. Second, the viral RNA genome is converted into DNA and the integrated provirus is established. Third, the virally encoded RNAs are transcribed and translated into viral proteins, some of which are post-transcriptionally modified and processed proteolytically. Expression of the HIV genome is under complex control, and the details of these regulatory circuits are not yet entirely clear. There are several viral proteins involved, including TAT and ART/TRS. When they are better understood, these proteins may represent legitimate targets for antiviral drug therapy; however, they will not be discussed here.

The first two stages of the HIV life cycle appear quite similar to equivalent steps in the life cycle of other retroviruses.[1] The product of the viral *env* gene, the envelope glycoprotein, binds specifically to a host receptor on the outer membrane of the cell. In the case of HIV, the host protein recognized by the HIV envelope is known,[2] and attempts are under way to study this reaction in detail and to develop reagents that interfere with it.[3-6]

The mechanisms by which the RNA genomes of retroviruses are copied into DNA are largely understood,[1,7,8] and will not be repeated here. What is relevant is that one of the products of the viral *pol* gene, RT, has two distinct enzymatic functions. The first is a DNA-polymerizing function that is responsible for making a DNA copy of the RNA genome found in the virion, giving rise to an RNA–DNA hybrid. The second activity, RNase H, specifically degrades the RNA in this RNA–DNA hybrid, so that the DNA-polymerizing activity can make the second DNA strand. The actual integration event, in which the DNA copy of the viral genome is inserted into host DNA, is still somewhat mysterious. A viral protein that also derives from the *pol* gene, the integration protein, is required at some step in the integration reaction. The recent development of an *in vitro* integration assay holds promise in demystifying the integration process.[9]

Of the viral proteins that are candidates for antiviral drug development, we have chosen to begin with RT. Reverse transcription is a prerequisite for viral replication and, because copying viral RNA into DNA is the first step in viral replication following penetration of the cell, interruption of reverse transcription blocks the establishment of a provirus in the genome of the host. Reverse transcriptases from other retroviruses have been studied intensively and show considerable homology to the enzyme found in HIV.[10] The reactions catalyzed by the enzyme both in copying RNA into DNA and in degrading the RNA template in the RNA–DNA hybrid are well understood and, more important, are readily assayed in simple, quantitative *in vitro* assays. This key feature can be exploited in *in vitro* drug screening and will be discussed later. In addition, reverse transcription appears to have no direct counterpart in the life of normal cells except that most, if not all, cells have endogenous retrotransposons that encode similar proteins.[11] It is generally thought that these endogenous retroviruses (or retrotransposons) are not essential to the life of normal cells. It should therefore be possible to interrupt reverse transcription and thus inhibit viral replication without harm to the host, although it will be important to avoid inhibiting host enzymes with related substrates (*e.g.,* the host DNA-dependent DNA polymerases and host RNase H). The only drug now recognized as effective against HIV is azidothymidine (AZT), a nucleotide analogue that either directly or indirectly interferes with viral replication at the level of reverse transcription.[12,13] AZT's principal drawback is that it is also toxic to the host (probably by interfering with host DNA-dependent DNA polymerase).

A number of laboratories, including our own, are engaged in studies designed to reveal the HIV RT in molecular detail, with the goal of providing information relevant to the design of drugs specifically intended to inhibit this enzyme.

Expression of HIV Reverse Transcriptase in *Escherichia coli* ■

"Alpha to Omega" ■

During viral infections, retroviral RTs (including HIV RT) are initially synthesized as part of a larger polyprotein. They are released from this polyprotein by a viral protease during virion maturation. Only relatively small amounts of RT are found within the virion, so that large-scale purification of the enzyme from virions is impractical. Recombinant DNA technology provides an alternate approach: large amounts of the HIV RT can be prepared by producing it in genetically engineered cells without the concomitant synthesis of other viral proteins. Because the viral RT is released from the interior of a polyprotein precursor by proteolytic cleavage, the segment of the viral genome that encodes it does not begin with an initiation codon, nor does it end with a termination codon. This makes the task of overexpressing the RT more difficult, and the various laboratories that have approached this problem have used three different expression techniques. The simplest is to fuse part or all of the RT open reading frame to another gene that supplies both a translational initiator and a terminator.[14-17] However, the proteins produced by such constructions have amino and carboxy termini that differ from the viral enzyme. Because the goal is to produce a protein that faithfully mimics the viral protein, this strategy has substantial drawbacks.

A second approach is to synthesize a sufficiently large portion of the polyprotein so that it will contain the viral protease in addition to a complete copy of the HIV RT. This apparently allows the proteolytic processing that normally occurs in virions to proceed in the genetically engineered cell.[18-20] Unfortunately, the amount of RT made by constructions of this type is not large. Moreover, it is difficult to prove unambiguously that the proteolytic cleavages that take place in the genetically engineered cell (usually yeast or *E. coli*) occur at exactly the same sites as in virions.

The third approach, used both by us[21,22] and by others,[23] is to modify the region encoding RT in such a fashion that an initiation and a termination codon are introduced into the HIV genome at positions that would normally encode the protein segment recognized by the viral protease (Figs. 2–1 and 2–2). Although it is possible to introduce a termination codon precisely at the proteolytic recognition site that creates the carboxy terminus of the HIV reverse transcriptase, it is not possible to do this at the amino terminus. Reverse transcriptase molecules isolated from HIV virions have an amino-terminal proline. Because translation always initiates with a methionine, an

FIG. 2–1 Construction of the plasmid that causes the expression of HIV reverse transcriptase (RT) in *E. coli.* That portion of the HIV genome encoding the RT is designated by "HIV" at the top of the figure. The region encoding the RT lies between positions 2129 and 3808. That portion of the DNA between the *Bal*I site (*Bal*) and the second *Kpn*I site (*Kpn*) was introduced into the *E. coli* expression plasmid pUC12N (see Ref. 22). The regions encoding the amino (between *Nco*I and *Bal*I) and carboxy (between *Kpn*I and *Sal*I) termini were prepared as synthetic double-stranded DNA segments. In the completed plasmid (*lower section*) sequences deriving from pUC12N are shown in black, synthetic segments are hatched, and the segment deriving from cloned HIV DNA is shown as an open box.

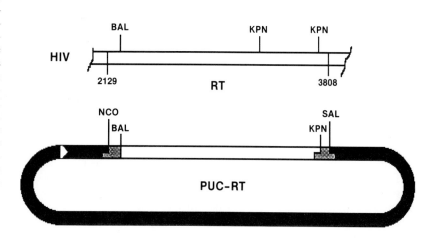

amino-terminal methionine is required. For convenience, we routinely embed the codon for the initiator methionine of our DNA constructs within the recognition site for the restriction enzyme *Nco*I, which is CCATGG (see Fig. 2–2). This sequence can function as an efficient site for translational initiation in *E. coli,* yeast, and higher eukaryotes, and allows us to express precisely the same unfused protein in each of these hosts.[24] This is possible because there are *Nco*I/ATG expression vectors for all three systems. Having created an appropriate genetically engineered

segment beginning with an *Nco*I/ATG, it is simple to move the segment from one expression system to another. The only drawback to using an *Nco*I/ATG is that if the *Nco*I site is to be conserved, the first base of the second codon is also specified (as a G). This precludes the use of certain codons in the second position (including proline), and the modified HIV RT segment we have made encodes methionine and valine as the first two amino acids, followed by the proline normally found at the amino terminus (see Fig. 2–2). When the amino acid at the second position is

FIG. 2–2 Modifications of the sequences of HIV RT for expression in *E. coli.* (Synthetic DNA segments are open boxes, pUC12N segments are black and the portion deriving directly from the HIV genome is hatched.) The DNA sequence of the original HIV clone and the amino acids encoded near the sites of proteolytic processing (PROT) are given, as are those for the synthetic DNA segments at the joints between the synthetic DNA and pUC12N (pUC).

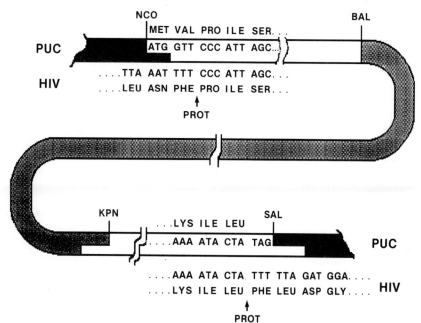

critical to the structure and function of the protein, it is possible to use the technology just described with an oligonucleotide that will ligate to (but not re-create) an *Nco*I site. Under these conditions, any base can be inserted at the first base of the second codon. In addition, there are certain proteins from which *E. coli* removes one or two of the amino-terminal amino acids. We have not yet subjected our *E. coli*-synthesized HIV RT to amino-terminal protein sequencing, so we do not yet know the fate of the two extra amino-terminal amino acids. However, we do have direct evidence (discussed below) that, whatever the status of the amino terminus, the protein made in *E. coli* has an active site whose structure closely resembles the viral enzyme.

There is no evidence that HIV RT is modified posttranscriptionally; therefore, we have chosen to express the protein in *E. coli.* If it had proved necessary to express the protein in another host to produce an appropriately modified protein, the presence of an *Nco*I site at the initiator ATG would have made it simple to move the modified segment to yeast and higher eukaryotic expression plasmids. Such a yeast expression plasmid has been prepared, and strains carrying this expression plasmid make significant amounts of enzymatically active HIV reverse transcriptase (McGill C, Hizi A, Garfinkel D, Hughes S, Strathern J: Unpublished observations). For expression in *E. coli,* the modified segment encoding RT was introduced into the expression plasmid pUC12N, a derivative of pUC12 that has two bases near the *lac*Z ATG mutated to create an *Nco*I site[25,26] (see Figs. 2–1 and 2–2; also see Ref. 22). Introduction of the pUC12N plasmid containing HIV RT into *E. coli* results in the synthesis of large amounts of a new protein of 66 kDa, the size of the HIV RT (Fig. 2–3). Lysis of this strain with Triton X-100 releases approximately half of the 66 kDa protein present in the *E. coli* in a soluble form; extracts of this strain contain large amounts of RT enzymatic activity, which is not found in extracts prepared from control strains of *E. coli.*[22]

The observation that the 66 kDa protein has RNA-dependent DNA polymerase activity suggests that it has a structure that approximates the viral reverse transcriptase. However, we wished to demonstrate directly that the active site for the HIV RNA-dependent DNA polymerase made in *E. coli* is essentially identical to the active site of the viral enzyme. We probed the active site with the competitive inhibitors dideoxy guanidine triphosphate (ddGTP) and dideoxy thymidine triphosphate (ddTTP). To validate the sensitivity of the assay, the effect of these inhibitors was tested not only with the two forms of HIV RT

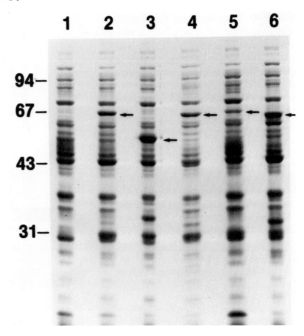

FIG. 2–3 HIV RT proteins made in *E. coli. E. coli* DH5 containing the parental plasmid pUC12N or derivatives that carry wild-type or mutant HIV RT were collected by centrifugation, lysed, and the proteins fractionated on an SDS-polyacrylamide gel. Each lane was loaded with protein derived from 60 μl of liquid culture. Protein was visualized with Coomassie brilliant blue. The position of migration of protein molecular weight markers (in kDa) is given at the left of the figure. Lane 1 shows the proteins from DH5 carrying the parental plasmid pUC12N; lane 2, the proteins from a strain carrying pUC12N with the wild-type HIV polymerase inserted; lane 3, the mutant CT-133; lane 4, CT-23; lane 5, CT-16; lane 6, AT-23. The proteins expected to be synthesized by each mutant are described in Table 2–2. The HIV RT-related proteins are designated by arrows.

(prepared from virions and from *E. coli*), but also with murine leukemia virus (MuLV) RT. In this assay, the two HIV RTs were indistinguishable but were clearly distinguished from the MuLV enzyme, demonstrating that the assay can detect small differences in the active sites of RNA-dependent DNA polymerases (Fig. 2–4).

We are now purifying the HIV RT to provide material for structural, biochemical, and immunologic experiments. For these purposes, it is important to be able to prepare substantial quantities of essentially pure protein. Under optimal growth conditions, the bacteria contain (judged by gel electrophoresis and staining with Coomassie blue) the HIV RT as several percent of the total protein. (see Fig. 2–3). We have been working closely with Program Resources, Inc. (PRI) on the development of large-scale growth and

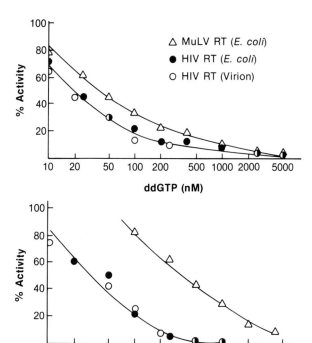

FIG. 2-4 Effect of inhibitors of the polymerizing function of MuLV and HIV RT. Extracts of *E. coli* strains that make the HIV RT and MuLV RT were passed over Sephadex G-25 and assayed for polymerizing activity in comparison with HIV RT from disrupted virions. Increasing amounts of either ddGTP (*top*) or ddTTP (*bottom*) were added to standard *in vitro* polymerization reactions (see Ref. 22). The template used to study ddTTP inhibition was poly(rA); the template used to study ddGTP inhibition was poly(rC). Activity is expressed as percentage of the incorporation seen in the absence of added inhibitor. The concentration of the inhibitors is displayed on a logarithmic scale.

purification of the enzyme. Pat Clark of PRI has recently prepared approximately 50 mg of essentially pure 66 kDa HIV RT from *E. coli*. Most of this material is being used for structural studies, with a smaller amount being used for immunizations.

Structural Studies ■

"Know the Enemy" ■

Although RT is unique to retroviruses and retrotransposons, there are cellular enzymes that have activities related to both the DNA polymerizing activity, which can use either DNA or RNA as a substrate, and the RNase H enzymatic activities of RT. The

host employs DNA-dependent DNA polymerases to copy its genome, and host RNase H is believed to remove the RNA primers used in the replication of genomic DNA. A drug directed at HIV RT should be able to discriminate between the viral enzyme and host enzymes. The availability of large amounts of pure HIV RT will permit an in-depth biochemical analysis of the enzyme, as well as provide material for x-ray crystallographic analyses.

The biochemical analyses will be aimed at achieving a better understanding of the enzymatic properties of the RT. It is relatively straightforward to analyze the RNA-dependent DNA polymerizing activity in partially purified extracts, because *E. coli* DNA-dependent DNA polymerases do not use RNA templates effectively. The RNase H function is much more difficult to assay in *E. coli* extracts because of interference from the *E. coli* RNase H. *E. coli* strains deficient in RNase H are available,[27,28] and it is possible to assay RNase H in gels immediately following electrophoretic fractionation.[29,30] However, we intend to pursue the analyses of the enzymatic properties of the HIV RT using purified material. We also propose to probe the active sites of RT by direct chemical modification (see Ref. 31 for an example of chemical modification with MuLV reverse transcriptase), which, in conjunction with x-ray structural data and mutagenic studies (described below), should reveal those features of the active site important for drug design.

A clear understanding of the structure of the HIV RT should emerge from the x-ray crystallographic analyses. These are being carried out in the laboratories of Edward Arnold (Rutgers University) and Richard Dickerson (UCLA). Although the first attempts at crystallization will be done with the enzyme alone, it should also be useful to try to crystallize the enzyme in the presence of its substrates and inhibitors. Precise knowledge of the interaction of the enzyme with an inhibitor may suggest ways in which the structure of the inhibitor could be modified to make it interact more precisely with, and bind more strongly to, the active site.

Mutagenic Studies ■

"A Moving Target" ■

There are two distinct motivations for undertaking a comprehensive mutagenic analysis of the HIV RT. The more obvious is that mutagenic analyses, especially when linked with structural and biochemical analyses, may be quite revealing of the architecture of HIV RT and its active site. There is also a second reason: the HIV genome and the proteins it encodes are not static, fixed entities. Even if we are able to find an inhibitor that specifically blocks the particular form of the HIV RT we have expressed, that inhibitor may not block all possible forms of the HIV RT. It should be borne in mind that when a drug like AZT is used to treat large numbers of patients, the treatment itself provides a strong selection for drug-resistant variants, if such variants are compatible with RT function. We know from preliminary experiments with the inhibitors ddGTP and ddTTP that the Moloney murine leukemia virus RT is substantially more resistant to the inhibitor ddTTP than is the HIV enzyme.[22] The Moloney murine leukemia virus enzyme is a valid RT, and it is possible that variant forms of the HIV enzyme could arise that would be more resistant to ddTTP. Although ddTTP is not used as an antiviral drug for HIV, the argument applies with equal force to compounds that are.

What we really need to determine is not the structure of the active sites of particular variants of the HIV RT but the possible limits that the active site can assume. With this knowledge, it may be possible to synthesize an inhibitor that the enzyme cannot evade. There are two pathways that can be used to explore the limits on the structure of the active site. The first is to analyze evolutionary variants of RT.

Although there are differences in the amino acid sequences of the RTs of different retroviruses, all of these enzymes have similar enzymatic activities. This implies some conservation of the structure of the active sites. Closer examination of the amino acid sequences of the various known RTs reveals substantial regions of significant homology,[10] reinforcing the idea that the three-dimensional structures of the catalytic sites are quite similar.

A clear understanding of the structural features of at least some of these enzymes will probably be quite useful in understanding the acceptable limits on the structure of RT active sites. To this end, we have already expressed the Moloney murine leukemia virus RT in *E. coli,* using the same protocol we used to express the HIV enzyme,[21] and x-ray crystallographic analyses are planned.

It is also possible to analyze permissible variation in the structure of the HIV RT by making mutant forms of the enzyme using the *E. coli* system. Three types of procedures are planned: deletion, site-directed, and random mutagenesis. Deletion mutants have been used to define the regions of the enzyme that are necessary to produce a correctly folded, active enzyme (Table 2–1; see also Ref. 22). In addition, a nested set of amino- and carboxy-terminal deletions can be used to map the binding sites for monoclonal antibodies directed against the HIV RT. Carrying the HIV RT on a small plasmid makes the mutagenesis relatively simple. Deletion mutants can be prepared using convenient restriction sites. Site-directed mutants can be made by using mismatched oligonucleotide primers, by insertion of short DNA segments at defined restriction sites, or by replacing individual segments of the HIV RT coding region with double-stranded synthetic DNA. Random mutagenesis can be done by direct chemical treatment of the purified plasmid DNA or by passing the plasmid through a mutator strain of *E. coli.*

Our group (Ref. 23 and unpublished data) and others[32] have already begun to make site-directed mutants of the HIV RT. However, such experiments are most efficient when substantial structural information is available. In planning these experiments we have been guided by sequence comparisons with the RTs of other retroviruses. In the future, the results

Table 2–1
Relative Reverse Transcriptase Activities of Carboxy- and Amino-Terminal Deletion Mutants*

HIV RT Construct	Sequence	Activity (%)
Wild-type (p66)	Two additional amino-terminal amino acids, Met-Val, compared with the virion enzyme	100
CT-133 (p51)	133 amino acids deleted from the carboxy-terminus; the last 11 amino acids derive from the +1 reading frame, giving a sequence leu-trp-tyr-gln-his-thr-lys-glu-leu-glu-glu-met-asn-lys at the carboxy terminus	0.4
CT-23	Ends tyr-leu-ala-trp-val-leu	4.1
CT-16	Ends his-lys-gly-ile-gly-ile-gly-gly	45
CT-8	Ends asp-lys-leu-val	60
AT-23	Deletion of 23 amino terminal amino acids, but retains the two extra amino acids present in the wild-type enzyme; sequence begins with met-val-trp-pro-leu-thr	0

* HIV RT constructs in *E. coli* were assayed for reverse transcriptase activity in bacterial extracts. The various clones are named for the mutations they express. *CT* = deletions from the carboxy terminus of the molecule followed by the number of amino acids deleted; *AT* = deletions from the amino acid terminus of the reverse transcriptase followed by the number of amino acids deleted.

of chemical modification experiments and, more important, of x-ray structural analyses, will also be used in planning site-directed mutants. For some of the mutations we have tested, the mutated form of the HIV RT does not accumulate in *E. coli*. The significance of this observation is unclear, although we have assumed that grossly misfolded forms of the protein are much more susceptible to proteolysis than is the properly folded protein. If this interpretation is correct, the issue is moot, because only those mutations that give rise to relatively subtle alterations in structure (particularly of the active site) are of interest.

We also expect to proceed with random mutagenesis. Attempts will be made to directly screen lysed colonies of *E. coli* for mutations in the RNA-dependent DNA polymerase function. This would permit the screening of sufficiently large numbers of mutants so that relatively rare mutations could be sought. If such screens are possible, we then should be able to screen in *E. coli* for drug-resistant mutants of the sort that could arise from the genetic selection imposed by the treatment of large numbers of AIDS patients with particular drugs. We plan to use the *E. coli* system to screen for AZT-resistant mutants of the HIV RT. If such variant forms of the HIV RT are obtained, it will be especially important to employ them in drug screening and drug design experiments because they would be able to evade the only drug now available. When mutants are obtained by random mutagenesis, it will be important to be able to identify the responsible mutation rapidly. A series of oligonucleotides has been prepared that corresponds to sequences found at intervals of approximately 200 base pairs on both strands of the DNA encoding the HIV RT. By using these oligonucleotides to prime dideoxy sequencing reactions, the sequence of each mutant can be determined rapidly.

Any interesting mutants derived by either site-directed or random mutagenesis protocols will be analyzed biochemically. It would be helpful if a protocol for the rapid purification (on at least a modest scale) of large numbers of independent mutant proteins could be developed. We hope that antisera (discussed in a later section) prepared against the HIV RT made in *E. coli* will provide antibodies that can be used to prepare immunoaffinity columns for this purpose. The purified material will be especially important in analyzing the effects of mutations on RNase H function, which is difficult to assay in crude *E. coli* lysates. If the purification of large numbers of samples proves difficult, there are assay systems for both RNase H[29,30] and the RNA-dependent DNA polymerizing functions[33,34] of RT that can be done directly on material fractionated by gel electrophoresis. A small subset of the available mutants may ultimately be

candidates for x-ray structural analyses; however, because this process is quite labor intensive, the total number of proteins that can be analyzed in this fashion will be relatively small.

Drug Screening and Drug Design ∎

"Separate the Wheat from the Chaff" ∎

The goal of all the experiments described here is the development of new drugs effective against HIV. The information obtained from the structural, enzymatic, and biochemical studies may be useful in directed drug design, and the purified RT can also be employed in primary drug screens. Dealing with the purified RT in isolation has several distinct advantages over assays that rely on the inhibition of viral replication in a tissue culture system. The RNA-dependent DNA polymerase and the RNase H assays are completely safe, because neither employs live virus. They are rapid, taking only a few hours, and relatively simple and inexpensive. The assays are quantitative, and large numbers of samples can be analyzed in a single day. However, there are also drawbacks. Using the purified RT, it will be possible to screen for only two of the viral enzymatic functions. Although drugs that inhibit other steps in the viral life cycle would be missed when screened by the assays for RNA-dependent DNA polymerase and RNase H, similar *in vitro* assays could be set up for the other viral enzymes.

Any of the *in vitro* assays that rely directly on purified viral enzymes will not be sensitive to the permeability of the host cell to the drug, the drug's toxicity for the cell, or to modifications that the cell might make to the drug. Despite these drawbacks, the *in vitro* assays for RNA-dependent DNA polymerase and RNase H may provide an extremely useful primary screen. The simplicity of these assays will permit the screening of many more compounds than can be screened with the same amount of effort using a viral replication assay. Any compound that showed promise in an *in vitro* assay would have to undergo further testing in a viral replication assay system. However, the elimination of numerous ineffective compounds in the primary screening process could reduce the total time necessary to define an effective new drug. It may also be possible, at least in some instances, to anticipate the modifications that cells could make on a potential inhibitor. For example, large numbers of nucleotide analogues should be tested as inhibitors of the RNA-dependent DNA polymerase. In addition to testing the free bases and the nucleotides (which would most likely be the form administered to patients), the nucleoside triphosphates could be tested in the *in vitro* assay. An additional advantage of this kind of *in vitro* screening is that it can begin immediately, using the purified protein now at hand.

In the future, a complete three-dimensional picture of the HIV RT should come from the x-ray structure work. This should provide a molecular map of the surface of the active sites of the protein. With this information, it may be possible to design drugs that exactly "fit" the active sites. Such drugs could be tested for binding to the RT, using the purified enzyme, and for inhibition of its enzymatic functions, both in the *in vitro* assays and in the viral replication assay. If these results are promising, it may be possible to cocrystallize a promising inhibitor with the HIV RT to measure the degree to which an exact fit has been achieved. Because the degree of the inhibition is likely to be correlated with the precision of the molecular fit between the inhibitor and the three-dimensional surface of the corresponding active site, the importance of understanding the features of the active site in detail should be apparent. As noted earlier, it will also be extremely important to determine the mutational changes that can alter the surface of the active sites without perturbing the enzyme's function. The structure of active sites of other retroviral RTs and variants of the HIV RT must be kept in mind in planning the structure of a drug designed to inhibit the HIV RT.

Generation of Immunologic Reagents ■

"The Tools of the Trade" ■

An additional use of the HIV RT made in *E. coli* is that it can be used to generate a battery of monoclonal antibodies. These antibodies will certainly be useful as tools for investigating the RT, and may have broader relevance in clinical settings. The pure *E. coli* HIV RT that has already been prepared is now being used to generate antisera. It is reasonable to expect to obtain monoclonal antibodies that recognize epitopes found throughout the RT molecule. The *E. coli* expression system provides a relatively simple means to map the approximate binding sites for at least some of the monoclonal antibodies. We are preparing a nested set of amino- and carboxy-terminal deletions of the HIV RT by making appropriate deletions in the cloned DNA that encodes the protein. The relative position of the epitopes recognized by monoclonal antibodies that can bind to denatured

forms of the enzyme can be determined by identifying which monoclonal antibodies bind which of the deleted HIV RTs in a simple Western transfer assay (Fig. 2–5).

It may be possible, among the monoclonal antibodies that recognize the native form of the enzyme, to find antibodies that react directly with the active site. Knowledge of the structure of these antibodies could provide structural clues relevant to drug design. Antibodies covalently linked to columns may also provide a rapid method to purify HIV RT. Although this may or may not prove useful in providing material for the initial studies, the availability of a rapid and simple method to purify the proteins from a large number of different mutants will be invaluable when

FIG. 2–5 Mapping the recognition sites for monoclonal antibodies. A set of amino- and carboxy-terminal deletions of the HIV RT is being prepared (*e.g.*, CT-8 and CT-133 in Table 2–1 and Fig. 2–2). The full-length protein is schematically represented by the open box at the top. The next four smaller boxes represent carboxy-terminal deletions (see Table 2–1) generated by excising portions encoding various amounts of the carboxy portion of the enzyme. The bottom three boxes represent amino-terminal deletions. To obtain an in-frame amino-terminal deletion, a new synthetic DNA segment is inserted between the *Nco*I/ATG and convenient internal restriction sites. The binding site of a monoclonal antibody is determined by fractionating the various mutant proteins by acrylamide gel electrophoresis, transferring them to nitrocellulose filters, and probing with the antibody (Western blot). In this hypothetic example, a particular monoclonal reacts with most, but not all, of the deleted forms of HIV RT, as indicated by (+) or (−) at the left in the drawing. The region containing the epitope recognized by this hypothetical monoclonal is indicated by a small bar at the top.

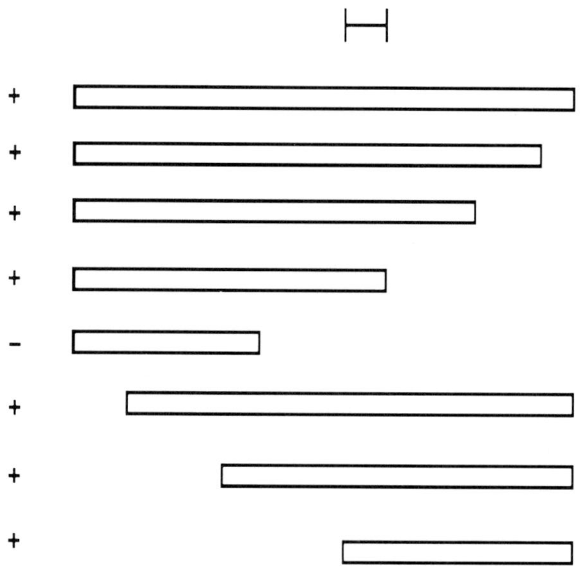

we proceed to the biochemical analyses of substantial numbers of mutants.

The monoclonal antibodies could be used to screen patients for the presence of the virus, although methods that detect the viral genome will probably be more sensitive and more useful. A well-defined set of monoclonal antibodies may have another use, however. A large amount of genetic variation in the HIV envelope is well-documented. Although the RT appears to be less variable than the envelope, variation should be anticipated. If an appropriate battery of monoclonal antibodies existed, they could be used to survey viruses isolated from patients for the presence and absence of individual epitopes. Such surveys may be useful in epidemiologic studies.

General Implications for Chemotherapy ■

"A Hawk from a Handsaw" ■

We have used a strategy similar to that used to express the HIV and MuLV RTs to express the HIV and MuLV integration proteins (Hizi A, Hughes SH: Unpublished observations), and several other laboratories are using recombinant DNA techniques to produce a variety of proteins from HIV and other retroviruses. However, the logic that has led to a molecular dissection of HIV has implications that go beyond this virus and the disease it causes. We have already suggested that the principal difficulty in developing antiviral drugs is the relative rarity of viral proteins that provide targets that allow a chemotherapeutic agent to distinguish viral functions from host functions. For this reason, it has been essentially impossible to identify antiviral drugs by random screening protocols. It is obvious that the type of molecular dissection currently being applied to HIV can be applied to other pathogenic viruses, and such work has already begun in several laboratories.

It may be possible, although substantially more difficult, to use similar techniques in developing specific drugs effective against human cancers. Currently, most of the chemotherapies that are effective against cancer rely on drugs that are toxic to rapidly growing cells. Although considerable progress has been made in effective therapies, most anticancer drugs are still quite toxic to the patient. As with all chemotherapies, the goal is to discover drugs that distinguish the host from the pathogen. What makes this a particularly difficult task in cancer chemotherapy is that, compared with bacterial or even with viral pathogens,

cancer cells provide no truly foreign proteins that can serve as specific targets.

The derangement of normal cells that leads to the development of cancer appears to involve the mutation of normal cellular genes known as oncogenes (for a comprehensive review, see Ref. 35). The mutations now known perturb the function of the protein encoded by the oncogene, the regulation of the expression of the oncogene, or both. It is likely that both types of oncogene activation produce proteins closely related to the oncogene protein in its normal form. When activation results in the overproduction of the oncogene protein, this is obvious. However, even when the oncogene is activated by mutation in the region encoding the oncogene protein itself (as opposed to a region regulating levels of expression), the structure of the activated oncogene is likely to resemble closely the structure of the normal protein.

In their normal form, oncogenes appear to play key roles in the regulation of cellular growth control and differentiation. Their ability in altered form to cause a cell to escape from growth control is almost certainly directly related to their normal roles. It is simplest to think of the oncogene proteins as being able, under certain conditions, to induce the cell to grow and divide, and of the activating mutation as one that permanently locks the oncogene protein in this activated configuration.

The recent x-ray structural analyses of the normal and activated *ras* proteins conform to this hypothesis. The overall structures of the two proteins are quite similar.[36] Nevertheless, there are *always* differences, either in the structure of the protein (as in the case of the activated *ras* protein) or in the amount of the oncogene protein made. These differences are subtle, but it is precisely such subtle differences that only directed drug design can hope to exploit.

However, this type of approach will place considerable additional burden on both the researcher and the clinician. For the researcher, it will be necessary to identify and solve the structure of all of the oncogenes that play roles in the initiation and progression of human cancer. The number of known oncogenes is still expanding rapidly, with no obvious end in sight. Even if this job were complete, and specific drugs were available that could block each of the individual oncogene proteins, it still would remain for the clinician to decipher which oncogenes were activated in a particular patient before trying to administer a specific (and appropriate) drug.

Fortunately, it appears, both in animal model systems and in patients, that particular types of cancer are closely correlated with the activation of particular oncogenes. In addition, there is both direct evidence (from model systems) and indirect evidence (from data gathered in patients) to suggest that multiple events (presumably the activation of different oncogenes) are required to produce a fully pathogenic cancer cell. Although this will probably make the task of understanding (and properly diagnosing) the different forms of cancer more difficult, it also holds the possibility that drugs directed at more than one oncogene can be given simultaneously to individual patients. It may also be possible to use conventional chemotherapy in combination with drugs specifically designed to interact with and inhibit particular oncogenes.

Whether or not either this particular view of the cancer cell or the proposal to design and direct drugs at particular oncogenes is correct in detail, the scientific approach it implies is correct in its general form. To defeat cancer cells, we must strive to better understand these cells in molecular detail. The realization that many human diseases were caused by pathogenic bacteria led to the isolation of the bacteria, which were then used to screen for drugs that inhibited their growth and, thereby, to develop effective antibiotics.

We are now in a position to try a more sophisticated approach to the more difficult problem of developing drugs designed to inhibit particular steps in the viral life cycle. We must first isolate viral enzymes to provide materials for drug screens. The next, and more difficult step is elucidation of the precise structure of the viral protein, which could lead to the design of drugs whose structures precisely match the target viral protein.

It is our hope that this type of approach, or extensions thereof, can eventually be applied to an even more difficult problem than the development of specific antiviral drugs: the design and development of specific anticancer drugs.

References ■

1. Weiss R, Teich N, Varmus HE, Coffin J (eds): RNA Tumor Viruses. Cold Spring Harbor, NY, Cold Spring Harbor Laboratory, 1985
2. Maddon PJ, Dalgleish AG, McDougal JS et al: The T4 gene encodes the AIDS virus receptor and is expressed in the immune system and the brain. Cell 47:333–348, 1986
3. Lasky LA, Groopman JE, Fennie CW et al: Neutralization of the AIDS retrovirus by antibodies to a recombinant envelope glycoprotein. Science 233:209–212, 1986
4. Pert CB, Hill JM, Ruff MR et al: Octapeptides deduced from the neuropeptide receptor-like pattern of antigen T4 in brain potently inhibit human immunodeficiency virus receptor binding and T-cell infectivity. Proc Natl Acad Sci USA 83:9254–9258, 1986
5. Lasky LA, Nakamura G, Smith DH et al: Delineation of a region of the human immunodeficiency virus type 1 gp120 glycoprotein critical for interaction with the CD4 receptor. Cell 50:975–985, 1987
6. Willey RL, Smith DH, Lasky LA et al: In vitro mutagenesis identifies a region within the envelope gene of the human immunodeficiency virus that is critical for infectivity. J Virol 62:139–147, 1988
7. Varmus HE: Form and function of retroviral proviruses. Science 216:812–820, 1982
8. Hughes SH: Synthesis, integration and transcription of the retroviral provirus. In Vogt P, Koprowski H (eds): Current Topics in Microbiology and Immunology, Vol 10, pp 23–49. New York, Springer-Verlag, 1983
9. Brown PO, Bowerman B, Varmus HE et al: Correct integration of retroviral DNA in vitro. Cell 49:347–356, 1987
10. Johnson MS, McClure A, Feng D-F et al: Computer analysis of retroviral *pol* genes: Assignment of enzymatic functions to specific sequences and homologies with nonviral enzymes. Proc Natl Acad Sci USA 83:7648–7652, 1986
11. Baltimore D: Retroviruses and retrotransposons: The role of reverse transcription in shaping the eukaryotic genome. Cell 40:481–482, 1985
12. Mitsuya H, Broder S: Strategies for antiviral therapy in AIDS. Nature 325:773–778, 1987
13. Furman PA, Fyfe JA, St Clair MH et al: Phosphorylation of 3'-azido-3'-deoxythymidine and selective interaction of the 5'-triphosphate with human immunodeficiency virus reverse transcriptase. Proc Natl Acad Sci USA 83:8333–8337, 1986
14. Kotewicz M, D'Alessio M, Driftmier M et al: Cloning and over-expression of Moloney murine leukemia virus reverse transcriptase in *Escherichia coli.* Gene 35:249–258, 1985
15. Tanese N, Roth M, Goff S: Expression of enzymatically active reverse transcriptase in *Escherichia coli.* Proc Natl Acad Sci USA 82:4944–4948, 1985
16. Hu S, Court D, Zweig M et al: Murine leukemia virus *pol* gene products: Analysis with antisera generated against reverse transcriptase and endonuclease fusion proteins expressed in *Escherichia coli.* J Virol 60:267–274, 1986
17. Tanese N, Sodroski J, Haseltine W et al: Expression of reverse transcriptase activity of human T-lymphotropic virus type III (HTLV III/LAV) in *Escherichia coli.* J Virol 59:743–745, 1986
18. Farmerie WG, Loeb DD, Casavant NC et al: Expression and processing of the AIDS virus reverse transcriptase in *Escherichia coli.* Science 236:305–308, 1987
19. Le Grice S, Benck V, Mous J: Expression of biologically active T-cell lymphotropic virus type III reverse transcriptase in *Bacillus subtilis.* Gene 55:95–103, 1987
20. Mous J, Heimer EP, LeGrice S: Processing protease and reverse transcriptase from human immunodeficiency virus type I polyprotein in *Escherichia coli.* J Virol 62:1433–1436, 1988
21. Hizi A, Hughes SH: Expression in *Escherichia coli* of a Moloney murine leukemia virus reverse transcriptase whose structure closely resembles the viral enzyme. Gene 66:319–323, 1988
22. Hizi A, McGill C, Hughes SH: Expression of soluble, enzymatically active, human immunodeficiency virus reverse transcriptase in *Escherichia coli* and analysis of mutants. Proc Natl Acad Sci USA 85:1218–1222, 1988
23. Larder B, Purifoy D, Powell K et al: AIDS virus reverse transcriptase defined by high level expression in *Escherichia coli.* EMBO J 6:3133–3137, 1987

24. Hughes SH, Greenhouse JJ, Petropoulos CJ et al: Adaptor plasmids simplify the insertion of foreign DNA into helper-independent retroviral vectors. J Virol 61:3004–3112, 1987
25. Vieira J, Messing J: The pUC plasmids, an M13 mp7-derived system for insertion mutagenesis with synthetic universal primers. Gene 19:259–268, 1982
26. Norrander J, Vieira J, Rubenstein I et al: Manipulation and expression of the Maize Zein storage protein in *Escherichia coli.* J Biotech 2:157–175, 1985
27. Kanaya S, Crouch RJ: DNA sequence of the gene coding for *Escherichia coli* ribonuclease H. J Biol Chem 258:1276–1281, 1983
28. Ogawa T, Pickett GG, Kogoma T et al: RNase H confers specificity in the dnaA-dependent initiation of replication at the unique origin of the *Escherichia coli* chromosome *in vivo* and *in vitro.* Proc Natl Acad Sci USA 81:1040–1044, 1984
29. Rucheton M, Lelay MN, Jeanteur PH: Evidence from direct visualization after denaturing gel electrophoresis that RNase H is associated with MSV-MuLV reverse transcriptase. Virology 97:221–223, 1979
30. Tanese N, Goff SP: Domain structure of the Moloney murine leukemia virus reverse transcriptase: Mutational analyses and separate expression of the DNA polymerase and RNase H activities. Proc Natl Acad Sci USA 85:1777–1781, 1988
31. Basu A, Nanduri V, Gerard GF et al: Substrate binding domain of Murine leukemia virus reverse transcriptase. J Biol Chem 26:1648–1653, 1988
32. Larder B, Purifoy D, Powell K et al: Site-specific mutagenesis of AIDS virus reverse transcriptase. Nature 327:716–717, 1987
33. Spanos A, Sedgwick SG, Yarranton GT et al: Detection of the catalytic activities of DNA polymerases and their associated exonucleases following SDS-polyacrylamide gel electrophoresis. Nucleic Acids Res 9:1825–1839, 1981
34. Hansen J, Schulze T, Mellert W et al: Identification and characterization of HIV-specific RNase H by monoclonal antibody. EMBO J 7:239–243, 1988
35. Bishop JM: Viral oncogenes. Cell 42:23–38, 1985
36. deVos A, Tong L, Milburn M, et al: Three-dimensional structure of an oncogene protein: Catalytic domain of human C-H-*ras* p21. Science 239:888–893, 1988

Berton Zbar

Chromosomal Deletions in Lung Cancer and Renal Cancer

3

Introduction ■

A consistent genetic change—the loss of DNA sequences on the short arm of chromosome 3 (3p)—is present in almost all tumor samples we have studied from patients with renal cell carcinoma[1] and small cell lung carcinoma.[2] The consistency of these findings suggests that loss of DNA sequences on chromosome 3p may be of fundamental importance in the origin or evolution of these tumors. Specifically, these findings raise the possibility that elimination of the normal function of a single gene pair leads to these two types of carcinoma. Evidence supporting these observations, and their potential applications for studies of the etiology and diagnosis of renal cell carcinoma (RCC) and small cell lung carcinoma (SCLC), is discussed in this chapter.

Review of Basic Biologic Principles ■

DNA Polymorphism ■

Understanding these findings requires a review of the principles and techniques of molecular biology used in our work.[1,2] Human somatic cells contain 46 chromosomes: 22 pairs of chromosomes (autosomes) and the two sex chromosomes. One member of each chromosome pair is inherited from each parent. This pairing of chromosomes ensures a redundancy of genetic material (there are two copies of each autosomal gene). The maternal and paternal members of a chromosome pair are not identical: about 1%–4% of the nucleotide sequences on homologous chromosomes are different.[3] These chemical differences, generally located in regions of chromosomes that do not encode genetic information, are of three major types: single nucleotide changes, differences in the number of tandemly repeated nucleotide sequences, and insertions or deletions of blocks of nucleotides.

These nucleotide differences between homologous chromosomes may create (or destroy) a site for cleavage of DNA by an enzyme (*i.e.,* restriction endonuclease), or they may shorten (or increase) the distance between two restriction endonuclease sites. The net result is that DNA fragments of different size are produced after digestion of DNA with restriction endonucleases. In Figure 3–1, the arrows indicate the location of sites for restriction endonuclease cleavage; a cleavage site present on one chromosome is absent at the corresponding location on the homologous chromosome. This accounts for the difference in DNA fragment size. These differently sized DNA fragments are markers that characterize and distinguish each member of a chromosome pair. As shown in Figure 3–2, differences in DNA fragment size (restriction fragment length polymorphisms, or RFLPs) are detected by digesting the DNA with enzymes, separating the DNA fragments by agarose gel electrophoresis, transferring the DNA fragments to a filter membrane, and reacting the filter membrane with a radioactive human DNA fragment (probe). Filter membranes are then placed with a piece of film to produce an autoradiograph.

These polymorphic DNA fragments represent an invaluable "tool kit" for the cancer researcher because they permit identification of genetic changes in tumors that were previously undetectable. Data from studies of DNA polymorphisms may ultimately supplement pathologic analysis of tumor tissues and provide new understanding of cancer etiology.

A

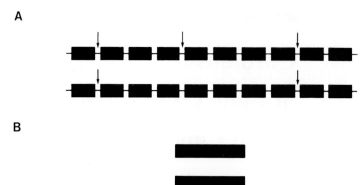

B

FIG. 3–1 DNA polymorphism. (*A*) A locus on a pair of homologous chromosomes; arrows indicate sites for cleavage by a restriction endonuclease. The additional site for restriction endonuclease cleavage present on one homologous chromosome accounts for the difference in DNA fragment size. (*B*) The size of DNA fragments, detected by Southern transfer, hybridization, and autoradiography.

Probes and Determination of Genotype ■

The probes that detect polymorphisms were isolated by investigators whose major objective was to provide a set of genetic markers that would identify the chromosomal location of genes responsible for inherited diseases.[4] They were isolated empirically from li-

FIG. 3–2 Schematic of Southern transfer analysis. (From Vande Woude GF, Gilden RV, in DeVita VT Jr, et al (eds): Cancer: Principles and Practice of Oncology. Philadelphia, J B Lippincott, 1985, p 28)

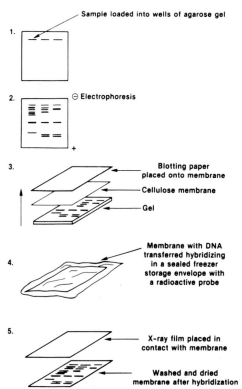

braries of human DNA, which contain the total human genome divided into bite-sized portions and inserted into individual bacteriophages (books). The first step in identifying and isolating polymorphic DNA fragments is screening the library to identify DNA sequences that are present as single copies in the genome. Single-copy DNA fragments are then screened against a panel of human DNA samples; each panel is digested with a different restriction endonuclease to locate DNA fragments that detect bands of different size. Candidate probes are tested against DNA extracted from leukocytes of three-generation families to determine whether the markers behave, as expected, as Mendelian codominant alleles.

In principle, the number of these genetic markers is unlimited. The location for each probe is determined (mapped) with somatic cell hybrid panels, by linkage to known probes or by *in situ* hybridization. This analysis establishes a location for the genetic marker on a specific region of a chromosome.

The classic probes were two-allele systems based on single nucleotide differences;[5] current probes are multiallele systems based on a variable number of tandemly repeated (VNTR) nucleotide sequences.[6] The high degree of polymorphism of VNTR probes makes them the tools of choice.

The constitutional genotype is determined by analysis of DNA extracted from normal tissue. This DNA is digested with an appropriate restriction endonuclease and tested with suitable probes according to the procedure outlined in Figure 3–2. By convention, the larger DNA fragment is referred to as allele 1 (A1) and the smaller DNA fragment or fragments as A2. A person with both alleles is by definition heterozygous (1,2) at that locus; an individual with one type of allele is by definition homozygous (1,1 or 2,2) at that locus. The frequency of heterozygosity of each genetic marker is a characteristic that can be determined by population studies.

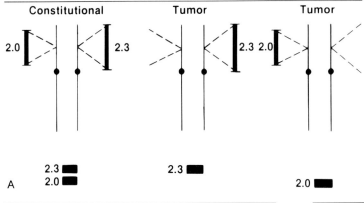

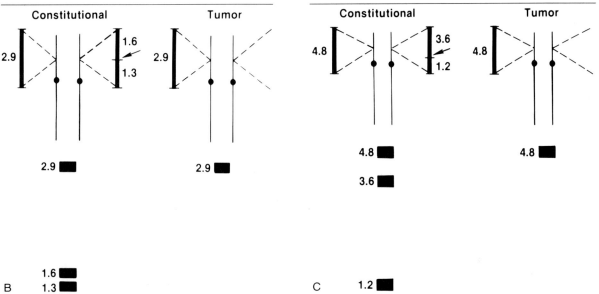

FIG. 3-3 Detection of genetic changes in tumors by RFLP analysis. Schematics illustrate hypothetic test results with three probes—DNF15S2 (*A*), D3S2 (*B*), and D3S3 (*C*)—that detect RFLP on chromosome 3p. In contrast to the normal (constitutional) tissue, there is only one allele in DNA extracted from the patient's tumor.

Detecting Genetic Changes in Solid Tumors ■

RFLP ANALYSIS □

Cavenee and associates devised a test for loss of specific DNA sequences in human tumors based on DNA polymorphism (Fig. 3–3).[7] DNA polymorphisms in a patient's normal tissue are compared with those in the patient's cancer. (Heterozygous persons are required for this analysis.) Figure 3–3 shows the normal and tumor tissues of a hypothetical patient tested with three probes to chromosome 3p. Figure 3–4 illustrates probe binding sites. In contrast to the normal tissue, there is only one allele in the DNA extracted from this patient's tumor. Thus, the tumor genotype differs from the normal genotype at this locus; the part of the chromosome that carries this DNA fragment has,

in some manner, been deleted from the cell. The phrase "loss of heterozygosity" is used to describe this genetic change. Detection of loss of heterozygosity in tumors of a particular type points to the location of genes that may be abnormal in that form of cancer.

OTHER METHODS □

Other methods for detecting change in heterozygosity in human tumors can be used when samples of a patient's normal tissues (DNA) are not available. One method involves comparing the frequency of heterozygosity at particular loci in tumor samples of a particular histologic type, in normal tissues of patients with that form of cancer, and in the general population. In the absence of a genetic change at that locus, the frequency of heterozygosity in a tumor panel should be similar to that in normal tissues from which the tumor population was derived: a significantly lower frequency suggests that there is a process operating that has led to a loss of heterozygosity. Note that this is a population comparison; it is not possible to say that in an individual patient an allele has been lost.

An approach that can be used with unpaired samples of rare tumors is to determine the numerical value and 95% tolerance limits for the ratio of signal intensities of alleles 1 and 2.[8] The allele ratio for a locus is a constant that, once determined, can be used by other laboratories. When the allele ratio for a tumor sample is outside the 95% tolerance limits for the normal population at that locus, it is likely that there is loss of heterozygosity.

Linkage Analysis ■

The tool kit of polymorphic DNA probes not only provides valuable reagents for detecting loss of heterozygosity but is useful in determining the chromosomal location of diseases caused by mutations at single loci. The principle of this form of genetic anal-

ysis is to identify a polymorphic DNA marker "linked" to the disease, that is, invariably present in affected family members but absent from unaffected family members. Mendel's law of independent assortment describes the fact that genetically determined phenotypic traits are inherited independently of one another. When the genes that determine two traits are located close together on the same chromosome, the genes are *not* sorted independently of one another, and inheritance of the traits is linked. Because the chromosomal location of the genetic markers is known, the demonstration that disease inheritance is linked to a particular genetic marker establishes the chromosomal location of the gene that

FIG. 3–5   Banding pattern of human chromosome 3. *Left:* chromosome 3 at a haplotype karyotype of 400 bands. *Right:* chromosome 3 at a haplotype karyotype of 550 bands.[9] (Reprinted with permission of *Cytogenetics and Cell Genetics,* from Cytogenet Cell Genet 31:1–23, 1981)

FIG. 3–4   Probe binding sites for three chromosome 3p probes: DNF15S2 (*A*), D3S2 (*B*), and D3S3 (*C*). Restriction endonuclease cleavage sites are indicated by arrows. *Solid arrows* indicate cleavage sites present in all people (invariant); *Dashed arrows* indicate cleavage sites that are present in some, but not all, people.

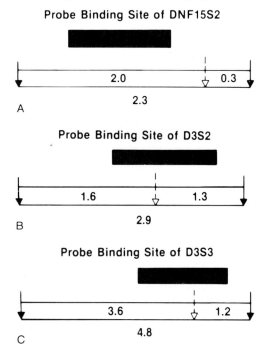

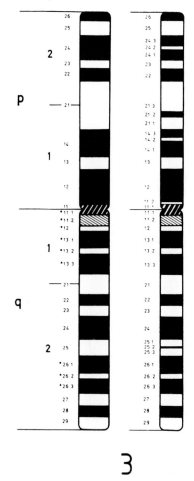

3

predisposes to that disease. This method involves a statistical analysis of genotyping data and correlation of the genotypic information with the presence (or absence) of the disease.

Chromosome 3 Abnormalities ■

Cytogenetic Analyses in RCC and SCLC ■

Cytogenetic analysis has suggested that abnormalities of chromosome 3 may be important in the origin or evolution of RCC and SCLC. To understand the data gained from these analyses, it is necessary to refer to Figure 3–5, which shows a schematic version of the banding pattern (the physical map) of human chromosome 3.[9] The chromosome is divided by the centromere into the short (p) and long arms (q), which in this case are about the same size. The p and q arms are further divided into regions 1 and 2, which are in turn subdivided.

Renal cell carcinoma,[10–21] and small cell lung carcinoma[22–26] show a consistent abnormality of the short arm of chromosome 3 in the region 3p13-3p23. Samples from both hereditary and sporadic cases of RCC and from sporadic SCLC have been examined for genetic changes. In hereditary cases, inherited

(constitutional) cytogenetic abnormalities provide clues to the location of cancer genes. In one large family with renal cell carcinoma, affected family members had a constitutional, balanced reciprocal translocation between chromosomes 3 and 8 (Figs. 3–6 and 3–7).[18] The short arm of chromosome 3 from 3p14.2 to the 3p terminus was translocated to the long arm of chromosome 8; part of the long arm of chromosome 8 was translocated to the short arm of chromosome 3. Of the family members with the t(3;8), 90% developed RCC by age 60. The close correlation between inheritance of the translocation chromosome and disease development suggests that a gene predisposing to renal cancer is located on chromosome 3 (or 8) at the point where the chromosome was broken. In another family, the proband had a translocation confined to the tumor between the short arm of chromosome 3 and chromosome 11.[17] The common feature in these families is a rearrangment of chromosome 3, suggesting that this is the location of the gene that predisposes to RCC. In sporadic RCC, rearrangements of chromosome 3p are the most frequently observed cytogenetic abnormality. Kovacs and coworkers showed that 22 of 25 primary RCCs showed rearrangements of 3p.[10] The only cytogenetic abnormality in several sporadic RCCs was a structural abnormality of chromosome

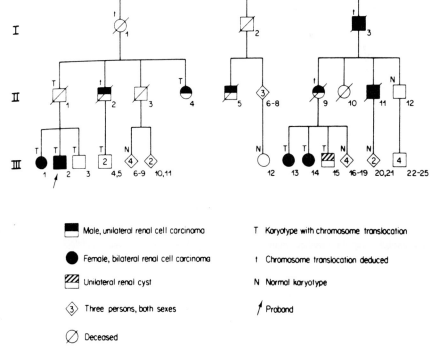

FIG. 3–6 Pedigree of family with chromosome 3;8 balanced translocation and RCC. (Reprinted with permission of *The New England Journal of Medicine,* from Cohen AJ et al: N Engl J Med 301:592–595, 1979)

■ Male, unilateral renal cell carcinoma

● Female, bilateral renal cell carcinoma

▨ Unilateral renal cyst

◇ Three persons, both sexes

⊘ Deceased

T Karyotype with chromosome translocation

t Chromosome translocation deduced

N Normal karyotype

⟋ Proband

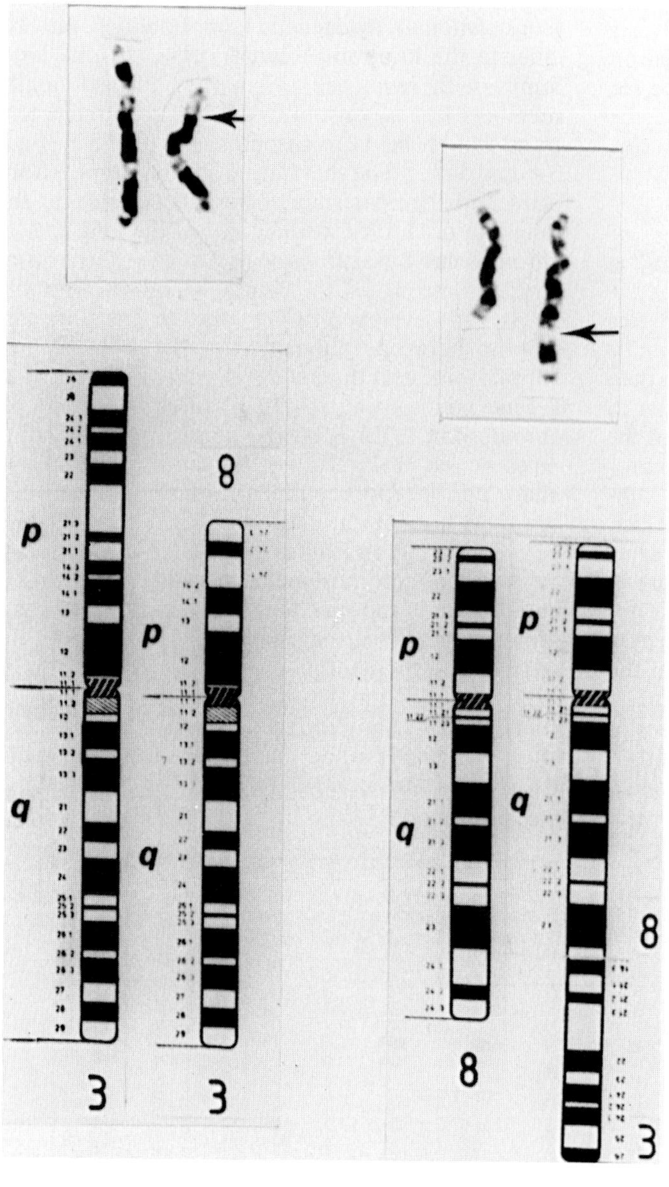

FIG. 3-7 Detailed diagram of chromosome 3;8 balanced translocation associated with familial RCC.[19] (Reprinted with permission of *Cancer Genetics and Cytogenetics,* from Wang N et al: Cancer Genet Cytogenet 11:479–481, 1984)

3p, suggesting that the change on chromosome 3 in these renal tumors was primary, that is, essential to their origin.

Work by Whang-Peng and colleagues has focused attention on deletions of chromosome 3p in SCLC.[22,23] Although cytogenetic analysis of SCLC lines showed structural changes in a number of chromosomes, Whang-Peng detected a structural abnormality of chromosome 3 in every SCLC sample examined. The abnormality detected was a deletion of one chromosome 3p; the extent of the chromosome 3 loss varied from sample to sample. The region of

chromosome 3 that was consistently lost (*i.e.,* the shortest region of overlap) was located between 3p14 and 3p21. The consistency of 3p deletion in SCLC lines is controversial, as is the size of the deletion. The Dartmouth group was unable to detect 3p deletion in the majority of SCLC lines examined.[27] Buys's group recently reported that the minimal region deleted in SCLC was 3p21-p23.[25] A report by Waters and associates suggested 3p21-p24 as the common region of overlap.[26]

These cytogenetic observations suggested that changes at chromosome 3p were a characteristic genetic change in SCLC and RCC and further indicated a tentative location for the aberrant gene or genes. The complexity of the cytogenetic findings in most RCCs and SCLCs hindered confirmation of these observations. It is possible that in some tumor samples genetic material was not deleted but translocated to other chromosomes. Also, in some samples the deletion may have been too small to be detected by cytogenetic methods. More sensitive methods for detecting loss of DNA sequences were needed to confirm and extend the cytogenetic observations.

Recombinant Human DNA Probes ■

The RFLP analysis developed by Cavenee and coworkers[7] provided the requisite tools to address the questions raised by cytogenetic analysis. This method is more sensitive (the minimum deletion detectable by cytogenetics is about 5000 kilobases [kb]; RFLP analysis can detect a 1 kb deletion) and can be performed on primary tumors, without the possible artifacts introduced by the cytogenetic requirement for

growth in cell culture. RFLP analysis samples the genome of numerous tumor cells rather than a few cells in mitosis, and can be performed by persons with skills in molecular biology, not just those with training in sophisticated cytogenetic techniques.

Probes that detect polymorphisms on chromosome 3p were needed to perform this study. For a patient to be evaluable, the normal (constitutional) tissues had to be heterozygous at chromosome 3p. Because only a fraction of the population analyzed will be heterozygous at any chromosome locus, we used several chromosome 3 probes to increase the probability of finding people who were heterozygous for at least one locus at 3p.

Table 3-1 lists currently available probes for the short arm of chromosome 3, the restriction enzymes used to detect the polymorphisms, DNA fragment size for each allele, the frequency of heterozygosity, and, where known, the assigned location of the sequence on the physical map of chromosome 3.[5,6,28-37] When our work began, three polymorphic probes were available: D3S2, D3S3, and DNF15S2. Results of RFLP analysis with RCC and SCLC are

Table 3–1
Polymorphic Probes for Chromosome 3p*

Symbol	Probe	Enzyme	HZG	Constant Bands	Allele	Length	Location	Ref.
D3S2	pHF12-32	Msp I	0.42		A1	2.9	3p14-3p21	5, 30
					A2	1.3, 1.3		
D3S3	pMS1-37	Msp I	0.08		A1	4.9	3p14	5, 31
					A2	3.7, 1.2		
DNF15S2	pH3H2	Hind III	0.48	2	A1	2.3	3p21	32, 33
					A2	2.0		
D3S30	pYNZ86.1	Msp I	0.50	2	A1	2.6	3p	34
					A2	2.1		
D3S32	pEFD145.1	Rsa I	0.50		A1	2.4	3p	28
					A2	1.3, 1.1		
		Taq I			B1	6.0		
					B2	4.0		
D3S4	B67	Taq I	0.24		A1	13	3p	28
					A2	12		
		Msp I	0.27	3	B1	4.8		
					B2	1.6		
RAF1	p627	Taq I	0.38	8	A1	6.8	3p24-3p25	35, 59
					A2	6.3		
		Bgl I	0.50	5	B1	4.0		
					B2	3.3		
ERBA2	pBH302	Hind III	0.43		A1	7.0	3p21-3p24	36, 37
					A2	5.5		
D3S12	CRI-R59	Msp I	0.67		Six alleles		3p	29
D3S13	CRI-R96	Msp I	0.64		Three alleles		3p	29
D3S23	CRI-P112	Msp I	0.40		Two alleles		3p	29
D3S18	CRI-L162	Taq I	0.19		Two alleles		3p	29
D3S22	CRI-R532	Msp I	0.62		Six alleles		3p	29
D3S17	CRI-L892	Taq I	0.71		Five alleles		3p	29

* HZG = frequency of heterozygosity; lengths are in kilobases (kb).

illustrated here with these three probes. Since that time, additional chromosome 3p probes have been isolated, and it is predicted that within 1 or 2 years, this number will be increased 100-fold. Note the location of two oncogenes: c-*raf*-1 at 3p24-3p25 and c-*erb*A beta at 3p21-p24.

For studies aimed at isolating a disease gene located on 3p, it is important to know the linear order of the loci on the chromosome. This information has been generated by White and coworkers for one set of chromosome 3p markers[28] and by Donis-Keller and coworkers for a second set (Fig. 3–8).[29] These markers were arranged in a linear fasion by studying the frequency of recombination in large three-generation families. The distance between these markers is determined by the frequency of their recombination. Their arrangement on the linkage map is supplemented by studies of somatic cell hybrids with different 3p deletions or translocations to provide a location of the probe that corresponds to the cytogenetically determined chromosomal bands (physical map).

Renal Cell Carcinoma ■

Biology ■

Renal cell carcinoma, the most common cancer of the kidney, accounts for 2% of cancer deaths in the United States; there are about 18,000 new cases in the United States each year. Electron microscopic studies indicate that RCC originates from the proximal renal tubule epithelial cell. Cigarette smoking is thought to play a role in the etiology of sporadic RCC.

Although the vast majority of cases of RCC are of the sporadic type, there are occasional families with many affected members. These rare families with heritable RCC are of extraordinary importance because the disease behaves like a single autosomal dominant gene disorder. Thus, identification of the abnormal gene in hereditary RCC offers insight into common sporadic RCCs. The hallmarks of a familial cancer (early age of onset, bilateral involvement of a paired organ, and multiple independent primary tumors) are present in familial RCC. The condition occurs in two, apparently distinct, clinical forms: a "pure" form, in which RCC is the only inherited disease manifestation,[38] and von Hippel–Lindau disease,[39–47] in which this carcinoma is one of several inherited disease manifestations, including retinal angiomas, cerebellar hemangioblastomas, and cysts of the kidney, pancreas, and epididymis. Because sophisticated medical techniques are required to detect cerebellar hemangioblastomas (*i.e.,* magnetic resonance imaging) and retinal angiomas (*i.e.,* funduscopy) some families previously regarded as having pure RCC may actually be examples of von Hippel–Lindau disease. The possibility that von Hippel–Lindau disease and familial RCC are different manifestations of the same gene must be considered. The frequency of the von Hippel–Lindau syndrome mutation has been estimated to be 1.8×10^{-7} (number of mutants per 10^6 gametes = 0.18).[47] Von Hippel–Lindau syndrome is inherited as an autosomal dominant disease. It is possible that RCC in von Hippel–Lindau disease may be pathologically distinguished from pure RCC by the presence of renal cysts lined with clear cells.[42]

The total number of reported cases of families with pure familial RCC is about 28.[38] Because of this small

FIG. 3–8 Linkage maps for chromosome 3 and 3p, showing the linear relationships of chromosome 3 probes mapped by the Collaborative Research group[29] and the Howard Hughes Medical Institute group.[28] (Adapted from Leppert M et al: Cytogenet Cell Genet 46:648, 1987; and Donis-Keller H et al: Cell 51:319–337, 1987)

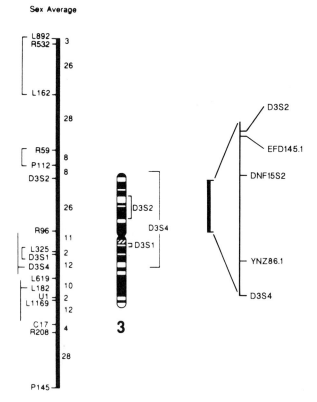

number, the mode of inheritance is not known. For the RCC family with the 3;8 balanced translocation (described earlier), the mode of inheritance was consistent with that of an autosomal dominant disease, with the translocation chromosome as the marker of disease phenotype. Attempts to find additional examples of constitutional abnormalities of chromosome 3 in individuals with RCC were unsuccessful.[48]

Renal oncocytomas, renal tumors that originate from the proximal renal tubule, are distinguished from RCC by morphology and, usually, by the absence of metastases.[49-53] These tumors are usually asymptomatic and are discovered incidentally. Flow cytometery studies of renal oncocytomas by Lieber and coworkers showed that the DNA content of oncocytomas was not uniformly diploid, suggesting the possibility of underlying genetic abnormalities.[53] A few case reports of oncocytomas showed cytogenetic changes. Renal oncocytoma may represent a *forme fruste* of RCC—a slice in the evolution of renal malignancy and, as such, worthy of RFLP analysis.

A model of hereditary RCC has been developed in Wistar rats.[54] The disease originates in the proximal renal tubule and depends on an autosomal dominant gene. Parabiosis experiments suggested that the gene has a direct effect on the kidney. The question raised by this animal model is whether there are similarities between the gene responsible for hereditary RCC in rats and humans. Hereditary renal cell carcinoma in humans is unusual in having a closely related animal model.

Loss of Alleles at Chromosome 3p Loci in Primary Sporadic RCC ■

We analyzed primary tumors of 31 untreated patients with sporadic RCC; we found a loss of alleles at loci on the short arm of chromosome 3 in 19 of 22 evaluable patients.[1] Figures 3–3A and 3–9 illustrate the results of an RFLP analysis with the probe DNF15S2. The schematic (Fig. 3–3A) illustrates the polymorphism obtained with this probe. A DNA fragment of either 2.0 or 2.3 kb is produced by digestion with the restriction endonuclease Hind III. The 2.0 kb fragment is produced when there is an additional site for Hind III digestion. Either allele can be lost in a tumor (the loss is random). The schematic in Figure 3–4A also illustrates the probe binding site; the probe does not extend over the variable Hind III restriction endonuclease site. The results from four patients are presented in Figure 3–9. In patients 5 and 15, there was a loss of allele 1; in patients 13 and 18, there was

a loss of allele 2 (shown by significant reduction in signal intensity).

Figures 3–3B and 3–10 illustrate the results with the probe D3S2. The polymorphism is illustrated in Figures 3–3B. When genomic DNA was digested with the restriction endonuclease Msp I, either a 2.9 kb fragment or a 1.6 kb and 1.3 kb doublet fragment was produced. The polymorphism was the result of a variable Msp I site (indicated in Fig. 3–3B by the arrow). Figure 3–10 shows the results from paired samples from five patients with this probe. Signal intensity was reduced for allele 1 in patient 13 and for allele 2 in patients 14, 15, 16, and 18. These differences were quantitated by densitometry (see below).

The reduction but not complete elimination of signal from one allele probably reflects contamination of primary renal tumors with host leukocytes. Belldegrun and colleagues,[55,56] in a study of 36 primary RCCs, found that disaggregated primary RCCs contained a mean of 40% tumor cells and 60% leukocytes, primarily lymphocytes (Fig. 3–11). One approach to determining whether the residual signal observed

FIG. 3–9 Southern hybridization of 3p probe DNF15S2 to normal kidney (*N*) and RCC (*T*) DNA. T* indicates a renal tumor (first passage) grown in an immunodeficient mouse. Patient numbers are shown below the blots, and the size of the polymorphic bands (in kb) on the right. Alleles at each locus are designated 1 or 2 according to decreasing length; C indicates a constant band.[1] (Reprinted with permission of *Nature,* from Zbar B et al: Nature 327: 721–724, 1987)

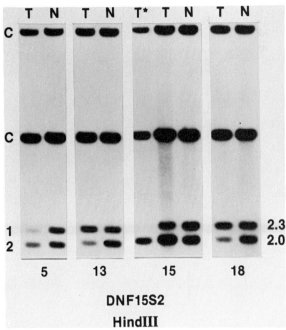

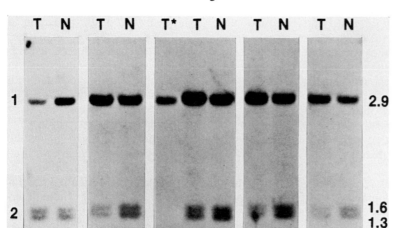

FIG. 3–10   Analysis as in Figure 3–9, using probe D3S2.[1] (Reprinted with permission of *Nature,* from Zbar B et al: Nature 327:721–724, 1987)

FIG. 3–11   Percent tumor cells in 36 primary RCCs. Differential cell counts were performed after disaggregation by enzymatic digestion.[56] (Reprinted with permission of *Journal of Urology,* from Belldegrun A: J Urol 150–155, 1988)

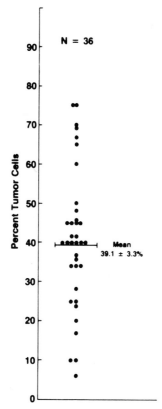

on autoradiographs originates from nonmalignant stromal tissue is to test renal tumors growing in immunodeficient mice. The proliferative advantage of the tumor cells would be expected to select for pure populations of tumor cells. A renal tumor grown from tissue from patient 15 in an immunodeficient mouse (xenograft) was available. The results (Figs. 3–9 and 3–10) show a complete loss of the allele that was diminished in the primary renal tumor. When tested with a probe for DNF15S2, the primary renal tumor showed a 32% decrease in A1; no A1 signal is present in the xenograft. When tested with a probe for D3S2, the primary renal tumor showed a 29% decrease in intensity of A2; A2 was completely lost in the xenograft.

These findings do not eliminate the possibility that the residual signal observed on autoradiographs reflects heterogeneity of loss at chromosome 3p in the primary renal tumors. It is possible that some but not all renal tumor cells have chromosome 3p deletion. Growth of primary RCCs in immunodeficient mice might select for those RCCs with the chromosome 3p deletion. This possibility was evaluated in unpublished experiments by Linehan and colleagues. These workers removed host leukocytes from disaggregated primary human renal tumors by panning with a monoclonal antibody to human leukocyte antigens, extracted genomic DNA from separated and unseparated tumor cell suspensions, and then used RFLP analysis to test for chromosome 3p allele loss. The purified primary renal tumor cells showed results consistent with those obtained in immunodeficient mice. The conclusion is that primary RCCs are homogeneous in terms of loss of DNA sequences on chromosome 3p.

Evaluation of RFLP Data by Densitometry ■

To establish objective criteria for significant decreases in allele signal intensity, it was necessary to quantitate the decrease in allele signal intensity and to evaluate the results statistically. As noted above, the ratio of allele signal intensity at a locus is a constant that can be determined by densitometric analysis of samples from a panel of normal individuals. The mean and 95% tolerance limits were determined for the DNF15S2 locus with DNA extracted from nine normal kidneys (Figs. 3–12 and 3–13). It is clear from previous autoradiographs (Fig. 3–9) that the intensities of the larger (2.3 kb) and smaller (2.0 kb) alleles are about equal. Visual inspection is corroborated by the results of densitometry; the ratio of the A1 and A2 alleles for this probe is about 1.0. This ratio agrees well with the value determined for this probe by Buys and coworkers.[57] For 15 of 16 primary renal tumors, the DNF15S2 allele ratio fell outside the defined 95% tolerance limits. This is a reflection of the loss of one allele in the primary tumor and the presence of residual normal tissue in the sample. (An alternative explanation for the change in allele ratio, chromosome 3 trisomy in the renal tumors, was not detected.)

Other Studies and Summary of Data on Chromosome 3p Allele Loss ■

The allele loss on chromosome 3p in RCC detected in this laboratory has been confirmed by Kovacs and colleagues,[58] who found that 18 of 21 cytogenetically

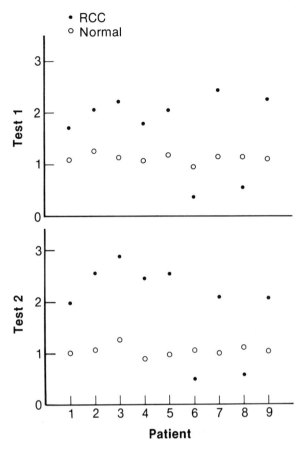

FIG. 3–12 Densitomety analysis of replicate DNA polymorphism analyses. Intensities of alleles 1 and 2 were quantitated in normal tissues (○) and primary RCCs (●) from patients who were heterozygous at the DNF15S2 locus. The Y axis represents the ratio of signal intensity for alleles 1 and 2; the X axis represents individual patients. Tests 1 and 2 were conducted on separate occasions by restriction endonuclease digestion of new aliquots of DNA, followed by agarose gel electrophoresis, Southern transfer, and hybridization to the probe DNF15S2. Note that the allele ratio for DNF15S2 in normal kidney is about 1.

FIG. 3–13 Mean and 95% tolerance limits[8] of the DNF15S2 allele ratio in normal kidney, based on data presented in Figure 3–12. *Open circles* indicate normal kidney; *solid circles* indicate primary RCCs. Note that each primary RCC sample falls outside the 95% tolerance limits.

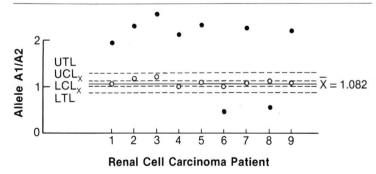

Table 3–2
**Frequency of Allele Loss at Specific Chromosome 3p Loci
in Primary Renal Cell Carcinomas***

| Probe | Study | | | | |
	Zbar et al[1]	Zbar et al (unpublished)	Kovacs et al[10]	Buys et al (unpublished)	Total
D3S3	1/2	1/2	0/9		2/14 (14%)
DNF15S2	9/9	6/7	16/21	3/3	34/40 (85%)
D3S2	7/8	3/3	2/11	1/1	13/23 (57%)

* Number with allele loss/number heterozygous. Of the 31 RCCs studied in our laboratory, 28 were tested at three loci and 3 were tested at one locus (DNF15S2).

examined RCCs had an abnormality of chromosome 3p distal to band 3p11.2-p13. RFLP analysis showed loss of heterozygosity at the DNF15S2 locus in 16 of 21 cases (76%); D3S2 heterozygosity was lost in 2 of 11 cases (18%). On the basis of combined cytogenetic and molecular genetic data, Kovacs and colleagues suggested a location for the gene that predisposes to RCC on the telomeric side of DNF15S2 on the short arm of chromosome 3.

Examination of the data from our laboratory and from Kovacs and coworkers indicates that DNF15S2 is the probe that most consistently detected chromosome 3p allele loss in RCC (Table 3–2). If this observation does not reflect technical problems (such as readier detection of allele loss with this probe), the results suggest that the RCC gene would be closer to the DNF15S2 locus than to D3S3 or D3S2.

Allele Loss on Other Chromosomes ■

A limited amount of work has been done to determine whether allele loss in RCC is limited to chromosome 3. Our group found evidence for allele loss (c-Ha-*ras*) on chromosome 11p in 1 of 9 informative RCC samples.[1] Anglard and colleagues, in a comprehensive analysis of 11p changes in primary RCCs, found a frequency of 11p loss of about 40% (unpublished data).

Significance of the Chromosome 3p Loss in RCC ■

The cytogenetic and molecular genetic data on chromosome 3 changes in nonhereditary and familial primary RCC can be summarized as follows:

- Rearrangement or deletion of chromosome 3p is the most consistent abnormality observed in cytogenetic studies of sporadic renal cell carcinomas.
- In some sporadic and hereditary RCCs, rearrangement or deletion of the short arm of chromosome 3 is the only cytogenetic abnormality.
- In one large family with hereditary RCC, a constitutional balanced 3;8 translocation was consistently associated with the development of RCC.
- Molecular genetic analysis indicates that virtually all evaluable RCC samples have loss of alleles at loci on chromosome 3p.
- The gene that predisposes to von Hippel–Lindau disease has been linked to a genetic marker located on the chromosome 3p.[59]
- Unpublished studies of a small nuclear family with RCC as the major manifestation of von Hippel–Lindau disease indicate that the chromosome 3 retained in the renal tumors was from the affected parent.

Taken together, these data provide compelling evidence that there is a gene located on chromosome 3p that is involved in the origin of RCC.

The Two-Mutation Theory ■

The changes detected on chromosome 3p in primary RCC may best be interpreted in terms of the two-mutation theory of cancer. Knudson concluded, based on an epidemiologic analysis of retinoblastoma and Wilms' tumor, that two mutations at allelic loci within a single cell were necessary and sufficient for tumor origin (Fig. 3–14).[60–62] He postulated that hereditary and nonhereditary forms of a given cancer were caused by mutations at the same locus. In he-

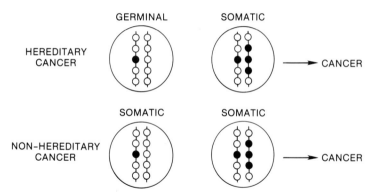

FIG. 3–14 Two-mutation theory of cancer. Each cell contains a pair of homologous chromosomes; *solid circles* indicate sites of mutations. The first mutation usually is a structural change in a specific cancer gene (*single solid circle*). The second mutation usually involves a much larger region of the chromosome by mitotic errors (*multiple solid circles*).

reditary tumors, the first mutation is transmitted in the germ line and involves structural changes in specific cancer genes; the second mutation is in somatic cells and arises from mitotic errors that may involve entire chromosomes. In nonhereditary tumors, both mutations are in somatic cells. The only difference between the hereditary and nonhereditary forms of a cancer is that in nonhereditary tumors both mutations are somatic. The two mutations are "null" mutations; they eliminate a protein essential for differentiation from the cell. Genes that lead to cancer when the functions of both copies have been eliminated by mutation are referred to as recessive oncogenes, or tumor suppressor genes.[63–65]

Reduced to its essentials, the two-mutation hypothesis of cancer regards sporadic human tumors as the cellular equivalents of hereditary diseases. In hereditary diseases like Huntington's disease, a single abnormal gene is sufficient to cause the disease. In tumors like hereditary and nonhereditary retinoblastoma, abnormalities at a single genetic locus within a retinal cell are sufficient to produce cancer.

The two-mutation concept has proven extraordinarily useful in unifying and simplifying concepts about cancer etiology. There is now convincing evidence that this theory applies to human retinoblastoma, Wilms' tumor,[66–68] multiple endocrine neoplasia (MEN) types I and II,[69,70] bilateral acoustic neurofibromatosus,[71] and hereditary polyposis.[72] The evidence accumulated in this report strongly supports the suggestion that the chromosome 3p allele loss detected in RCC represents the second mutation of the two-mutation process and that this carcinoma should be added to the list of human tumors that originate through this process.

Cavenee and coworkers provided molecular genetic support for this concept by discovering that the second mutation in retinoblastoma takes the form of abnor-

mal mitotic (chromosomal) events.[7] These events included nondisjunction, nondisjunction plus reduplication, and mitotic recombination. The net effect of these chromosomal mechanisms is to deprive the cell of the normal wild-type allele at a particular locus. Loss of heterozygosity is the hallmark of the second mutation; it is difficult to detect the first mutation.

Criteria for Identifying a Human Recessive Oncogene ■

To determine whether the chromosome 3p allele loss observed in RCC (and SCLC) reflects the presence of a recessive oncogene, it may be useful to review the criteria for a recessive oncogene. Identification of consistent loss of heterozygosity at a particular locus in a group of tumors suggests the presence of a recessive oncogene at that locus. The correlation of loss of heterozygosity at a particular locus with the presence of a recessive oncogene is complicated by the fact that some adult solid tumors are characterized by loss of alleles at loci on multiple chromosomes. In at least one neoplasm, MEN II, the locus identified by loss of heterozgyosity (chromosome 1)[73] did not correspond to the locus identified by linkage analysis (chromosome 10).[70]

The second criterion for a recessive oncogene is the identification by linkage analysis of a chromosomal location linked to predisposition to cancer. Combining these two criteria, the two-mutation theory predicts that, in a hereditary neoplasm, loss of heterozygosity occurs at the locus of the disease gene (identified by linkage analysis) on the chromosome inherited from the nonaffected parent.

The genetic changes identified on chromosome 3p in RCC fit all the criteria for a recessive oncogene. Linkage analysis in von Hippel–Lindau disease has identified chromosome 3p as the site of the disease gene. In a small nuclear family with RCC as the major manifestation of von Hippel–Lindau disease, the chromosome 3p lost in the tumors of the proband was from the nonaffected parent (unpublished data).

Specific Genetic Predisposition to von Hippel–Lindau Disease ■

Convincing evidence is now available that a gene that predisposes to RCC is located on chromosome 3p. The von Hippel–Lindau disease gene has been linked to a gene, c-*raf*-1, located on the terminal portion of 3p (3p25).[59] The major question raised by this observation is whether the von Hippel–Lindau disease gene is the only gene located on chromosome 3p that predisposes to RCC. Several pieces of evidence suggest that it is not. The first piece of evidence is clinical; there are families in which the only inherited disease manifestation is RCC. Second, the location of the breakpoint in the t(3;8) family is distinct from the gene location derived from the linkage study. Third, RCC in von Hippel–Lindau disease has pathologic features that are distinct from those in familial RCC.[74] Still, the possibility must be considered that the von Hippel–Lindau disease gene is responsible for sporadic RCC and pure familial RCC, and that the different inherited disease manifestations represent differences in the same gene at the molecular level.

Some Considerations on Germinal and Somatic Mutations ■

One question with hereditary tumors is when the second, somatic, mutation occurs. The observation that this mutation is often a mitotic error suggests that it is temporally related to maximal proliferation of that organ. In retinoblastoma, both mutational events must occur before the age of onset of the tumor, which places them temporally during embryonic development of the retina or shortly after birth. By analogy, in hereditary RCC, the onset of the somatic mutational events would be expected during embryonic development and differentiation of the kidney. It should be noted in this context that mitotic errors appear to be far more frequent than small structural (point) mutations.[75,76]

Small Cell Lung Carcinoma ■

Biology ■

Cancer of the lung is the leading cause of cancer deaths in men and the second leading cause in women.[77] Small cell lung carcinoma, a histologically distinct form of lung cancer, represents about 25% of lung carcinomas. There are about 35,000 new cases of SCLC in the United States each year. The cell of origin of this neoplasm is thought to be a neuroendocrine cell located in the basal layer of the bronchial mucosa (the Kulchitsky cell). Smoking is strongly associated with disease development. In contrast to RCC, there is no known familial form of SCLC.

Advances in cell culture techniques, along with the development of selective growth media, have made it possible to grow SCLC lines *in vitro*.[78–80] These cell lines have proven to be a valuable resource for the biochemical, morphologic, antigenic, and genetic characterization of SCLC, the cells of which secrete a characteristic group of molecules.

Extrapulmonary small cell carcinomas, histologically and biochemically indistinguishable from SCLC, originate in a variety of tissues outside the lung.[81–84] We and others have examined SCLC, non-small cell

Table 3–3
Frequency of Heterozygosity at 3p in Small Cell Lung Carcinoma: Paired and Unpaired Samples

Probe	Frequency		
	Predicted*	Found	*p* Value
DNF15S2	24/51 (26/51)	0/51	<0.00001 (<0.00001)
D3S2	21/50 (19/50)	3/50	0.00002 (0.00009)
D3S3	4/51 (13/51)	1/51	0.18 (0.00043)

* The predicted frequency is the number of samples tested (denominator) multiplied by the frequency of the allele in a reference population, or in the normal tissues of a population with lung cancer (in parentheses).

lung, and extrapulmonary small cell cancers for evidence of allele loss on chromosome 3p and other chromosomes. This section will present the results of tests for allele loss in these carcinomas.

RFLP Analyses ■

In our laboratory, a total of 50 paired and unpaired SCLC samples have been tested for chromosome 3p allele loss.[2] Because SCLC is usually not treated by surgical excision of the primary tumor, we analyzed cell lines established from biopsy specimens of primary tumors and from metastases. In a few cases, tissue was available from autopsy or biopsy specimens of tumor-bearing lymph nodes. The probes used for analysis of SCLC samples were identical to those used to study primary RCC. In our series of paired SCLC samples, there were 13 patients who were heterozygous for one or more loci on chromosome 3p. In every tumor sample, there was a loss of alleles at loci on chromosome 3p. No tumor samples remained heterozygous at the 3p loci tested. We analyzed 35 unpaired SCLC cell lines and found a frequency of heterozygosity for all three 3p probes of 3 in 35. This result is significantly different from the expected frequency of 25 in 35. As shown in Table 3–3, there is a striking reduction in the frequency of heterozygosity at chromosome 3p in SCLC samples.

The results of this analysis are illustrated in Figures 3–15 through 3–17. (For schematics of the RFLPs, see Fig. 3–3.) Figure 3–15, the results with the probe for DNF15S2, shows complete loss of signal corre-

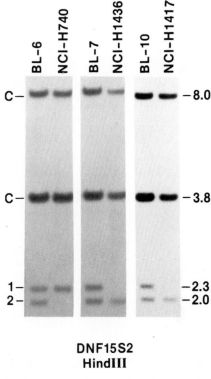

FIG. 3–15 Autoradiographs of Southern blots for paired samples from patients with SCLC, probed by DNF15S2 *left,* normal tissue; *right,* tumor tissue. Allele 1 is the longer DNA fragment; allele 2 is the smaller fragment. The allele number is indicated at the left of figure and the size of the DNA fragment is at the right. (C = constant band). Probe DNF15S2. (Reprinted with permission of *The New England Journal of Medicine,* from Brauch H et al: N Engl J Med 317:1109–1113, 1987)

FIG. 3–16 Autoradiographs, as in Figure 3–5, with probe D3S2.[2] (Reprinted with permission of *The New England Journal of Medicine,* from Brauch H et al: N Engl J Med 317:1109–1113, 1987)

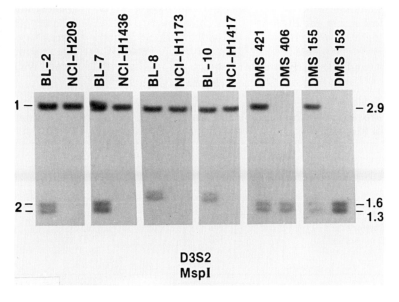

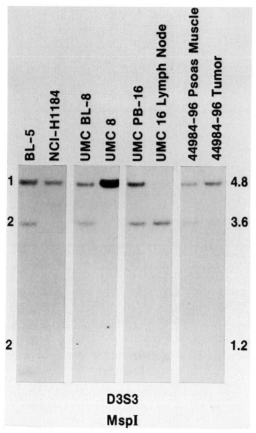

FIG. 3–17 Autoradiographs, as in Figure 3–15, with Probe D3S3.[2] (Reprinted with permission of *The New England Journal of Medicine,* from Brauch H et al: N Engl J Med 317:1109–1113, 1987)

D3S3: there is a complete loss of signal corresponding to allele 1 in patient UMC PB-16; A2 is lost in patients BL-5, B1-8, and 44984-96. The complete loss of signal reflects the fact that the SCLC lines, in contrast to the primary RCCs, did not contain admixed normal cells.

Loss of alleles at loci on chromosome 3p was observed in cell lines, autopsy samples, and biopsy samples and in samples collected both before and after treatment. These results indicate that the 3p allele loss is not an artifact associated with growth of SCLC in cell culture and is not a consequence of treatment of patients with mutagenic drugs.

Deletion of DNA sequences on the short arm of chromosome 3 in SCLC has been documented by several groups,[57,85–87] (see Table 3–4). Given the consistency of this observation, chromosome 3p deletion in SCLC can be considered to be a characteristic of these tumors in the United States, Europe, and Japan.

Size of the 3p Deletion ■

Analysis of the extent of 3p deletion with a battery of chromosome 3p probes indicates that in most SCLC cell lines the deletion is quite large and includes most of the short arm of chromosome 3. Cytogenetic analysis suggests that, by shortest region of overlap analysis, the minimal region of the chromosome 3p deletion is 3p21-3p24.

Consistent Loss of Heterozygosity at Loci on Chromosomes 13 and 17 ■

Yokota and colleagues[86] found a consistent loss of heterozygosity on chromosomes 13 and 17 in SCLC lines. Naylor and coworkers[85] found loss of heterozygosity at 13q (probe pIE8) in 9 of 12 evaluable patients. We have confirmed the results of Yokota and

sponding to A1 in patients BL-7 and BL-10; A2 is lost in patient BL-6. In Figure 3–16 (probe D3S2), there is complete loss of A1 in patients DMS 421 and DMS 155; allele 2 is lost in patients BL-2, BL-7, BL-8, and BL-10. Figure 3–17 shows the results with

Table 3–4
Frequency of Chromosome 3p Loss in SCLC: Summary of Experience in Five Series*

| | Locus | | |
Series	D3S3	DNF15S2	D3S2
Brauch et al[2]	4/4	5/5	6/6
Kok et al[57]	ND	7/7	ND
Naylor et al[85]	6/6	5/5	7/7
Yokota et al[86]	ND	ND	7/7
Johnson et al[87]	6/7	16/17	10/11
Total	16/17	33/34	30/31

* Data are number with allele loss/number heterozygous. NBD = not broken down by probe; ND = not done.

coworkers by finding loss of heterozygosity at chromosome 17p in all evaluable SCLC samples (unpublished data).

Extrapulmonary Small Cell Carcinomas ■

During the studies on SCLC, several samples were analyzed that appeared to be exceptions to the generalization regarding loss of alleles at loci on chromosome 3p (Table 3–5). Two of these exceptions were extrapulmonary small cell carcinomas.[2,88] The data gathered so far suggest that these two types of neuroendocrine neoplasms can be distinguished at the DNA level by the absence of a deletion at chromosome 3p in extrapulmonary small cell carcinomas.[88] Considering the high frequency of deletion at chromosomes 13 and 17 in SCLC, it is possible that a profile of chromosomal deletions may be an even more powerful analytic tool to characterize and distinguish extrapulmonary small cell carcinomas from SCLC. That is, extrapulmonary small cell carcinomas may be distinguished by their retention of heterozygosity at loci on chromosomes 3p, 13q, and 17p. This observation has several implications. First, the availability of such a genetic marker for extrapulmonary small cell carcinomas permits the clinician to distinguish those tumors from metastases of an occult primary SCLC. This improved diagnostic precision may improve design of treatment trials for this uncommon tumor. Second, the fact that tumors that are histologically and biochemically indistinguishable can be differentiated at the DNA level suggests differences in mechanisms of carcinogenesis.

Non-Small Cell Lung Carcinoma ■

There is controversy about the frequency of loss of heterozygosity at loci on 3p in non-small cell lung carcinoma (NSCLC; summarized in Table 3–6). Kok

Table 3–5
Frequency of Heterozygosity in Extrapulmonary Small Cell Carcinomas[2,88]

Site of Origin	Probe		
	D3S3	DNF15S2	D3S2
Prostate		1/1	1/1
Cervix	1/1	1/1	
Uterus			1/1
Axilla		1/1	
Cervical lymph node			0/1

and colleagues found loss of heterozygosity at loci on chromosome 3p in all NSCLC samples examined.[57] Yokota and associates[86] found loss at 3p in 6 of 6 evaluable adenocarcinomas of the lung. We detected chromosome 3p allele loss in about 25% of samples of primary NSCLCs.[2] The problem in arriving at a correct estimate of the frequency of loss of alleles at 3p in primary NSCLC samples arises from the presence of intimately admixed normal cells in proportions that can obscure 3p deletion in tumor cells. If tumor samples contained less than 20% to 40% tumor cells, our methods would not be sensitive enough to reliably detect loss of chromosome 3p alleles. In future studies, the tumors used for DNA extraction should be monitored by the frozen section technique,[89] and results should be reported with an estimate of the proportion of normal cells in the tumor sample. Alternatively, host cells can be separated from tumor by growth in cell culture or immunodeficient mice, or by immunologic techniques.

Mechanism of Loss of Heterozygosity ■

In contrast to retinoblastoma, Wilms' tumor and rhabdomyosarcoma, the commonest mechanism for loss of heterozygosity observed in primary RCC and SCLC was chromosomal deletion. Chromosomal nondisjunction, nondisjunction with duplication, or

Table 3–6
Frequency of Loss of Heterozygosity at 3p in Non-small Cell Lung Carcinoma

Tumor Type	Study			Total
	Brauch et al[2]	Kok et al[57]	Yokota et al[86]	
Adenocarcinoma	2/7	7/7	5/6	14/20
Squamous cell	1/3	4/4	0/1	5/8
Large cell	0/2	1/1	0/1	1/3
Bronchioalveolar	1/3			1/2

somatic recombination as mechanisms for loss of heterozygosity were either not observed or observed infrequently.

Conclusion ■

Loss of DNA sequences on chromosome 3p is found in virtually every sample of RCC and SCLC. This genetic change is not related to drug treatment or cell culture. The major question is, What is the significance of this genetic change for tumor etiology and diagnosis?

The evidence indicates that in RCC there is a recessive oncogene located on chromosome 3p, and that 3p deletion represents the second step of a two-mutation process. The net result is to uncover a null mutation on the corresponding chromosome 3 homologue. In other words, genetic changes at chromosome 3p are essential to the origin of RCC. The recent discovery that the von Hippel–Lindau gene locus is on chromosome 3p fits wells with this conclusion and indicates that there is a locus for a gene that predisposes to RCC located on chromosome 3p. One major question is whether the von Hippel–Lindau disease gene is the only gene on chromosome 3p that predisposes to RCC.

Stanbridge and coworkers, using somatic cell genetic techniques, were able to demonstrate suppression of the malignant phenotype in a Wilms' tumor line by transfer of a normal chromosome 11.[90] It should be possible to adapt these techniques to determine whether transfer of a normal chromosome 3 would modify the malignant phenotype of RCC lines. Finally, it should be possible to use the techniques of reverse genetics to isolate a large number of fragments from human chromosome 3 and to eventually isolate the RCC gene.

Isolation of the RCC gene—like isolation of the retinoblastoma gene—will revolutionize genetic counseling by identifying family members at risk and will provide reagents to determine whether the 3p gene in pure RCC is different from the von Hippel–Lindau disease gene. The cloned RCC gene will permit studies of gene transcription to determine if this gene is involved in the pathogenesis of SCLC.

The precise role of 3p deletion in the origin or evolution of SCLC is uncertain, in part because of the lack of a suitable familial context in which to study the disease. The possible role of 3p deletion in SCLC can be analyzed only by inference, that is, by comparison with other cancers in which familial forms are available for study. The simplest explanation of the data is that two mutations at allelic loci on chromosome 3 may be sufficient to trigger SCLC formation and that the RCC and SCLC genes are, in fact, identical. More complicated explanations of the data would include a separate chromosome 3p gene involved in SCLC origin, or RCC gene involvement in SCLC evolution rather than origin. As in RCC, somatic cell genetic techniques may be valuable in assessing the significance of the observed genetic changes. The model would predict that transfer of a normal chromosome 3 into an SCLC would reverse some of the features of the neoplastic phenotype.

The results summarized in the chapter may be viewed in the more general context of the value of RFLP analysis as a new approach for the study of cancer etiology and diagnosis. The identification of sites in the genome that are consistently deleted in a particular tumor type suggests that the site identified may be a locus for a recessive oncogene. This suggestion can be tested by linkage studies, an approach recently used to identify a new recessive oncogene linked to MEN I.[69] The finding of genetic differences between extrapulmonary small cell cancer and small cell lung carcinoma illustrates that RFLP analysis can distinguish between tumors with similar morphology. Genetic differences between tumors of similar morphology raise questions about carcinogenesis and tumor homogeneity/heterogeneity. Conversely, RFLP analysis can identify tumors of different histology that may have a common genetic abnormality (*e.g.,* RCC and SCLC).

This form of analysis has a practical application in cancer diagnosis, and is now being used to identify persons at risk in families with retinoblastoma. The results to date raise the possibility that each type of solid tumor may have a characteristic pattern of chromosomal deletion and that such tumor genotypes may be useful in distinguishing benign from malignant tumors and in distinguishing tumor types.

References ■

1. Zbar B, Brauch H, Talmadge C, Linehan M: Loss of alleles at loci on the short arm of chromosome 3 in renal cell carcinoma. Nature 327:721–724, 1987
2. Brauch H, Johnson B, Hovis J et al: Molecular analysis of the short arm of chromosome 3 in small-cell and non-small-cell carcinoma of the lung. N Engl J Med 317:1109–1113, 1987
3. Ayala FJ, Kiger JA Jr: Modern Genetics, 2nd ed, pp 760–763. Menlo Park, CA, Benjamin/Cummings Co, 1984
4. White R, Lalouel J-M: Chromosome mapping with DNA markers. Sci Am 258:40–48, 1988
5. Barker D, Schafer M, White R: Restriction sites containing CpG show a higher frequency of polymorphism in human DNA. Cell 36:131–138, 1984
6. Nakamura Y, Leppert M, O'Connell P et al: Variable number of tandem repeat (VNTR) markers for human gene mapping. Science 235:1616–1622, 1987

7. Cavenee WK, Dryja TP, Phillips RA et al: Expression of recessive alleles by chromosomal mechanisms in retinoblastoma. Nature 305:779–784, 1983

8. Dixon WJ, Massey FJ Jr: Introduction to Statistical Analysis, 3rd ed. New York, McGraw-Hill, 1969

9. An international system for human cytogenetic nomenclature—High resolution bonding. Cytogenet Cell Genet 31:1–23, 1981

10. Kovacs G, Szucs S, De Riese W, Baumgartel H: Specific chromosome aberration in human renal cell carcinoma. Int J Cancer 40:171–178, 1987

11. de Jong B, Oosterhuis JW, Idenburg VJS et al: Cytogenetics of 12 cases of renal adenocarcinoma. Cancer Genet Cytogenet 30:53–61, 1988

12. Teyssier JR: What is the genetic mechanism underlying the recurrent 3p rearrangement in human renal cell carcinoma? Cancer Genet Cytogenet 25:179–181, 1987

13. Teyssier JR, Ferre D, Adnet JJ et al: Recurrent deletion of the short arm of chromsome 3 in human renal cell carcinoma: Shift of the c-raf-1 locus. JNCI 77:1187–1195, 1986

14. Yoshida MA, Ohyashiki K, Ochi H et al: Cytogenetic studies of tumor tissue from patients with nonfamilial renal cell carcinoma. Cancer Res 46:2139–2147, 1986

15. Szucs S, Muller-Brechlin R, DeRiese W, Kovacs G: Deletion 3p: The only chromosome loss in a primary renal cell carcinoma. Cancer Genet Cytogenet 26:369–373, 1987

16. Carroll PR, Murty VVS, Reuter V et al: Abnormalities of chromosome region 3p12-3p14 characterize clear cell renal carcinoma. Cancer Genet Cytogenet 26:253–259, 1987

17. Pathak S, Strong LC, Ferrell RE, Trinidade A: Familial renal cell carcinoma with a 3;11 chromosome translocation. Science 217:939–940, 1982

18. Cohen AJ, Li FP, Marchetto DJ et al: Hereditary renal cell carcinoma associated with a chromosomal translocation. N Engl J Med 301:592–595, 1979

19. Wang N, Perkins KL: Involvement of band 3p14 in t(3;8) hereditary renal carcinoma. Cancer Genet Cytogenet 11:479–481, 1984

20. Kovacs G, Hoene E: Loss of der(3) in renal carcinoma cells of a patient with a constitutional t(3;12). Human Genet 78:148–150, 1988

21. King CR, Schimke RN, Arthur T et al: Proximal 3p deletion in renal cell carcinoma cells from a patient with von Hippel-Lindau disease. Cancer Genet Cytogenet 27:345–348, 1987

22. Whang-Peng J, Bunn PA Jr, Kao-Shan CS et al: A nonrandom chromosomal abnormality del 3p(14-23) in human small cell lung cancer (SCLC). Cancer Genet Cytogenet 6:119–134, 1982

23. Whang-Peng J, Kao-Shan CS, Lee EC et al: Specific chromosome defect associated with human small-cell lung cancer: Deletion 3p(14-23). Science 215:181–182, 1982

24. Morstyn G, Brown J, Novak U et al: Heterogeneous cytogenetic abnormalities in small cell lung cancer cell lines. Cancer Res 47:3322–3327, 1987

25. De Leij L, Postmus PE, Buys CHCM et al: Characterization of three new variant type cell lines derived from small cell carcinoma of the lung. Cancer Res 45:6024–6033, 1985

26. Waters JJ, Ibson JM, Twentyman PR et al: Cytogenetic abnormalities in human small cell lung carcinoma: cell lines characterized for *myc* gene amplification. Cancer Genet Cytogenet 30:213–223, 1988

27. Wurster-Hill DH, Cannizzaro LA, Pettengill OS et al: Cytogenetics of small cell carcinoma of the lung. Cancer Genet Cytogenet 13:303–330, 1984

28. Leppert M, O'Connell P, Nakamura Y et al: Two linkage groups on chromosome 3. Cytogenet Cell Genet 46:648, 1987

29. Donis-Keller H, Green P, Helms C et al: A genetic linkage map of the human genome. Cell 51:319–337, 1987

30. Harris P, Morton CC, Guglielmi P et al: Mapping by chromosome sorting of several gene probes including c-myc to the derivative chromosomes of a 3;8 translocation associated with familial renal cancer. Cytometry 7:589–594, 1986

31. Gerber MJ, Miller YE, Drabkin HA, Scoggin CH: Regional assignment of the polymorphic probe D3S3 to 3p14 by molecular hybridization. Cytogenet Cell Genet 42:72–74, 1986

32. Donlon TA, Magenis RE: Localization of the cloned segment λ/Ch4A to chromosome 1 band p36: A confirmation of locus *D1S1.* Cytogenet Cell Genet 37:454–455, 1984

33. Carritt B, Welch HM, Parry-Jones NJ: Sequences homologous to the human D1S1 locus present on human chromosome 3. Am J Hum Genet 38:428–436, 1986

34. Nakamura Y, Culver M, Gillilan S et al: Isolation and mapping of a polymorphic DNA sequence pYNZ86.1 on chromosome 3 (D3S30). Nucleic Acids Res 15:10079, 1987

35. Bonner T, O'Brien SJ, Nash WG et al: The human homologs of the raf (mil) oncogene are located on human chromosomes 3 and 4. Science 223:71–74, 1984

36. Rider DH, Gorman PA, Shipley JM et al: Localization of the oncogene c-erbA2 to human chromosome 3. Ann Hum Genet 51:153–160, 1987

37. Dobrovic A, Houle B, Belouchi A, Bradley WEC: erbA-related sequence coding for DNA-binding hormone receptor localized to chromosome 3p21-3p25 and deleted in small cell lung carcinoma. Cancer Res 48:682–685, 1988

38. Li FP, Marchetto DJ, Brown RS: Familial renal carcinoma. Cancer Genet Cytogenet 7:271–275, 1982

39. Green JS, Bowmer MI, Johnson GJ: Von Hippel-Lindau disease in a Newfoundland kindred. Can Med Assoc J 134:133–146, 1986

40. Horton WA, Wong V, Eldridge R: Von Hippel-Lindau disease: Clinical and pathological manifestations in nine families with 50 affected members. Arch Intern Med 136:769–777, 1976

41. Lauritsen JG: Lindau's disease: A study of one family through six generations. Acta Chir Scand 139:482–486, 1973

42. Spencer WF, Novick AC, Montie JE et al: Surgical treatment of localized renal cell carcinoma in von Hippel-Lindau's disease. J Urol 139:507–509, 1988

43. Melmon KL, Rosen SW: Lindau's Disease. Review of the literature and study of a large kindred. Am J Med 36:595–617, 1964

44. Silver ML: Hereditary vascular diseases of the nervous system. JAMA 156:1053–1056, 1954

45. Christoferson LA, Gustafson MB, Petersen AG: Von Hippel-Lindau's disease. JAMA 178:280–282, 1961

46. Hardwig P, Robertson DM: von Hippel Lindau disease: A familial, often lethal, mutli-system phakomatosis. Opthalmology 91:263–270, 1984

47. Vogel F, Motulsky AG: Human Genetics. Problems and Approaches, 2nd ed, pp 350–352. Berlin, Springer-Verlag, 1986

48. Kantor A, Blattner WA, Blot WJ et al: Hereditary renal cell carcinoma and chromosome defects. N Engl J Med 307:1403–1404, 1982

49. Psihramis KE, Althausen AF, Yoshida MA et al: Chromosome anomalies suggestive of malignant transformation in bilateral renal oncocytoma. J Urol 136:892–895, 1986

50. Lieber MM, Hosaka Y, Tsukamoto T: Renal oncocytoma. World J Urol: 5:71–79, 1987

51. Psihramis KE, Cin PD, Dretler SP et al: Further evidence that renal oncocytoma has malignant potential. J Urol 139:585–587, 1988

52. Case 51-1985. Case records of the Massachusetts General Hospital. N Engl J Med 313:1596–1603, 1985

53. Rainwater LM, Farrow GM, Lieber MM: Flow cytometry of renal oncytoma: Common occurrence of deoxyribonucleic acid polyploidy and aneuploidy. J Urol 135:1167–1171, 1986

54. Eker R, Mossige J, Johannessen JV, Aars H: Hereditary renal adenomas and adenocarcinomas in rats. Diagnost Histopathol 4:99–110, 1981

55. Belldegrun A, Muul LM, Rosenberg SA: Interleukin 2 expanded lymphocytes in human renal cell cancer: Isolation, characterization and antitumor activity. Cancer Res 48:206–214, 1988

56. Belldegrun A, Uppenkamp I, Rosenberg SA: Anti-tumor reactivity of human lymphokine activated killer cells (LAK) against fresh and cultured preparations of renal cell cancer. J Urol 139: 150–155, 1988

57. Kok K, Osinga J, Carritt B et al: Deletion of a DNA sequence at the chromosomal region 3p21 in all major types of lung cancer. Nature 330:578–581, 1987

58. Kovacs G, Erlandsson R, Boldog F et al: Consistent chromosome 3p deletion and loss of heterozygosity in renal cell carcinoma. Proc Natl Acad Sci USA 85:1571–1575, 1988

59. Seizinger BR, Rouleau GA, Ozelius LJ et al: Von Hippel Lindau disease maps to the region of chromosome 3 associated with renal cell carcinoma. Nature 332:268–269, 1988

60. Knudson AG Jr: Mutation and cancer: A model for Wilms' tumor of the kidney. JNCI 48:313–324, 1972

61. Knudson AG: Hereditary cancer, oncogenes and antioncogenes. Cancer Res 45:1437–1443, 1985

62. Knudson AG Jr: Genetics of human cancer. Annu Rev Genet 20:231–251, 1986

63. Hansen MF, Cavenee WF: Genetics of cancer predisposition. Cancer Res 47:5518–5527, 1987

64. Klein G: The approaching era of the tumor suppressor genes. Science 238:1539–1545, 1987

65. Murphee AL, Benedict WF: Retinoblastoma: Clues to human oncogenesis. Science 223:1028–1033, 1984

66. Fearon ER, Vogelstein B, Feinberg AP: Somatic deletion and duplication of genes on chromosome 11 in Wilms' tumors. Nature 309:176–178, 1984

67. Koufos A, Hansen MF, Lampkin BC et al: Loss of alleles at loci on human chromosome 11 during genesis of Wilms' tumor. Nature 309:170–172, 1984

68. Orkin SH, Goldman DS, Sallan SE: Development of homozygosity for chromosome 11p markers in Wilms' tumor. Nature 309:172–174, 1984

69. Larsson C, Skogseid B, Oberg K et al: Multiple endocrine neoplasia type 1 gene maps to chromosome 11 and is lost in insulinoma. Nature 332:85–87, 1988

70. Matthew CGP, Chin KS, Easton DF: A linked genetic marker for multiple endocrine neoplasia type 2A on chromosome 10. Nature 328:527–528, 1987

71. Seizinger BR, Martuza RL, Gusella JF: Loss of genes on chromosome 22 in tumorigenesis of human acoustic neuroma. Nature 322:644–647, 1986

72. Bodmer WF, Bailey CJ, Bodmer J et al: Localization of the gene for familial adenomatous polyposis on chromosome 5. Nature 328:614–616, 1987

73. Mathew CGP, Smith BA, Thorpe K et al: Deletion of genes on chromosome 1 in endocrine neoplasia. Nature 328:524–526, 1987

74. Christenson PJ, Craig, JP, Bibbo MC, O'Connell KJ: Cysts containing renal cell carcinoma in von Hippel Lindau's disease. J Urol 128:798–800, 1982

75. Rabin MS, Gottesman MM: High frequency of mutation to tubercidin resistance in CHO cells. Somat Cell Genet 5:571–583, 1979

76. Siminovitch L: Mechanisms of genetic variation in Chinese hamster ovary cells. In Gottesman MM (ed): Molecular Cell Genetics, pp 869–879. New York, Wiley-Interscience, 1985

77. Silverberg E, Lubera J: Cancer statistics: 1987. CA 37:2–19, 1987

78. Carney DN, Gazdar AF, Bepler G et al: Establishment and identification of small cell lung cancer lines having classic and variant features. Cancer Res 45:2913–2923, 1985

79. Gazdar AF, Carney DN, Nau MM, Minna JD: Characterization of variant subclasses of cell lines derived from small cell lung cancer having distinctive biochemical, morphological and growth properties. Cancer Res 45:2924–2930, 1985

80. Gazdar AF, Carney DN, Russell EK et al: Establishment of continuous, clonable cultures of small-cell carcinoma of the lung which have amine precursor uptake and decarboxylation cell properties. Cancer Res 40:3502–3507, 1980

81. Pittman S, Russell PJ, Jelbart ME et al: Flow cytometric and karyotypic analysis of a primary small cell carcinoma of the prostate: a xenografted cell line. Cancer Genet Cytogenet 26: 165–169, 1987

82. Ibrahim NBN, Briggs JC, Corbishley CM: Extrapulmonary oat cell carcinoma. Cancer 54:1645–1661, 1984

83. Wick MR, Weatherby RP, Weiland LH: Small cell neuroendocrine carcinoma of the colon and rectum: Clinical, histologic and ultrastructural study and immunohistochemical comparison with cloacogenic carcinoma. Hum Pathol 18:9–21, 1987

84. Ulbright TM, Roth LM, Stehman FB et al: Poorly differentiated (small cell) carcinoma of the ovary in young women: Evidence supporting a germ cell origin. Human Pathol 18:175–184, 1987

85. Naylor SL, Johnson BE, Minna JD, Sakaguchi AY: Loss of heterozygosity of chromosome 3p markers in small-cell lung cancer. Nature 329:451–454, 1987

86. Yokota J, Wada M, Shimosato Y et al: Loss of heterozygosity on chromosomes 3, 13 and 17 in small-cell carcinoma and on chromosome 3 in adenocarcinoma of the lung. Proc Natl Acad Sci USA 84:9252–9256, 1987

87. Johnson BE, Sakaguchi AY, Gazdar AF et al: Restriction fragment length polymorphism studies show consistent loss of chromosome 3p alleles in small cell lung cancer patients tumors. J Clin Invest (in press)

88. Johnson BE, Naylor SL, Zbar B et al: Restriction fragment length polymorphism (RFLP) studies show loss of chromosome 3p alleles in small cell lung cancer (SCLC) but not in extrapulmonary small cell cancer (EXSCC) (abstr). Proc Am Soc Clin Oncol 7:999, 1988

89. Bos JL, Fearon ER, Hamilton SR et al: Prevalence of ras gene mutations in human colorectal cancers. Nature 327:293–297, 1987

90. Weissman BS, Saxon PJ, Pasquale SR et al: Introduction of a normal human chromosome 11 into a Wilms' tumor cell line controls its tumorigenic expression. Science 236:175–180, 1987

91. Vande Woude GF, Gilden RV: Principles of cancer biology: Molecular biology. In DeVita VT Jr, Hellman S, Rosenberg S (eds.): Cancer: Principles and Practice of Oncology, 2nd ed, p 28. Philadelphia, JB Lippincott, 1985

Nancy A. Jenkins

Neal G. Copeland

Transgenic Mice in Cancer Research

4

Introduction ■

For years mice have constituted the ideal mammalian model system because of their well-defined genetics, convenient size, fertility, short gestation period, ease of maintenance, and variable susceptibility and resistance to diseases. Their study has provided a wealth of information about normal cell processes, including growth and differentiation, and about abnormal processes culminating in neoplastic disease. Mouse strains with a high spontaneous incidence of heritable neoplastic disease are particularly valuable for cancer research. These strains develop disease at reproducible times and frequencies and have uniform genetic backgrounds, which greatly simplifies the interpretation of experimental results. Other mouse tumor models have been developed by treating strains with low tumor incidence using a variety of mutagens. However, the latter approach is limited because the resultant increased tumor susceptibilities are usually not heritable.

Within the last few years, powerful new techniques for producing heritable alterations in the mouse genome have made it possible to derive an essentially limitless number of high tumor incidence strains. In these approaches, exogenous, or foreign, DNA is incorporated into the mouse genome such that it is represented in both somatic and germ-cell lineages. The mice are referred to as "transgenic" and the foreign DNA is referred to as a "transgene." The transgene can be a gene linked to its own normal regulatory (promoter/enhancer) sequences, or it can be a hybrid gene composed of the promoter/enhancer sequences of one gene linked to the coding sequences of another gene of interest. When this DNA is incorporated into the genome of separate mice of the same inbred strain, these mice are isogenic. Comparisons can then be made between different transgenic lines of mice carrying the same transgene, because the genetic back-

ground is the same in all cases. Similarly, the effects of different transgenes can readily be compared by incorporating them into the same inbred strain. In practice, it is often difficult to generate isogenic transgenic mice. Therefore, transgenic mice are usually made on F_1 or F_2 hybrid inbred or randomly bred backgrounds. The transgene can subsequently be placed on an inbred strain background by genetic crosses.

From the perspective of cancer research, oncogenes (genes that are causally associated with neoplastic diseases) are the most valuable test genes. Transgenic mice are particularly well-suited for studying the consequences of oncogene expression in the whole animal. By varying the promoter/enhancer directing expression of the oncogene, the pattern of expression of the oncogene can be easily altered. In this manner, the transforming activity of an oncogene and the consequences of its expression on growth and differentiation can be analyzed in a variety of tissues and at various stages of development. Finally, by crossing transgenic mice expressing different oncogenes, the ability of these genes to cooperate in oncogenesis can be explored and multi-step models of carcinogenesis can be created and studied.

Creation of Transgenic Mice by Pronuclear Injection ■

The most common method for producing transgenic mice involves the microinjection of linear DNA into the pronucleus of the mouse zygote. This technique was pioneered by several investigators in the early 1980s[1-4] (see Ref. 5 for a review). The overall scheme by which microinjection is accomplished is diagrammed in Figure 4–1. Linear double-stranded DNA (Fig. 4–1A) is injected into the male pronucleus

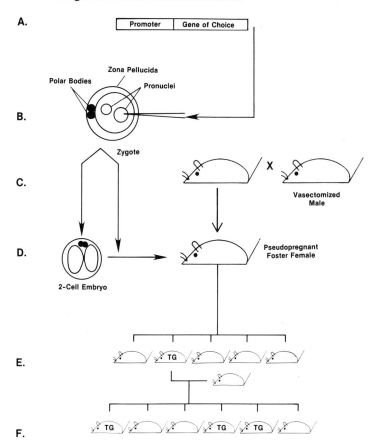

FIG. 4-1   Derivation of transgenic mice by microinjection of zygotes. (From Hogan B, Constantini F, Lacy E: Manipulating the Mouse Embryo; A Laboratory Manual, pp 151–203. Cold Spring Harbor, NY, Cold Spring Harbor Laboratory, 1986)

of the mouse zygote (Fig. 4–1*B*). Microinjected zygotes, or two-cell embryos produced by overnight culture of microinjected zygotes, are transferred to the oviducts of pseudopregnant female hosts (Fig. 4–1*D*), produced by prior mating to vasectomized male mice (Fig. 4–1*C*). Progeny derived from microinjected zygotes are born after a normal gestation period (Fig. 4–1*E*).

The mechanism of DNA integration is unknown. However, integration usually occurs before the onset of DNA replication in the zygote, so that the transgene is carried in every cell of the mouse. In most cases, more than one copy of the transgene integrates into the genome. When this occurs, the copies are usually integrated at the same chromosomal site in a tandem, head-to-tail array. Integration can occur at many sites; there is no evidence for preferred sites of integration. Mice carrying the transgene can be identified by Southern blot analysis of genomic DNA isolated from tail biopsies of progeny: they are referred to as "founder mice" and generally represent 25% of the progeny (Fig. 4–1*E*). Founder mice are bred to wild-type mice (Fig. 4–1*F*) and, ultimately, lines homozygous for each transgene can be established.

One of the important attributes of transgenic mice is that most (but not all) transgenes are expressed in an appropriate tissue-specific and developmental fashion (reviewed in Ref. 5). This is true whether the gene is normally expressed in one or many cell types. This implies that transcriptional regulatory proteins involved in establishing tissue-specific gene expression are capable of functioning regardless of the chromosomal location of their target sequences. However, the level of expression of a transgene often varies widely in different founder animals. These variations may reflect differences in transgene copy number (F. Costantini, personal communication),[6,7] as well as integration sites. Correct tissue-specific and developmental expression of transgenes derived from several mammalian species has been reported, indicating that signals for the regulation of expression of these genes are evolutionarily well-conserved.

Mouse Models Derived from Microinjection of Simian Virus 40 DNA ■

Choroid Plexus Tumors in Transgenic Mice Harboring SV40 Early Region Genes ■

The first report of tumors in transgenic mice resulting from pronuclear injection of a known transforming gene was made by Brinster and coworkers.[8] They microinjected the early region of simian virus 40 (SV40), which included the genes for both large and small T-antigen under the control of their natural promoter/enhancer. SV40 is a papovavirus that induces a subclinical infection in rhesus monkeys and that grows lytically in African green monkey cells in culture. SV40 transforms both rodent and human cells in culture. Transgenic mice harboring SV40 T-antigen transgenes developed brain tumors of the choroid plexus epithelial cells (Table 4–1) (choroid plexus tumors had previously been observed after intracerebral inoculation of SV40 virus into newborn hamsters[9]). Thymic hyperplasia, glomerulosclerosis, and renal cysts were also observed in some mice (Table 4–1).[8,10] The frequency of obtaining transgenic mice with this DNA did not differ significantly from that in studies employing other transgenes, indicating that SV40 early region genes are not detrimental to mouse development.

SV40 T-antigen mRNA and protein were readily detected in affected tissues. SV40 T-antigen expression was either not detected or detected only at low levels in unaffected tissues or in susceptible tissues prior to the development of overt pathology, suggesting that tumorigenesis depends on high levels of SV40 gene expression.[8,11,12] The thymic hyperplasia and kidney pathology that develop in some transgenic mice may represent secondary sites of T-antigen gene activation in which cellular conditions do not readily support tumor development. Alternatively, the lower levels of T-antigen expression observed in kidney and thymic tissue relative to brain tissue may not be sufficient for complete transformation *in vivo*. The SV40 genes were frequently amplified in tumor tissue, further indicating that high levels of SV40 gene expression are intimately involved in tumorigenesis.[8]

This construct also contained a metallothionein (MT) fusion gene in addition to the SV40 early region genes encoding small and large T-antigen. Subsequent studies showed that large T-antigen alone was sufficient for tumorigenesis and that the MT fusion gene was not necessary for choroid plexus tumor formation (Table 4–1).[10,13] Transgenic mice carrying a mutant SV40 large T-antigen gene, designated SV40 (cT), that was defective for transport of large T-antigen from

Table 4–1
Tumors in Transgenic Mice Harboring SV40 Early Region Fusion Genes

Transgene	Pathology	Ref.
SV40 early region (small and large T-antigen)	Choroid plexus tumors, thymic hyperplasia, glomerulosclerosis, renal cysts	8, 10, 13, 119
SV40 large T-antigen	Choroid plexus tumors, thymic hyperplasia, glomerulosclerosis, renal cysts	10, 13
SV40 large cT-antigen (transport-defective T-antigen)	Choroid plexus tumors, thymic hyperplasia, glomerulosclerosis, renal cysts	14
SV40Δe/MTGH (metallothionein enhancer)	Demyelinating peripheral neuropathies, hepatocellular carcinomas, pancreatic β-cell tumors	16
Elastase/SV40 early region	Pancreatic acinar cell tumors	17
Insulin/SV40 early region	Pancreatic β-cell tumors	21
Vasopressin/SV40 early region	Pancreatic β-cell tumors, anterior pituitary tumors	22
αA crystallin/SV40 early region	Lens tumors	33
ANF/SV40 early region	Right atrial hyperplasia, cardiac arrhythmias	34
hPNMT/SV40 early region	Adrenal gland tumors, eye tumors	35
Protamine/SV40 early region	Right atrial rhabdomyosarcomas, osteosarcomas	36
GRF/SV40 early region	Thymic hyperplasia	37
MMTV/SV40 early region	Ductal epithelial cell tumors, lymphoma (B-cell), Leydig cell tumors	52
Ig/Tp/SV40 early region	Choroid plexus tumors, lymphoma (B-cell, histiocytic)	69
H-2K^b/SV40 early region	Choroid plexus tumors, thymic hyperplasia, multiple endocrine neoplasia	71

the cell cytoplasm into the nucleus also developed tumors similar to those occurring in transgenic mice carrying a wild-type large T-antigen gene (Table 4–1).[14] Surprisingly, this mutant gene exhibited a markedly decreased ability to transform primary cells in culture and to induce tumors in newborn hamsters.[15] These experiments emphasize the importance of extranuclear forms of SV40 large T-antigen in tumor formation and indicate that *in vitro* cell transformation assays do not always accurately reflect the oncogenic potential of a transforming gene *in vivo.*

Studies involving transgenic mice carrying SV40 early region deletion mutants show that the SV40 enhancer (72-base repeat region) plays an important role in choroid plexus tumor specificity. The overall frequency of pathology, including the choroid plexus tumors, was significantly reduced when the enhancer was deleted.[13] When the SV40 enhancer was deleted from a construction that also contained an MT/ growth hormone fusion gene (SV40Δe/MTGH), a new pattern of pathology was observed (see Table 4–1).[16] Transgenic mice carrying this construction developed demyelinating peripheral neuropathies, hepatocellular carcinomas, and pancreatic β-cell tumors. These pathologies may result from an enhancing effect of the MT sequences on large T-antigen gene expression, made possible by the removal of an otherwise dominant SV40 enhancer. The MT genes are "housekeeping" genes expressed in many cell types. Thus, the basis of the tissue distribution of tumors is unclear; it may result from tissue-specific differences in levels of expression or, alternatively, from differences in tissue susceptibility to SV40 transformation.

To further clarify the role of SV40 early gene expression in tumorigenesis, lines of transgenic mice carrying SV40 early region genes were established that differed in their disease incidence. In the initial experiments described by Brinster and coworkers, 16 of 25 founder transgenic mice died within 3 to 6 months of age[8]; several had tumors of the choroid plexus. However, 9 of the 25 mice never developed tumors. The transgenes and genetic background were similar or identical in both classes of progeny. Therefore, these differences in tumor phenotypes may result from variations in the level of SV40 T-antigen expression resulting from differences in the chromosomal integration site of the transgene. This has generally been confirmed in subsequent studies.[11,12] The availability of transgenic lines that differ in T-antigen expression and tumor incidence provides an important model system for the identification of host factors regulating these events.

Pancreatic Neoplasia Induced by SV40 T-antigen Fusion Genes ■

SV40 T-antigen expression can lead to tumor development in a variety of organs. In other studies, the pancreas has served as a target site for studying the consequences of SV40 gene expression. By fusing the promoter and enhancer of the rat elastase I gene to the SV40 early region genes, Ornitz and coworkers[17] succeeded in inducing T-antigen expression and tumors in the acinar cell compartment of the exocrine pancreas. Elastase is one of several pancreatic serine proteases synthesized in the exocrine cells of the pancreas and secreted into the gut. Elastase expression normally begins at day 14 of mouse development, when the acinar cells begin to differentiate. Elastase expression levels plateau a few weeks after birth. Not surprisingly, 17-day-old transgenic fetuses could be distinguished from their normal littermates by the increased size and firm texture of their pancreases. T-antigen expression was also detected in most transgenic mice by this point, and, as expected, was restricted to pancreatic acinar cells. However, pancreatic tumors did not develop until 12 to 28 weeks after birth, suggesting that secondary genetic events are required. Ornitz and coworkers[17] suggested that these secondary events are related to chromosome loss. They found that tumor progression proceeded from a preneoplastic state, characterized by increased numbers of tetraploid cells, to frank tumor nodules containing primarily aneuploid cells. This observation is consistent with reports that nonmalignant neoplasms are typically euploid, whereas approximately 90% of malignant neoplasms are aneuploid.[18–20] The transition from euploidy to aneuploidy may be associated with chromosome loss and the uncovering of recessive tumor suppressor genes similar to those postulated to be uncovered in retinoblastoma and Wilms' tumor.

Transgenic mice that carried rat insulin II promoter/SV40 early region fusion genes were also generated (Table 4–1).[21] T-antigen expression and pancreatic tumors were detected exclusively in the β-cells of the endocrine pancreas, where the insulin gene is normally expressed. Again, tumor progression proceeded through various distinct phases. In young mice, the islets were normal in size but contained increased numbers of β-cells and decreased numbers of α- and δ-cells. Dense packing and disorganization of islets was followed by their expansion (hyperplasia). Solid tumors eventually developed between 10 and 20 weeks after birth. Secondary genetic events appeared necessary for tumor development. For example, most islets showed hyperplasia of the β-cells, but no more than 4 or 5 of the approximately 100 islets in the pancreas developed into β-cell tumors. Furthermore, the β-cells seemed to express the transgene well before the development of hyperplasia and tumors. Whether the secondary events result from chromosome loss or the activation of other oncogenes is unknown.

Another report describes tumorigenesis in the endocrine pancreas of transgenic mice resulting from the abnormal expression of a vasopressin promoter/SV40 early region gene construct (see Table 4–1).[22] This hybrid oncogene contained 1.25 kilobases (kb) of 5′ upstream sequences derived from the bovine arginine-vasopressin (AVP) gene linked to the SV40 early region genes. AVP expression is normally observed in the vasopressinergic cells of the hypothalamus. However, the AVP/SV40 fusion gene was not expressed there; instead, expression and oncogenicity was limited to the β-cells of the pancreas and to cells of the anterior pituitary. These results suggest that some regulatory signals controlling AVP expression are missing from this hybrid transgene construct. In contrast to the expression patterns observed with elastase/SV40 and insulin/SV40 fusion genes, AVP/SV40 expression appeared to be confined to, or activated in, a small number of cells that expanded clonally to give rise to tumors. It is unclear whether secondary genetic events are required for AVP/SV40-induced tumor formation. Similarities have been noted in the tumors induced in transgenic mice carrying AVP-SV40 fusion genes and those occurring in patients with familial human multiple endocrine neoplasia type I (Wermer's syndrome).[22] AVP/SV40 transgenic mice may thus provide a useful model system for the study of this genetic disease.

One gene implicated in SV40 T-antigen-induced tumorigenesis *in vivo* is the cellular gene encoding the transforming protein p53. The p53 protein is present in a wide variety of transformed cells but is present in only very low amounts in normal cells. In cells transformed by SV40 virus, the p53 protein is specifically associated with large T-antigen.[23–25] Significant levels of p53 protein were detected in pancreatic β-cells of transgenic mice harboring insulin/SV40 T-antigen fusion genes, whereas p53 was not detectable in normal β-cells.[26] Further, in pancreatic β-cell tumors, the two proteins were found in a complex.[26] However, these results cannot readily explain the progression of a small fraction of these cells into solid tumors because p53 was expressed in all β-cells expressing large T-antigen, including the earliest stages of tumor development.

The ability to mount an immune response to SV40 T-antigen has been implicated in the control of SV40-induced tumors in normal, immunocompetent mice.[27–30] This ability may also affect tumor progression in different SV40 transgenic lines of mice. Some SV40 transgenic mice appear to be specifically tolerant to SV40 T-antigen, whereas others exhibit an autoimmune response. This difference appears to result from the delayed onset of T-antigen expression during development of some transgenic lines.[31,32] These observations suggest that tolerance, as well as an autoimmune response to a transgenic self-antigen, can occur, and that the nature of this response may play an important role in tumor development in transgenic mice.

These transgenic mice should serve as useful models for the study of pancreatic cancer, a leading cause of cancer-related deaths in the U.S. population. Cell lines have been derived from some of these tumors which retain both pancreatic and neoplastic properties,[17] and should also be of value.

Other Tumors Produced by SV40 Early Region Fusion Genes ■

Many other transgenic tumor models have been created using SV40 early region fusion genes (see Table 4–1). The murine αA-crystallin promoter fused to the SV40 early region induced lens tumors.[33] αA-crystallin is one of the major structural components of the lens. An atrial natriuretic factor (ANF) promoter directed tumors to the right atrium of the heart.[34] ANF is a peptide hormone that is synthesized and stored in the cardiac atria. Although the ANF/SV40 fusion gene was expressed in both atria, only the right atria developed tumors. A human phenylethanolamine N-methyltransferase (hPNMT) promoter directed tumors to the adrenal glands and eyes,[35] locations consistent with the known pattern of expression of the hPNMT gene in transgenic mice.

Mice carrying a hybrid gene composed of the SV40 early region fused to the 5′ and 3′ flanking sequences of the mouse protamine 1 gene (mP1) developed rhabdomyosarcomas of the right atrium as well as bilateral osteosarcomas.[36] Because the endogenous mP1 gene is transcribed exclusively in haploid round spermatids, these tumors were unexpected. Although the mP1/SV40 fusion gene was also expressed in round spermatids, T-antigen protein was not detected and no pathology was observed. Because the mP1 sequences contained within this fusion gene have previously been shown to contain all the sequences necessary for testis-specific expression, the unusual expression of the construct in transgenic mice may reflect the presence of novel regulatory elements generated by the fusion of mP1 and SV40 sequences. Similarly, unexpected thymic hyperplasia has been observed in transgenic mice harboring a neuronal promoter—hypothalamic peptide growth hormone-releasing factor (GRF) promoter—linked to SV40 early region genes.[37]

In a recent review, a number of other tumors produced by SV40 early region fusion genes have been described.[5] These tumors include hepatic tumors induced by fusion to the albumin promoter; pituitary tumors induced by fusion to the growth hormone, prolactin, or glycotropin promoters; and glial cell tumors induced by fusion to the adenovirus EIA promoter. These mice, as well as mice carrying other SV40 early region fusion genes that are likely to be produced in the future, should provide investigators with an extensive and valuable collection of model systems for cancer research.

Tumors Induced by Other SV40-Related Papovaviruses ■

The papovaviruses, of which SV40 is but one example, are a group of small, double-stranded DNA tumor viruses that have been isolated from a variety of different species (reviewed in Ref. 38). These viruses differ widely in their tropism and oncogenicity, and comparisons *in vitro, in vivo,* and in transgenic mice may help identify regions of the viral genomes that contribute to these differences.

JC virus (JCV) and BK virus (BKV), although structurally related to SV40, have different host ranges, tissue tropisms, and pathology.[38,39] Both viruses are ubiquitous in humans; 70% to 80% of the adult population is seropositive for each virus. BKV is found predominantly in the kidney, where it induces subclinical infections; JCV is associated with a fatal demyelinating disease, progressive multifocal leukoencephalopathy, in patients whose cellular immunity is impaired.[39] Multiple glial tumors have also been observed in cases of progressive multifocal leukoencephalopathy. Both JCV and BKV transform hamster cells in culture and induce tumors in newborn rats.[38] JCV induces tumors in tissues of neural origin, whereas BKV induces brain tumors of ventral surfaces, insulinomas, and osteosarcomas.

Transgenic mice harboring the JCV or BKV early region genes developed tumors at sites consistent with their tissue specificity and disease spectrum in humans. Transgenic mice carrying JCV developed adrenal neuroblastomas,[40,41] whereas those carrying BKV developed hepatocellular carcinomas and renal tumors (Table 4–2).[40] Virus-related tumor antigens were expressed in these transgenic mice. Thus, transgenic mice harboring human viruses will be useful models for virally induced human diseases.

Bautch and coworkers[42] have derived transgenic mice carrying early region genes derived from polyoma (Py) virus, a mouse papovavirus. Py virus infection in adult mice is asymptomatic. In contrast, infection of newborns results in tumor formation in a broad range of tissues (reviewed in Refs. 43 and 44). The Py early region encodes three genes: large T-antigen, which is required for virus replication; middle T-antigen, a membrane protein with transforming activity; and small T-antigen, a protein of undefined function.[38] Large T-antigen is capable of immortalizing primary cells *in vitro,* whereas middle T-antigen confers the transformed phenotype to immortalized cells. These two oncogenes can therefore cooperate to transform primary cells in culture.[45,46]

In transgenic mice, Py large T-antigen was not tumorigenic, but Py middle T-antigen induced multifocal tumors of the vascular endothelium (hemangiomas, see Table 4–2).[42] Both genes were expressed under the control of the normal Py early region gene sequences. This distribution was different from the broad spectrum of tumors generated by infection of

Table 4–2
Tumors Induced in Transgenic Mice by SV40-Related Papovavirus Genes

Transgene	Pathology	Ref.
JCV early region	Adrenal neuroblastomas	40, 41
BKV early region	Hepatocellular carcinomas, renal tumors	40
Py large T-antigen	None	42
Py middle T-antigen	Vascular endothelial tumors	42
BPV-I	Fibrosarcomas	47

newborn mice with intact Py virus. Although endothelial tumors are occasionally observed in virally infected mice, tumors of the salivary gland, thymus, mammary gland, and bone are far more prevalent.[43,44] Therefore, viral components required for tumorigenesis in nonendothelial tissues may be missing in the transgenes carried by these transgenic mice. The distinct phenotypes induced by Py, SV40, JC, and BK viruses in transgenic mice suggest that further experiments, including the introduction of other viral components or hybrid molecules derived from two or more viruses differing in their oncogenic spectrum, will ultimately allow the identification of those sequences required for virus tropism and pathology.

Finally, Lacey and coworkers[47] have derived transgenic mice carrying a tandemly duplicated bovine papillomavirus 1 (BPV-1) genome. BPV-1 is a member of the papovavirus family that induces benign fibropapillomas with proliferative squamous epithelial and dermal fibroblast components following cutaneous tissue infection in cattle. Transgenic mice harboring the BPV-1 genome developed heritable fibrosarcomas of the skin, a phenotype analogous to that observed following natural BPV-1 infection in cattle (see Table 4–2). Tumors developed after a long latency (8 to 9 months of age), usually in areas prone to wounding. Irritation and wounding are also cofactors in BPV-induced fibropapillomas in cows.[47]

BPV-1 replicates as a stable extrachromosomal element in a variety of cultured mouse fibroblasts and can morphologically transform cells in culture. In transgenic mice, extrachromosomal BPV-1 DNA was detected in all tumors, whereas only integrated BPV-1 DNA was detected in normal tissues. The similarities between BPV-1-induced tumors in transgenic mice and cattle suggest that transgenic mice will be useful for studying BPV-1 oncogenesis.

Transgenic Mice Harboring MMTV/*onc* Fusion Genes: Models for Studying Mammary Tumors and Oncogene Cooperativity ■

Shortly after the initial report describing the high incidence of choroid plexus tumors in SV40 transgenic mice,[8] a study was published describing a high incidence of mammary adenocarcinomas in transgenic mice carrying mouse mammary tumor virus/*Myc* fusion genes (Table 4–3).[48] These fusion genes contained a mouse mammary tumor virus (MMTV) long terminal repeat (LTR) linked to normal c-*myc* proto-oncogene sequences. MMTV is an endogenous mouse retrovirus causally associated with the development of mouse mammary adenocarcinomas.[49] MMTV transcription is regulated by steroid hormones, with viral RNA expression highest in the lactating mammary gland.[50] Therefore, it was not surprising that mammary adenocarcinomas were the predominant tumor identified in MMTV/*Myc* transgenic mice. In one line, all females inheriting an MMTV/*Myc* gene developed mammary adenocarcinomas during their second or third pregnancies. Secondary genetic changes appeared to be required for tumor formation.

In most transgenic lines derived in these studies, expression of the fusion gene was restricted to breast, salivary gland, and, occasionally, testis. However, one line showed anomalous widespread expression of *Myc* (see Table 4–3).[48,51] The basis for this unusual expression pattern is unknown but may result from differences in the transgene integration site or from undetected rearrangements in the transgene. The consequences of this expression were increased incidences of testicular, breast, lymphocytic (B- and T-cell), and mast cell tumors. However, there was no obvious disturbance of normal development and

Table 4–3
Tumors in Transgenic Mice Harboring MMTV/*onc* Fusion Genes

Transgene	Pathology	Ref.
MMTV/*Myc*	Mammary adenocarcinomas, testicular tumors, lymphoma (B- and T-cell), mast cell tumors	48, 51
MMTV/SV40 early region (small and large T-antigen)	Ductal epithelial cell tumors, lymphoma (B-cell), Leydig cell tumors	52
MMTV/H*ras*	Mammary adenocarcinomas, salivary gland adenocarcinomas, lymphoma, harderian gland hyperplasia	53
MMTV/*Myc* + MMTV/H*ras*	Mammary adenocarcinomas, salivary gland adenocarcinomas, lymphoma (B-cell), harderian gland hyperplasia, seminal vesicle tumors	53
MMTV/SV40 large T-antigen	Lymphoma (pre-B, T-cell, histiocytic)	54

maturation in these mice. Interestingly, tumors were obvious disturbance of normal development and maturation in these mice. Interestingly, tumors were not observed in every tissue expressing high levels of *Myc*. This implies that either some cells lack additional cellular factors required for *Myc*-induced transformation, or *Myc* transformation requires the activation of other oncogenes, which are activated less efficiently in certain tissues. Nevertheless, these studies definitively show that *Myc* is capable of participating in the transformation of several different cell types.

Much less specificity has been observed for tumors in mice harboring MMTV/SV40 early region genes (see Table 4–3).[52] SV40 expression was detected in the epithelial cells of such organs as lungs, kidneys, prostate, salivary, and mammary glands; expression was also detected in Leydig cells and lymphoid tissue. The neoplastic diseases that developed in these mice include carcinomas of the kidney, lung, and prostate; lymphomas; Leydig cell tumors; and ovarian tumors. The differences observed in expression and tumor formation in MMTV/*Myc* and MMTV/SV40 transgenic mice may result from differences in transgene construction (*i.e.,* MMTV/*Myc* contains an additional 1.5 kb of MMTV envelope coding sequences, which are known to contain additional glucocorticoid regulatory elements), from the interaction of regulatory regions contained in the different components of these constructions, or from the differential ability of SV40 and *Myc* to transform cells *in vivo*.

The ability of two different oncogenes to cooperate in tumorigenesis of transgenic mice was also evaluated (see Table 4–3).[53] Transgenic mice carrying an MMTV promoter fused to the activated H*ras* oncogene were derived and mated with MMTV/*Myc* transgenic mice. MMTV/H*ras* transgenic mice, unlike MMTV/*Myc* transgenic mice, developed multiple pathologies, including Harderian gland hyperplasia, mammary and salivary gland adenocarcinomas, and lymphomas. The tumor distribution observed in MMTV/*Myc* and MMTV/H*ras* transgenic mice in some instances appears to result from the differential carcinogenic effects of *Myc* and H*ras*. For example, both the MMTV/*Myc* and MMTV/H*ras* transgenes are abundantly expressed in salivary glands of transgenic mice, but only MMTV/H*ras* mice develop tumors of the salivary glands. In F_1 hybrid mice expressing both *Myc* and H*ras,* there was a dramatic and synergistic acceleration of tumor formation. However, expression of *Myc* and H*ras* in the same tissue was not sufficient for tumor formation; additional somatic mutations appeared to be required.

Expression of these two transgenes also had profound effects on the incidence of certain tumors. For example, the incidence of B-cell lymphomas in MMTV/*Myc* or MMTV/H*ras* transgenic mice was 3%, whereas that in dual carriers was 30%.

The ability of SV40 small T-antigen to cooperate with SV40 large T-antigen to induce tumors in transgenic mice has also been explored.[54] As described above, transgenic MMTV/SV40 mice, which carry the complete SV40 early region and express both small and large T-antigen, developed B-cell lymphomas and ductal epithelial cell tumors.[52] In contrast, transgenic mice expressing only large T-antigen under the control of the MMTV promoter primarily developed malignant lymphomas; ductal epithelial tumors were never observed.[54] Epithelial cells divide slowly, whereas lymphoid cells divide rapidly. These results suggest that SV40 small T-antigen cooperates with large T-antigen to facilitate tumorigenesis in slowly dividing cells but is dispensable for transformation in rapidly dividing cells. This is consistent with studies indicating that SV40 viral mutants deleted for small T-antigen showed a reduced ability to transform growth-arrested fibroblasts that could be partially complemented by the addition of mitogens.[55–57] Transgenic mice carrying other MMTV/*onc* fusion genes analogous to those just described should be particularly valuable for the study of oncogene cooperativity and tumorigenesis.

Transgenic Mice as Models for Studying Hematopoietic Disease ■

It should be possible to create transgenic mouse models for hematopoietic diseases by fusing promoters/enhancers active in different hematopoietic cell lineages to biologically active oncogenes. This approach was recently used to create transgenic mice carrying a c-*Myc* gene fused to an immunoglobulin μ- or κ-chain enhancer.[58] Both immature and mature B-cell lymphomas were observed in these mice within a few months after birth.

The best characterized of these mice carry a c-*Myc* gene linked to an immunoglobulin heavy chain enhancer (Eμ/*Myc* mice). The Eμ/*Myc* transgene in these mice appears to be expressed exclusively in B-cells, which proliferate abnormally.[59,60] Pre-B-cells of polyclonal origin were overrepresented in number, even before birth, while mature B-cells were present in reduced numbers.[59] Interestingly, the immune responsiveness of Eμ/*Myc* animals did not appear to be greatly affected by the reduced number of mature

B-cells. The initial pre-B-cell proliferation was limited and benign.[58] However, by 5 months of age, 90% of the animals had died of B-cell lymphomas, which were monoclonal in origin.[61] Strain differences in tumor susceptibility of Eμ/Myc mice have also been observed.[61] This observation illustrates the importance of the host strain background in tumor development and provides a note of caution for investigators evaluating tumor incidence in transgenic mice.

Transgenic mice constitutively expressing growth factor or growth factor receptor genes have also been generated.[62,63] Abnormal expression of these classes of genes has been implicated in malignant transformation of hematopoietic cells. Transgenic mice carrying a murine granulocyte-macrophage colony stimulating factor (GM-CSF) gene fused to a Moloney murine leukemia virus (Mo-MuLV) LTR promoter developed pathologic lesions of the lens and retinal tissue, as well as macrophage accumulations in the pleural and peritoneal cavities. These mice also developed macrophage lesions in the striated muscle. In contrast, transgenic mice carrying a human interleukin-2 (IL-2) receptor light chain gene fused to a mouse $H\text{-}2K^d$ promoter demonstrated no overt pathology, even though they expressed functionally active IL-2 receptors on unstimulated spleen and thymus cells. The lack of overt pathology probably results from the fact that the human IL-2 receptor gene used in these experiments does not respond to murine IL-2. By substituting the mouse IL-2 receptor gene, it should be possible to study the pathologic consequences of its inappropriate expression in transgenic mice.

Transgenic mice may also be useful for elucidating the functions of lymphocyte-specific cell surface antigens in normal development and neoplastic disease. Although several of these antigens have been identified, they exhibit very complex expression patterns in many cases, and their role in normal development and neoplastic disease is poorly understood. One of these genes, Thy-1, is a cell surface glycoprotein expressed on mouse T-lymphocytes, neurons, and hematopoietic stem cells. Transgenic mice carrying wild-type human or mouse Thy-1 genes generally expressed the transgenes in a pattern characteristic of normal human or mouse tissues.[64] In contrast, a hybrid gene composed of the 5' region of the mouse Thy-1 gene combined with the 3' untranslated sequences from the human gene was expressed abnormally in kidney podocytes, resulting in severe proteinuria and death of founder mice.[65] Another hybrid gene containing the coding region of the human gene flanked by mouse 5' and 3' sequences was expressed abnormally

in the kidney tubular epithelia, resulting in a proliferative kidney disorder.[65] Finally, a mouse Thy-1 gene fused to a mouse immunoglobulin heavy chain enhancer (Eμ) was expressed on B-lymphocytes, resulting in a heritable lymphoid hyperplasia of the bone marrow and lymph nodes.[66] The various phenotypes associated with abnormal Thy-1 expression suggest that the Thy-1 protein can play an important role in the activation, proliferation, and differentiation of many cell types.

Specificity and Mechanisms of Action of Oncogenes in Transgenic Mice ∎

Tissue-Specificity of Oncogene Action ∎

Several studies indicate that tissues vary in their susceptibility to neoplastic transformation by oncogenes. For example, MMTV/Myc and MMTV/Hras transgenic mice are susceptible to different tumors, even though these mice express both oncogenes in the same tissues.[53] This was also found in transgenic mice expressing Wap/Myc and Wap/Hras fusion genes.[67,68] The Wap (whey acid protein) promoter, like the MMTV LTR promoter, is expressed in mammary epithelial cells in response to lactogenic hormones. In addition, Suda and coworkers[69] reported that different tumors develop in transgenic mice expressing three different oncogenes (Hras, Myc, and the SV40 early region genes) fused to the same human immunoglobulin heavy chain enhancer (Ig) and SV40 early region promoter (Tp). Ig/Tp/SV40 mice developed choroid plexus tumors, B-cell lymphomas, and histiocytic lymphomas, whereas Ig/Tp/Myc mice developed pre-B-cell lymphomas, and Ig/Tp/Hras mice developed lung adenocarcinomas. Finally, Quaife and coworkers[70] reported that expression of Hras, under the control of the rat elastase I promoter, leads to neoplasia of the fetal exocrine pancreas, whereas a comparable elastase/Myc construct produced no pancreatic tumors in transgenic mice. These phenotypes were different from those observed in elastase/SV40 mice, where pancreatic tumors developed 12 to 28 weeks after birth.[17]

Tumors Induced by the Promiscuous Expression of an Oncogene ∎

The tissue specificity of SV40 transformation has been assayed by creating transgenic mice harboring an SV40 early region linked to the promiscuous $H\text{-}2K^b$

enhancer.[71] The H-$2K^b$ gene is known to be expressed in most cell types in the mouse, although levels vary from tissue to tissue.[72] H-$2K^b$/SV40 transgenic mice developed choroid plexus tumors, thymic hyperplasia, and multiple endocrine neoplasia (see Table 4–1). Endocrine tumors developed later in life than other tumors and primarily involved the pancreas, pituitary, thyroid, adrenals, and testes. The development of thymic hyperplasia was preceded by elevated levels of T-antigen expression in susceptible cells. This was not true, however, in endocrine tumors. Several other tissues analyzed expressed T-antigen, yet most of these tissues did not develop tumors. This model seems well-suited for studying tissue-specific differences in susceptibility to neoplastic transformation by an oncogene.

Interference with Normal Development by the Deregulated Expression of Proto-oncogenes ■

In addition to tumor formation, deregulated expression of oncogenes in transgenic mice can result in abnormal development. This finding was not unexpected, since proto-oncogenes are thought to have important functions in normal development. It may be possible to gain further insights into these normal functions by analyzing the consequences of deregulated proto-oncogene expression in transgenic mice. Two studies describing the effects of the proto-oncogenes *Fos* and *Mos* on mouse development have been reported.

The *Fos* oncogene was originally identified in two mouse sarcoma viruses, FBJ-MSV and FBR-MSV. Both viruses induce osteosarcoma-like tumors in newborn mice. The c-*fos* proto-oncogene appears to be involved in multiple normal cell processes, including control of growth and differentiation as well as signal transduction. Transgenic mice carrying c-*fos* were derived by introducing a fusion gene consisting of a human MT promoter linked to c-*fos*.[73] High levels of c-*fos* mRNA were detected in a variety of tissues and specifically interfered with normal bone development, without inducing malignant tumors. c-*fos*-Induced lesions were first detected at the onset of bone development. The lesions were slowly progressive thickenings, usually located at the ends of the long bones. Growth of the lesions ceased a few weeks after birth; they were not invasive and consisted primarily of differentiated bone-synthesizing cells. It is unlikely that secondary genetic changes were required to produce these lesions. The virally induced tumors and the transgenic bone lesions showed some similarities: the target tissue in both cases was bone and the lesions involved bone precursor cells that were closely associated with blood vessels.

Deregulated expression of c-*mos* in transgenic mice has been shown to interfere with normal lens development.[74] The *Mos* oncogene was first identified in the mouse sarcoma virus Mo-MSV, and is a member of the *src* kinase family of oncogenes. The highest levels of c-*mos* expression have been detected in normal testes and ovaries[75,76]; however, the role of c-*mos* in normal development is poorly understood. Transgenic mice carrying the c-*mos* coding region linked to the MSV LTR expressed c-*mos* in several tissues, yet hyperplasia and neoplasia were not observed. However, there were defects in the lens of the eye, which were associated with a massive overexpression of c-*mos* mRNA in the lens. These defects were characterized by insufficient elongation of differentiating lens fibers, which normally takes place soon after birth, and by the lack of basement membrane secretion, which resulted in breakdown of the posterior lens capsule. This condition leads to posterior protrusion and swelling of lens tissue. Although there is no direct evidence indicating that c-*mos* has a physiologic role in any of these processes, these findings nevertheless indicate that abnormal c-*mos* expression can affect normal differentiation. Continued study of c-*fos* and c-*mos* transgenic mice should provide additional insights into the role of these genes in development and disease.

Induction of Tumors in Transgenic Mice by the *tat* Gene of Human T-lymphotropic Virus Type 1 ■

Human T-lymphotropic virus type 1 (HTLV-I) is a suspected causative agent in human adult T-cell leukemia. In addition to the viral genes required for retrovirus replication, HTLV-I encodes several other genes, including *tat*, a transactivating protein that regulates HTLV-I expression. The *tat* gene is thought to play a prominent role in cell transformation induced by HTLV-I, perhaps by deregulating the expression of cellular genes involved in cell growth. Transgenic mice provide an opportunity to study the consequences of *tat* expression *in vivo* in the absence of other viral genes.

Among eight founder transgenic mice that expressed *tat* under the control of the HTLV-I LTR, all developed obvious pathologies.[77] Three mice expressed high levels of *tat* in muscle and developed mesenchymal tumors at 13 to 17 weeks of age. The remaining five mice expressed *tat* in the thymus and in muscle. The latter group exhibited extensive thymic depletion and growth retardation, and all died between 3 to 6 weeks of age. Thus, *tat* can act as an oncogene *in vivo* and HTLV-I can be a transforming virus. These findings have important implications for the study of other human retroviruses, including HTLV-II and human immunodeficiency virus types I and II (HIV-I and HIV-II).

A detailed analysis of *tat*-transgenic mice indicated that the tumors arose from the sheaths of peripheral nerves and were composed of perineural cells and fibroblasts.[78] Many parallels can be drawn between these tumors and human neurofibromatosis (von Recklinghausen's disease), the most common known single-gene disorder affecting the human nervous system. Although neurotropic properties of HTLV-I in humans have recently been documented, more evidence is needed to establish a link between HTLV-I infection and von Recklinghausen's disease.

Creation of Transgenic Mice Resistant to Chemotherapeutic Agents ■

Genes encoding resistance to chemotherapeutic agents can be incorporated into the mouse germline, providing models for genetic engineering of chemotherapy resistance in humans. Inbred mice carrying resistance genes can also be used for tumor transplantation studies. By transferring a tumor from a strain that does not carry drug resistance genes into a drug-resistant transgenic host, one could pursue more aggressive chemotherapies without destroying normal host cells. These results would also provide useful information for clinicians contemplating insertion of drug resistance genes into human bone marrow cells to enhance tumor-specific chemotherapy.

With this goal in mind, transgenic mice have been created that carry a mutant dihydrofolate reductase gene capable of conferring resistance to methotrexate.[79] The mutant enzyme results from a single nucleotide substitution that decreases the binding affinity for dihydrofolate and reduces substrate turnover 20-fold relative to the wild-type enzyme; the mutant enzyme is 270-fold more resistant to MTX than the wild-type enzyme. Among eight transgenic mouse lines studied, all were significantly more resistant to MTX than control mice.[80] Animals heterozygous for this transgene also exhibited an array of developmental abnormalities, including stunted growth, reduced fertility, pigmentation changes, and skeletal

defects.[79] Therefore, although genes conferring resistance to chemotherapeutic agents can produce systemic drug resistance in transgenic mice, expression of these mutant transgenes can induce adverse mutational effects.

Other Methods of Creating Transgenic Mice ■

Pluripotential Mouse Embryonic Stem Cell Lines ■

Transgenic mice can also be created using pluripotential mouse embryonic stem (ES) cell lines, derived from the inner cell mass (ICM) cells of preimplantation mouse embryos (Fig. 4–2*A*). When blastocysts, or ICM cells derived from blastocysts, are grown in culture under the appropriate conditions, stable pluripotential stem cell lines can be established (Fig. 4–2).[81,82] Upon return to a host embryo, usually by injection into the blastocoel cavity (Fig. 4–2*B*), and transfer of the injected blastocysts into the oviducts of a suitable pseudopregnant foster female (Fig. 4–2*C*), ES cells can differentiate normally to give rise to mosaic (or chimeric) mice. These mice represent a mixture of ES cells and normal host cells (Fig. 4–2*D*). Some ES cell lines have been shown to reproducibly colonize the somatic and germ cell lineages in chimeric mice (Fig. 4–2*E*).[83] These ES cell lines thus provide useful vehicles for creating transgenic mice. Foreign DNA can be incorporated into these cells while in culture by a variety of techniques including transfection, electroporation, or infection with retroviral vectors.[84–86]

At present, the main disadvantage to this approach is that, in practice, it is often difficult to derive and maintain ES cell lines that remain karyotypically normal and pluripotent, and can repopulate the mouse germline in chimeras. However, these difficulties should be resolved as techniques improve and better culture conditions are established.

ES cell lines offer several advantages for creating transgenic mice compared with the more standard approach involving microinjection of DNA into zygotes. One of the main advantages is that genetically altered and clonally isolated cell lines can be selected before their reintroduction into the embryo. In this way, only ES cells carrying the gene of interest are reintroduced into the mouse embryo. An application of this approach has recently been reported by Williams and coworkers, who established ES cell lines that expressed the Py virus middle T-antigen under

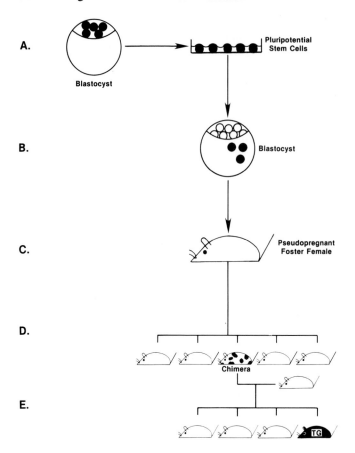

FIG. 4-2 Derivation of transgenic mice by manipulation of pluripotential embryonic stem cells. (From Hogan B, Constantini F, Lacy E: Manipulating the Mouse Embryo; A Laboratory Manual, pp 205–218. Cold Spring Harbor, NY, Cold Spring Harbor Laboratory, 1986)

the control of a thymidine kinase gene promoter.[87] Chimeric embryos obtained by blastocyst injection of these clones were developmentally arrested at mid-gestation, when multiple hemangiomas disrupted blood vessel formation. These results suggest that Py virus middle T-antigen can act as a single-step oncogene in endothelial cells. Transgenic mice produced by microinjection of the Py virus middle T-antigen gene coupled to its own regulatory elements also developed hemangiomas,[42] however, the tumors did not appear until 2.5 to 6.5 months after birth. The reason for the differences in tumor susceptibilities observed in these studies is not clear but may result from differences in the levels of middle T-antigen expressed by the different promoters used in these experiments.

A second important application of ES cell lines is their potential for introducing mutations into the mouse germline. By selecting clonal lines that carry mutations in a gene of interest, it should then be possible to introduce the mutant gene into the mouse germline by blastocyst injection. These mice are initially heterozygous for the mutation, and recessive lethal mutations can be maintained in the heterozygous state. By intercrossing heterozygous mice, the mutation can be made homozygous and its effects on development can be studied; thus, it should be possible to derive mouse models containing almost any genetic lesion of interest.

The feasibility of this approach was recently demonstrated by several investigators who selected and transferred ES cells carrying mutations in the mouse X-linked hypoxanthine-guanosine phosphoribosyl transferase (HPRT) gene with the hope of creating animal models for the Lesch–Nyhan syndrome in humans.[88,89] These mutations were either spontaneous or generated following retroviral infection of ES cell lines. A number of other investigators have recently succeeded in altering an endogenous ES cell HPRT gene by homologous recombination.[90,91] In one case, a normal HPRT gene was mutated by homologous recombination;[91] in another, a mutant HPRT gene was corrected by homologous recombination.[90] These results suggest that it will soon be possible to generate mouse models for virtually any human genetic disease in which the molecular basis is understood.

The ability to mutate the mouse germline by homologous recombination affords a unique opportunity to directly study the role of proto-oncogenes in normal cell processes and therefore better understand their function in neoplastic disease. Despite much research effort, these functions largely remain elusive. This failure has largely resulted from our inability to mutate these genes in the whole organism and to study the ensuing consequences. It should be possible in the near future to derive mice carrying mutations in this interesting family of genes by using the ES cell technology, in conjunction with mutation by homologous recombination. Thus, our understanding of the functions of proto-oncogenes will be greatly facilitated.

Introduction of Genes into the Mouse Germline by Infection of Preimplantation Mouse Embryos with Retroviral Vectors ■

Several investigators have reported the successful transfer of foreign DNA sequences into the mouse germline by infection of preimplantation mouse embryos with retroviral vectors.[86,92–94] However, this approach to gene transfer is limited for several reasons: the amount of foreign DNA that can be incorporated into a retroviral vector is relatively small, so the introduced gene is often not expressed;[92,94] also the vector sequences are sometimes rearranged during virus propagation,[95] and tissue-specific or inducible gene expression has yet to be demonstrated in this system. Thus, the current methods of choice for producing transgenic mice involve microinjection of DNA into zygotes or injection of genetically altered ES cell lines into the blastocyst.

Applications for Transgenic Mice Beyond Cancer Research ■

Transgenic mice have provided useful models for several endeavors aside from cancer research. Although these are only indirectly relevant to the subject of this chapter, we thought it important to briefly mention some of these applications.

Heart Disease □ A cDNA encoding the human low-density lipoprotein (LDL) receptor under the control of a mouse MT-1 promoter has been expressed in transgenic mice.[96] Overexpression of this receptor led to a dramatic lowering of plasma concentrations of apoproteins B-100 and E, the two ligands of the LDL receptor.

Down's Syndrome □ This syndrome, which results from human trisomy 21, is thought to be induced by a 1.5-fold increase in the expression of genes on human chromosome 21. Through the use of transgenic mice that express genes isolated from human chromosome 21, the consequences of increased dosage of these genes can be studied and their potential involvement in Down's syndrome addressed.[97]

Hemophilia B □ Hemophilia B is a bleeding disorder caused by a functional deficiency of clotting factor IX. Transgenic mice containing a full-length human factor IX cDNA expressed high levels of factor IX mRNA and biologically active factor IX clotting activity.[98]

Gene Therapy □ Several hereditary genetic deficiencies of mice have been totally or partially corrected by gene transfer in transgenic mice.[99–106]

Osteogenesis Imperfecta Type II □ Substitutions of glycine residues in α_1-collagen lead to an inherited disorder in humans, osteogenesis imperfecta type II. Transgenic mice harboring similar mutant collagen genes display a phenotype similar to the human disease.[107]

Hepatitis B □ Several investigators have succeeded in producing transgenic mice expressing hepatitis B surface antigen genes.[108–113] These mice provide models for the chronic hepatitis B carrier state in humans.

Diabetes □ Insulin-dependent diabetes is caused by the loss of insulin-producing β-cells in the pancreas. High levels of expression of class II major histocompatibility complex genes in β-cells of transgenic mice impaired β-cell function, resulting in diabetes.[114,115]

Cell Ablation □ A method of deleting specific cell lineages has been developed. Transgenic mice were created that carry a toxic gene, diphtheria toxin A, linked to a tissue-specific promoter.[116–118] This method provides new approaches for studying cell-lineage relationships and for analyzing cellular interactions during development.

Conclusion ■

The future for the use of transgenic mice in cancer research seems especially bright. In the 4 years since the first transgenic tumor models were reported, a wealth of information has been collected regarding the role of oncogenes in neoplastic disease. The specificity and regularity with which these transgenic lines develop tumors will continue to provide cancer researchers with an enormous reservoir of tumors useful for drug screening and other studies pertaining to clinical intervention. Finally, with the expected advances in germline gene-targeting by homologous recombination in ES cell lines, the roles of proto-oncogenes in normal growth and development can be explored and potential models for virtually any human disease can be developed.

The authors thank Linda Brubaker and Robin Handley for typing the manuscript, and Arthur Buchberg, Jeff Ceci, Monica Justice, David Kingsley, Leslie Lock, John Mercer, Karen Moore, Luis Parada, Michael Rosenberg, Peter Seperack, Linda Siracusa, Sally Spence, and Marjorie Strobel for helpful comments. This work was supported by the National Cancer Institute under Contract N01-C0-74101 with Bionetics Research, Inc.

References ■

1. Gordon JW, Scangos GA, Plotkin DJ et al: Genetic transformation of mouse embryos by microinjection of purified DNA. Proc Natl Acad Sci USA 77:7380–7384, 1980
2. Wagner TE, Hoppe PC, Jollick JD et al: Microinjection of a rabbit β-globin gene into zygotes and its subsequent expression in adult mice and their offspring. Proc Natl Acad Sci USA 78:6376–6380, 1981
3. Palmiter RD, Brinster RL, Hammer RE: Dramatic growth of mice that develop from eggs microinjected with metallothionein-growth hormone fusion genes. Nature 300:611–615, 1982
4. Palmiter RD, Chen HY, Brinster RL: Differential regulation of metallothionein-thymidine kinase fusion genes in transgenic mice and their offspring. Cell 29:701–710, 1982
5. Palmiter RD, Brinster RL: Germline transformation of mice. Ann Rev Genet 20:465–499, 1986
6. Swift GH, Hammer RE, MacDonald RJ et al: Tissue-specific expression of the rat pancreatic elastase I gene in transgenic mice. Cell 38:639–646, 1984
7. Grosveld F, van Assendelft GB, Greaves DR et al: Position-independent, high-level expression of the human β-globin gene in transgenic mice. Cell 51:975–985, 1987
8. Brinster RL, Chen HY, Messing A et al: Transgenic mice harboring SV40 T-antigen genes develop characteristic brain tumors. Cell 37:367–379, 1984
9. Janisch W, Schrieber D: In Binger DD, Swenberg JA (eds): Experimental Tumors of the Central Nervous System, p 36. Kalamazoo, MI, Upjohn Company, 1977
10. MacKay K, Striker LJ, Pinkert CA et al: Glomerulosclerosis and renal cysts in mice transgenic for the early region of SV40. Kidney Int 32:827–837, 1987
11. Van Dyke T, Finlay C, Levine AJ: A comparison of several lines of transgenic mice containing the SV40 early genes. Cold Spring Harbor Symp Quant Biol 50:671–678, 1985
12. Van Dyke TA, Finlay C, Miller D et al: Relationship between simian virus 40 large tumor antigen expression and tumor formation in transgenic mice. J Virol 61:2029–2032, 1987
13. Palmiter RD, Chen HY, Messing A et al: SV40 enhancer and large T-antigen are instrumental in development of choroid plexus tumors in transgenic mice. Nature 316:457–460, 1985
14. Pinkert CA, Brinster FL, Palmiter RD et al: Tumorigenesis in transgenic mice by a nuclear transport-defective SV40 large T-antigen gene. Virology 160:169–175, 1987
15. Lanford RE, Wong C, Butel JS: Differential ability of a T-antigen transport-defective mutant of simian virus 40 to transform primary and established rodent cells. Mol Cell Biol 5:1043–1050, 1985
16. Messing A, Cehn HY, Palmiter RD et al: Peripheral neuropathies, hepatocellular carcinomas and islet adenomas in transgenic mice. Nature 316:461–463, 1985
17. Ornitz DM, Hammer RE, Messing A et al: Pancreatic neoplasia induced by SV40 T-antigen expression in acinar cells of transgenic mice. Science 238:188–193, 1987
18. Barlogie B, Drewinko B, Schumann J et al: Cellular DNA content as a marker of neoplasia in man. Am J Med 69:195–203, 1980
19. Friedlander ML, Hedley DW, Taylor IW: Clinical and biological significance of aneuploidy in human tumors. J Clin Pathol 37:961–974, 1984
20. O'Hara MF, Bedrossian CW, Johnson TS et al: Flow cytometry in cancer diagnosis. Prog Clin Pathol 9:135–153, 1984
21. Hanahan D: Heritable formation of pancreatic β-cell tumours in transgenic mice expressing recombinant insulin/simian virus 40 oncogenes. Nature 315:115–122, 1985
22. Murphy D, Bishop A, Rindi G et al: Mice transgenic for a vasopressin-SV40 hybrid oncogene develop tumors of the endocrine pancreas and the anterior pituitary. Am J Pathol 129:552–566, 1987
23. Linzer DIH, Levine AJ: Characterization of a 54K dalton cellular SV40 tumor antigen present in SV40-transformed cells and uninfected embryonal carcinoma cells. Cell 17:43–52, 1979
24. Lane DP, Crawford LV: T-antigen is bound to a host protein in SV40-transformed cells. Nature 278:261–263, 1979
25. McCormick F, Harlow E: Association of a murine 53,000-dalton phosphoprotein with simian virus 40 large-T antigen in transformed cells. J Virol 34:213–224, 1980
26. Efrat S, Baekkeskov S, Lane D et al: Coordinate expression of the endogenous p53 gene in β cells of transgenic mice expressing hybrid insulin-SV40 T-antigen genes. EMBO J 6:2699–2704, 1987
27. Tevethia SS, Balsecki JW, Waneck G et al: Requirement of thymus-derived θ-positive lymphocytes for rejection of DNA virus (SV40) tumors in mice. J Immunol 113:1417–1423, 1974
28. Gooding LR: Characterization of a progressive tumor from C3H fibroblasts transformed in vitro with SV40 virus. Immunoresistance in vivo correlates with phenotypic loss of H-2K^k. J Immunol 129:1306–1312, 1982
29. Pan S, Knowles BB: Monoclonal antibody to SV40 T-antigen blocks lysis of cloned cytotoxic T-cell line specific for SV40 TASA. Virology 125:1–7, 1983
30. Abramczuk J, Pan S, Maul G et al: Tumor induction by simian virus 40 in mice is controlled by long-term persistence of the

viral genome and the immune response of the host. J Virol 49:540–548, 1984

31. Adams TE, Alpert S, Hanahan D: Non-tolerance and auto-antibodies to a transgenic self antigen expressed in pancreatic cells. Nature 325:223–228, 1987

32. Faas SJ, Pan S, Pinkert CA et al: Simian virus 40 (SV40)-transgenic mice that develop tumors are specifically tolerant to SV40 T-antigen. J Exp Med 165:417–427, 1987

33. Mahon K, Chepelinsky AB, Khillan JS et al: Oncogenesis of the lens in transgenic mice. Science 235:1622–1628, 1987

34. Field LJ: Atrial natriuretic factor-SV40 T antigen transgenes produce tumors and cardiac arrhythmias in mice. Science 239:1029–1033, 1988

35. Baetge EE, Behringer RR, Messing A et al: Transgenic mice express the human phenylethanolamine N-methyltransferase gene in adrenal medulla and retina. Proc Natl Acad Sci USA 85:3648–3652, 1988

36. Behringer RR, Peschon JJ, Messing A et al: Heart and bone tumors in transgenic mice. Proc Natl Acad Sci USA 85:2648–2652, 1988

37. Botteri FM, van der Putten H, Wong DF et al: Unexpected thymic hyperplasia in transgenic mice harboring a neuronal promoter fused with simian virus 40 large T antigen. Mol Cell Biol 7:3178–3184, 1987

38. Tooze J: Molecular Biology of Tumor Viruses: Part 2, DNA Tumor Viruses. Cold Spring Harbor, NY, Cold Spring Harbor Laboratory, 1981

39. Johnson RT: Evidence for polyomaviruses in human neurological disease. In Sever JC, Madden DL (eds): Polyomaviruses and Human Neurological Diseases, pp 183–190. New York, Alan R Liss, 1983

40. Small JA, Khoury G, Jay G et al: Early regions of JC virus and BK virus induce distinct and tissue-specific tumors in transgenic mice. Proc Natl Acad Sci USA 83:8288–8292, 1986

41. Small JA, Scangos GA, Cork L et al: The early region of human papovavirus JC induces dysmyelination in transgenic mice. Cell 46:13–18, 1986

42. Bautch VL, Toda S, Hassell JA et al: Endothelial cell tumors develop in transgenic mice carrying polyoma virus middle T oncogene. Cell 51:529–538, 1987

43. Gross L: The parotid tumor (polyoma) virus. In Oncogenic Viruses, 2nd ed, pp 651–750. Oxford, Pergamon Press, 1970

44. Eddy BE: Polyomavirus. In Foster HL, Small JD, Fox JG (eds): The Mouse in Biomedical Research, Vol II, pp 293–311. New York, Academic Press, 1982

45. Treisman R, Novak U, Favaloro J et al: Transformation of rat cells by an altered polyoma virus genome expressing only the middle-T protein. Nature 292:595–600, 1981

46. Rassoulzadegan M, Cowie A, Carr A et al: The roles of individual polyoma virus early proteins in oncogenic transformation. Nature 300:713–718, 1982

47. Lacey M, Alpert S, Hanahan D: Bovine papillomavirus genome elicits skin tumours in transgenic mice. Nature 322:609–612, 1986

48. Stewart TA, Pattengale PK, Leder P: Spontaneous mammary adenocarcinomas in transgenic mice that carry and express MTV/myc fusion genes. Cell 38:627–637, 1984

49. Weiss R, Teich N, Varmus H et al: Molecular Biology of Tumor Viruses: RNA tumor viruses, 2nd ed. Cold Spring Harbor, NY, Cold Spring Harbor Laboratory, 1982

50. Yamamoto KR: Steroid receptor regulated transcription of specific genes and gene networks. Annu Rev Genet 19:209–252, 1985

51. Leder A, Pattengale PK, Kuo A et al: Consequences of widespread deregulation of the c-myc gene in transgenic mice:

Multiple neoplasms and normal development. Cell 45:485–495, 1986

52. Choi Y, Henrard D, Lee I et al: The mouse mammary tumor virus long terminal repeat directs expression in epithelial and lymphoid cells of different tissues in transgenic mice. J Virol 61:3013–3019, 1987

53. Sinn E, Muller W, Pattengale P et al: Coexpression of MMTV/v-Ha-ras and MMTV/c-myc genes in transgenic mice: Synergistic action of oncogenes in vivo. Cell 49:465–475, 1987

54. Choi Y, Lee I, Ross S: A requirement for the simian virus 40 small tumor antigen in tumorigenesis in transgenic mice. Mol Cell Biol (in press)

55. Sleigh MJ, Topp WC, Hanich R et al: Mutants of SV40 with an altered small t protein are reduced in their ability to transform cells. Cell 14:79–88, 1978

56. Martin RG, Setlow VP, Edwards CAF et al: The roles of the simian virus 40 tumor antigens in transformation of Chinese hamster lung cells. Cell 17:635–643, 1979

57. Seif R, Martin RG: Simian virus 40 small t antigen is not required for the maintenance of transformation but may act as a promoter (cocarcinogen) during establishment of transformation in resting rat cells. J Virol 32:979–988, 1979

58. Adams JM, Harris AW, Pinkert CA et al: The c-myc oncogene driven by immunoglobulin enhancers induces lymphoid malignancy in transgenic mice. Nature 318:533–538, 1985

59. Langdon WY, Harris AW, Cory S et al: The c-myc oncogene perturbs B lymphocyte development in Eμ-myc transgenic mice. Cell 47:11–18, 1986

60. Alexander WS, Schrader JW, Adams JA: Expression of the c-myc oncogene under control of an immunoglobulin enhancer in Eμ-myc transgenic mice. Mol Cell Biol 7:1436–1444, 1987

61. Harris AW, Pinkert CA, Crawford M et al: The Eμ-myc transgenic mouse: A model for high-incidence spontaneous lymphoma and leukemia of early B cells. J Exp Med 167:353–371, 1988

62. Lang RA, Metcalf D, Cuthbertson RA et al: Transgenic mice expressing a hemopoietic growth factor gene (GM-CSF) develop accumulations of macrophages, blindness, and a fatal syndrome of tissue damage. Cell 51:675–686, 1987

63. Nishi M, Ishida Y, Honjo T: Expression of functional interleukin-2 receptors in human light chain/Tac transgenic mice. Nature 331:267–269, 1988

64. Gordon JW, Chesa PG, Nishimura H et al: Regulation of Thy-1 gene expression in transgenic mice. Cell 50:445–452, 1987

65. Kollias G, Evans DJ, Ritter M et al: Ectopic expression of Thy-1 in the kidneys of transgenic mice induces functional and proliferative abnormalities. Cell 51:21–31, 1987

66. Chen S, Botteri FM, van der Putten H et al: A lymphoproliferative abnormality associated with inappropriate expression of the Thy-1 antigen in transgenic mice. Cell 51:7–19, 1987

67. Andres A-C, Schonenberger C-A, Groner B et al: Ha-ras oncogene expression directed by a milk protein gene promoter: Tissue specificity, hormonal regulation, and tumor induction in transgenic mice. Proc Natl Acad Sci USA 84:1299–1303, 1987

68. Schonenberger C-A, Andres A-C, Groner B et al: Targeted c-myc gene expression in mammary glands of transgenic mice induces mammary tumours with constitutive milk protein gene transcription. EMBO J 7:169–175, 1988

69. Suda Y, Aizawa S, Hirai S et al: Driven by the same Ig enhancer and SV40 T promoter ras induced lung adenomatous tumors, myc induced pre-B cell lymphomas and SV40 large T gene a variety of tumors in transgenic mice. EMBO J 6:4055–4065, 1987

70. Quaife CJ, Pinkert CA, Ornitz DM et al: Pancreatic neoplasia induced by *ras* expression in acinar cells of transgenic mice. Cell 48:1023–1034, 1987

71. Reynolds RK, Hoekzema GS, Vogel J et al: Multiple endocrine neoplasia induced by the promiscuous expression of a viral oncogene. Proc Natl Acad Sci USA 85:3135–3139, 1988

72. Bieberich C, Scangos G, Tanaka K et al: Regulated expression of a murine class I gene in transgenic mice. Mol Cell Biol 6:1339–1342, 1986

73. Ruther U, Garber C, Komitowski D et al: Deregulated c-*fos* expression interferes with normal bone development in transgenic mice. Nature 325:412–416, 1987

74. Khillan JS, Oskarsson MK, Propst F et al: Defects in lens fiber differentiation are linked to c-*mos* overexpression in transgenic mice. Genes and Develop 1:1327–1335, 1987

75. Propst F, Vande Woude GF: Expression of c-*mos* proto-oncogene transcripts in mouse tissues. Nature 315:516–518, 1985

76. Propst F, Rosenberg MP, Iyer A et al: c-*mos* proto-oncogene RNA transcripts in mouse tissues: Structural features, developmental regulation, and localization in specific cell types. Mol Cell Biol 7:1629–1637, 1987

77. Nerenberg M, Hinrichs SH, Reynolds RK et al: The *tat* gene of human T-lymphotropic virus type 1 induces mesenchymal tumors in transgenic mice. Science 237:1324–1329, 1987

78. Hinrichs SH, Nerenberg M, Reynolds RK et al: A transgenic mouse model for human neurofibromatosis. Science 237:1340–1343, 1987

79. Gordon JW: A foreign dihydrofolate reductase gene in transgenic mice acts as a dominant mutation. Mol Cell Biol 6:2158–2167, 1986

80. Isola LM, Gordon JW: Systemic resistance to methotrexate in transgenic mice carrying a mutant dihydrofolate reductase gene. Proc Natl Acad Sci USA 83:9621–9625, 1986

81. Evans MJ, Kaufman MH: Establishment in culture of pluripotential cells from mouse embryos. Nature 292:154–156, 1981

82. Martin GR: Isolation of a pluripotent cell line from early mouse embryos cultured in medium conditioned by teratocarcinoma stem cells. Proc Natl Acad Sci USA 78:7634–7638, 1981

83. Bradley A, Evans M, Kaufman MH et al: Formation of germline chimaeras from embryo-derived teratocarcinoma cell lines. Nature 309:255–256, 1984

84. Gossler A, Doetschman T, Korn R et al: Transgenesis by means of blastocyst-derived embryonic stem cell lines. Proc Natl Acad Sci USA 83:9065–9069, 1986

85. Robertson E, Bradley A, Kuehn M et al: Germ-line transmission of genes introduced into cultured pluripotential cells by retroviral vector. Nature 323:445–448, 1986

86. Stewart CL, Ruther U, Garber C et al: The expression of retroviral vectors in murine stem cells and transgenic mice. J Embryol Exp Morph 97(Suppl):263–275, 1986

87. Williams RL, Courtneidge SA, Wagner EF: Embryonic lethalities and endothelial tumors in chimeric mice expressing polyoma virus middle T oncogene. Cell 52:121–131, 1988

88. Hooper M, Hardy K, Handyside A et al: HPRT-deficient (Lesch-Nyhan) mouse embryos derived from germline colonization by cultured cells. Nature 326:292–295, 1987

89. Kuehn MR, Bradley A, Robertson EJ et al: A potential animal model for Lesch-Nyhan syndrome through introduction of HPRT mutations in mice. Nature 326:295–298, 1987

90. Doetschman T, Gregg RG, Maeda N et al: Targeted correction of a mutant HPRT gene in mouse embryonic stem cells. Nature 330:576–578, 1987

91. Thomas KR, Capecchi MR: Site-directed mutagenesis by gene targeting in mouse embryo-derived stem cells. Cell 51:503–512, 1987

92. Huszar D, Balling R, Kothary R et al: Insertion of a bacterial gene into the mouse germ line using an infectious retrovirus vector. Proc Natl Acad Sci USA 82:8587–8591, 1985

93. van der Putten H, Botteri FM, Miller AD et al: Efficient insertion of genes into the mouse germ line via retroviral vectors. Proc Natl Acad Sci USA 82:6148–6152, 1985

94. Stewart CL, Schuetze S, Vanek M et al: Expression of retroviral vectors in transgenic mice obtained by embryo infection. EMBO J 6:383–388, 1987

95. Joyner AL, Bernstein A: Retrovirus transduction: Segregation of the viral transforming function and the Herpes Simplex virus *tk* gene in infectious Friend spleen focus-forming virus thymidine kinase vectors. Mol Cell Biol 3:2191–2202, 1983

96. Hofmann SL, Russell DW, Brown MS et al: Overexpression of low density lipoprotein (LDL) receptor eliminates LDL from plasma in transgenic mice. Science 239:1277–1281, 1988

97. Epstein CJ, Avraham KB, Lovett M et al: Transgenic mice with increased Cu/Zn superoxide dismutase activity: Animal model of dosage effects in Down's Syndrome. Proc Natl Acad Sci USA 84:8044–8048, 1987

98. Choo KH, Raphael K, McAdam W et al: Expression of active human blood clotting factor IX in transgenic mice: Use of a cDNA with complete mRNA sequence. Nucleic Acids Res 15:871–884, 1987

99. Hammer RE, Palmiter RD, Brinster RL: Partial correction of murine hereditary growth disorder by germ-line incorporation of a new gene. Nature 311:65–67, 1984

100. LeMeur M, Gerlinger P, Benoist C et al: Correcting an immune-response deficiency by creating E$_\alpha$ gene transgenic mice. Nature 316:38–42, 1985

101. Costantini F, Chada K, Magram J: Correction of murine thalassemia by gene transfer into the germ line. Science 233:1192–1194, 1986

102. Mason AJ, Pitts SL, Nikolics K et al: The hypogonadal mouse: Reproductive functions restored by gene therapy. Science 234:1372–1378, 1986

103. Nishimoto H, Kikutani H, Yamamura K-I et al: Prevention of autoimmune insulitis by expression of I-E molecules in NOD mice. Nature 328:432–434, 1987

104. Readhead C, Popko B, Takahashi N et al: Expression of a myelin basic protein gene in transgenic shiverer mice: Correction of the dysmyelinating phenotype. Cell 48:703–712, 1987

105. Popko B, Puckett C, Lai E et al: Myelin deficient mice: Expression of myelin basic protein and generation of mice with varying levels of myelin. Cell 48:713–721, 1987

106. Cavard C, Grimber G, Dubois N et al: Correction of mouse ornithine transcarbamylase deficiency by gene transfer into the germ line. Nucleic Acids Res 16:2099–2110, 1988

107. Stacey A, Bateman J, Choi T et al: Perinatal lethal osteogenesis imperfecta in transgenic mice bearing an engineered mutant pro (I) collagen gene. Nature 332:131–136, 1988

108. Babinet C, Farza H, Morello D et al: Specific expression of hepatitis surface antigen (HBsAg) in transgenic mice. Science 230:1160–1163, 1985

109. Chisari FV, Pinkert CA, Milich DR et al: A transgenic mouse model of the chronic hepatitis B surface antigen carrier state. Science 230:1157–1160, 1985

110. Chisari FV, Filippi P, McLachlan A et al: Expression of hepatitis B virus large envelope polypeptide inhibits hepatitis B surface antigen secretion in transgenic mice. J Virol 60:880–887, 1986

111. Chisari FV, Filippi P, Buras J et al: Structural and pathological effects of synthesis of hepatitis B virus large envelope polypeptide in transgenic mice. Proc Natl Acad Sci USA 84:6909–6913, 1987

112. Farza H, Salmon AM, Hadchouel M et al: Hepatitis B surface antigen gene expression is regulated by sex steroids and glucocorticoids in transgenic mice. Proc Natl Acad Sci USA 84:1187–1191, 1987

113. Burk RD, DeLoia JA, Elawdy MK et al: Tissue preferential expression of the hepatitis B virus (HBV) surface antigen gene in two lines of HBV transgenic mice. J Virol 62:649–654, 1988

114. Sarvetnick N, Liggitt D, Pitts SL et al: Insulin-dependent diabetes mellitus induced in transgenic mice by ectopic expression of class II MHC and interferon-gamma. Cell 52:773–782, 1988

115. Lo D, Burkly LC, Widera G et al: Diabetes and tolerance in transgenic mice expressing class II MHC molecules in pancreatic beta cells. Cell 53:159–168, 1988

116. Palmiter RD, Behringer RR, Quaife CJ et al: Cell lineage ablation in transgenic mice by cell-specific expression of a toxin gene. Cell 50:435–443, 1987

117. Breitman ML, Clapoff S, Rossant J et al: Genetic ablation: Targeted expression of a toxin gene causes microphthalmia in transgenic mice. Science 238:1563–1565, 1987

118. Behringer RR, Mathews LS, Palmiter RD et al: Dwarf mice produced by genetic ablation of growth hormone-expressing cells. Genes and Development 2:453–461, 1988

119. Small JA, Blair DG, Showalter SD et al: Analysis of a transgenic mouse containing simian virus 40 and v-*myc* sequences. Mol Cell Biol 5:642–648, 1985

C. A. Stein
Jack S. Cohen

Antisense Compounds: Potential Role in Cancer Therapy

5

Introduction ■

The majority of drugs used in chemotherapy are natural products or derivatives that either block enzyme pathways or randomly interact with DNA. Screening procedures designed to select such drugs have become increasingly inefficient. A new approach is based upon the concept of using messenger RNA (mRNA) as the primary drug target (Fig. 5–1). Either another mRNA molecule or a synthetic oligodeoxynucleotide (Fig. 5–2) with the complementary base sequence to the target mRNA forms a hybrid duplex by hydrogen-bonded base pairing. This hybridization can be expected to prevent expression of the target mRNA's protein product (Fig. 5–3). This process is termed "translation arrest," and because the mRNA sequence expressed by the gene is called the "sense base sequence," the complementary sequence is the "antisense" sequence. These molecules can also be referred to as "antimessengers." Antimessenger inhibition of mRNA would be more efficient than inhibition of an enzyme active site because one mRNA molecule gives rise to multiple protein copies. Further, the selective inhibition of expression of a gene product required for normal cellular function yields the desired goal of chemotherapy: selective cell death.

This approach varies in difficulty depending on whether the antimessenger compound employed is an mRNA or an oligodeoxynucleotide (oligo). If an antisense mRNA is used to inhibit gene expression by hybridizing with its natural complement (Fig. 5–4), the incorporation of the new DNA fragment into the genome of the cell and the control of its expression in conjunction with the natural sense mRNA become major considerations. Although this approach has major implications for studies of the mechanism of gene expression, its complexity makes it unlikely that

the intracellular expression of antisense mRNA[1] will become a viable drug option.

By contrast, oligos of any base sequence can be readily synthesized in milligram quantities by an automated process (Fig. 5–5).[2,3] Such compounds, when added to cells grown in culture, selectively inhibit the expression of a particular gene. In cancer cells, this inhibition could cause cell death, and in virally infected cells it could result in inhibition of viral replication. These hypotheses rest on three basic assumptions: [a] that oligos will be stable *in vivo,* [b] that oligos will penetrate into cells, and [c] that oligos will hybridize effectively with the target sense mRNA sequence once inside the cell. Each of these points is considered separately below.

In addition, there are other questions that arise regarding the use of oligos *in vivo.* If the base sequence of a target gene specific for various tumor types is identified, will the antisense oligo indeed affect the growth properties of the cell? Will the target sequence be accessible on the mRNA of choice (Fig. 5–6)?[4] Will there be other similar gene sequences present in cells that can cause unexpected inhibitions? Will the oligos bind to proteins necessary for DNA/RNA synthesis or degradation? These questions raise a series of considerations that are discussed in the subsequent sections on applications of oligos and analogues.

Stability of Oligos *in Vivo* ■

Oligodeoxynucleotides, as the basic building blocks of DNA, are chemically stable compounds that retain the essential base sequence for the genetic expression of the cell. The deoxyribose derivatives are more resistant to hydrolysis than the ribose derivatives of

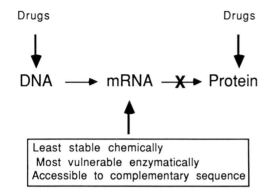

Drugs   Drugs

DNA ——→ mRNA —X→ Protein

Least stable chemically
Most vulnerable enzymatically
Accessible to complementary sequence

FIG. 5–1 Rationale for the use of antisense oligodeoxynucleotide as a drug to prevent translation of mRNA into protein.

RNA, because the 2'-hydroxyl group facilitates phosphodiester bond cleavage in the latter (Fig. 5–7). Nevertheless, the phosphodiester bond in deoxynucleotides is readily cleaved by the many deoxyribonucleases (DNases) that occur in cells. Enzymes known as exonucleases cleave from the end of a DNA chain, whereas endonucleases cleave anywhere along the chain (Fig. 5–8). Some enzymes have both capabilities, and some cleave both DNA and RNA phosphodiester bonds, but usually with different rates. Thus, oligos cannot be expected to survive long in the cellular milieu because of enzymatic degradation. Various estimates of the viability of an oligo in growth media and cellular supernatant place the half-life anywhere from a few minutes to a few days. This is particularly devastating for a method that depends on the sequence or length of a chain molecule, because a single cleavage may render the oligo useless. In fact, the breakdown of the oligo into high concentrations of mononucleotides can be toxic to the cell.

To overcome this disadvantage, several synthetic analogues have been proposed (Figs. 5–2 and 5–5). The rationale is that a chemical change in the phosphodiester group will render it impervious to nuclease cleavage. Generally this is the case, and methylphosphonates (M-oligos, containing P-CH$_3$),[5] phosphorothionates (S-oligos, containing PS),[6,7] and phosphoramidates (containing P-NR$_2$)[3] are known to be resistant to nucleases. However, they are susceptible to slow cleavage, and other enzyme activities, such as depurination, eventually lead to the degradation of the synthetic oligo. Nevertheless, these oligo analogues exhibit increased longevity in the cell.

Another class of analogues of the naturally occurring nucleotides are the α-oligos, in which the orientation of the bases on the deoxyribose ring is opposite to that in the normal β-configuration (Fig. 5–9). These analogues are nuclease-resistant because of this abnormal orientation of the base.[8]

Synthetic oligo analogues may cause problems because of their antigenicity. This concern arises partly because of the well-known antigenicity of poly(IC); however, there is a major difference between a polyribonucleotide and an oligodeoxynucleotide in terms of their antigenic stimulation. At present, there is no firm evidence on which to base an evaluation of the biologic effects of these compounds.

Cellular Uptake of Oligos ■

The mechanisms whereby oligos enter cells are unknown. Initially, there was skepticism that poly-anions such as oligos could cross cell membranes and enter cells. The first results showing selective inhibi-

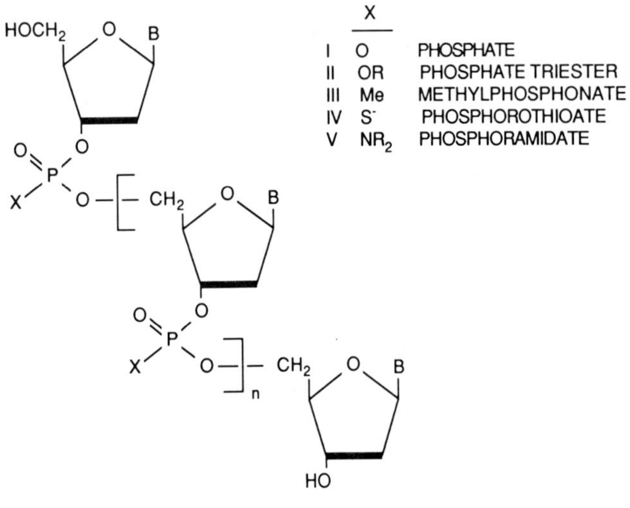

	X	
I	O	PHOSPHATE
II	OR	PHOSPHATE TRIESTER
III	Me	METHYLPHOSPHONATE
IV	S$^-$	PHOSPHOROTHIOATE
V	NR$_2$	PHOSPHORAMIDATE

FIG. 5–2 Structures of normal (I) and modified (II–V) oligos. B is adenine, guanine, cytosine, or thymine; Modified phosphate analogues are II, phosphotriester; III, methylphosphonate (M-oligo); IV, phosphorothioate (S-oligo); V, phosphoramidate. Analogues II, III, and V are neutral, whereas IV retains a negative charge like the normal phosphate group. N is usually in the range of 3–30.

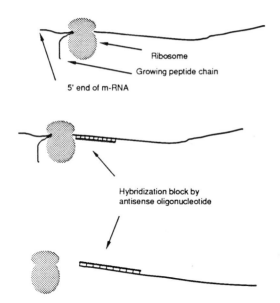

FIG. 5–3 Representation of the hybridization of complementary nucleic acids with mRNA, thus preventing ribosomal translation to protein.

explored by Neale and associates[13] and Ruby and co-workers,[14] who found just such a system in prokaryotes. Bennett and associates,[15] found that white blood cells bind exogenous DNA in a saturable and competitive fashion that is not inhibited by RNA, poly(dA-dT), or mononucleotides. A protein of molecular weight 30 kDa was identified as the putative binding protein.

In contrast, uptake of fluorescent labeled oligos into HL60 cells was strongly inhibited by deoxynucleotide mono-, di-, and triphosphates when the sugar was phosphorylated in the 5′ position. 2′- and 3′-Phosphorylated nucleotides were less effective, as were nucleosides, monosaccharide-6-phosphates, and deoxyribose-5-phosphate. Methylphosphonate oligos also did not block the cellular uptake of these tagged materials. On the other hand, oligos containing 3 to 20 deoxynucleotides (3- to 20-mers) of any sequence were strong inhibitors of uptake. Homopolymers or monomers of adenosine, cytidine, guanosine, thymidine or uridine (A, C, G, T, or U) were also effective, as was double-stranded DNA (plasmid pCD) and transfer RNA (tRNA). The potency of the inhibition was proportional to the length of the oligo (*i.e.,* longer

tion of gene expression, using the antisense approach of Zamecnik and Stephenson,[9,10] implied that oligos can indeed penetrate cells. Although other results indicated that oligos enter cells, until recently there was no clear-cut proof. One of the most direct approaches to studying the kinetics of cellular uptake is the use of an oligo with a covalently linked fluorescent group (Fig. 5–10), which can then be monitored by fluorescence measurements as it is taken up by cells. Some elegant work of this kind has been done by Helene and associates, who showed the uptake of a fluorescent acridine-linked oligo into trypanosomes (Fig. 5–11).[11] However, there is always some ambiguity in such measurements—the highly aromatic covalently linked group could change the membrane permeability of the oligo, and the fluorescent group could be cleaved from the oligo by nucleases. To address these problems, we have investigated the uptake of fluorescently linked oligos into HL60 cells. A temperature study showed that although the uptake of the acridine linker alone is temperature-independent, that of the linked-oligo is highly temperature-dependent (Fig. 5–12).[12] This suggests an energy-dependent process is involved in the transmembrane transport of oligos; formal proof would require demonstration of intracellular uptake of oligomer against a concentration gradient. Such proof is currently lacking, although the appropriate experiments are in progress.

The suggestion that there is a cell surface receptor for large or small pieces of DNA has recently been

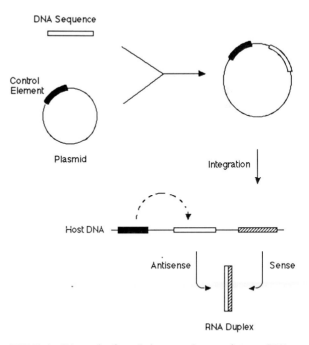

FIG. 5–4 Schematic of translation arrest by an antisense mRNA. Incorporation of the appropriate DNA sequence into a plasmid or other vector is followed by integration into the host DNA, expression of the mRNA sequence antisense to the natural mRNA, and formation of a hybrid duplex.

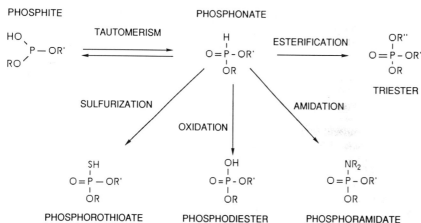

FIG. 5-5 Methods for automated synthesis of oligos. (*A*) Stepwise synthesis producing normal or phosphorothioate oligo at each cycle by oxidation or sulfurization, respectively. Methylphosphonate is likewise formed using a methylphosphonamidite (P-CH$_3$ instead of a P-OCH$_3$ group). (*B*) Single-step processing of the product of hydrogen phosphonate synthesis. Chemical processes can replace the P-H bond to obtain the appropriate products.

oligos are better inhibitors), and the rate of uptake of an oligo was inversely proportional to its length.[12]

These developments regarding the kinetics of cellular uptake of oligos lead to several interesting conclusions. For example, the rate of uptake in cellular systems will most likely be a function of many factors, including the ambient concentration of nucleotide phosphodiesters. This, in turn, will vary with the serum used and the age of the cell culture.

One rationale for using methylphosphonate analogues was that these uncharged molecules should, unlike the normal phosphodiesters, enter cells more effectively.[16] It now appears that these hydrophobic compounds may cross the cell membrane by a passive diffusion process, because they show no competition

for the transport mechanism observed for normal oligos.[12] Thus, the question of cellular uptake may become important in relation to the effectiveness of any particular oligo analogue that is being considered for biologic activity.

Hybridization of Oligos ■

The process of hybridization involves the binding of two complementary base sequences according to the Watson–Crick base-pairing scheme (A with T or U; G with C). For an oligo to be an effective antisense inhibitor, it must be able to hybridize efficiently with its mRNA target to yield an oligo:RNA hybrid. This

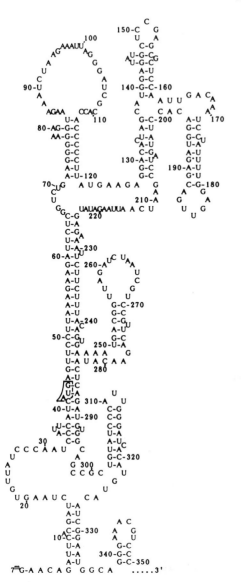

FIG. 5-6   Calculated secondary structure of the 5' 350-nucleotide segment of VSV M mRNA, with the initiation codon (AUG) outlined. Residues 17–31 appear as a single-stranded bulge, and are a potential target for translation arrest. (Wickstrom E et al: Biophys J 49:15–17, 1986)

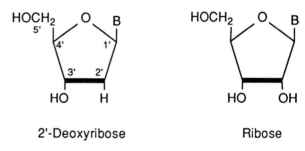

FIG. 5-7   Structure of the carbohydrate components of DNA (2'-deoxyribose), and RNA (ribose). The 2'-hydroxyl group in RNA confers its greater hydrolytic instability.

cific. This can significantly affect the ability of the synthetic analogue to hybridize efficiently with its target, because for an oligo of n internucleotide linkages there will be 2^n stereoisomers. The effect on hybridization will of course depend on the size of the group that is substituted for one of the oxygens of the phosphate group.

The hybridization efficiency can be estimated from the melting temperature (T_m) of the oligo, with either a complementary oligo or a polyribonucleotide present. The T_m is determined from the inflection point of the melting curve generated by measuring a spectroscopic parameter (such as ultraviolet absorption) as a function of temperature (Fig. 5–14A). Some examples of melting curves and T_ms are shown in Figure 5–14B. A sharply defined melting curve with high slope indicates a cooperative two-state transition between a duplex that is stable at low temperature and the single-stranded random coil, which is formed at high temperature. A very low T_m, or a very shallow or broadened melting curve, indicates that a stable duplex is not present (Fig. 5–14A). The T_m is an important measurement to ensure that any particular analogue will be a useful antisense compound.

In α-oligos, their opposite base orientation relative to the sugar gives a novel parallel duplex rather than the usual antiparallel duplex (Fig. 5–15). This apparently results in an even higher T_m for an α–β duplex than the natural β–β duplex,[17] although it does not seem to mean that these analogues are improved antisense inhibitors.

Applications of Oligos as Inhibitors of Gene Expression ■

In this section, we consider the applications of oligos and their analogues in the inhibition of gene expression.[18] This is not an exhaustive survey of the literature, but rather a discussion of examples of appli-

is expected to occur readily for an oligo with normal phosphodiester linkages, but a synthetic analogue may have altered hybridization capability.

When a phosphorus atom has four different groups attached in a tetrahedron, it becomes a chiral center (Fig. 5–13), just like a tetrahedral carbon atom. This results in the possibility of two nonsuperimposable mirror images, or enantiomers. Thus, there are two stereoisomers for each phosphorus atom in a synthetic oligo for which the synthetic method is nonstereospe-

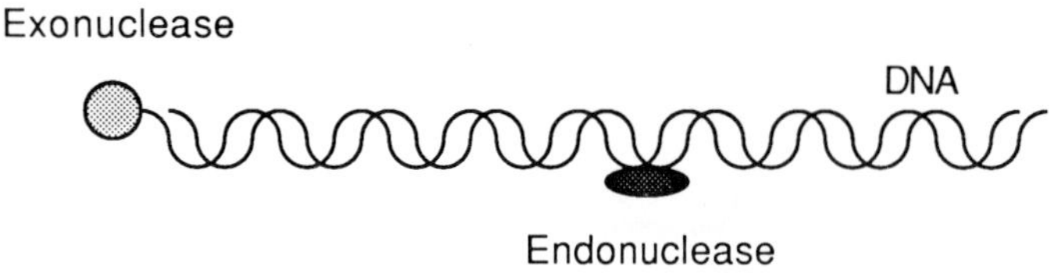

Exonuclease

DNA

Endonuclease

FIG. 5–8 Schematic representation of the function of exonuclease, which cleaves phosphodiester bonds only at the end of a DNA molecule, and of endonuclease, which cleaves anywhere along the length.

cations in each area: cell-free systems, viral systems, and expression of normal cellular genes and oncogenes. Some question may arise as to the relevance of these results, particularly those obtained in cell-free systems, to potential clinical applications. However, the value of systems that permit monitoring of the comparative and quantitative measures of inhibition of expression of a particular gene product should not be underestimated.

Inhibition of Viral Gene Expression ■

The earliest efforts to show inhibition of gene expression by oligos were carried out by Zamecnik and Stephenson.[9,10] These workers, by a laborious manual procedure, synthesized a 13-mer complementary to the reiterated 5'- and 3'-terminal sequences of the Rous sarcoma virus 35S RNA. They assayed the media of infected chick embryo fibroblast cells and found a 99% decrease in reverse transcriptase (RT) activity several days after administering 10 μM of oligomer. No cellular toxicity was observed, and the decreased

RT levels were thought to correlate with decreased cellular transformation. It is important to note that the media used in these studies were heat-treated to destroy nuclease activity.

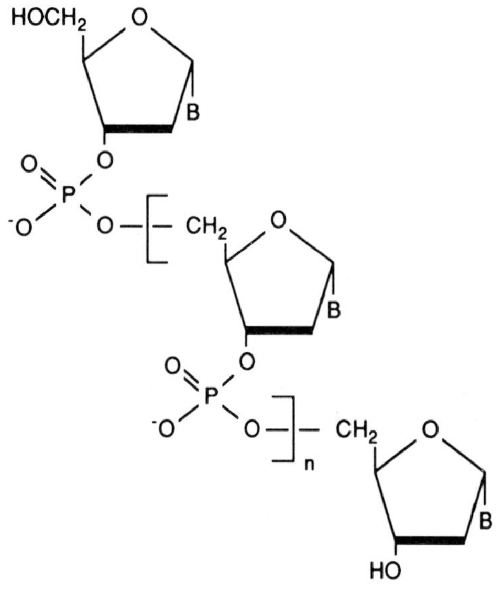

Several years later, Agris and colleagues[19,20] synthesized a series of M-oligos directed against the initiation codon regions of a group of vesicular stomatitis virus (VSV) mRNAs. These messages control the synthesis of a number of viral proteins, known as L, G, NS, N, and M. In infected mouse L-cells, treatment with oligo caused a global decrease in viral protein synthesis and a 10-fold decrease in viral titer. There was no effect on L-cell protein synthesis, nor was there any cytotoxicity. Lemaitre and coworkers[21] synthesized normal oligos with a poly-L-lysine (14 kDa, 66 amino acid residues) covalently attached to the 3' terminus through a morpholine ring. One oligo (a 15-mer) was complementary to the 5' end of an mRNA coding for the VSV N-protein. The other, a 13-mer, was complementary to a sequence located in the middle of the message. The average oligo:lysine molar ratio was 0.5. After incubation of infected L929 cells with oligomer, a dose-dependent reduction of VSV titer was seen with the 5' complementary sequence, whereas no effect was seen with the internally directed sequence. Cellular protein synthesis increased, presumably resulting from a reversal of VSV-induced shutoff of host protein synthesis.

These experiments raise questions regarding the optimal location of targets for inhibitory oligos. The secondary structure for the 5' half of a VSV mRNA was calculated by Wickstrom and colleagues.[4] Nucleotides 17–31 formed a single-strand bulge, and nucleotides 37–46, which contained the initiation co-

FIG. 5–9 Structure of α-oligodeoxynucleotide, in which the orientation of the bases is opposite to the β-configuration of naturally occurring DNA (see Fig. 5–2).

FIG. 5–10 Representation of an oligo (*wavy line*) to which a fluorescent acridine (Acr) derivative is attached by a linker to the terminal 5'-phosphate group. *m* Indicates the number of methylene groups contained in the linker.

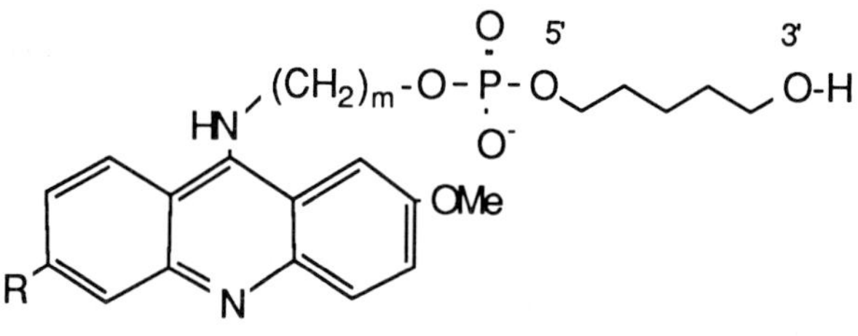

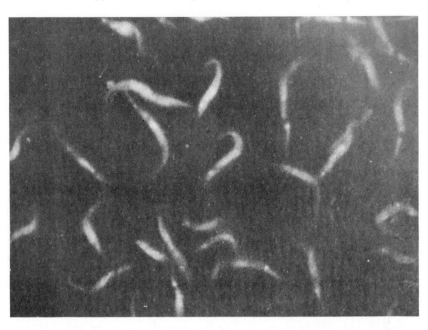

FIG. 5-11   Fluorescence micrograph (1000×) of *Trypanosoma brucei* showing uptake of Acr-linked oligo.[11]

don, formed another, smaller bulge (see Fig. 5–6). An oligo complementary to the former was inhibitory in a translation system and also nonspecifically inhibited Brome mosaic virus mRNA translation in the same system. The issue is clearly one of considerable import, namely, whether or not all messages will have sequences that are accessible to oligos for hybridization, particularly those adjacent to the initiation codon region. It should be remembered that the secondary structures of these mRNAs are based on simple base-pairing and energy-minimization calculations.[22] In addition, the preponderance of evidence indicates that sequences directed against the initiation codon regions are most successful at inhibiting gene expression.

Other viral systems have been studied by Miller, Ts'o, and colleagues, using M-oligos.[23,24] Sequences complementary to the splice junction site of the SV40 large T-antigen produced by infected African green monkey kidney cells were tested. A 6-mer showed

FIG. 5-12   The effect of temperature on the cellular uptake of free acridine and 5'-Acr-dT$_{12}$. Cells were incubated and cellular uptake was analyzed by flow cytometry.[12]

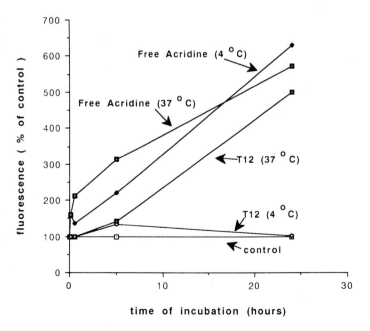

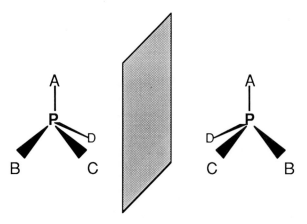

FIG. 5–13 Representation of a chiral tetrahedral phosphorus atom, to which four groups A, B, C, D are attached. The two stereoisomers are mirror images that cannot be superimposed, and therefore are two physically distinct substances.

30% inhibition of antigen production, whereas a 9-mer (25 μM) inhibited production by perhaps as much as 45%.[23] Two 6-mers were constructed that are complementary to the 5'-terminal sequences of U1 RNA (a molecule associated with the splicing of mammalian and viral pre-mRNAs). Again, the production of the large T-antigen was significantly inhibited. These results, while interesting and provocative, are difficult to understand in terms of sequence-specific inhibition, because the T_m of a 6-mer M-oligo–RNA duplex must be less than the assay temperature of 37°.

These authors[24] also synthesized an 8-mer M-oligo complementary to the acceptor splice junction of the HSV type 1 immediate-early pre-mRNAs 4 and 5. Infected Vero cells were incubated with this oligo. Virus titers were decreased one order of magnitude at 75 μM and the effect was dose-dependent, but the decrease was not as dramatic if the oligo was added 1 hour after infection. The synthesis of viral functional and structural proteins was shown to be inhibited, as was virus-fraction DNA, as measured by tritiated thymidine incorporation. The normal cellular DNA fraction was increased; in untreated cells, no labeled cellular DNA could be observed at all.

Inhibition of HIV Gene Expression ∎

In studying HIV, it is important to remember that although the basic antisense strategy presumes interaction of an oligo with the mRNA target, there are several life cycle stages (Fig. 5–16) that might enable hybridization to occur with single-stranded viral spe-

cies (including the viral RNA itself). Thus, one should keep an open mind regarding the potential interaction of oligos with HIV-infected systems. In addition, the presence of RT is an important difference between retroviral and other systems.

Zamecnik and associates[25] recognized that DNA synthesis catalyzed by RT is initiated at the lysine-tRNA primer binding site near the 5' end.[26] They constructed normal oligos complementary to this region, termed (a), as well as to a sequence including the primer binding site and a region 5' to it, (b). In addition, they synthesized oligos complementary to the splice site regions of the pre-mRNA that express the 3' open reading frame. This included both splice acceptor and splice donor sites (c).

The oligos that were complementary to (a) and (b) included: a 12-mer, which contained a 3'-terminal dideoxythymidine (ddT); a 20-mer; and a 26-mer with a 3'-terminal noncomplementary tail of (Poly-A)$_3$. The RT activity and the production of HIV-encoded 15 kDa and 24 kDa proteins (p15 and p24) was examined in H9 cells. Inhibition was noted for all constructs but was most pronounced for a 20-mer complementary to the splice acceptor site for the *tat*-III gene. The concentration of the oligo was 9 μM. The authors note 67% inhibition of RT activity, as well as 95% and 88% inhibition of p15 and p24 levels, respectively. The oligo containing the 3' ddT moiety [(b) category] was not particularly effective in H9 cells, but did have some effect on RT expression when tested in infected peripheral blood cells.

More recently, S-oligos have been shown to be effective inhibitors of HIV gene expression. S-oligos will form stable double-stranded duplexes with RNA, although in each case the T_m will be lower than that of the duplex formed with the normal oligo.[27] This effect is particularly pronounced with S-oligos of <50% GC content. They are nuclease-resistant[27] but not totally inert, being degraded slowly. Their solubilities are similar to those of the normal congeners, and these properties, coupled with their relative ease of preparation, make S-oligos attractive candidates for gene-specific inhibitors. However, as mentioned above, their rate of cellular uptake appears to be quite slow.

In their initial experiments, Matsukura and coworkers[28] synthesized a series of S-oligos complementary to sequences of the *art/trs* (now termed *ren*) genes of HIV (Fig. 5–17). The protein product of the *trs* gene acts posttranscriptionally to increase levels of unspliced viral mRNA and to direct it away from splicing and into the cytoplasm. It also appears to increase the stability of the unspliced message and is essential for viral replication. These researchers ex-

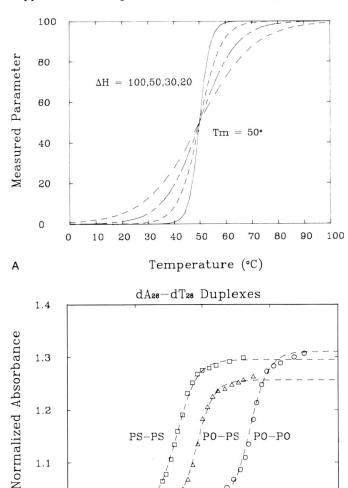

FIG. 5–14 Melting curves of oligodeoxynucleotides. (*A*) Theoretical curves. Duplexes are more stable at low temperature; at high temperature they melt to single-stranded random coils. In between they pass through the melting temperature (T_m; defined as the inflection point at which half of the sample has melted). The examples have $T_m = 50°$. The slope depends on the physical properties of the sample, including the length of the oligo, its concentration, and the salt concentration, and is a measure of the heat of melting (enthalpy, indicated by ΔH). In sharper transitions the melting process is more cooperative and ΔH is higher. In shallower melting curves the process is less cooperative and ΔH is lower. A shallow curve may indicate many melting transitions because of different lengths of oligos, or different stereoisomers in a mixture. (*B*) Examples of experimental melting curves of duplexes $dA_{28} \cdot dT_{28}$ in which both strands are normal (all PO), one strand is all-PS and the other normal, or both strands are all-PS. Note that T_m decreases with substitution of PS for PO, but the slope of the curves remains essentially constant, indicating a good two-state transition. *Dotted lines* are theoretical fits of experimental data for the two-state transition equation.[27]

amined normal as well as M-oligo counterparts to these sequences. ATH8 cells were used as targets for the cytopathic effect inhibition assay of HIV.[29] At 25 μM, a 14-mer S-oligo (ODN-1) complementary to the *art/trs* region inhibited the cytopathic effect of the virus by 95%, compared to 4% and 10% for the normal oligo and the M-oligo, respectively. Similar results were seen with an S-oligo directed 12 nucleotides downstream of the complement of ODN-1. When N-methylthymidine (which cannot form a Watson–Crick base pair with adenosine) was incorporated into ODN-1 instead of thymidine, no anti-HIV activity was observed. This seems to indicate that sequence-specific inhibition is occurring, at least under the operant conditions in this system.

In subsequent experiments with an *art/trs* sequence-specific S-oligo, a somewhat different assay was employed. In this viral expression inhibition assay, chronically HIV-infected and HIV-producing T-cells, which are relatively resistant to the cytopathic effect of HIV, were cultured with or without the S-oligo (usually a 28-mer). On day 5, culture supernatants were assayed for HIV p24 *gag* protein levels by enzyme-linked immunosorbent assay (ELISA) or radioimmunoassay (RIA).[30] A marked diminution in the levels of p24 *gag* protein (from 25 ng/ml to about 5 ng/ml) was seen at an antisense oligo concentration of 10 μM. The effect was highly concentration-dependent. Tritiated thymidine uptake was not affected, indicating little if any cellular cytotoxicity due to the

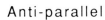

Anti-parallel　　　　Parallel

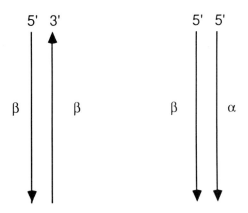

FIG. 5–15 Antiparallel double strand alignment of natural DNA in the β-configuration compared to the unusual parallel alignment of a duplex of strands in both the α- and β-configurations.

S-oligo. Both sense and antisense constructs of normal oligos were entirely ineffective in inhibiting p24 *gag* protein expression, as was an antisense construct to the *gag* message itself. In the presence of this 28-mer antisense S-oligo directed at the *art/trs* region, it was

no longer possible (by Northern blotting) to detect the 9.4 kb genomic mRNA of HIV. Reduction of the viral burden by such an approach may be clinically attractive should sufficient quantities of the oligos become available.

The factors of base composition and chain length were evaluated with the homopolymers dA, dC, and dT in three lengths (Fig. 5–18).[28] Unexpectedly, S-dC_{28} was one of the most potent of all compounds tested, sequence-specific or otherwise. The compound had no measurable cytotoxicity, with virtually 100% inhibition of the viral cytopathic effect at a concentration as low as 5 μM, and substantial protection was still observed at a concentration an order of magnitude lower. Inhibition was also observed for S-dA_{28} and S-dA_{14}, but to a lesser extent. S-dA_5 and S-dC_5, as well as all homo-oligos of T, were ineffective. For both homo-oligos and sequence-specific constructs, longer sequences were, on a molar basis, more effective than shorter ones (28 = 21 > 14 ≫ 5). We observed similar results in Tahr cells infected with caprine encephalitis arthritis virus (Dahlberg and coworkers: Unpublished results).

Matsukura and associates[28] have also shown, by Southern blotting, that S-dC_{28} decreases the *de novo* synthesis of viral DNA at concentrations as low as 1

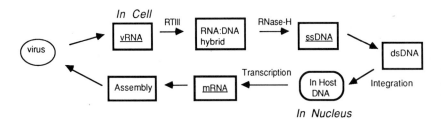

FIG. 5–16 Life cycle of the human immunodeficiency virus (HIV). The single-stranded sites vulnerable to hybridization with an oligo are viral RNA (*vRNA*), single-stranded DNA (*ssDNA*), and messenger RNA (*mRNA*). Double-stranded DNA is labelled *dsDNA*.

FIG. 5–17 Sequences of the coding exon I of the *art/trs* gene of HIV and the oligos used for testing.[28]

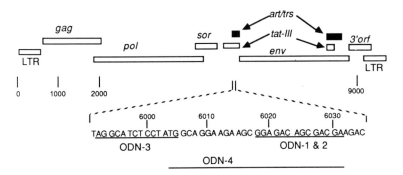

Anti-sense:	ODN-1:	5'-TCG TCG CTG TCT CC-3'
	ODN-3:	5'-CAT AGG AGA TGC CT-3'
	ODN-4:	5'-TCG TCG CTG TCT CCG CTT CTT CCT GCC A-3'
Sense:	ODN-2:	5'-GGA GAC AGC GAC GA-3'
Random:	ODN-5:	5'-CTG GTT CGT CTC CC-3'
	Oligo-dC:	5'-(C)n -3'
	Oligo-dA:	5'-(A)n -3'

μM. S-dC$_{14}$ (5 μM), synergizes with 2',3' dideoxy-adenosine (2 μM) in providing complete protection against the viral cytopathic effect, although each alone was only marginally effective.

Recently, Majumdar and colleagues showed that S-dC$_{28}$ can directly inhibit the RT of HIV, with an inhibition constant (K$_i$) of about 3 nM. The K$_i$ for the normal (all PO) congener is about 800 nM.[32a] The inhibition is noncompetitive, and there appears to be one high-affinity site and a larger number of lower affinity binding sites on the RT molecule. Cytidine homo-oligos that contain alternating blocks (9 individual consecutive PS or PO linkages) placed either at the 5' or 3' ends of the molecule seem to have intermediate inhibitory properties, but tend to behave, with regard to enzyme inhibition, more like the all-PS compound. The effect of oligo length on inhibition is identical to that described by Matsukura and coworkers[28] in the cytopathic effect inhibition assay. Direct inhibition of RT provides a convenient expla-

nation for the effectiveness of these compounds (Fig. 5–19), but it may not be the entire story. As a class, homopyrimidines (*e.g.*, C$_{28}$), are capable of forming triple helices with DNA by non-Watson–Crick base pair formation. Such structures could conceivably form at regulatory sites, with a consequent decrease in synthesis of viral proteins.

S-dC$_{28}$, however, is only one of a class of GC-rich S-oligos that all seem to be equally effective in the cytopathic effect inhibition assay. This class includes, among others, dC$_{21}$, d(GGC)$_7$, d(CCA)$_7$, d(CCT)$_7$, d(5-methyl-C)$_{28}$, and the self-complementary sequence d(GC)$_{10}$G. It is not clear whether all these molecules can directly inhibit RT, and this is currently under evaluation. Finally, we have observed S-dC$_{28}$, in unpublished preliminary experiments, to be a potent inhibitor of DNA α- and γ-polymerases (Gao and colleagues: Unpublished results).

Inhibition of mRNA Expression in Cell-Free and Bacterial Systems ∎

The most commonly used cell-free systems utilize reticulocyte lysate from rabbits or wheat germ. Both suffer from the drawback of artificiality—effects seen

FIG. 5–18 Comparison of anti-HIV activity for three lengths of S-dC and S-dA. The target cells (2 × 10^5 ATH8 cells) were pretreated with the stated concentrations of each oligomer for 16 h and incubated with polybrene for 45 min. Following centrifugation, each set of pelletted cells was exposed to HIV (500 virions per cell) and incubated for 1 h.[28]

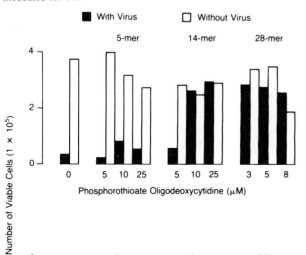

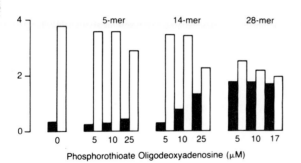

FIG. 5–19 Proposed mechanism of inhibition of HIV gene expression by non-sequence-specific S-oligo. (*A*) Presumed normal function of the reverse transcriptase (RT-III) of HIV, with viral RNA (vRNA) transcribed into viral DNA and broken down by the RNase H activity. (*B*) Supposed effect of S-oligo (S-ODN) in binding to RT-III, presumably at the primer binding site, blocking retrotranscription of the vRNA. Whether nonspecific base pairing between the S-oligo and the vRNA occurs is not known. A distinct antisense mechanism is also operative for sequence-specific S-oligo, but at higher concentrations than the non-sequence-specific mechanism illustrated here.

A. Normal Function

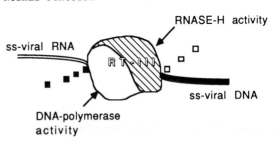

B. In presence of S-ODN

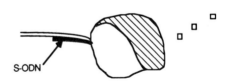

may bear little or no relationship to what actually occurs within living cells. On the other hand, if a particular oligo fails to inhibit mRNA translation in such a system, it is unlikely to do so in cellular systems. Also, the cell-free systems can be used to test large numbers of mRNAs for oligo binding and inhibition.

Miller and coworkers[31,32] synthesized and characterized a variety of antisense M-oligos complementary to sequences in the rabbit globin message and compared their inhibitory effects with the normal congeners. These oligos were complementary to both α- and β-chain regions; most included the AUG initiation site, and some included sequences near the initiation codon. Translation was studied in the reticulocyte lysate and wheat germ systems. A 12-mer (to α 28–39) at 100 μM inhibited 97% of the α-chain and 96% of the β-chain production in the reticulocyte system and 100% of both α and β in the wheat germ system. The inhibition was concentration-dependent, and greatly reduced at 5 μM. Antisense constructs of the area on the 3' side of the initiation codon region had little or no effect at any concentration used. In other experiments, even shorter oligos were found to be inhibitory, including a tetramer at 200 μM complementary to α 37–40, β 54–57. However, a thymidine hexamer and a random sequence had little or no inhibitory effect. The results with the tetramer are difficult to understand in light of the fact that the T_m of the putative M-oligo–RNA duplex is much less than 37°. M-oligos were no more effective at translation inhibition in these systems than were normal oligos.

One advantage to the use of M-oligos as inhibitors of gene expression is that the compounds are uncharged, nonpolar, and presumably enter cells by passive diffusion. Because of their enhanced lipophilicity, they are presumably soluble in intracellular lipid particles and membranes. However, M-oligos of more than 12 bases in length are virtually insoluble in water. This problem has been circumvented by incorporating polar 5'- or 3'-terminal phosphates or phosphodiester linkages, but it is unclear how this will affect the kinetics of cellular uptake. M-oligos are also difficult to synthesize in high yield (usually about 50% of the yield of a normal oligo). Further, steric hindrance caused by the methyl group contributes to destabilization of the double helix,[33] and to a decrease in T_m. These factors may explain in part why M-oligos usually require high concentrations to achieve their maximum effect.

Marcus-Sekura and associates[34] studied a plasmid containing the gene for expression of the enzyme chloramphenicol acetyl transferase (CAT) in bacteria.

Normal oligos, M-oligos, and S-oligos were compared for their effectiveness in inhibiting CAT activity. An S-oligo (30 μM) was most effective, followed by the M-oligo, with the normal oligo being minimally effective. All the 15-mers used included complementary sequences to the initiation region. In contrast to the results of Matsukura and coworkers,[28] an N-methyl-thymidine S-oligo also produced a significant inhibition of CAT activity. Eckstein and others[6,35] have shown that phosphorothioate nucleotides can inhibit a variety of enzymes, particularly nucleases. These facts, in addition to the recently observed noncompetitive inhibition of RT and inhibition of DNA α- and γ-polymerase, imply that S-oligos may interact with a host of cellular enzymes, as well as with specific nucleic acid sequences.

At the present time, it is not known with certainty whether M-oligos or S-oligos are more effective as synthetic analogues. In some systems, each class is effective, whereas in others, neither is effective. It may emerge that they are in fact complementary: M-oligos do not appear to use the same cellular uptake mechanism as do normal or S-oligos, and probably enter cells rapidly by diffusion. S-oligos are taken up slowly by cells, but far lower concentrations are needed. Combining the two in the same experiment might yield interesting data.

Oligos with Covalently Linked Groups ■

Helene and coworkers have synthesized oligos that have had organic molecules attached to either their 3' or 5' ends. Initially, these were preponderantly acridine derivatives, which were not only fluorescent but also intercalated into a double-stranded structure (Fig. 5–20). Intercalation stabilizes the double-stranded structure (increases the T_m), and theoretically allows a shorter oligo to be used for inhibition of gene expression. However, the shorter the oligo, the less the sequence specificity.

Asseline and associates[36] prepared a series of oligos of the type $(Tp)_n(CH_2)_mAcr$, where the acridine is linked at the 3' end of the molecule, and m = 5 or 6, and found a large increment in T_m for the acridine-linked compounds. This effect diminishes with increasing oligo length. Toulme and colleagues,[37] using this approach, synthesized oligos complementary to the UUAAA triple tandem repeat sequences contained in a specific mRNA from phage T4 (r_1 = UUAAA, r_2 = UUAAAUUAAA, r_3 = UUAAAUUAAAUUAAA). Each oligo contained a covalently linked 3'-acridine (Acr) derivative. r_3-Acr was the most effective construct in inhibiting protein syn-

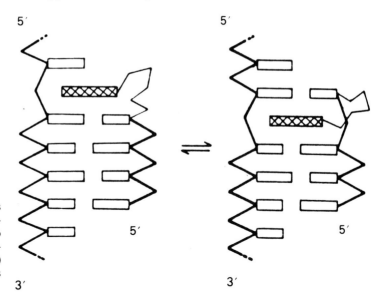

5′   5′

⇌

5′   5′

FIG. 5–20 Representation of the complexes formed when a planar ring molecule such as an acridine (*hashed box*) is covalently linked to an oligo that forms a duplex with its complement. The acridine can either stack on top of the last base pair (*left*) or can intercalate between adjacent base pairs (*right*).[38]

3′   3′

thesis in a cell-free system (78% decrease, as compared to 35% in the presence of r_3 alone). The order of inhibition was r_1-Acr $<$ r_2-Acr $<$ r_3-Acr, which parallels the orders of melting temperatures, although the T_m difference between r_3 and r_3-Acr is only 4°C. Higher concentrations of acridine alone also inhibited translation. Similar observations have been made in other systems.[38] Parenthetically, these types of molecules may, in a cell-free system, be directed against the common 5′ terminal sequences found in all *Trypanosoma brucei* mRNAs.[11,39,40] When used against cultured trypanosomes, an acridine-linked sequence-specific nonamer was lethal to the parasite.

This work was expanded on by Cazenave and co-workers,[41] who synthesized a variety of oligos with acridine linked at the 3′ end. These oligos were directed against various sequences in the rabbit globin mRNA, and the oligo plus the message was then injected into frog oocytes. An 11-mer complementary to globin sequence 44–54 could be shown to inhibit β-globin synthesis by 50%. Injections of acridine alone, at the same concentration (50 μM), and of the oligo without the acridine were ineffective. This last observation was explained in light of the increased T_m for the acridine-linked species (36°) versus the unlinked 11-mer (31°). In the wheat germ system, however, although the Acr-11-mer at 1 μM decreased β-globin synthesis by 90%, the acridine derivative was no more effective at translation inhibition. The differences in the frog oocyte and wheat germ systems forced the authors to conclude that perhaps duplex stability was not as important as they initially sup-

posed. α-Oligos have also been linked to an intercalating group.[42] These molecules were shown to be highly nuclease-resistant. Both linked and unlinked α-oligos formed more stable duplexes with ribopolymers than did β-DNA.

The group of Knorre, Vlassov, Zarytova, and co-workers have developed several new synthetic methods for linking organic groups to either the 3′ or 5′ termini of oligonucleotides.[43] They also describe molecules with both 3′- and 5′-linked groups (Fig. 5–21). Oligos of different lengths (14-, 12-, 10-, 8-, and 6-mers) were directed against positions 261–274 of the sequence of the tick-borne encephalitis virus.[44] At the 5′ end, the alkylating group N-(2-chloroethylamine) was attached, while an intercalating phenazine ring was covalently bound to the 3′ end. For comparative purposes, a series of oligos of similar length were synthesized that contained only the alkylator, placed at either the 5′ or 3′ end. In experiments using the 5′ alkylator, the first nucleotide adjacent to the DNA–RNA duplex was the predominant site of alkylation. When 3′-linked alkylators were employed, the site of alkylation was somewhat more diffuse, and included a guanosine residue 80 nucleotides from the target site. The authors suggested that this residue may abut the target site due to secondary structure.

Addition of an intercalating capacity by the presence of a phenazine ring increased the stability of the duplexes. Thus, the authors were able to show that even 6- and 8-mers were capable of alkylating the DNA fragment, and of doing so with high efficiency even at 40°. In these experiments, however, small

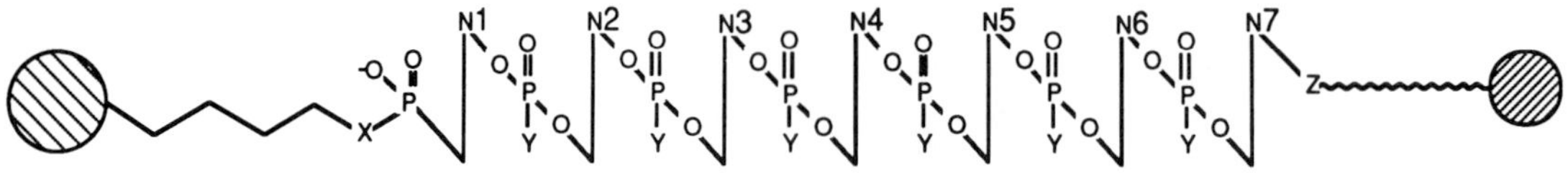

FIG. 5-21 Representation of an oligo with different groups linked at the 3′ and 5′ ends. The linkages can be by phosphate (PO), phosphoramidate (PN), or phosphonate bonds (PC). The two groups can be intercalating groups, reactive groups (such as an EDTA moiety), or an alkylator.

amounts of products modified at other positions both upstream and downstream were also seen.

A modified base alkylator was synthesized by Webb and Matteucci.[45] They prepared 5-methyl-N4,N4-ethanocytosine, incorporated it into an oligo, and showed that the complementary strand would be alkylated on hybridization. Unfortunately, their synthesis is not trivial, and the entire process is not very efficient.

Mechanisms of Action of Oligos ■

A fascinating attempt to understand some of the mechanisms of inhibition of translation by oligos was made by Haeuptle and colleagues.[46] In an *in vitro* system, chicken lysozyme mRNA was transcribed from a plasmid. The transcribed message was translated in the wheat germ system in the presence or absence of a 5-, 10-, 15-, or 20-mer complementary to the mRNA sequence immediately adjacent to the 3′ side of the unique SstI restriction site. The 5-mer was unable to arrest translation; the others gave rise to truncated polypeptides. In addition, for each oligo, only one species of truncated polypeptide was observed. The authors favored the idea that ribosomes coming upon the blocked site may dissociate. This might allow the tailing ribosomes to continue translating until the blocked site is reached, causing repeated cycles of initiation and elongation. The position of the oligo with regard to the reading frame was unimportant, as oligos complementary to all three positions of the reading frame arrested translation. In all cases, only truncated polypeptides were synthesized.

These authors also constructed an Ii-CAT fusion protein that consisted of two fragments of the human invariant chain (209 amino acids each) fused out of frame to the CAT protein so that protein synthesis was terminated after 62 amino acids. (The human invariant chain is a structural protein that has been associated with the MHC locus.) An oligo was constructed that was complementary to the 3′ end of the Ii fragment. The fully arrested peptide is one Ii unit

(Ii-1). The first read-through product is an in-tandem Ii-Ii dimer (Ii-2). The full-fusion protein requires read-through of these two blocks. When the experiment was performed, it was found that Ii-1 was the predominant product. The Ii-2 product was seen in smaller amounts, but the double-read-through product was not seen at all. These experiments were performed in the wheat germ system; in the reticulocyte lysate system, 50% of the translated products were full-length polypeptides.

Cazenave and coworkers,[41] using the wheat germ system and sequences complementary to rabbit β-globin message, found that hybridization led to loss of intact mRNA. Shorter mRNA fragments were seen by Northern blotting. For example, when a 17-mer complementary to the 3–19 base sequence was employed, an mRNA shortened by some 60 nucleotides relative to the native message was observed. A 500-nucleotide mRNA fragment was detected by a probe complementary to the 3′ end of the β-globin message following incubation with a 17-mer complementary to the sequence 113–129. In the frog oocyte system, injection of a mixture of this 17-mer with rabbit β-globin message led to a slow decrease of the intact message with time. No fragments were observed; the authors suggest this may be due to the rapid degradation of fragments inside the oocyte. Similar results were observed when acridine was end-linked to the oligo. Therefore, RNase H activity, which cleaves the mRNA strand of the RNA–DNA duplex (Fig. 5–22), may explain the so-called translation arrest effect of oligos. As the level of RNase H activity varies in test systems, so may the inhibitory ability of exogenous oligos. This may further complicate variability due to other factors, including different intrinsic rates of

FIG. 5-22 Diagram of RNase H activity. The RNA molecule is cleaved (*arrow*) where a DNA · RNA duplex is formed, in this case with an S-oligo.

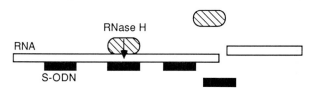

cellular uptake, the availability for binding of appropriate sites on the message, the presence of blocking materials in the extracellular media (*e.g.*, nucleotide 5' monophosphates), and the effectiveness of any nucleases present.

Oligos and Cancer ■

To inhibit the growth of malignant cells, there are several strategies that employ sequence-specific oligos. For example, a variety of cancers are sensitive to methotrexate, which exerts its antineoplastic effects by inhibition of the enzyme dihydrofolate reductase. Unfortunately, cancer cells invariably become resistant to the effects of the drug with time. Maher and Dolnick[47] constructed normal oligos (11- to 20-mers) complementary to the 5' end of the dihydrofolate reductase (DHFR) mRNA. A 5-fold reduction in the synthesis of DHFR was observed in the reticulocyte lysate system at an oligo concentration of 200 μM. In-tandem contiguous oligos seemed to inhibit translation better than each alone, and two contiguous 14-mers, each at 25 μM, inhibited translation as did a 20-mer complementary to the same region at 200 μM. These results are provocative, but may not be applicable to a cellular system because of the kinetics of uptake. Messages related to multi-drug resistance may be particularly attractive choices with respect to inhibition of expression by oligos.

Neckers and coworkers have recently been using oligos to inhibit the expression of oncogenes. They have focused their efforts on the c-*myc* oncogene and have constructed a 15-mer complementary to the initiation codon region.[48] Employing normal T-lymphocytes, they noted that the oligo inhibited mitogen-induced c-*myc* protein expression and prevented the cells from entering S phase. Transcriptional activation of either the IL-2 or transferrin receptor genes was not affected. In HL60 cells, a line that contains a 16–20-fold amplification of c-*myc* mRNA levels, a dose- and time-dependent decrease in c-*myc* protein levels was observed.[49] With the normal oligos, this effect was noted within hours and persisted for 24–36 hours. Similar conclusions with regard to the normal oligo were also reached by Wickstrom and associates,[50] although at far lower concentrations of oligo. Holt and associates[51] noted phenotypic differentiation in HL60 cells treated with a 15-mer at a concentration of 4 μM. These authors detected an S1 nuclease-resistant dimer whose length corresponded to that of a 15-mer, indicating intracellular duplex formation.

Parallel c-*myc* inhibition studies with an analogous antisense S-oligo 15-mer found variable results when the oligo was added to the cell supernatant, but when it was added in liposomes, consistent c-*myc* inhibition was observed (although this was greatly reduced after 24 hours; Fig. 5–23).[52] This antisense S-oligo also inhibited DNA synthesis and cell growth. Empty liposomes, or those containing non-sense oligos, were in-

FIG. 5–23 Inhibition of c-*myc* gene expression by a 15-mer S-oligo. Fluorescence activated cell sorter analysis of c-*myc* protein content of a population of cells (fused with liposomes containing either no oligo, non-sense S-oligo, or antisense S-oligo) is shown as a function of time.[52]

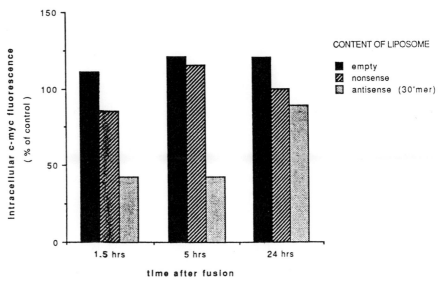

effective. However, this work is still in its preliminary phases.

In studies of the *ras* oncogene in a cell-free system, Cheng and colleagues[53] have observed that S-oligos are more effective than normal or M-oligos in inhibiting *ras* expression, although they found that the effect was relatively non-sequence-specific except at very low concentrations of antisense S-oligo.

Toward a New Chemotherapy? ■

As discussed above, only a few chemically modified oligo analogues have been used to selectively inhibit gene expression: phosphotriesters, methylphosphonates, phosphorothioates, and α-oligos. Many other chemical analogues can be conceived (such as the seleno-phosphate oligos[7]; Mori and coworkers: Unpublished results), but consideration of these four structures leads to several conclusions:

Ethyl phosphotriesters are readily deesterified enzymatically,[16] which might be an advantage as a prodrug if the normal oligo product is not broken down too readily. (A less hydrolyzable phosphotriester, such as tBu, might be useful in this respect.)
Methylphosphonates are difficult to synthesize, and the steric hindrance of the methyl group apparently causes major lowering of the T_m; these compounds are also relatively insoluble in water with $n > 10$.
Phosphorothioates are a relatively conservative substitution at P that appear to provide the highest potency in inhibition of HIV[28] and also inhibit an oncogene by an antisense mechanism,[49] but they

appear to be transported across the cell membrane more slowly than normal oligos.[12]
The α-oligos would be very expensive to produce, given that the synthesis has to start at the nucleoside level, and although they give parallel rather than antiparallel duplexes with normal β-DNA, the duplexes with RNA are not susceptible to RNase H cleavage.[54,55]

Many other chemical modifications of the phosphate group are possible in oligos: alkylated-thio (P-SR); hydrogen phosphonate, which might be expected to be reactive and oxidized *in vivo;* bridging methylenephosphonate (P-CH$_2$-R) linked to the 3' or 5' position of deoxyribose in place of the normal ester bonds, which might be less sterically hindering than the nonbridging methylphosphonate but is much harder to synthesize; or combinations of modifications. However, all of these would probably decrease the hybridizability and increase the difficulty of synthesis (and cost) of these compounds. Another approach could alternate normal phosphodiester and modified groups singly or as block copolymers (Fig. 5–24). This would have the virtue of increasing the potency without decreasing the hybridizability of the putative antimessenger drug molecule.

Attachment of active groups provides a means to expand the function of an oligo drug. As indicated above, only a few such substances have actually been synthesized to date, starting with the intercalators of Helene and coworkers[36] and extending to the reactive radical-producing groups, such as EDTA-Fe(II).[56,57] However, it was found that an EDTA-attached oligo is transported very slowly across the cell membrane.[12] Thus, the potential value of the reactivity of such

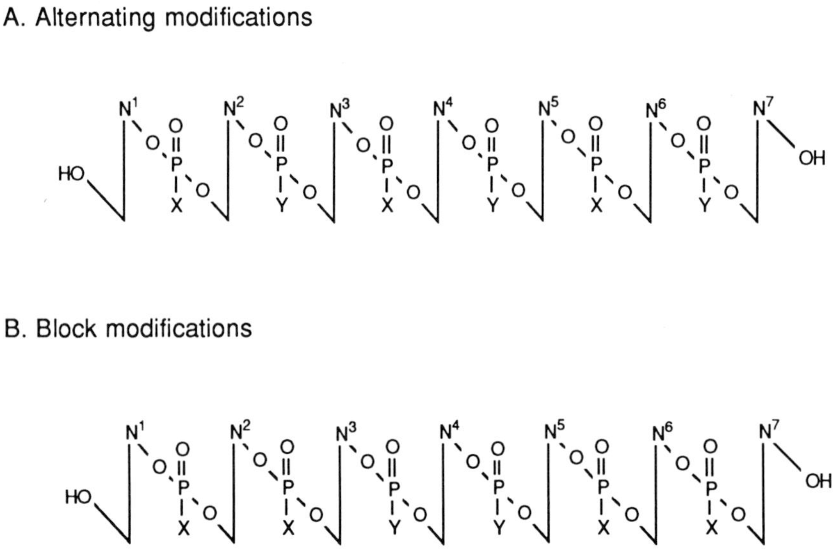

A. Alternating modifications

B. Block modifications

FIG. 5–24   Possible chemical structures of oligos. (*A*) Alternate modified phosphate groups (X, Y); (*B*) block modifications. Modifications can also be restricted to 3' or 5' termini to reduce exonuclease activity.

groups must be tested for all the required drug properties. One of these properties is the need for nuclease resistance, and a combination of a S-oligo with a linked group is a specific goal that has recently been achieved.[12] Another molecule that has been attached to a normal oligo is a protein[58] (Fig. 5–25). This approach provides an interesting, if technically difficult, way of linking a nuclease activity to an oligo of specific sequence, and, in effect, converting a DNA molecule into an enzyme that could selectively destroy its own complement DNA or RNA. Unfortunately, such a combined oligo-protein might also be expected to have greatly reduced cell transport rates, as well as being more expensive to produce. Another means of obtaining an oligo-nuclease activity would be to attach a hydrolytic group to the oligo. Experiments to realize this are under way in our laboratory, notably with the attachment of imidazole, which is known to be a major hydrolytic group in RNase activity.[59]

To improve the cellular uptake of these potential drug molecules, it might be possible to attach other chemical groups designed specifically for this purpose, such as a poly-lysine[21] or a detergent group that could assist the oligo in "punching" its way through the cellular membrane. However, the latter might be too general a property to allow for the desired specificity. Other possibilities include a specific surface receptor group that could be hydrolyzable once the oligo reaches the cell surface. This receptor group could be designed to increase the rate of oligo uptake if it is related to the properties of the transport mechanism for oligos, now being characterized.[12]

A further relevant area of specific interaction involves chemical specificity with double-stranded DNA. Dervan has "engineered" some very interesting drugs that are designed to bind to the major or minor groove of double-standed B-form DNA.[60] It should be possible to link such compounds to oligos to obtain interesting, potentially biologically active compounds. Combining the binding capacity of a specific base sequence with a joined group that would attach to the chosen groove of either DNA or RNA could form a stable complex or a chemically active drug species.

It is known that oligo-pyrimidines bind to poly-purine-rich sequences of double-standed DNA, and this has been used to study the selective breakdown of double-stranded DNA by EDTA-[61] or azidopro-flavine-[62]linked oligo-pyrimidines. This is similar to the use of an oligo with an attached reactive group to attack its complementary strand, as has been done with alkylating agents,[47] EDTA,[44,45,63] phenanthro-line-copper (II) complexes,[64] and iron porphyrins.[65] But in this case, the oligo is designed to bind to double-stranded DNA to form a triple helix (Fig. 5–26).

Other classes of potential nuclease-resistant oligos include sugar-modified analogues, as well as simpler chemical substances. An example is internucleoside linkages that are not phosphodiesters but may be based on carboxyl esters.[66]

Conclusion ■

Although the above discussion is speculative, and its direct application to anticancer drugs is as yet unclear, it is based on firm observations. These suggest that specific sequence oligos that have value in studies on the mechanisms of cellular processes may also have

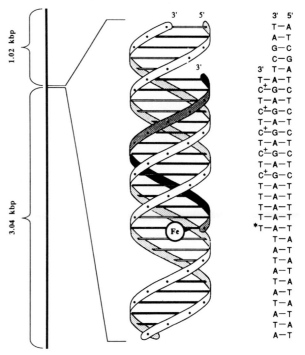

FIG. 5–26   Triple helix formation between double-stranded DNA (in the B-form) and an oligo with an EDTA group attached to the 5′ end. *Left:* the point of cleavage of the plasmid DNA, due to chemical reaction of the EDTA moiety with Fe(II) ions. *Right:* the actual base sequences employed (C^+–G–C represent base tripling with a protonated cytidine).[60]

FIG. 5–25   Attachment of a protein, staphylococcal nuclease, by a disulfide bond to an oligo. The linker is attached to the 3′-terminal nucleotide by a 3′-sulfur bond.[58]

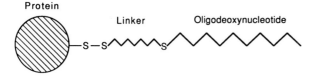

potential therapeutic properties. Before these properties can be realized, much more research is necessary. Areas of interest that must be elucidated before human studies can be conducted include novel chemical synthesis and purification methods, biochemical and cellular testing for desired specific drug effects, and biologic testing (including necessary pharmacologic and toxicologic testing). This also presumes that the methods of synthesis for such complex compounds can be scaled up to the range required for drug production (*i.e.,* gram and kilogram quantities).[66] New methods of chemical and microbiologic synthesis of such compounds are now being considered. It is hoped that the vast range of potential molecular architecture possible in an oligo will in the future be exploited for the development of a range of potential anticancer drugs.

References ■

1. Green PJ, Pines O, Inouye M: The role of antisense RNA in gene regulation. Annu Rev Biochem 55:569–97, 1986
2. Caruthers MH: Gene synthesis machines: DNA chemistry and its uses. Science 230:281–285, 1985
3. Froehler BC, Ng PG, Matteucci MD: Synthesis of DNA via deoxynucleoside H-phosphonate. Nucleic Acids Res 14:5399–5407, 1986
4. Wickstrom E, Somonet W, Medlock K, Ruiz-Robles I: Complementary oligonucleotide probe of vesicular stomatitis virus matrix protein mRNA translation. Biophys J 49:15–17, 1986
5. Murakami A, Blake K, Miller PS: Characterization of sequence-specific oligodeoxynucleoside methylphosphonates and their interaction with rabbit globin mRNA. Biochemistry 24:4041–4046, 1985
6. Eckstein F: Investigation of enzyme mechanisms with nucleoside phosphorothioates. Anal Biochem, 1985
7. Stec W, Zon G, Egan V, Stec B: Automated solid-phase synthesis, separation and stereochemistry of phosphorothioate analogues of oligodeoxyribonucleotides. J Am Chem Soc 106:6077–6079, 1984
8. Morvan F, Rayner B, Imbach JL et al: α-DNAII: Synthesis of unnatural α-anomeric oligodeoxyribonucleotides containing the four usual bases and study of their substrate activity for nucleases. Nucleic Acids Res 15:3421–3437, 1987
9. Zamecnik P, Stephenson M: Inhibition of Rous sarcoma virus replication and cell transformation by a specific oligodeoxynucleotide. Proc Natl Acad Sci USA 75:280–284, 1978
10. Stephenson M, Zamecnik P: Inhibition of Rous sarcoma viral RNA translation by a specific oligodeoxyribonucleotide. Proc Natl Acad Sci USA 75:285–288, 1978
11. Verspieren P, Cornellisen AWCA, Thuong T, Helene C, Toulme JJ: An acridine-linked oligodeoxynucleotide targeted to the common 5' end of trypanosome mRNAs kills cultured parasites. Gene 61:307–315, 1988
12. Stein CA, Mori K, Loke SL et al: Phosphorothioate and normal oligodeoxynucleotides with 5'-linked acridine: Characterization and preliminary kinetics of cellular uptake. Gene 72:333–342, 1988
13. Neale GAM, Mitchell A, Finch LR: Uptake and utilization of deoxynucleoside 5'-monophosphates by *Mycoplasma mycoides.* J Bacteriol 158:943–947, 1984
14. Ruby EG, McCabe JB, Barke JI: Uptake of intact nucleoside monophosphates by *Bdellovibrio bacteriovorus* 109J. J Bacteriol 163:1087–1094, 1985
15. Bennett RM, Kotzin BL, Merritt MJ: DNA receptor dysfunction in systemic lupus erythematosus and kindred disorders. J Exp Med 166:850–863, 1987
16. Miller P, McParland K, Jayaraman K, Ts'o P: Biochemical and biological effects of nonionic nucleic acid methylphosphonates. Biochemistry 20:1874–1880, 1981
17. Morvan F, Rayner B, Imbach JL, Chang DK, Lown JW: α-DNA I: Synthesis, characterization by high field 1H NMR, and base-pairing properties of the unnatural hexadeoxyribonucleotides α[dCCTTCC] with its complement β[GGAAGG]. Nucleic Acids Res 14:5019–5032, 1986
18. Stein CA, Cohen JS: Oligodeoxynucletides as inhibitors of gene expression: A review. Cancer Res 48:2659–2668, 1988
19. Miller PS, Agris C, Blake K et al: Nonionic oligonucleotide analogs as new tools for studies on the structure and function of nucleic acids inside living cells, In Pullman B and Jortner J (eds): Nucleic Acids: The Vectors of Life, pp 521–535. Boston, D. Reidel, 1983
20. Agris CH, Blake K, Miller P, Reddy M, Ts'o P: Inhibition of vesicular stomatitis virus protein synthesis and infection by sequence-specific oligodeoxyribonucleoside methylphosphonates. Biochemistry 25:6268–6275, 1986
21. Lemaitre M, Bayard B, Lebleu B: Specific antiviral activity of a poly(L-lysine)-conjugated oligodeoxyribonucleotide sequence complementary to vesicular stomatitis virus N protein mRNA initiation site. Biochemistry 84:648–652, 1987
22. Jacobson AB, Good L, Simonetti J, Zucker M: Some simple computational methods to improve the folding of large RNAs. Nucleic Acids Res 12:45–52, 1984
23. Miller PS, Agris C, Aurelian L et al: Control of ribonucleic acid function by oligonucleoside methylphosphonates. Biochemie 67:769–776, 1985
24. Smith C, Aurelian L, Reddy M, Miller P, Ts'o P: Antiviral effect of an oligo (nucleoside methylphosphonate) complementary to the splice junction of herpes simplex virus type 1 immediate early pre-mRNAs 4 and 5. Proc Natl Acad Sci USA 83:2787–2791, 1986
25. Zamecnik PC, Goodchild J, Yaguchi Y, Sarin P: Inhibition of replication and expression of human T-cell lymphotropic virus type III in cultured cells by exogenous synthetic oligonucleotides complementary to viral RNA. Proc Natl Acad Sci USA 83:4143–4146, 1986
26. Goodchild J, Letsinger RL, Sarin PS, Zamecnik M, Zamecnik P: Inhibition of replication and expression of HIV-1 tissue culture by oligodeoxynucleotide hybridization competition. Human Retroviruses, Cancer, and AIDS 1988:423–438
27. Stein CA, Subasinghe C, Shinozuka K, Cohen JS: Physicochemical properties of phosphorothioate oligodeoxynucleotides. Nucleic Acids Res 16:3209–3221, 1988
28. Matsukura M, Shinozuka K, Zon G et al: Phosphorothionate analogs of oligodeoxynucleotides: Novel inhibitors of replication and cytopathic effects of human immunodeficiency virus (HIV). Proc Natl Acad Sci USA 84:7706–7710, 1987
29. Mitsuya H, Broder S: Inhibition of in vitro infectivity and cytopathic effect of HTLV-III/LAV by 2',3'-dideoxynucleosides. Proc Natl Acad Sci USA 83:191–1915, 1986
30. Matsukura M, Zon G, Shinozuka K et al: Phosphorothioate oligodeoxynucleotides as inhibitors of the replication of HIV. Gene 72:343–348, 1988
31. Blake K, Murakami A, Miller PS: Inhibition of rabbit globin mRNA translation by sequence-specific oligodeoxyribonucleotides. Biochemistry 24:6132–6138, 1985
32. Blake K, Murakami A, Spitz S et al: Hybridization arrest of globin synthesis in rabbit reticulocyte lysates and cells by oli-

godeoxyribonucleoside methylphosphonates. Biochemistry 24: 6139–6145, 1985

32a. Majumdar C, Stein CA, Subasinghe S, Cohen JS, Broder S, Wilson S: Studies on the mechanism of HIV reverse transcriptase: Primer recognition as revealed by phosphorothioate oligodeoxynucleotides. Biochem (in press)

33. Bower M, Summers MF, Powell C et al: Oligodeoxyribonucleotide methylphosphonates: NMR and UV spectroscopic studies of Rp-Rp and Sp-Sp methylphosphonate modified duplexes of d[GGAATTCC]. Nucleic Acids Res 15:4915–4930, 1987

34. Marcus-Sekura C, Woerner A, Shinozuka K, Zon G, Quinnas G: Comparative inhibition of chloramphenicol expression by antisense oligonucleotide analogs having alkylphosphotriester, methylphosphonate, and phosphorothioate linkages. Nucleic Acids Res 15:5749–5763, 1987

35. Ott J, Eckstein F: Protection of oligonucleotide primers against degradation by DNA polymerase I. Biochemistry 26:8237–8241, 1987

36. Asseline U, Delarue M, Lancelot G et al: Nucleic acid-binding molecules with high affinity and base sequence specificity: Intercalation agents covalently linked to oligodeoxynucleotides. Proc Natl Acad Sci USA 81:3297–3301, 1984

37. Toulme J, Krisch H, Loreau N, Helene C: Specific inhibition of mRNA translation by complementary oligonucleotides covalently linked to intercalating agents. Proc Natl Acad Sci USA 83:1227–1231, 1986

38. Helene C, Montenay-Garestier T, Saison T et al: Oligodeoxynucleotide covalently linked to intercalating agents: A new class of gene regulatory substances. Biochemie 67:777–783, 1985

39. Cornelissen A, Verspieren M, Toulme JJ, Swinkels B, Bobst P: The common 5' terminal sequence on trypanosome mRNAs: A target for anti-messenger oligodeoxynucleotides. Nucleic Acids Res 14:5605–5614, 1986

40. Walder JA, Eder PS, Engman et al: The 35-nucleotide spliced leader sequence is common to all trypanosome mRNAs. Science 233:569–571, 1986

41. Cazenave C, Loreau N, Thuong NT, Toulme JJ, Helene C: Enzymatic amplification of translation inhibition of rabbit β-globin mRNA mediated by anti-message oligodeoxynucleotides covalently linked to intercalating agents. Nucleic Acids Res 15: 4717–4736, 1987

42. Thuong NT, Asseline U, Roig V, Takasugi M, Helene C: Oligo (α-deoxynucleotides) covalently linked to intercalating agents: Differential binding to ribo- and deoxyribo-polynucleotides and stability towards nuclease digestion. Proc Natl Acad Sci USA 84:5129–5133, 1987

43. Knorre D, Vlassov V, Zarytova V: Reactive oligonucleotide derivatives and sequence-specific modification of nucleic acids. Biochemie 67:785–789, 1985

44. Vlassov V, Zarytova V, Kutiavin I, Mamaev S, Podyminogen M: Complementary addressed modification and cleavage of a single stranded DNA fragment with alkylating oligonucleotide derivatives. Nucleic Acids Res 14:4065–4076, 1986

45. Webb TR, Matteucci MD: Hybridization triggered cross-linking of deoxyoligonucleotides. Nucleic Acids Res 14:7661–7674, 1986

46. Haeuple M, Frank R, Dobberstein B: Translation arrest by oligodeoxynucleotides complementary to mRNA coding sequences yields polypeptides of predetermined length. Nucleic Acids Res 14:1427–1448, 1986

47. Maher L, Dolnick B: Specific hybridization arrest of dihydrofolate reductase mRNA in vitro using anti-sense RNA or anti-sense oligonucleotides. Arch Biochem Biophys 253:214–220, 1987

48. Heikkila R, Schwab G, Wickstrom E et al: The role of c-myc in lymphocyte proliferation: Inhibition of S phase entry but not G_0 to G_1 traversal by a c-myc antisense oligodeoxynucleotide. Nature 328:445–449, 1987

49. Loke SL, Stein CA, Cohen JS, Jaffe E, Neckers LM: Role of c-myc in HL-60 growth and differentiation: Studies with oligodeoxynucleotides complementary to c-myc mRNA (abstr). Leukemia Society of America, March 16–19, 1988

50. Wickstrom EL, Bacon TA, Gonzalez A, Freeman DL, Lyman GH, Wickstrom E: Human promyelocytic leukemia HL-60 cell proliferation and c-myc protein expression are inhibited by an antisense pentadecanucleotide targeted against c-myc mRNA. Proc Natl Acad Sci USA 85:1028–1032, 1988

51. Holt JT, Redner RL, Nienhuis AW: An oligomer complementary to c-myc mRNA inhibits proliferation of HL-60 promyelocytic cells and induces differentiation. Molec Cell Biol 8:963–973, 1988

52. Loke SL, Stein CA, Zhang X, Avigan M, Cohen JS, Neckers LM: Delivery of c-myc antisense phosphorothioate oligodeoxynucletide to hematopoeitic cells in culture by liposomes. Curr Topics Microbiol Immunol (in press)

53. Cheng L, Zon G et al: Inhibition of ras oncogene by oligos in cell free system. Unpublished results, 1988

54. Gagnor C, Bertrand JR, Thenet S et al: α-DNA VI: comparative study of α- and β-anomeric oligodeoxynucleotides in hybridization to mRNA and in cell free translation inhibition. Nucleic Acids Res 15:10419–10436, 1988

55. Cazenave C, Chevrier M, Thuong T, Helene C: Rate of degradation of [α-] and [β-]oligodeoxynucleotides in Xenopus oocytes. Implications for anti-messenger strategies. Nucleic Acids Res 15:10507–10521, 1987

56. Boutorin A, Vlassov V, Kazakov S, Kutiavin I, Podyminogen M: Complementary addressed reagents carrying EDTA-Fe(II) groups for directed cleavage of single-stranded nucleic acids. FEBS Lett 172:43–46, 1984

57. Dreyer G, Dervan P: Sequence-specific cleavage of single-stranded DNA: Oligodeoxynucleotide-EDTA-Fe(II). Proc Natl Acad Sci USA 82:968–972, 1985

58. Corey DR, Schultz PG: Generation of hybrid sequence-specific single-stranded deoxyribonuclease. Science 238:1401–1403, 1987

59. Borah B, Chen C, Egan W, Miller M, Wlodawer A, Cohen J: Nuclear magnetic resonance and neutron diffraction studies of the complex of ribonuclease A with uridine vanadate, a transition-state analogue. Biochemistry 24:2058–2067, 1985

60. Dervan PB: Design of sequence-specific DNA-binding molecules. Science 232:464–471, 1986

61. Moser HE, Dervan PB: Sequence-specific cleavage of double-helical DNA by triple helix formation. Science 238:645–650, 1987

62. Praseuth D, Perrouault L, LeDoan T, Chassignol M, Thuong N, Helene C: Sequence-specific binding and photocrosslinking of a and b oligodeoxynucleotides to the major groove of DNA via triple helix formation. Proc Natl Acad Sci USA 85:1349–1353, 1988

63. Chu B, Orgel L: Nonenzymatic sequence-specific cleavage of single-stranded DNA. Proc Natl Acad Sci USA 82:963–967, 1985

64. Chi-hong B, Sigman D: Nuclease activity of 1,10-phenanthroline-copper: Sequence-specific targeting. Proc Natl Acad Sci USA 83:7147–7151, 1986

65. LeDoan T, Perrouault L, Chassignol M, Thuong T, Helene C: Sequence-targeted chemical modifications of nucleic acids by complementary oligonucleotides covalently linked to porphyrins. Nucleic Acids Res 15:8643–8659, 1987

66. Zon G: Oligonucleotide analogs as potential chemotherapeutic agents. Pharm Res 5:539–549, 1988

James J. Mulé
Steven A. Rosenberg

Immunotherapy With Lymphokine Combinations

6

Introduction ■

Rapid progress is being made in the development of immunotherapeutic approaches to the treatment of established cancer by utilizing two rapidly developing fields of knowledge—cellular immunology and recombinant DNA technology.

Information is accumulating on the importance of the cellular immune response in tumor regression. It is now well accepted that much of the host immunologic defense against neoplasms is cell-mediated. Experimental animal models indicate that T-cells may play a large role in this process because they can adoptively transfer tumor immunity, cause regression of established tumor following systemic administration, and kill tumor cells *in vitro* in a major histocompatibility complex (MHC)-restricted fashion.[1-3] There is also evidence that natural killer (NK) cells, macrophages, and, under certain circumstances, B-cells have an antitumor effect, the latter probably by producing lymphocyte-dependent or cytotoxic antibodies.[4] In addition, in 1980, we described a potent antitumor effector cell, the lymphokine-activated killer (LAK), that has the capacity to lyse a broad spectrum of fresh NK-resistant tumor cells, but not fresh normal cells, in an MHC-unrestricted fashion. LAK cells are generated by the incubation of lymphocytes solely in the lymphokine interleukin-2 (IL-2).[3,5-7] An increased understanding of the role of lymphokines and monokines in immunoregulation; the characteristics of MHC-restricted and MHC-unrestricted tumor cell lysis; and the isolation, genetic cloning, and expression of recombinant lymphokines, monokines, and growth factors has permitted more selective approaches to stimulating antitumor immune reactions in tumor-bearing hosts.

In the past, the limited availability of the native form of lymphokines and monokines hampered attempts to evaluate their potential value in cancer therapy. The ability to use antitumor effector cells, such as LAK cells, *in vivo* in adoptive immunotherapy depended on the availability of sufficient quantities of the necessary purified cytokine. For example, large quantities of IL-2 were required not only to activate and expand antitumor effector cells in vitro but also to maintain functional activity and survival of these cells once administered systemically to tumor-bearing hosts.[3,8,9] Recombinant DNA technology has overcome the problem of quantity and has permitted thorough examinations *in vivo* of the antitumor efficacy of these proteins.[3,8-10] Through this technology, a growing list of recombinant cytokines has become available that includes interleukins 1, 2, 3, 4, 5, 6, and 7, interferons (IFNs), colony-stimulating factors, and tumor necrosis factor (TNF) alpha and beta.

It is now documented that selective manipulation of the immune system by recombinant cytokines results in the regression of advanced metastatic cancer in mice and in humans. For example, in murine models, the systemic administration of recombinant IL-2 alone at high doses or at lower doses in combination with LAK cells mediates the regression of established lung and liver metastases from a variety of tumors.[3,8,9,11,12] In a study of 157 patients who had failed standard effective therapy, the adoptive transfer of LAK cells plus IL-2 or IL-2 alone mediated the complete or partial regression of advanced metastatic cancer in selected patients.[13,14] Although substantial reduction in tumor size can be achieved following single-modality treatment with TNF-α,[15,16] IL-2,[12,13,17] or IFN-α[18-20] alone, these responses are generally transient, and few patients are actually cured of disease. Often, dose-limiting toxicities from high-dose administration of a cytokine preclude any attempts to continue treatment.[12,13,21,22] Further, many patients do not respond to immunotherapy in clinical

99

trials, and efforts are under way to increase the effectiveness of these approaches while reducing toxicity.

In animal models, substantial improvements in experimental cancer therapies have been made by combining biologic response modifiers to augment the actions of these therapies and permit reduction of the doses necessary to achieve the same or better antitumor effect. In this chapter, we review recent efforts to improve cancer treatment based on immunotherapies using combinations of recombinant cytokines. We will also discuss possible mechanisms by which synergistic antitumor effects are achieved by cytokine combinations *in vivo*.

Augmentation of Antitumor Effects by Combining IL-2 and Chemotherapeutic Agents ■

Results from animal models have shown that treatment with chemotherapeutic agents, particularly cyclophosphamide (Cytoxan; CTX), can enhance specific adoptive immunotherapy, presumably by eliminating tumor-induced suppressor cells, altering the *in vivo* distribution of the transferred cells, or by direct tumoricidal activity.[23-25] Therapy with large doses of IL-2 alone can cause the regression of both murine and human tumors of various histologies and at several different sites.[12,13,17,26,27] This therapy is associated with marked toxicity, which is its prime limitation.[13,21,22,28] Toxicity is expressed primarily as a capillary leak syndrome and appears to be immunologically mediated, as immunosuppressed mice show decreased toxicity to IL-2.[22,29] Previous studies using ^{125}I-albumin to measure capillary permeability showed that CTX was able to decrease the toxic effects of IL-2.[29] Further studies revealed that CTX at doses of 100 mg/kg and 150 mg/kg completely protected mice from a 100% lethal dose of IL-2, and doses of 50 mg/kg and 150 mg/kg allowed administration of a median of 4.5 and 10.0 more doses of IL-2, respectively, before death from IL-2 toxicity occurred.[30] Because the mechanisms of action and toxicities of chemotherapeutic agents and lymphokines appear quite different, the antitumor efficacy of chemotherapeutic agents plus IL-2 was compared to treatment with either therapy alone in a mouse model of advanced pulmonary metastases.[30] Results of replicate survival experiments are shown in Figure 6–1. In mice harboring pulmonary metastases from a weakly immunogenic MCA-105 sarcoma, administration of recombinant IL-2 alone, 50,000 or 100,000 U thrice daily, improved survival slightly, with an increased

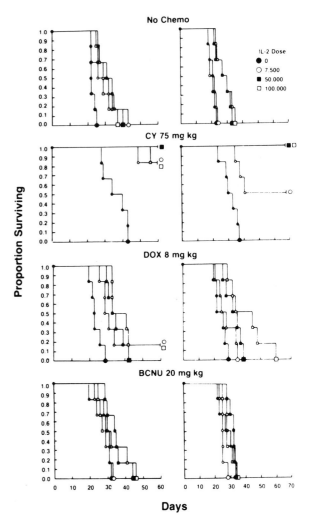

FIG. 6–1   Treatment of mice bearing 10-day pulmonary metastases with varying doses of recombinant IL-2 and either no chemotherapy or chemotherapy with cyclophosphamide (Cy), doxorubicin (DOX), or BCNU.[30] Note that all mice in both series of experiments died of tumor when treated with any dose of IL-2 alone. No mice were cured when treated with Cy alone, although there were substantial numbers of cures when Cy was combined with IL-2.

mean survival time (MST) of 9 and 7 days, respectively ($p < 0.002$). Similarly, treatment with CTX, doxorubicin (dox), or 1,3-bis(2-chloroethyl)-1-nitrosourea (BCNU) alone increased the MST by 11, 1, or 8 days, respectively. However, CTX in conjunction rIL-2, 7500, 50,000, and 100,000 U intraperitoneally (IP) thrice daily, resulted in substantial improvement of survival and long-term cures (MST $\geq$ 60 days for all IL-2 doses, with a cure rate of 31/36 mice for all combinations of IL-2 and CTX; $p < 0.02$ compared to CTX alone or IL-2 alone). Similar enhancement of antitumor effects of IL-2 plus CTX was obtained against the murine colon adenocarcinoma MC-38.[30]

Because the greatest effects were seen when IL-2 was combined with CTX, this interaction was studied in more detail. The doses of CTX and IL-2 were independently varied to determine the optimal dose of each. Recombinant IL-2 doses of 0, 7500, 50,000, and 100,000 units IP thrice daily were used with CTX doses of 0, 25, 75, and 150 mg/kg. CTX was given on day 10, and IL-2 was given on days 11–16. Figure 6–2 shows the results of two experiments using the MCA-105 sarcoma. In animals bearing 10-day MCA-105 pulmonary metastases, treatment with CTX alone at doses of 75 mg/kg or greater had some impact on survival (MST = 25 days in experiment 1 and 31 days in experiment 2; $p < 0.002$ compared to no treatment), but all animals were dead by day 58 unless IL-2 was also used. IL-2 alone had some survival benefit at the highest dose (MST = 26 days for 100,000 U of IL-2 in experiment 1 and 22 days in experiment 2; $p < 0.002$ compared to controls), but again there were no long-term survivors. At each dose of CTX, the addition of increasing doses of IL-2 resulted in an increasing survival benefit. Following CTX doses of 75 mg/kg and 150 mg/kg, the addition of IL-2 at all doses resulted in cure (animals alive at day 120) of the majority of mice ($p < 0.002$ compared to CTX alone for each IL-2 group).

Similar effects were seen in animals with MCA-106 and MC-38 tumors (summarized in Table 6–1), with long-term survivors seen only when CTX and IL-2 were combined. In mice bearing the nonimmunogenic MCA-101 sarcoma, the highest survival rate resulted when the largest dose of each agent was administered, although no long-term survivors were seen. Thus, pretreatment with CTX followed by high-dose IL-2 contributed to enhanced antitumor effects compared to either modality alone.

The combination of CTX and IL-2 in the treatment of cancer patients is currently being studied. Mitchell and colleagues[31] evaluated the effectiveness and tolerability of low-dose CTX plus low-dose intravenous (IV) IL-2 in the treatment of 27 patients with disseminated melanoma. Patients received IL-2, 3.6 million U/m² IV daily for 5 days on 2 successive weeks, starting 3 days after an IV dose of 350 mg/m² CTX. Six of 24 patients who received more than one 2-week cycle of therapy had a remission. Regression of metastases was observed at various sites, including liver, subcutaneous tissue, lymph node, and lungs; one complete and five partial responses were obtained. Although clinically significant cancer regressions occurred, it is difficult to compare the relative effec-

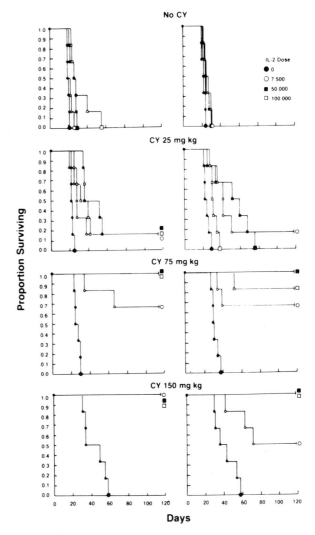

FIG. 6-2 Treatment of mice bearing 10-day pulmonary metastases with varying doses of IL-2 and varying doses of cyclophosphamide (Cy) given alone.[30] With increasing doses of Cy, the combination of Cy and IL-2 produced cures.

tiveness and duration of these responses with responses to IL-2 alone, administered more intensively.[32] It is also not clear that CTX added to the antitumor activity of IL-2. However, it represented a modification of the original regimen that was intended to reduce toxicity.

Rosenberg and colleagues at the National Cancer Institute treated 15 patients with metastatic melanoma with IL-2, 100,000 U/kg every 8 hours beginning 36 hours after a single IV dose of CTX ranging from 10 to 50 mg/kg. Only two partial responses were seen in these patients. Thus, although the number of treated patients was small, the response rate did not

Table 6–1
Effect of Increasing Doses of CTX and IL-2 on Survival of Mice with Experimentally Induced Pulmonary Metastases[30]*

CTX Dose (mg/kg)	IL-2 Dose (units)	MCA-106		MCA-101		MCA-38	
		MST†	Percent Cured	MST†	Percent Cured	MST†	Percent Cured
0	0	25	0	21	0	25	0
	7,500	28	0	20	0	26	0
	50,000	27	0	23	0	29‡	0
	100,000	30‡	0	18	0	29‡	0
25	0	25	0	21	0	26	0
	7,500	27	0	24§	0	44§	16
	50,000	35§	0	24	0	41§	16
	100,000			21§	0	67§	50
75	0	24	0	24§	0	34§	0
	7,500	29§	0	29§	0	65§	33
	50,000	36§	33	32§	0	80§	50
	100,000	>54§	66	33§	0	>90§	100
150	0	28§	0	24§	0	60§	16
	7,500	35§	0	31§	0	>90§	66
	50,000	42§	50	32§	0	>90§	100
	100,000			33§	0	>90§	83

* CTX was given IV on Day 10, and IL-2 in varying doses was given IP thrice daily on days 11 to 16. The three types of tumor cells were injected IV (tail vein) on day 0.

† Median survival time for six mice per group, in days; cured mice were alive without tumor at Day 120.

‡ Group survival significantly different from no-IL-2 control group ($p < 0.05$).

§ Group survival significantly different from that of no-CTX group receiving the same dose of IL-2 ($p < 0.05$).

appear to be higher than that expected from the use of IL-2 alone (Rosenberg and coworkers: Unpublished observations). Further studies of the combination of chemotherapeutic agents and IL-2 in humans are needed.

Augmentation of Antitumor Efficacy by Combining IL-2 and Monoclonal Antibody ■

Multiple efforts are under way to use specific antitumor monoclonal antibodies (moAbs) in the immunotherapy of established cancer.[33–39] The most straightforward application of this approach is the administration of antibody alone, without further modification.[33–36] In this approach, the antitumor moAb may act directly on target cells, mediating tumor destruction by binding complement, or through effector cells by antibody-dependent cellular cytotoxicity (ADCC) responses.[40,41]

Prior *in vitro* studies established that a specific moAb to the murine B16 melanoma, of the IgG2b isotype, could mediate ADCC reactions against fresh B16 melanoma cells using LAK effector cells (Table 6–2).[42] The ability of anti-B16 moAb to cause ADCC of B16 melanoma targets *in vitro* was tested with two allogeneic (DBA/2 and C3H) and a syngeneic (C57BL/6) LAK cell as effectors. LAK cells were generated by 3-day incubation of mouse splenocytes solely in IL-2. LAK cells from all three strains mediated ADCC. The increase of lytic activity in the presence of anti-B16 moAb was between 1.4-fold and 2.5-fold (in lytic units/10^6 cells) compared with the LAK cells alone. Fresh splenocytes or those cultured for 3 days without IL-2 did not mediate ADCC.[42]

Regression of hepatic metastases has been achieved using LAK cells and recombinant IL-2 in mice and in humans.[13,26] The ability of moAbs to augment these responses, based on ADCC reactions *in vivo,* has been investigated. In animal models, a specific moAb has been used to treat established 3-day hepatic metastases from the B16 melanoma.[43] Mice received the combination of anti-B16 moAb and IL-2, given three times daily for 5 days after the first antibody treatment. As illustrated in Table 6–3, there was a synergistic effect of anti-B16 melanoma moAb and IL-2 on the reduction of liver metastases. The effect was significant when 25,000 U of recombinant IL-2 was

Table 6–2

ADCC of Fresh B16 Melanoma Cells Mediated by LAK with Specific B16 Melanoma Monoclonal Antibody[42]

LAK Effectors	Anti-B16 Antibody*	Percent Lysis (Mean ± SE)†			LU/10⁶ Cells‡
		100:1	20:1	4:1	
Expt. 1					
DBA/2	−	36 ± 8	11 ± 4	−8 ± 3	1.4
	+	52 ± 8	21 ± 7	5 ± 3	2.9
C3H	−	41 ± 8	8 ± 5	3 ± 8	1.7
	+	56 ± 4	28 ± 6	11 ± 2	4.3
Expt. 2					
C3H	−	37 ± 7	25 ± 3	19 ± 4	2.9
	+	53 ± 4	30 ± 5	18 ± 2	5
Expt. 3					
C57BL/6	−	36 ± 3	18 ± 1	0 ± 0	2.2
	+	45 ± 2	23 ± 1	3 ± 1	3

* Ten μg was added to the target cells and incubated for 30 min at 37°C before addition of the effectors.

† Values for quadruplicate wells in 4-hr chromium-release assay.

‡ Lytic units, defined as the number of effector cells mediating 30% specific lysis of 10^4 target cells.

administered at each dose of moAb. No reduction in the number of metastases was noted when antigenically unrelated tumor or nonspecific immunoglobulin was employed.[43] Collectively, these results demonstrate that established B16 melanoma liver metastases can be significantly reduced by treatment with anti-B16 moAb, and that this therapeutic effect can be further improved by the systemic administration of IL-2.

In contrast to the results obtained with hepatic metastases, anti-B16 moAb given alone or together with IL-2 had no effect on 3-day established pulmonary metastases from B16 melanoma.[44] However, when IL-2 was combined with the IV administration of LAK cells that could mediate ADCC *in vitro*, there was a significant reduction in the number of lung metastases (Fig. 6–3). Two injections of LAK cells mixed with 1 mg of anti-B16 moAb were necessary to achieve the enhanced antitumor effect on established B16 melanoma lung metastases.

Augmentation of antitumor effects by the combination of specific moAb and recombinant IL-2 has

Table 6–3

Synergistic Effect of Anti-B16 Melanoma Monoclonal Antibody and IL-2 on B16 Melanoma Liver Metastases in Groups of Six Mice[43]*

Treatment	Number of Metastases (Mean ± SE)		
	Expt. 1	Expt. 2	Expt. 3
HBSS	86.6 ± 17.5	164.8 ± 27.0	188.8 ± 19.4
Anti-B16 antibody†	23.0 ± 5.0	31.0 ± 7.2‡	111.5 ± 12.4
25,000 U IL-2	61.6 ± 25.1	154.0 ± 20.6	144.0 ± 5.8
Anti-B16 + 25,000 U IL-2	6.2 ± 2.6§	6.8 ± 1.9‖	33.5 ± 11.1¶

* Anti-B16 melanoma moAb was administered on days 4 and 7 after tumor cell inoculation. IL-2 was given thrice daily on days 4 to 9 after tumor cell inoculation.

† Total amounts of anti-B16 antibody, given in two injections, were 2 mg in experiment 1; 1.2 mg in experiment 2; and 1 mg in experiment 3.

‡ $p < 0.005$ compared to HBSS-treated group.

§ $p < 0.01$ compared to IL-2 group; $p < 0.05$ compared to anti-B16 group.

‖ $p < 0.01$ compared to IL-2; $p < 0.01$ compared to anti-B16.

¶ $p < 0.005$ compared to IL-2; $p < 0.01$ compared to anti-B16

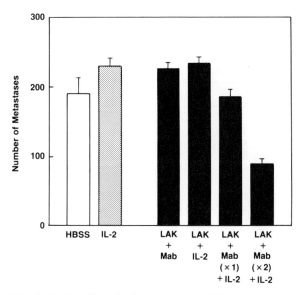

FIG. 6–3 The effect of a single versus two C3H LAK and anti-B16 monoclonal antibody (Mab) injections on established B16 melanoma lung metastases.[44] Mice were injected with 5×10^7 C3H LAK cells, with or without 1 mg of anti-B16 Mab, on either day 3 or days 3 and 6 after tumor cell inoculation; IL-2, 25,000 U IP, was given thrice daily from day 3 to 8. Each bar represents the mean number (±SE) of metastases for six mice. Mice that received LAK + Mab × 2 followed by IL-2 had significantly fewer metastases ($p < 0.05$) than those given either LAK + Mab in one injection + IL-2 or LAK + IL-2 alone.

been demonstrated in tumor models other than B16 melanoma. For example, Berinstein and Levy[45] reported a marked additive and, at times, synergistic effect (as measured by tumor incidence and survival) with the addition of IL-2 to monoclonal anti-idiotype antibodies in the therapy of a murine B-cell lymphoma. In these experiments, therapy with moAb, with or without IL-2, began on the same day as tumor injection. Recent studies by Kawase and colleagues[46] demonstrated that cells of the MH 134 murine hepatoma line are relatively resistant to lysis by LAK cells *in vitro*. However, LAK cells readily lysed this tumor line in the presence of an anti-MH 134 moAb of the IgG1 isotype. Combined therapy of C3H mice bearing MH 134 ascitic tumor with IP injection of IL-2 and specific moAb resulted in greater suppression of tumor growth than either agent alone. In this study, therapy was initiated 1 day after the injection of tumor cells. More stringent experiments are required to determine the potency of combination therapy with IL-2 and specific antitumor moAb in animals with large tumor burdens and established tumors.

Synergistic Antitumor Effects by Combining IL-2 and Interferons ■

The interferons have both antiviral and antitumor activities in murine and human studies.[19,20,47–52] IFN-α has shown promise as an antitumor agent in human trials, particularly against hematologic malignancies such as hairy cell leukemia.[53] Solid tumors may also respond, but the response rate is disappointingly low in most circumstances.[54] The exact mechanisms of *in vivo* IFN antitumor effects are currently unknown, but the IFNs have been shown in both murine and human systems to directly inhibit tumor growth,[55,56] promote a partial reversal of the malignant phenotype,[57–59] and enhance expression of surface molecules including β_2-microglobulin, Fc receptors, tumor antigens, and histocompatibility antigens.[60–66] Interferons also augment NK activity,[67,68] modulate B-cell function,[69,70] inhibit T-cell suppressor activity,[71] and activate macrophages.[72,73]

cDNA from IFN-α, IFN-β, and IFN-γ has been isolated, cloned, and expressed in *Escherichia coli*. Because of the possible additive or synergistic combination of the antitumor activity of IL-2 and the multiple immunomodulatory effects of IFNs, *in vivo* studies to determine the antitumor efficacy of these two cytokines administered in combination have been performed in tumor-bearing mice.[18,74–76]

Major homologies between the individual human leukocyte interferons permitted the construction of hybrid DNA recombinants with quantitatively different activities on human and mouse cells.[77] One such hybrid, IFN-$\alpha_{A/D}$ (Bg1), is highly active on mouse cells.[77] The antitumor effects of combined immunotherapy with IL-2 and the IFN-$\alpha_{A/D}$ hybrid have been investigated in the treatment of mice with established single or multiple hepatic metastases,[18] multiple pulmonary metastases,[78] and subcutaneous tumor.[79]

Mice with established 3-day liver metastases were treated with IL-2 alone, IFN-$\alpha_{A/D}$ alone, or the combination. Two different doses (25,000 and 75,000 U) of each lymphokine were administered IP thrice daily for 3 consecutive days. This dosage regimen was chosen to minimize the antitumor effects of IL-2 as a single agent. On day 17, the mice were killed and the number of liver metastases counted. As shown in Table 6–4, neither lymphokine alone at either dose significantly reduced the number of metastases when compared to control mice injected with Hanks balanced salt solution (HBSS). However, in all four groups treated with combinations of IL-2 and IFN-$\alpha_{A/D}$, a >90% decrease in the mean number of me-

Table 6–4
Results of IL-2/IFN-α Treatment of 3-day MCA-106
Hepatic Micrometastases[18]*

Dose of IFN-α	Dose of IL-2		
	0	25,000 U	75,000 U
None			
No. metastases	208 ± 42	207 ± 30	170 ± 32
Reduction	0	<1%	18%
25,000 U			
No. metastases	163 ± 39	14 ± 6†	2 ± 1‡
Reduction	22%	93% (22%)	98% (46%)
75,000 U			
No. metastases	113 ± 43	5 ± 3‡	4 ± 2†
Reduction	46%	99% (46%)	98% (66%)

* 5×10^5 MCA-106 sarcoma cells were injected intrasplenically. Number of metastases is the mean (±SE) for six animals; percent reduction is in comparison to controls; in combination groups, predicted values based on an additive effect are given in parentheses. Treatments were given IP thrice daily for 3 consecutive days.

† $p < 0.02$ vs. HBSS, IL-2 alone, and IFN-α alone.

‡ $p < 0.05$ vs. HBSS, IL-2 alone, and IFN-α alone.

tastases was observed ($p < 0.02$). This reduction was greater than that predicted by addition of the independent effects of each lymphokine given alone (93% reduction versus predicted 22% with 25,000 U IL-2 and 25,000 U IFN-$\alpha_{A/D}$; 98% reduction versus predicted 66% with 75,000 U of each lymphokine). Representative livers from each group are shown in Figure 6–4. Thus, in this weakly immunogenic micrometastasis model, therapeutic synergy between IL-2 and IFN-$\alpha_{A/D}$ was evident.

The effects of combined therapy in a 10-day macrometastatic tumor model were also evaluated. Multiple MCA-106 liver metastases were induced in mice and, 10 days later when tumor nodules were readily identified on the liver surface, immunotherapy was begun with IL-2 alone, IFN-$\alpha_{A/D}$ alone, or the combination. Two similar doses (20,000 and 100,000 U) of each lymphokine were given IP thrice daily for 4 consecutive days. Mice were killed and their livers harvested on day 18. Findings are summarized in Table 6–5. As in the 3-day MCA-106 model, no effect was noted when either lymphokine was used alone. With combination immunotherapy, however, the number of hepatic metastases was significantly reduced (by 66%–99%) relative to control HBSS-injected mice ($p < 0.05$). This reduction was again greater than that predicted by an additive model (66% reduction versus <1% predicted with 20,000 U IL-2 and 20,000 U IFN-$\alpha_{A/D}$; 99% and 68% reduction in two experiments versus 5% and 22% predicted with 100,000 U of each lymphokine). This decrease in the

number of metastases resulted in a dose-dependent survival benefit in the combination therapy group.[18]

To determine the efficacy of combined immunotherapy with IL-2 and IFN-$\alpha_{A/D}$ in the treatment of

FIG. 6–4 Gross pathologic appearance of representative liver specimens from mice treated with IL-2, IFN-α, or both.[18] Mice were injected with 5×10^5 MCA-106 tumor on day 0. On day 3, therapy was begun with HBSS (*upper left*), IL-2 (*upper right*), IFN-α (*lower left*), or both lymphokines (*lower right*).

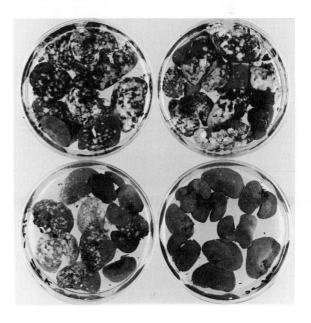

Table 6–5
IL-2/IFN-α Treatment of 10-day MCA-106 Hepatic Metastases[18]*

Dose IFN-α†	No IL-2		20,000 U IL-2†		100,000 U IL-2†	
	No. Metastases	Reduction	No. Metastases	Reduction	No. Metastases	Reduction
Expt. 1						
None	190 ± 46	0	ND	ND	180 ± 49	5%
20,000 U	ND	ND	ND	ND	ND	ND
100,000 U	192 ± 47	<1%	ND	ND	0.7 ± 0.3‡	>99% (<5%)
Expt. 2						
None	122 ± 34	0	211 ± 32	<1%	108 ± 37	12%
20,000 U	133 ± 36	<1%	41 ± 16§	66% (<1%)	16 ± 10‖	87% (11%)
100,000 U	107 ± 43	12%	5 ± 3‖	96% (12%)	39 ± 24¶	68% (22%)

* MCA-106 sarcoma cells (5 × 10⁵) were injected intrasplenically. No. of metastases is mean (±SE) for six animals/group; reduction in metastases is in comparison to controls. For combination-treatment groups, the predicted values based on an additive effect are given in parentheses. ND indicates not done.

† Doses were given IP thrice daily for 3 consecutive days.

‡ $p < 0.01$ vs. HBSS, IL-2 alone, and IFN-α alone.

§ $p < 0.05$ vs. IL-2 alone, and $p > 0.05$ vs. IFN-α alone.

‖ $p < 0.05$ vs. HBSS, IL-2 alone and IFN-α alone.

¶ $p > 0.05$ vs. IL-2 alone and IFN-α alone.

a large localized visceral tumor deposit, single large MCA-106 hepatic metastases were induced in mice, and immunotherapy was begun 10 days later. Two different doses of each lymphokine were used alone and in combination; doses were given IP thrice daily for 4 consecutive days. On day 17, the mice were killed and the tumor nodules weighed (Table 6–6). Synergy similar to that seen in the multiple liver metastases model was observed. Treatment with each lymphokine alone at low doses had no significant effect; treatment with either IL-2 or IFN-$\alpha_{A/D}$ alone at the highest doses was only modestly successful in re-

ducing tumor weight (54% and 41% with IL-2; 36% and 28% with IFN-$\alpha_{A/D}$ in two experiments; $p > 0.05$). In contrast, combination treatment at the highest doses reduced tumor weight by 87% and 84%, respectively ($p < 0.05$). Again, this was greater than would be predicted if the two therapies were merely additive (71% and 58% predicted). Even the reductions seen at low doses (61% and 50%) significantly exceeded those of each lymphokine alone and could not be attributed to an additive mechanism (predicted reductions = 40% and 24%, respectively).

Experiments were performed comparing the com-

Table 6–6
IL-2/IFN-α Treatment of 10-day Single Large MCA-106 Hepatic Metastases[18]*

Dose IFN-α†	No IL-2		25,000 U IL-2†		75,000 U IL-2†	
	Weight of Metastases	Reduction	Weight of Metastases	Reduction	Weight of Metastases	Reduction
Expt. 1						
None	983 ± 58	0	828 ± 56	16%	448 ± 80	54%
25,000 U	697 ± 129	29%	383 ± 131‡	61% (40%)	440 ± 55‡	55% (68%)
75,000 U	634 ± 79§	36%	309 ± 75‡	69% (46%)	127 ± 28‡	87% (71%)
Expt. 2						
None	1104 ± 91	0	981 ± 119	17%	647 ± 110§	41%
25,000 U	1002 ± 78	9%	549 ± 92‡	50% (24%)	390 ± 72‡	65% (46%)
75,000 U	791 ± 94	28%	487 ± 69‡	66% (40%)	179 ± 36‡	84% (58%)

* MCA-106 sarcoma cells (1 × 10⁶) were injected subcapsularly in the liver. Weight of metastases (in mg) is the mean ± SE for at least 6 animals/group. Reduction in weight is in comparison to controls; for combination-treatment groups, the predicted values based on an additive effect are given in parentheses.

† Doses were given IP thrice daily for 4 consecutive days.

‡ $p < 0.05$ vs. HBSS, IL-2 alone, and IFN-α alone.

§ $p < 0.05$ vs. HBSS.

Table 6–7
IL-2 and IFN-α or IFN-γ Treatment of 10-Day MCA-106 Hepatic Macrometastases[18]*

Dosage	Experiment 1		Experiment 2		Experiment 3	
IL-2/IFN-α/IFN-γ	No. Metastases	Mortality*	No. Metastases	Mortality	No. Metastases	Mortality
—/—/—	199 ± 24	0%	29 ± 7	0%	181 ± 21	0%
100,000 U/—/—	142 ± 41	0%	72 ± 33	0%	168 ± 32	0%
—/100,000 U/—	120 ± 38	0%	25 ± 8	0%	74 ± 26	0%
—/—/100,000 U†	129 ± 45	0%	30 ± 8	17%	95 ± 35	0%
100,000 U/100,000 U/—	9 ± 6‡	0%	1 ± 0.6§	0%	1.7 ± 1.5‡	0%
100,000 U/—/100,000 U†	99 ± 30	17%	80 ± 29	0%	63 ± 46‖	17%
—/100,000 U/100,000 U†	49 ± 25	67%	32 ± 8	50%	94 ± 45	17%
100,000 U/100,000 U/100,000 U†	12 ± 6¶	67%	2 ± 1	50%	14 ± 9#	0%

* Mice were injected intrasplenically with 5×10^5 MCA-106 sarcoma cells. Doses were given IP twice daily for 4 days. Mortality is defined as deaths occurring during or immediately after treatment.

† In experiments 2 and 3, only 50,000 U of IFN-γ was used.

‡ $p < 0.05$ vs. HBSS, IL-2 alone, IFN-α alone, and IFN-γ alone.

§ $p < 0.05$ vs. HBSS, IL-2 alone, and IFN-α alone; $p > 0.05$ vs. IFN-α alone.

‖ $p < 0.05$ vs. IL-2 alone; $p > 0.05$ vs. IFN-α alone.

¶ $p > 0.05$ vs. IL-2 and IFN-α combination; $p < 0.05$ vs. IL-2 alone and IFN-γ alone.

# $p < 0.05$ vs. HBSS, IL-2 alone, and IFN-γ alone; $p > 0.05$ vs. IFN-α alone and IL-2 and IFN-α combination.

bination of IL-2 and either IFN-$\alpha_{A/D}$ or IFN-γ to determine if the synergy observed with IFN-$\alpha_{A/D}$ could be generalized to other IFNs. Multiple MCA-106 hepatic metastases were induced in mice, and after 10 days immunotherapy was begun with IL-2, IFN-$\alpha_{A/D}$, IFN-γ, and combinations of the three lymphokines. In the first experiment, 100,000 U of each lymphokine was administered IP twice daily for 4 consecutive days; in the subsequent two experiments the dose of IFN-γ was reduced to 50,000 U because of toxicity. The number of metastases was counted on day 18 and mortality rates from treatment were determined (Table 6–7). Synergy was demonstrated between IL-2 and IFN-$\alpha_{A/D}$ in all three experiments, with 95%, 98%, and 99% reduction in metastases, respectively, compared to ≤60% in controls treated with

either lymphokine alone ($p < 0.05$). However, when IFN-γ was substituted for IFN-$\alpha_{A/D}$, the number of metastases was not reduced below that seen with IL-2 or IFN-γ alone. Thus, synergy was demonstrated in the therapeutic interaction of IL-2 and IFN-$\alpha_{A/D}$ but not that of IL-2 and IFN-γ. Similar results were obtained in the treatment of established pulmonary metastases (Table 6–8).

Substantially greater antitumor efficacy against both primary tumors and metastases of the murine reticulum cell sarcoma M 5076 was obtained when mice were treated with the combination of IFN-$\alpha_{A/D}$ and IL-2 than with either lymphokine alone.[74] Iigo and colleagues[75] compared the combination therapies of IL-2 and IFN-$\alpha_{A/D}$, IFN-β, and IFN-γ in various established murine subcutaneous tumor systems. The

Table 6–8
IL-2 and IFN-α or IFN-γ Treatment of 10-day MCA-106 Pulmonary Macrometastases*

Dosage IL-2/IFN-α/IFN-γ	No. Metastases at Day 17†	Mean	*p* Value
—/—/—	250, 250, 250, 250, 250, 250	250	—
100,000 U/—/—	250, 250, 250, 250, 250, 250	250	1.00
—/100,000 U/—	250, 250, 250, 250, 250, 218	245	>0.05
—/—/100,000 U	250, 250, 250, 250, 250, 250	250	1.00
100,000 U/100,000 U/—	4, 97, 18, 166, 47, 83	69	<0.01
100,000 U/—/100,000 U	250, 250, 250, 250, 164	233	>0.05

* Mice were injected IV with 5×10^5 MCA-106 sarcoma cells. Doses were given IP twice daily for 4 days.

† When metastases were too numerous to count reliably, an arbitrary value of 250 was assigned; each number represents an individual animal.

combination of IL-2 with either IFN-$\alpha_{A/D}$ or IFN-β was markedly effective (as measured by tumor size reduction and cure rate) in mice inoculated subcutaneously with solid tumor cells (adenocarcinoma 755, colon adenocarcinomas 26 and 38, and B16-F10 melanoma). Interferon-γ had little, if any, effect when combined with IL-2. Successful immunotherapy of early (1 to 3 day) subcutaneous or intraperitoneal B16 melanoma clone B$_5$59 in syngeneic mice has been reported with subcutaneous perilesional injections or IP injections, respectively, of IL-2 and IFN-γ. Over a 28-day period, in which IL-2 and IFN-γ were injected 14 times, this combination appeared to mediate additive therapeutic effects with subcutaneous tumors and synergistic effects with intraperitoneal tumors.[76] It is unclear from this particular study whether the combination of IL-2 and IFN-γ would be effective when administered systemically and what effect, if any, would be obtained with more advanced local tumors or metastases.

Synergistic Antitumor Interactions of IL-2, IFN-α, and Tumor-Infiltrating Lymphocytes ■

Yron and colleagues[5] described a method for isolating and expanding lymphocytes that were infiltrating into growing solid cancers. These tumor infiltrating lymphocytes (TIL) are capable of mediating potent antitumor effects *in vivo*. TIL appear to be 50–100 times more potent than LAK cells on a per cell basis when used for adoptive immunotherapy, and the administration of low levels of IL-2 can enhance their therapeutic activity.[80,81] This requirement for lower levels of IL-2 could potentially reduce the toxic effects associated with IL-2 administration. TIL can be readily

grown from a variety of human cancers, and clinical trials of TIL are in progress.[82-85]

The lysis of tumors cells by TIL is restricted by the recognition of MHC antigens, and the effectiveness of IL-2 therapy may be related to MHC expression by tumors.[86,87] Because the interferons can up-regulate MHC expression, the combined application of therapy with interferon, IL-2, and TIL in the treatment of established murine pulmonary metastases has been examined.[78]

These experiments were performed in mice that had received 500 cGy total body irradiation before the IV injection of tumor cells from the MC-38 murine colon adenocarcinoma. This sublethal irradiation eliminated the direct antitumor effects of the lymphokines alone mediated through activation of host radiosensitive lymphocytes.[18,88] Three days after tumor cell injection, mice received a single injection of TIL derived from the MC-38 tumor and immediately began treatment with either HBSS, IL-2, IFN-$\alpha_{A/D}$, or IL-2 plus IFN-$\alpha_{A/D}$. Because the administration of TIL in combination with IL-2 could mediate potent antitumor effects, small numbers of TIL and low doses of IL-2 (7500 U) were used so that the synergistic effects of TIL would be evident. This had the further advantage of decreasing toxicity from IL-2 administration.

A summary of four experiments is shown in Table 6–9. The adoptive transfer of TIL in conjunction with both IL-2 and IFN-$\alpha_{A/D}$ provided a marked increase in therapeutic benefit compared to the transfer of TIL with IL-2 alone or IFN-$\alpha_{A/D}$ alone. In a characteristic experiment (Table 6–9, experiment 4), the adoptive transfer of 2×10^6 TIL either alone or with IFN-$\alpha_{A/D}$, IL-2, or both lymphokines mediated tumor reductions (compared to controls) of 0, 0, 22 ($p = 0.007$), and 98% ($p = 0.002$), respectively. In all four experiments, the reduction mediated by TIL plus

Table 6–9
Number of Lung Metastases at Day 15 After IL-2 and IFN-α ± TIL (Means ± SE)*

IFN-α	IL-2	Expt. 1 −TIL	Expt. 1 +TIL	Expt. 2 −TIL	Expt. 2 +TIL	Expt. 3 −TIL	Expt. 3 +TIL	Expt. 4 −TIL	Expt. 4 +TIL
−	−	≥250	≥250	230	≥250	≥250	150	≥250	≥250
+	−	≥250	≥250	236	220	229	98	248	≥250
−	+	≥250	198	≥250	135	≥250	23	≥250	195
+	+	≥250	1	212	14	201	6	≥250	5

* Mice bearing 3-day lung metastases from the MCA-106 sarcoma were treated with varying combinations of TIL, IL-2, and IFN-α. Before injection of tumor cells, mice received 500 cGy of total body irradiation followed 2–4 h later by injection of MCA-106 tumor cells, 4–5 $\times$ 10^5 IV. At day 3, TIL was given IV (experiment 1, 10^6; experiment 2, 0.7 $\times$ 10^6; experiments 3 and 4, 2 $\times$ 10^6) along with 7500 U IL-2 and/or 50,000 U IFN-α IP thrice daily for 5 days.

IL-2 and IFN-$\alpha_{A/D}$ was significantly greater than that mediated by TIL plus IL-2 (*p* values = 0.003, 0.002, 0.03, and 0.01, respectively) or by any other treatment group.

In several adoptive immunotherapy models, the capacity of tumor-specific T-cell clones to mediate tumor regression has been demonstrated.[89–94] Recently, DeGraaf and colleagues[95] have obtained an increase in long-term survival of mice bearing an established retrovirus-induced T-cell leukemia by short-term adoptive chemoimmunotherapy with an antigen-specific Lyt-2+ cytotoxic T-cell clone and cyclophosphamide, only when combined with IFN-γ administration.

Thus, it is clear that cellular therapy and recombinant cytokine administration in combination can augment antitumor effects *in vivo* against established murine tumors.

Synergistic Antitumor Effects of Immunotherapy with Recombinant TNF and Lymphokines or Chemotherapeutic Agents ■

TNF-α, a cytokine secreted predominantly by macrophages, possesses a variety of biologic properties including potent antitumor activity *in vitro* and *in vivo*.[96,97] TNF isolated from human cells has a molecular weight of approximately 17,000 daltons and shares 79% homology with murine TNF.[98,99] First described by Carswell and colleagues[100] as a factor in the sera of mice treated with Bacillus Calmette–Guerin and endotoxin, TNF (both mouse and human) can now be obtained in large amounts in highly purified form from recombinant bacteria.[99,101,102]

Human and murine tumor lines have demonstrated degrees of susceptibility to recombinant TNF *in vitro*[103,104] and *in vivo*.[97,105–107] Recombinant TNF has recently been used alone *in vivo* in murine models for the treatment of several established tumors.[95,105–107] In Phase I clinical trials, systemic toxic effects have been seen at higher doses of TNF, and evaluations of clinical efficacy have, in general, been disappointing.[108,109] In mouse models, dose-limiting toxicity, degree of tumor immunogenicity, and rapid local regrowth of tumor after partial necrosis are major factors in cases where TNF fails. For example, Asher and coworkers[97] showed that mice bearing syngeneic MCA sarcomas were more susceptible to the toxic side-effects of TNF than were normal mice: 48% (41/86) of mice that received a single IV dose of TNF died within 48 hours after treatment compared

with no deaths in 28 normal animals receiving this dose. Thus, severe toxicity limits the amount of TNF that can be administered. Unfortunately, it is within this TNF dosage range (6–10 μg) that significant cures have been observed in animals surviving treatment; cure also appeared to be dependent on tumor immunogenicity. In these studies, TNF failed to mediate cures in mice bearing the nonimmunogenic MCA-101 and MCA-102 sarcomas. In contrast, of mice bearing the weakly immunogenic MCA-105 and MCA-106 sarcomas, which received 6–10 μg of TNF, 67% and 28%, respectively, were cured. In animals not cured by TNF administration, a viable rim of tumor often grew peripherally to the area of tumor necrosis by the second week; these tumors grew progressively and resulted in the death of animals. Thus, although substantial tumor reductions can be achieved following administration of TNF at subtoxic doses, few animals are actually cured of disease.[97] Efforts to minimize TNF toxicity while maintaining or increasing therapeutic efficacy would be of substantial benefit.

Synergistic antineoplastic effects (*e.g.,* antiproliferative) have been obtained *in vitro* against a variety of fresh and cultured tumor cells by the combination of TNF and IFN-α or IFN-γ.[110,111] More recently, *in vivo* studies in mice have been undertaken to examine the potential for synergistic (or additive) antitumor efficacy by combining recombinant TNF and recombinant lymphokines or chemotherapeutic agents in the treatment of established tumors.

Enhanced antitumor effects of systemic combination therapy with recombinant TNF and IFNs have been documented in syngeneic tumor models in animals. There are also published studies using para- or intralesional routes of administration.[112] Balkwill and colleagues[113] showed that a human ovarian cancer cell line growing intraperitoneally as a xenograft in athymic mice was highly sensitive to local therapy with the combination of TNF plus IFN-γ. In these experiments, all control (untreated) mice died by 42 days; therapy (starting 7 days after tumor cell injection) with 5×10^4 U of IFN-γ or 1 μg of TNF alone (each given daily for about 5 weeks) had no significant effect. In contrast, the combination of the two cytokines resulted in 85% survival at 150 days; significantly increased survival was also obtained when combination treatment was initiated as late as 21 days after tumor cell injection. Talmadge and colleagues[114] showed that TNF had additive therapeutic activity against experimental and spontaneous B16-BL6 melanoma metastases when administered in conjunction with suboptimal doses of IFN-γ. In their study, the combination of cytokines mediated reductions in the number of pulmonary metastases, but there were no complete cures.

In vivo synergistic antitumor effects have also been observed with the combination of TNF and IL-2. For example, Nishimura and colleagues[115] showed that with intratumoral injection of TNF plus IL-2 (given intradermally around the tumor site), more than 60% of MBL-2 lymphoma-bearing mice were cured of disease (compared to 0 and 25% with IL-2 alone and TNF alone, respectively). Cured mice could also reject a rechallenge of MBL-2 tumor cells. Winkelhake and coworkers[116] reported that simultaneous doses of TNF and IL-2, given systemically, exhibited synergy on Meth A sarcoma and four other subcutaneous experimental murine tumor types (B16 melanoma, EL-4 lymphoma, P815 mastocytoma, and L1210 leukemia).

To evaluate combined therapy with TNF and IL-2, we used subcutaneous tumors of the weakly immunogenic MCA-106 sarcoma, established over a 9-day period, that achieved a size of 5–6 mm in diameter.[117] Single doses (2, 4, 6, and 8 μg) of TNF (or excipient) were injected IV and IL-2 (25,000 U) was given IP thrice daily (4 hours after TNF) for 5 consecutive days. This dose of IL-2 was chosen because it did not mediate a significant antitumor response when administered alone.

As shown in Figure 6–5, significant sustained decreases of tumor area were seen at the lowest doses of TNF (2 μg) combined with IL-2, compared to TNF alone and excipient. No effects on tumor growth were

seen with IL-2 alone. Increasing doses of TNF plus IL-2 resulted in increasingly greater tumor reductions, with the 8 μg combination dose causing sustained disappearance of the tumor nodule within 2 weeks of initial therapy.

We next determined whether synergy in tumor reduction achieved by the combination of TNF and IL-2 resulted in prolonged survival and cure of the treated mice. Mice surviving without evidence of tumor for longer than 100 days were considered cured. Extended survival of mice bearing subcutaneous MCA-106 sarcomas was observed at all dosages of TNF given in association with IL-2 (Table 6–10). Cure was seen at all dosage levels of TNF with concurrent IL-2 therapy (2 μg TNF + IL-2 = 50%, NS; 4 μg TNF + IL-2 = 33%, NS; 6 and 8 μg TNF + IL-2 = 83%, $p < 0.05$ compared to mice treated with TNF alone). In addition, significant survival benefit was noted in groups in which IL-2 was delayed as much as 4 days after TNF injection.[117]

Therapy with a combination of TNF and IL-2 was assessed in mice bearing single hepatic tumors (4–5 mm). MCA-106 sarcoma cells were injected in the subcapsular surface of the liver and were allowed to grow for 10 days. At 10 days, a group of untreated mice were killed and the tumors were excised to evaluate baseline tumor size. Remaining groups received escalating IV doses of TNF (excipient, 2, 4, 6, or 8 μg). Half of these animals also received concurrent IL-2 therapy (25,000 U IP three times daily for 5 days). On day 17 after tumor cell injection, mice were

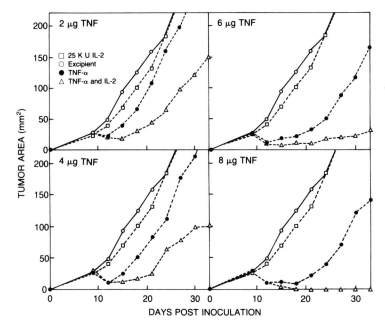

FIG. 6–5 Effect of concurrent TNF and IL-2 therapy on the growth of subcutaneous weakly immunogenic MCA-106 sarcoma.[117] Nine days after tumor inoculation, C57BL/6 mice (six per group) were treated with varying doses of TNF as a single IV injection (see *upper left* of each panel), and then excipient or IL-2 (25,000 U) was given IP for 5 days.

Table 6–10
TNF/IL-2 Synergy: Effect on Survival of Mice Bearing Established MCA-106 Subcutaneous Sarcoma[117]*

	Survival (Mean Days $\pm$ SE)	
TNF dose	No IL-2	IL-2
None	34 ± 3	44 ± 3
2 μg	40 ± 6	90 ± 5†
		$p < 0.002/p < 0.001$
4 μg	36 ± 4	73 ± 10
		$p < 0.006/p < 0.009$
6 μg	41 ± 4	94 ± 4
		$p < 0.001/p < 0.001$
8 μg	49 ± 14	85 ± 13
		$p < 0.05/p < 0.05$

* TNF was started on day 9 of tumor growth; IL-2 (25,000 U) was started on day 9. The p values are for comparison to excipient/to TNF alone at the same dose.

† Followed for >100 days.

Table 6–11
TNF/IL-2 Synergy: Effect on Weight of Single Hepatic Tumors of the Weakly Immunogenic MCA-106 Sarcoma[117]*

	Tumor Weight (mg)	
TNF Dose	No IL-2	IL-2
None	1407	1099
2 μg	642	295
		$p < 0.01/p < 0.05$†
4 μg	201	63
	$p < 0.05$‡	$p < 0.001/p < 0.005$†
6 μg	67	33
	$p < 0.01$‡	$p < 0.01/p < 0.01$†
8 μg	106	67
	$p < 0.05$‡	$p < 0.01/NS$†
Controls		110

* TNF was given as a single IV injection on day 10 after tumor cell inoculation; IL-2 was given IP thrice daily for 5 consecutive days beginning on day 10.

† The p values are for comparison to excipient/to TNF alone at the same dose.

‡ The p values are for comparison to no treatment group.

killed, and the liver tumors were excised and weighed in a blinded fashion. As shown in Table 6–11, substantial reductions in hepatic tumor weights were achieved with high-dose TNF (6 μg, $p < 0.01$; 8 μg, $p < 0.05$) as a single agent, as reported previously.[107] With the addition of concurrent IL-2 therapy, similar tumor reductions could be attained at a lower TNF dosage (4 μg, $p < 0.002$). High-dose TNF (6 and 8 μg), as well as the combination of TNF plus IL-2 therapy (4, 6, and 8 μg + IL-2) caused an actual tumor regression below the 10-day untreated control weights. No reduction in tumor weight was noted with IL-2 as a single agent at the suboptimal dose. The combination of TNF plus IL-2 resulted in significantly increased survival of the treated mice compared to either cytokine alone.[117] Thus, these experiments demonstrated the synergistic antitumor effects of combination therapy with TNF and IL-2 against a well-established, weakly immunogenic sarcoma growing in subcutaneous and visceral sites.

Most recently, McIntosh and colleagues,[118] using the tumor models described above, have shown that the addition of IFN-α to combined therapy with TNF plus IL-2 results in further enhancement of synergistic antitumor activities, as measured by tumor regression, survival benefit, and cure rates. The doses of both TNF and IL-2 could be substantially reduced by adding of IFN-α, with greater antitumor effects.

Several laboratories have demonstrated both *in vivo* and *in vitro* augmentation of the antitumor effects of TNF when combined with traditional antimetabolic chemotherapeutic agents.[119–121] We have evaluated the *in vivo* antitumor effects of the combination of TNF and doxorubicin (dox), 5-fluorouracil (5-FU), or CTX in a syngeneic murine tumor model.[122] Mice had established 10-day subcutaneous MCA-106 sarcoma at the initiation of systemic therapy. TNF plus dox or 5-FU showed a transient antitumor effect, whereas TNF plus CTX exhibited a synergistic antitumor response. As shown in Figure 6–6—a compendium of four separate experiments with TNF plus CTX—mice treated with CTX alone exhibited a reduction in average tumor area of 30% $\pm$ 12% by day 28 after tumor inoculation compared to untreated controls ($p < 0.001$). Those treated with 4 μg or 6 μg of TNF had a reduction in average tumor area of 35% $\pm$ 9% ($p < 0.02$) and 41% $\pm$ 9% ($p < 0.001$), respectively, compared to untreated controls. In contrast, mice treated with the combination of 4 μg or 6 μg TNF and CTX had substantially greater reductions in tumor size (70% $\pm$ 9%, $p < 0.005$ versus CTX and 4 μg TNF alone; and 94% $\pm$ 3%, $p < 0.005$ versus CTX and 6 μg TNF alone). Significant prolongation in survival was noted over animals treated with single agents (Fig. 6–7).

Comparisons of the numbers of tumor-free animals after treatment with TNF with or without CTX in mice bearing 10-day subcutaneous MCA 106 sarcoma, in four combined experiments, are shown in Table 6–12. Animals treated with CTX alone, or with 4 μg or 6 μg of TNF alone, had 10%, 0, and 14% cures at 90 days (all NS compared to untreated controls). In contrast, those treated with 4 μg or 6 μg of TNF plus CTX had significantly higher cure rates of 35% ($p < 0.02$) and 48% ($p < 0.04$), respectively.

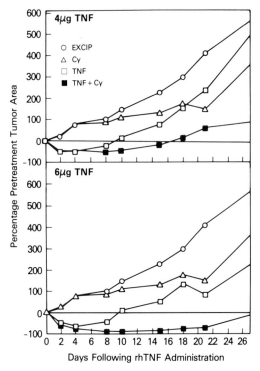

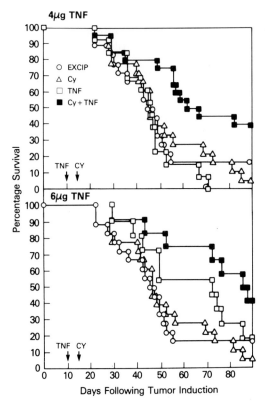

FIG. 6-6 Augmentation of antitumor effects by the combination of recombinant human TNF (rhTNF) and cyclophosphamide (Cy).[122] This compilation of four separate experiments shows percentage pretreatment tumor area at various time points following TNF (or excipient) administration. Mice bearing subcutaneous 10-day MCA-106 sarcoma were treated with 4 ug (*upper panel*) or 6 ug (*lower panel*) of TNF (or excipient) as a single IV injection, saline (HBSS) or Cy (100 mg/kg) was administered IV 48 hours later.

Possible Therapeutic Use of Combinations of Newly Cloned Interleukins ■

cDNA clones for both mouse and human lymphokines, namely IL-1 through IL-7, have been obtained and expressed in mammalian, bacterial, and yeast systems. These recombinant interleukins have broad biologic activities on hemopoietic progenitors, B-cells, mast cells, monocytes/macrophages, and T-cells. Interest in the possible therapeutic applications of these lymphokines stems mainly from their stimulatory actions on T-cells.

Table 6–13 summarizes the known T-cell activities of IL-1 through IL-6.[123-131] In particular, IL-4[127] and IL-6[130,131] may be of value in tumor immunotherapy; *in vitro* studies have demonstrated that these two lymphokines potentiate the proliferation and cytolytic activity of cytotoxic T-lymphocytes (CTL). IL-4 is also an endogenous T-cell growth factor during the immune response to a syngeneic murine retrovirus-induced tumor.[133]

FIG. 6-7 Enhanced survival of tumor-bearing mice by the combination of recombinant TNF and cyclophosphamide (Cy).[122] (See legend to Figure 6–6 for a description of experimental method.)

Because some of the functional activities of IL-4 and IL-2 overlap, the capacity of IL-4 to induce LAK activity was first examined in the mouse. We[134] and others[135] have reported that mouse IL-4 induced LAK activity in splenocyte cultures *in vitro*. Peace and coworkers[135] demonstrated IL-4 induced LAK activity against a variety of tumors including those of syngeneic (FBL leukemia, EL-4 thymoma, and B16 melanoma) and allogeneic (LSTRA leukemia, P815 mastocytoma, SL2 lymphoma, and YAC lymphoma) origin. In addition, mouse IL-4 augmented LAK activity in combination with IL-2 when measured against fresh syngeneic sarcoma targets.

We compared the capacity of mouse and human IL-4 to generate LAK activity from B6 mouse splenocytes.[136] Freshly prepared splenocytes were incubated in IL-4, IL-2, or the combination thereof for 5 days and then tested for the capacity to lyse fresh, MCA-102 and MCA-105 sarcoma targets in a 4 hour ^{51}Cr-release assay; the MCA-105 target is generally less LAK-susceptible than the MCA-102 target (Table 6–14). Murine IL-4 alone at 2000 U/ml induced LAK activity comparable to IL-2 alone and aug-

Table 6–12
Summary of Cure Rates for Tumor-bearing Mice Treated with TNF and Cyclophosphamide[122]*

Treatment		No. Treated	No. Surviving Treatment†	No. Cured‡	Percent Cured	p Value
CTX	TNF					
—	None	36	36	0	0	1.0
—	4 μg	36	20	0	0	1.0
—	6 μg	36	22	3	14	>0.05
100 mg/kg	None	42	40	4	10	>0.05
100 mg/kg	4 μg	44	34	12	35	<0.02
100 mg/kg	6 μg	42	23	11	48	<0.04

* Treatment consisted of single IV doses of TNF to mice bearing 10-day subcutaneous sarcoma, followed at 48 h by a single IV dose of CTX.

† Death within 36–48 h of TNF injection.

‡ Animals free of palpable tumor at 90 days.

mented this activity when combined with IL-2 at the suboptimal concentration of 200 U/ml. The LAK activity augmented by the combination of the two lymphokines was greater than that achieved by the optimal concentration of IL-2 alone (1000 U/ml). In contrast, human IL-4 alone, when used at concentrations as high as 20,000 U/ml, failed to generate LAK activity and to augment this activity when combined with IL-2. Thus, the LAK-inducing capacity of IL-4 observed with mouse splenocytes was species-specific.

We also examined the effects of IL-4 on IL-2-induced LAK cell expansion *in vitro.* B6 splenocytes were cultured in complete media (CM) containing IL-2 alone (1000 U/ml) for 5 days. These LAK cells were then replated and cultured in fresh CM containing varying amounts of IL-2, IL-4, or both for 4 additional days (*i.e.,* 9-day LAK). Table 6–15 shows the cell expansion data from two separate experiments. Recombinant IL-4 alone (2000 U/ml) maintained the viability and recovery of cells compared to those replated in CM alone. Increasing concentrations of IL-2 alone resulted in increasingly greater expansion in cell number.[137] The expansion, however, was increased at all IL-2 concentrations evaluated when IL-4 was added. Attempts to expand 5-day LAK

Table 6–13
Recombinant Interleukins with T-Cell Activities

Interleukin	Molecular Weight*	Effects on T-Cells	Ref.
IL-1 (α, β)	17,500	Costimulates; induces IL-2 production; increases IL-2 receptor number and binding, growth factor activation, and induction/release of cytokines	123
IL-2	15,000	Costimulates; activates cytotoxic response, chemotaxis, and induction/release of cytokines; induces non-MHC-restricted CTL killing	124
IL-3	25,000	Initiates growth of mature inducer T-cells (Thy-1+, Lyt-1+, Lyt-2−) and of Thy 1+, Lyt-1−, Lyt-2−, T3+ non-MHC-restricted CTL	125, 126
IL-4	20,000 (≥60,000 hyperglycosylated)	Costimulates (in proliferation of normal resting T-cells); stimulates thymocyte proliferation and differentiation to CTL (in presence of lectin or phorbol myristate acetate); helper factor for CTL generation in primary MLC and induces/amplifies *in vitro* primed MLC memory cells	127
IL-5	12,300 (18,000; 45–60,000)	As a cofactor, induces CTL differentiation; induces IL-2 receptor; causes release of soluble IL-2 receptor	128, 129
IL-6	26,000	Costimulates; induces IL-2 production; serves as CTL differentiation factor	130, 131
IL-7	25,000	T-cell activities yet to be determined	132

* Varies with degree of glycosylation.

Table 6–14
Species Specificity of IL-4 Induction and Augmentation of LAK Activity[136]*

Lymphokine (U/ml)			Cells/ml	$LU_{30}/10^7$ Cells	
IL-2	Murine IL-4	Human IL-4	($\times 10^6$)†	MCA-102	MCA-105
200	—	—	1.6	555	25
—	2000	—	0.8	800	50
—	—	2,000	0.9	<1	<1
—	—	20,000	1.1	<1	<1
200	2000	—	1.2	2174	476
200	—	2,000	1.3	800	31
200	—	20,000	1.3	769	42
1000	—	—	1.2	392	33

* B6 splenocytes were cultured at 2×10^6 cells/ml in 2 ml of CM containing varying amounts of lymphokine. After 5 days the cells were tested for cytolytic activity against ^{51}Cr-labeled fresh MCA-induced sarcoma cells in a 4 h assay.

† Viable cell recovery at day 5 of culture.

cultures that were initially induced with IL-4 alone failed when these cells were replated and cultured in varying concentrations of IL-2, IL-4, or both for 4 additional days (data not shown).

Aliquots of these same 9-day LAK cell cultures were also tested for cytotoxicity *in vitro* against MCA-105 sarcoma target cells (Table 6–16). Five-day IL-2-generated LAK recultured in IL-4 alone (2000 U/ml) showed significant cytotoxic activity compared to CM alone. Substantial augmentation of LAK activity was obtained from cell cultures containing both IL-4 and IL-2 (even at the optimal IL-2 concentration of 1000 U/ml) against this relatively LAK-insensitive MCA-105 target, in which IL-2 alone (up to 1000 U/ml) failed to elicit cytotoxicity. Thus, IL-4 was capable

of potent augmentation of both expansion and cytotoxic functions of IL-2-generated LAK effectors in short-term (9 day) cultures. Because combining IL-4 with IL-2 augments the short-term expansion of LAK cells as well as their cytolytic function on a per cell basis, a far greater number of lytic units per culture can be obtained. It will be of value to determine the *in vivo* therapeutic efficacy against sarcoma metastases of LAK effectors generated by the combination of IL-2 and IL-4.

In contrast, human IL-4 does not induce LAK activity, but rather inhibits IL-2 induction of LAK ac-

Table 6–15
IL-4 Augmentation of *in vitro* Expansion of LAK Cells in Combination with IL-2[136]*

IL-4 Dose (U/ml)	IL-2 Dose (U/ml)			
	0	10	100	1000
Expt. 1				
0	0.4	1.6	1.9	2.4
20	ND	1.8	2.1	3.4
200	ND	2.8	4.2	3.6
2000	1.3	3.6	5.2	5.9
Expt. 2				
0	0.5	1.6	4.6	5.3
20	ND	ND	ND	ND
200	ND	2.0	6.2	6.5
2000	0.9	4.4	9.7	9.0

* Day 5 LAK cells (B6 splenocytes cultured in CM containing 1000 U/ml IL-2 for 5 days) were replated at 2.5×10^5 cells/ml in 2 ml of CM containing varying amounts of lymphokine. Expansion is calculated as the ratio of the number of cells obtained on day 4 of expansion (*i.e.,* 9-day LAK cells) vs. the number of cells put into culture on day 0 of expansion.

Table 6–16
Augmentation of LAK Activity by IL-4: Dose Titration of IL-4 and IL-2 Versus Cytolytic Activity ($LU_{20}/10^7$ Cells) Against MCA-105 Targets[136]*

IL-4 Dose (U/ml)	IL-2 Dose (U/ml)			
	0	10	100	1000
Expt. 1				
0	<1	<10	ND	<10
20	ND	<10	ND	106
200	ND	145	ND	1137
2000	100	1087	ND	2381
Expt. 2				
0	<1	<1	<1	<10
20	ND	ND	ND	ND
200	ND	<10	<10	571
2000	133	909	2247	1852

* Day 5 LAK cells (C57BL/6 splenocytes cultured in CM containing 1000 U/ml IL-2 for 5 days; $LU_{30}/10^7$ vs. MCA-102 targets = 18 and 71 in expts. 1 and 2, respectively) were plated at 2.5×10^5 cells/ml in 2 ml CM containing varying amounts of lymphokine. After 4 days (day 9 LAK) the cells were tested for lytic activity against ^{51}Cr-labeled fresh MCA-induced sarcoma cells in a 4 h assay.

activity and cell proliferation from unstimulated lymphocytes of various lymphoid organs.[138] However, human IL-4 does, in fact, generate LAK activity and augments proliferation with IL-2 when the lymphocytes are preactivated with IL-2.[138]

Because IL-4 can amplify specific CTL responses in both the mouse[127] and human,[139] experiments have been done to determine recombinant IL-4 effects on TIL as part of the strategy of developing more potent antitumor immunotherapies for advanced cancers. In murine models, the transfer of 10- to 100-fold fewer tumor-specific T-cells than LAK cells for adoptive cellular immunotherapy results in comparable antitumor effects.[80,81] Our laboratory has recently demonstrated the existence and expansion of CTL lines and clones specific for autologous human melanoma,[82] and clinical trials using these TIL are in progress.[85] Selective accumulation of systemically administered, radiolabeled TIL into human tumors has also been noted.[140] Murine studies indicate that $>2 \times 10^{11}$ TIL would be required to effectively treat patients, and attempts to further expand these cells with specific antitumor activity are required. Therefore, study of human IL-4 effects on the growth of TIL specific for autologous melanoma is under way in our laboratory.[141]

Preliminary data suggest that human IL-4 can selectively grow T-cells with specificity for autologous melanoma in combination with low or high doses of IL-2 and augments the growth of these cells. The benefit, if any, of human IL-4 on TIL grown from tumors other than melanoma will be the subject of future experiments. IL-4 may be useful in cancer therapy, especially for the adoptive transfer of specific T-cells or in conjunction with IL-2 administration. Future efforts should also be directed toward analyses of the potential value of other recombinant lymphokines (*e.g.,* IL-6), singly or in combination, in tumor immunotherapy.

Mechanisms by Which Recombinant Cytokines Mediate Antitumor Effects *In Vivo* ■

Role of MHC Antigens and Tumor Immunogenicity ■

Tumor cell determinants may be recognized in an associative reaction with self MHC antigens to generate an immune response, and a role for MHC antigens in controlling tumor immune responses is suggested by experiments involving alteration of class I expression on tumor cells by selection[142,143] or gene transfection.[144-146] Increased class I expression by transfection of several virally transformed or carcinogen-induced murine tumors was shown to change metastatic potential,[144] tumorigenicity,[145] or immunogenicity.[146]

In addition to the antiproliferative effect of the interferons, these molecules can up-regulate MHC antigen expression; expression of class I antigens on tumors may be an important determinant of successful cytokine therapy. Tumor necrosis factor may have direct antitumor reactivity, may enhance immune function, and may be able to synergize with interferons in up-regulating MHC expression.

Table 6–17 shows that class I MHC molecules are present on two weakly immunogenic (MCA-105 and MCA-106) tumors that responded to high-dose IL-2 therapy, whereas macrometastases from two nonimmunogenic (MCA-101 and MCA-102) tumors that did not respond express little or no class I MHC antigen. To test whether or not modulation of MHC expression could render tumor cells sensitive to IL-2 immunotherapy, cell lines were derived from a murine melanoma, B16BL6, by transfection of the class I gene encoding K^b and the class II gene encoding Ia^k.[147] The original B16BL6 melanoma expressed little or no class I antigen and was not susceptible to therapy with IL-2. Pulmonary metastases were generated by IV injection of control line BL6-13 (a cell line derived from a subclone of B16BL6, transfected with a plasmid encoding the selectable marker for neomycin resistance) and class I transfectant CL8-2. Class I expression induced sensitivity of established 10-day macrometastases to therapy with high-dose IL-2 (Table 6–18) and sensitivity of 3-day micrometastases to high- and low-dose IL-2 (Table 6–19). Class II expression did not increase the sensitivity of B16BL6 melanoma to IL-2 therapy.[147]

Alteration of MHC expression in an established tumor by *in vivo* cytokine therapy may render that tumor more sensitive to concurrent IL-2 therapy. A possible explanation for the synergy between IFN-α and IL-2 in the treatment of pulmonary, hepatic, and subcutaneous tumors generated by murine sarcoma MCA-106 may be that IFN-α induced modulation of MHC antigens, rendering the tumor more susceptible to IL-2 therapy.

Using several murine sarcomas, we demonstrated that IFN-α and IFN-γ, when administered *in vivo*, can up-regulate class I but not class II expression on subcutaneous and pulmonary metastatic tumors.[148] Single-cell suspensions from subcutaneous tumors were prepared from mice treated with HBSS, IFN-α, IFN-γ, or IFN-γ + TNF-α. Flow cytometry analysis was performed using antibody 28-8-6 measuring class

Table 6–17
Correlation Between Class I MHC Expression on Murine Sarcomas and Susceptibility to IL-2 Therapy[147]

Tumor	Immunohistochemical Staining of Lung Tumor*		Immunofluorescence of Tumor Cells *in vitro*†		Susceptibility of Macrometastases to High-dose IL-2‡
	Class I	Class II	Class I	Class II	
MCA-101	−	−	−(0)	−	0
MCA-102	−	−	+(50)	−	0
MCA-105	+	−	++(95)	−	99%
MCA-106	+	−	++(80)	−	83%

* Mice were injected IV with 1–3 × 10⁵ tumor cells of nonimmunogenic (MCA-101, MCA-102) or weakly immunogenic (MCA-105, MCA-106) lines. Lungs were removed from animals killed on day 18 after injection, imbedded in OCT media, and quick-frozen; 6 μm sections were stained with an immunoperoxidase technique. Murine moAb 28-8-6 was used for K^b, a class I determinant and murine moAb 34-5-6 for IA^b, a class II determinant.

† Fresh tumor digested with hyaluronidase, collagenase, and DNase was passaged once in DMEM with 10% FCS until a homogeneous monolayer grew; cells were trypsinized and washed, then analyzed using a FACS II analyzer. Murine moAb 28-8-6 was used to detect K^b; 34-5-6 was used for IA^b. Numbers in parentheses represent percent fluorescence in the control subtracted from the experimental sample.

‡ Values are percent reduction of 10-day pulmonary metastases treated with 150,000 U IL-2 IP, thrice daily for 4 days, vs. treatment with no IL-2.

I K^b + D^b. The profiles and mean fluorescence values are shown in Figure 6–8 for the nonimmunogenic MCA-102 tumor and Figure 6–9 for the weakly immunogenic MCA-106 tumor. Untreated MCA-102 cells exhibit a modest amount of staining, with a mean channel fluoresence of 429. IFN-γ, 100,000 U/day IV for 4 days, raised mean fluoresence to 495. IFN-α, 100,000 U/day IV 4 days, raised mean fluoresence

Table 6–18
Increased Sensitivity of 10-day Pulmonary Metastases from a Transfected B16 Cell Line Expressing Class I Antigen to High-dose IL-2[147]*

Tumor†	Metastases (Mean ± SE) After Treatment with IL-2 in Doses of:		
	0	20,000 U/ml	100,000 U/ml
Expt. 1			
B16	271 ± 18	281 ± 18	284 ± 14
BL6-13	166 ± 15	142 ± 23	150 ± 27
CL8-2	152 ± 19	83 ± 29	27* ± 12
Expt. 2			
B16	238 ± 10	239 ± 10	218 ± 14
BL6-13	144 ± 23	157 ± 17	144 ± 21
CL8-2	126 ± 18	92 ± 11	71* ± 11

* 1–4.5 × 10⁵ tumor cells; IL-2 therapy, given IP every 8 h for 5 days, started on day 10 after tumor injection. Mice were killed on day 18 for counting of lung metastases. Each group contained 6–10 mice. Wilcoxon rank-sum test of treated groups compared with groups receiving HBSS alone, $p < 0.05$.

† BL6-13 contains the neomycin resistance plasmid only; CL8-2 contains both the neomycin resistance plasmid and the plasmid containing the DNA encoding K^b, a class I antigen. B16 is the parental line.

to 513, and 100,000 U every 8 hours IP for 4 days increased mean fluoresence further to 546. When 2 μg of TNF-α was added IV at the start of 4 days of IV IFN-γ therapy, mean fluoresence increased further to 582. TNF-α given alone at higher doses generally resulted in necrotic tumors that could not be analyzed.

The flow cytometry profiles and mean fluoresence values for MCA-106 tumor cells from animals treated with parenteral IFN-α and IFN-γ are shown in Figure 6–9. Untreated MCA-106 cells exhibit a modest amount of class I staining, with a mean fluoresence of 413. IFN-γ 100,000 U IP or IV given on the same schedule as in Figure 6–8 for the MCA-102 tumor, raised the mean fluoresence to 521 and 574, respectively. IFN-α, 100,000 U IP or IV in an identical schedule, increased the mean fluoresence to 497 and 449, respectively.

This work suggests that IFN-α alone may increase *in vivo* expression of MHC antigens and thus possibly render established tumors more immunogenic and more susceptible to destruction by the host immune system. However, IFN-γ is also capable of up-regulating tumor MHC expression *in vivo*, yet we have not been able to demonstrate that it has synergistic antitumor effects with IL-2 *in vivo*. Further, although IFN-α can up-regulate MHC class I molecules on MCA-102 sarcoma when administered *in vivo*, combination therapy with IL-2 plus IFN-α has failed to show synergistic antitumor efficacy against this nonimmunogenic tumor.[18] Therefore, increased expression of MHC antigens may be important for the synergistic activity of IL-2 and IFN-α against the weakly

Table 6–19
Increased Sensitivity of 3-day Pulmonary Metastases from a Transfected B16 Cell Line Expressing Class I Antigen to Low- and High-dose IL-2[147]*

Tumor	Metastases (Mean ± SE) after Treatment with IL-2 Dose of:			
	0	10,000 U	30,000 U	100,000 U
Expt. 1				
BL6-13	118 ± 17	120 ± 17	137 ± 28	102 ± 14
CL8-2	283 ± 16	108 ± 12†	17 ± 6‡	15 ± 5‡
Expt. 2				
BL6-13	187 ± 13	180 ± 20	162 ± 17	82 ± 12†
CL8-2	201 ± 24	34 ± 13	44 ± 33†	17 ± 9‡

* Mice were injected IV with $2–4.5 \times 10^5$ tumor cells; IL-2 therapy given every 8 h for 5 days, started on day 3 after tumor injection. Mice were killed on day 17 for lung metastases counting. Each group contains 6–10 mice. Comparisons of treatments are by Wilcoxon rank-sum test of treated groups compared with groups receiving HBSS alone.

† $p < 0.05$.

‡ $p < 0.005$.

immunogenic MCA-106 sarcoma, but it is not a complete explanation for the mechanism underlying this effect. Using cultured human tumor cells that produce tumors in nude athymic mice, Greiner and colleagues[64] have shown that IFN-α given *in vivo* can modulate expression of a human tumor antigen as well as MHC molecules. It is possible that IFN-α can up-regulate the expression of tumor-associated antigens that are not regulated by IFN-γ.

Pulmonary or subcutaneous tumors from mice treated with IFN-γ were shown to have a greater influx of class II positive inflammatory cells than tumors treated with IFN-α or other cytokines.[148] This finding suggests that IFN-γ priming of murine tumors before preparation of TIL[80,81] may increase the yield of immune cells as well as the immunogenicity of the tumor. Both IFN-α and IFN-γ may play different roles *in vivo* and *in vitro* in combination with IL-2 therapy to increase immune recognition, infiltrating lymphocyte yield, target immunogenicity, and reactivity of adoptively transferred cells.

Role of a Host Component ■

Initial studies in mice documented that high-dose IL-2 administered alone was capable of mediating the regression of established pulmonary and hepatic metastases and subcutaneous implants from a variety of experimentally induced tumors.[13,26,88] The immunotherapeutic effect of IL-2 was abrogated in hosts preirradiated with 500 cGy, strongly suggesting that the therapeutic action of IL-2 was not direct but was mediated through a relatively radiosensitive host component.[12,26,88]

Because it was unclear whether IFN-α modulated the host's immune response to the tumor or impacted directly on tumor growth, the effect of immunosuppression by sublethal total body irradiation was also investigated.[18] Just before induction of multiple MCA-106 sarcoma liver metastases, mice were exposed to 450 cGy of total body irradiation. Three days later, mice were treated with IL-2, IFN-α, or both. A single maximal dose of 100,000 U of either lymphokine was administered IP three times daily for 4 consecutive days. As seen in Table 6–20, IL-2 alone, IFN-α alone, and the two combined showed a substantial antitumor effect in nonirradiated mice ($p < 0.05$ versus saline-injected control mice). However, in irradiated mice, no significant reduction in the number of liver metastases was noted in groups treated with either cytokine alone; when IL-2 was combined with IFN-α, small, nonsignificant reduction of metastases (28%) was noted. Thus, abrogation of the antitumor activity mediated by the administration of IL-2 alone or IFN-α alone, as well as of the synergy normally seen with the combination, implicates a host radiation-sensitive component in the mechanism of action of both lymphokines.

Our further studies have shown that IL-2 mediates its antitumor effects through the *in vivo* generation of LAK cells as well as the stimulation of Lyt-2+ lymphoid cells with more selective antitumor reactivity.[27,147] To further define the mechanism of the synergistic therapeutic effect of IFN-α plus IL-2 we examined this combination in mice immunosuppressed as a result of selective depletion of Lyt-2+ cells by IV injection of 0.1 ml of ascitic fluid from a hybridoma producing a rat IgG2b moAb against the Lyt-2 T-cell antigen.[78] Results of two characteristic

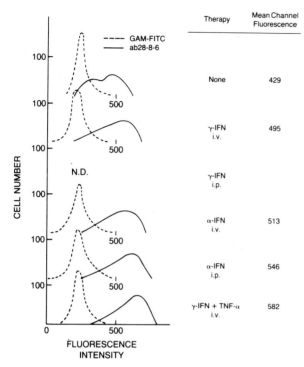

FIG. 6-8 Effect of *in vivo* cytokine treatment on MHC antigen expression by the MCA-102 sarcoma.[148] Flow cytometry profiles are shown with fluorescent channel number (measured logarithmically) on the abscissa and cell number on the ordinate. Mice bearing 10-day MCA-102 subcutaneous tumors were treated with 0.5 ml saline (HBSS) IP thrice daily; 100,000 U IFN-γ IV daily; 50,000 U IFN-γ IP thrice daily; 100,000 units IFN-α IV daily; 100,000 U IFN-α IP thrice daily; or a single dose of 2 ug TNF IV with 100,000 U IFN-γ IV daily (all given for 4 days). Mice were killed and tumors removed on day 15 after tumor cell injection and single cell suspensions were made. The profiles shown represent goat antimouse fluorescein isothiocyanate conjugated (FITC) alone with no primary antibody as a control, and antibody 28-8-6 recognizing K^b + D^b to measure class I expression. Mean channel fluorescence is shown for cells from tumor-bearing animals treated with each regimen.

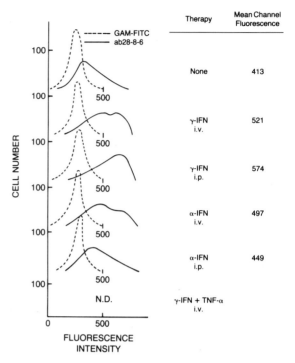

FIG. 6-9 Effect of *in vivo* cytokine treatment on MHC antigen expression by the MCA-106 sarcoma.[148] (See legend to Figure 6-8 for an explanation of experimental method.)

experiments are shown in Table 6-21. In normal mice, the combination of IFN-α and IL-2 showed synergistic therapeutic effect, with reduction of metastases of 85% (*p* = 0.001) and >99% (*p* < 0.001) in experiments 1 and 2, respectively; no significant reduction in metastases was seen in Lyt-2 depleted mice.

IFN-α can mediate a variety of biologic effects, including direct antiproliferative actions,[55,56] enhanced expression of histocompatibility antigens,[60-66] or tumor-associated antigens,[64] and augmentation of NK activity.[67,68] Our results indicate that host immune factors play a major role in the synergy of IFN-α and IL-2 because this synergy is eliminated in animals

depleted of Lyt-2+ cells and in those receiving sublethal total body irradiation.

Because tumor sensitivity to recombinant TNF appeared to correlate with relative tumor immunogenicity, we also examined the mechanism of TNF-induced regression of tumors in mice.[149] Mice bearing 8-day subcutaneous MCA-106 tumor were selectively depleted *in vivo* of T-cell subsets by the systemic administration of specific moAbs before TNF therapy. As shown in Figure 6-10, TNF-induced regression, but not early hemorrhagic necrosis, of the MCA-106 sarcoma was blocked in mice depleted of Lyt-2+ cells but not of L3T4+ cells. Treatment of all tumor-bearing animals with TNF resulted in a marked necrosis of the central portion of the tumor by 24 hours, with a reduction in average tumor area observed in the first few days after TNF administration. Over the course of the following week, normal mice and those depleted of Lyt-2+ T-cells (or both Lyt-2+ and L3T4+ T-cells) rapidly resumed their growth, and by 8 days after the injection of TNF, the size of tumors in these animals approximated that of tumors in mice receiving excipient alone.

The mechanism of the synergistic effects of TNF plus IL-2 remains to be determined; presumably, Lyt-

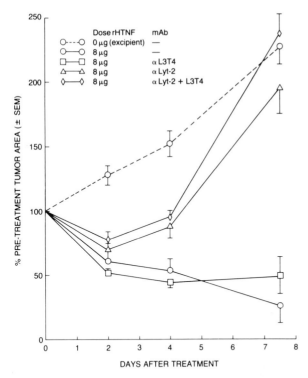

FIG. 6-10 Elimination of TNF-induced tumor regression by *in vivo* depletion of Lyt-2+ cells by monoclonal antibody.[149] C57BL/6 mice bearing 8-day subcutaneous MCA-106 sarcoma received IV antibody. Two days later, the animals received one IV injection of 8 μg TNF and were monitored for tumor progression/regression. Data are expressed as percentage of pretreatment tumor area.

2+ cells are involved. Neither TNF, IL-2, nor IFN-α exhibited antitumor effects on the nonimmunogenic MCA-102 tumor, which fails to induce Lyt-2+ effector cells in the host.[27] Partial necrosis of the MCA-102 sarcoma was observed shortly after TNF administration; however, these tumors soon recovered and regrew rapidly. Subcutaneous and single large hepatic tumors of the MCA-106 weakly immunogenic tumor undergo initial necrosis and a subsequent inflammatory response following the administration of TNF.[97,117] One action of IL-2 may involve the stimulation and proliferation of lymphoid cells with antitumor activity in this inflammatory infiltrate, resulting in further tumor destruction. Additional mechanisms may also be involved. For example, the combination of TNF and other biologic response modifiers (*i.e.,* IL-2, IFN) has been shown to augment the functional activities of T-cells,[150] NK cells,[151] macrophages,[152] polymorphonuclear leukocytes,[153] and B-cells *in vitro.*[154]

The *in vivo* mechanism responsible for the synergistic immunotherapeutic effect of the combination

Table 6-20
Radiation Effects on IL-2 and IFN-α in Reducing the Number (Mean ± SE) of 3-day MCA-106 Liver Metastases[18]

Dosage*			
IL-2	IFN-α	No Radiation	450 cGy†
—	—	99 ± 44	200 ± 37
100,000	—	1.3 ± 0.5‡	235 ± 5.7
—	100,000	4.3 ± 1.5‡	206 ± 30
100,000	100,000	4.0 ± 1.3‡	144 ± 36

* Treatment was given IP thrice daily for 4 days.
† Total body irradiation just prior to tumor cell injection.
‡ $p < 0.05$ vs. control (no treatment) group.

of chemotherapeutic agents (*i.e.,* cyclophosphamide) and IL-2 or TNF remains to be determined. Recombinant TNF causes early hemorrhagic necrosis of tumor and may act as a cytoreductive agent, thus reducing the overall tumor burden on which the chemotherapeutic agent must act. However, early hemorrhagic necrosis was also seen in the treatment of the nonimmunogenic MCA-102 sarcoma, and combined effects of TNF and chemotherapy were not seen in this model.[30] Cyclophosphamide, the most effective chemotherapeutic agent used in our studies, is known to reduce suppressor factors in mice, which may be important in dampening the immunologic reaction to the tumor.[23-25] Another potential mechanism may

Table 6-21
Loss of Therapeutic Effect in Lyt-2 Depleted Mice Receiving IFN-α, IL-2 or Both[78]

Treatment*		Lung Metastases (Mean ± SE)	
IFN-α	IL-2	Normal Mice	Lyt-2-Depleted Mice
		Experiment 1	
—	—	≥250	≥250
+	—	99 ± 38	≥250
—	+	217 ± 30	≥250
+	+	38 ± 12	≥250
		Experiment 2	
—	—	≥250	224 ± 22
+	—	195 ± 26	≥250
—	+	107 ± 31	236 ± 11
+	+	1 ± 1	174 ± 27

* Groups consist of 4–6 mice bearing 3-day pulmonary metastases from the MCA-106 tumor. Two hours before lymphokine therapy, the Lyt-2-depleted mice received 0.1 ml of ascites fluid from mice bearing a rat hybridoma (2.43) producing anti-Lyt-2 monoclonal IgG2b antibodies. IL-2 and IFN-α were administered at doses of 100,000 U IP thrice for 4 to 5 days.

involve an enhancement by CTX of the Lyt-2+ cell population, which is known to be effective in the secondary regressive phase of TNF activity.[149] Lyt-2+ cells have been shown to be involved in both TNF- and IL-2-mediated tumor regression *in vivo*.[27,147,149]

The combination of TNF and CTX resulted in significant cures for only the weakly immunogenic MCA-106 sarcoma. Only a very modest prolongation of survival was seen for the nonimmunogenic MCA-102 sarcoma. Further means to augment the therapeutic response of TNF to this tumor are needed.

The possible mechanisms by which CTX increases survival and cure rates when combined with IL-2 are numerous.[30] Most simply, IL-2 and CTX may be independently exerting direct antitumor effects, with the net result being merely the additive effect of two highly effective modalities. CTX may reduce tumor bulk to a sufficiently low level to enable IL-2 therapy to eliminate all residual tumor. The two modalities could thus appear to have synergistic effects on the endpoint of survival.

One way to separate the direct cytocidal effects of CTX from the effects of CTX on the tumor-bearing host would be to identify tumors that are resistant to CTX but responsive to therapy with IL-2. Efforts are under way to identify such a tumor system.

One attractive explanation for the enhanced antitumor effects of this combination is that CTX preferentially eliminates a suppressor cell population, thus allowing increased IL-2-driven antitumor responses to occur. Suppressor cell populations have been demonstrated in other highly immunogenic tumor models, but not in conjunction with *in vivo* IL-2 therapy.

Ultimately, the existence of CTX-sensitive suppressor cells in these tumor systems can be convincingly demonstrated only by the transfer of suppressor cell populations to CTX-treated animals, with the subsequent reversal of the effects of CTX. We have thus far failed to demonstrate suppressor populations in mice bearing syngeneic tumors, but this work is continuing.

The greater effectiveness of CTX on tumors with some degree of immunogenicity suggests that a portion of the effect of CTX alone may be immune-mediated. Moreover, the possibility that CTX inflicts nonspecific, sublethal damage on tumor cells, thus rendering them more susceptible to lysis by cytotoxic lymphocytes, cannot be conclusively excluded and requires further study.

Tumor Infiltrating Lymphocytes ■

In murine models, the combination of IFN-α and IL-2 showed synergy with Lyt-2+ TIL in mediating the reduction of established lung metastases.[78] In these experiments, any role for a host component in the response was eliminated by sublethal total body irradiation of the mice before cytokine and TIL administration. Thus, a logical assumption is that the antitumor properties of IFN-α and IL-2 reside at the effector level (*i.e.,* transferred TIL) or that the tumor cell surface may be the target. We have recently studied this synergy *in vitro*.

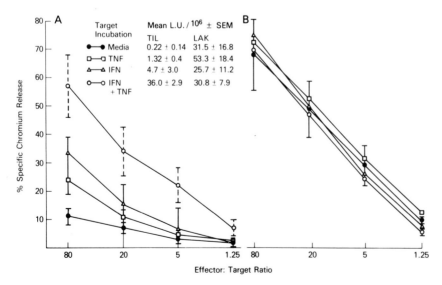

FIG. 6–11   Increased human tumor target susceptibility to TIL but not LAK lysis after cytokine treatment.[156] The renal adenocarcinoma TC 444 was cultured *in vitro* for 12 passages before treatment with recombinant cytokines for 3 days. Recovery of tumor cells was identical in all four groups. The results are a compilation of 4 h chromium[51] release assays from five experiments (mean ± SE). TIL 444 was cultured for 80–150 days in 1000 U/ml recombinant IL-2 without further antigenic stimulation.[83,87] LAK cells were generated by the *in vitro* incubation of peripheral blood mononuclear cells in 1000 U/ml of IL-2 for 3 days.

Tumor cell susceptibility to lysis *in vitro* by TIL is markedly increased following target treatment with IFN and TNF.[155,156] The combined results of five separate experiments are shown in Figure 6–11. Treatment *in vitro* of the human renal adenocarcinoma TC444 with IFN alone for 3 days significantly increased the tumor's susceptibility to lysis by autologous 444 TIL (Fig. 6–11*A*) but not by autologous 3-day LAK cells (Fig. 6–11*B*) when compared to media controls. Target cell susceptibility to TIL lysis was substantially increased by combined treatment with TNF and IFN; however, no increase was observed in LAK cell lysis. Further studies are under way to determine whether cytokine-induced enhancement of tumor susceptibility to lysis is observed with other human tumors; whether it is antigen-specific (*i.e.,* whether tumor-associated antigens increase) with restriction to the autologous TIL only; and whether cytokine up-regulation of MHC antigens on the tumor cell surface plays a role in heightened TIL lysis.

Conclusion ■

The recent availability of large quantities of recombinant lymphokines and monokines (cytokines) has permitted the examination *in vivo* of the efficacy of these reagents in cancer therapy. Interleukin-2 alone in high doses or combined at lower doses with LAK cells or TIL results in the regression of established pulmonary and hepatic metastases from certain tumors in murine models. Recent clinical trials have shown that therapy with high-dose IL-2 alone or in combination with LAK cells can mediate the regression of established metastatic disease in selected patients with advanced malignancy. These studies showed that the regression of established, growing cancer can be mediated by manipulating the immune system.

Recombinant cytokines are toxic when administered at high doses *in vivo*. Although substantial tumor size reductions can be achieved by single-modality treatments, few patients are actually cured of disease. Thus, efforts to minimize cytokine toxicity while maintaining or increasing therapeutic efficacy would be of substantial benefit.

As reviewed in this chapter, significant improvements in experimental cancer therapies have been made by combining recombinant lymphokines and monokines to augment their action and reduce the doses necessary to achieve the same or better antitumor effects. Immunotherapy studies in animals using recombinant cytokine combinations have shown

augmentation of antitumor effects and provide a rationale for clinical trials in patients with advanced cancers. It is hoped that these improvements will result in the development of immunotherapies with increased therapeutic benefit and reduced toxicity.

References ■

1. Rosenberg SA, Terry W: Passive immunotherapy of cancer in animals and man. Adv Cancer Res 25:323–388, 1977
2. Hellström KE, Hellström I: Lymphocyte-mediated cytotoxicity and blocking serum activity to tumor antigens. Adv Immunol 18:209, 1974
3. Rosenberg SA: Adoptive immunotherapy of cancer using lymphokine activated killer cells and recombinant interleukin-2. In DeVita VT, Hellman S, Rosenberg SA (eds): Important Advances in Oncology 1986, pp 55–91. Philadelphia, JB Lippincott, 1986
4. Kiessling R, Petranyi G, Karre K, Jondal M, Tracey D, Wigzell H: Killer cells: A functional comparison between natural, immune T-cell, and antibody-dependent in vitro systems. J Exp Med 143:772, 1976
5. Yron I, Wood TA, Spiess P, Rosenberg SA: In vitro growth of murine T-cells: V. The isolation and growth of lymphoid cells infiltrating syngeneic solid tumors. J Immunol 125:238–245, 1980
6. Lotze MT, Grimm E, Mazumder A, Strausser JL, Rosenberg SA: In vitro growth of cytotoxic human lymphocytes. IV. Lysis of fresh and cultured autologous tumor by lymphocytes cultured in T cell growth factor (TCGF). Cancer Res 41:4420–4425, 1981
7. Grimm EA, Rosenberg SA: The human lymphokine-activated killer cell phenomenon. In Pick E, Candy M (eds): Lymphokines, Vol 9, pp 279–311. New York, Academic Press, 1983
8. Rosenberg SA: Editorial: Lymphokine activated killer cells: A new approach to the immunotherapy of cancer. JNCI 75:595–603, 1985
9. Mulé JJ, Rosenberg SA: Successful adoptive immunotherapy of established metastases with lymphokine activated killer cells and recombinant interleukin-2. In Herberman RB, Wiltrout RH, Gorelik E (eds): Immune Responses to Metastases, pp 69–94. Boca Raton, FL, CRC Press, 1987
10. Rosenberg SA, Grimm EA, McGrogan M, Doyle M, Kawasaki E, Koths K, Mark DF: Biological activity of recombinant human interleukin-2 produced in E. coli. Science 223:1412–1415, 1984
11. Mulé JJ, Shu S, Schwarz SL, Rosenberg SA: Adoptive immunotherapy of established pulmonary metastases with LAK cells and recombinant interleukin-2. Science 225:1487–1489, 1984
12. Rosenberg SA, Mulé JJ, Spiess PJ, Reichert CM, Schwarz S: Regression of established pulmonary metastases and subcutaneous tumor mediated by the systemic administration of high dose recombinant IL-2. J Exp Med 161:1169–1188, 1985
13. Rosenberg SA, Lotze MT, Muul LM, Chang AE, Avis FP, Leitman S, Linehan WM, Robertson CN, Lee RE, Rubin JT, Seipp CA, Simpson CG, White DE: A progress report on the treatment of 157 patients with advanced cancer using lymphokine activated killer cells and interleukin-2 or high dose interleukin-2 alone. N Engl J Med 316:889–905, 1987

14. Rosenberg SA: The immunotherapy of cancer using interleukin-2: Current status and future prospects. Immunol Today 9:58–62, 1988

15. Asher A, Mulé JJ, Reichert CM, Shiloni E, Rosenberg SA: Studies on the anti-tumor efficacy of systemically administered recombinant tumor necrosis factor against several murine tumors in vivo. J Immunol 138:963–974, 1987

16. Mulé JJ, Asher A, McIntosh J, Lafreniere R, Shiloni E, Lefor A, Reichert CM, Rosenberg SA: Antitumor effects of recombinant tumor necrosis factor-alpha against murine sarcomas at visceral sites: Tumor size influences the response to therapy. Cancer Immunol Immunother 26:202–208, 1988

17. Lotze MT, Chang AE, Seipp CA, Simpson C, Vetto JT, Rosenberg SA: High dose recombinant interleukin-2 in the treatment of patients with disseminated cancer: Responses, treatment related morbidity and histologic findings. JAMA 256:3117–3124, 1986

18. Cameron RB, McIntosh JK, Rosenberg SA: Synergistic antitumor effects of combination immunotherapy with recombinant interleukin-2 and a recombinant hybrid interferon-alpha in the treatment of established murine hepatic metastases. Cancer Res 48:5810–5817, 1988

19. Quesada JR, Reubin JR, Manning JT: Alpha interferon for induction of remission in hairy cell leukemia. N Engl J Med 310:15–18, 1984

20. Spiegel RJ: The alpha interferons: Clinical overview. Semin Oncol 14(Suppl 2):1–12, 1987

21. Matory Y, Chang AE, Lipford N, Braziel R, Hyatt CL, McDonald HD, Rosenberg SA: The toxicity of recombinant human interleukin-2 in rats following intravenous infusion. J Biol Res Mod 4:377–390, 1985

22. Rosenstein M, Ettinghausen SE, Rosenberg SA: Extravasation of intravascular fluid mediated by the systemic administration of recombinant interleukin-2. J Immunol 137:1735–1742, 1986

23. Evans R: Combination therapy by using cyclophosphamide and tumor sensitized lymphocytes: A possible mechanism of action. J Immunol 130:2511, 1983

24. Greenberg PD, Kern KE, Cheever MA: Therapy of disseminated murine leukemia with cyclophosphamide and immune Lyt-1+, 2− T-cells. J Exp Med 161:1122–1134, 1985

25. North RJ: Cyclophosphamide-facilitated adoptive immunotherapy of established tumor depends on elimination of tumor induced suppressor cells. J Exp Med 155:1063–1074, 1982

26. Lafreniere R, Rosenberg SA: Adoptive immunotherapy of murine hepatic metastases with lymphokine activated killer (LAK) cells and recombinant interleukin-2 (RIL-2) can mediate the regression of both immunogenic and non-immunogenic sarcomas and an adenocarcinoma. J Immunol 135:4273–4280, 1985

27. Mulé JJ, Yang JC, Lafreniere R, Shu S, Rosenberg SA: Identification of cellular mechanisms operational in vivo during the regression of established pulmonary metastases by the systemic administration of high-dose recombinant interleukin-2. J Immunol 139:285–294, 1987

28. Rosenberg SA: Immunotherapy of patients with advanced cancer using interleukin-2 alone or in combination with lymphokine activated killer cells. In DeVita V, Hellman S, Rosenberg SA (eds): Important Advances in Oncology 1988, pp 217–257. Philadelphia, JB Lippincott 1988

29. Ettinghausen SE, Puri RK, Rosenberg SA: Increased vascular permeability in organs mediated by the systemic administration of lymphokine activated killer cells and recombinant interleukin-2 in mice. JNCI 80:177–188, 1988

30. Papa MZ, Yang JC, Vetto JT, Shiloni E, Eisenthal A, Rosenberg SA: Combined effects of chemotherapy and interleukin-2 in the therapy of mice with advanced pulmonary tumors. Cancer Res 48:122–129, 1988

31. Mitchell MS, Kempf RA, Harel W, Shau H, Boswell WD, Lind S, Bradley EC: Effectiveness and tolerability of low-dose cyclophosphamide and low-dose intravenous interleukin-2 in disseminated melanoma. J Clin Oncol 6:409–424, 1988

32. Rosenberg SA: Cancer therapy with interleukin-2: Immunologic manipulations can mediate the regression of cancer in humans. J Clin Oncol 6:403–406, 1988

33. Bernstein ID, Tam MR, Nowinski RC: Mouse leukemia therapy with monoclonal antibodies against thymus differentiation antigen. Science 207:68–71, 1980

34. Herlyn DM, Steplewski Z, Herlyn MF, Koprowski H: Inhibition of colorectal carcinoma in nude mice by monoclonal antibody. Cancer Res 40:717–721, 1980

35. Hellström I, Brankovan V, Hellström KE: Strong antitumor activities of IgG3 antibodies to a human melanoma-associated ganglioside. Proc Natl Acad Sci USA 82:1499–1502, 1985

36. Kirch ME, Hammerling U: Immunotherapy of murine leukemias by monoclonal antibody. I. Effect of passively administered antibody on growth of transplanted tumor cells. J Immunol 127:805–810, 1981

37. Weinstein JN, Parker RJ, Holton OD, Keenan AM, Covell DG, Black CDV, Sieber SM: Lymphatic delivery of monoclonal antibodies: Potential for detection and treatment of lymph node metastases. Cancer Invest 3:85–96, 1985

38. Krolick KA, Uhr JW, Slavin S, Vitetta ES: In vivo therapy of murine B cell tumor (BCL1) using antibody-ricin A chain immunotoxins. J Exp Med 155:1797–1809, 1982

39. Hwang KM, Foon KA, Cheung PH, Pearson JW, Oldham RK: Selective antitumor effect on L10 hepatocarcinoma cells of a potent immunoconjugate composed of the A chain of Abrin and a monoclonal antibody to a hepatoma-associated antigen. Cancer Res 44:4578–4586, 1984

40. Schulz G, Bumol TF, Reisfeld RA: Monoclonal antibody-directed effector cells selectively lyse human melanoma cells in vitro and in vivo. Proc Natl Acad Sci USA 80:5407–5411, 1983

41. Lovchik JC, Hong R: Antibody dependent cell mediated cytolysis (ADCC): analysis and projections. Prog Allerg 22:1–44, 1977

42. Shiloni E, Eisenthal A, Sachs D, Rosenberg SA: Antibody dependent cellular cytotoxicity mediated by murine lymphocytes activated in recombinant interleukin-2. J Immunol 138:1992–1998, 1987

43. Eisenthal A, Lafreniere R, Lefor AT, Rosenberg SA: The effect of anti B16 melanoma monoclonal antibody on established murine B16 melanoma liver metastases. Cancer Res 47:2771–2776, 1987

44. Eisenthal A, Cameron RC, Rosenberg SA: The effect of combined therapy with lymphokine activated killer (LAK) cells, interleukin-2 and specific monoclonal antibody on established B16 melanoma lung metastases. Cancer Res (in press)

45. Berinstein N, Levy R: Treatment of a murine B cell lymphoma with monoclonal antibodies and IL-2. J Immunol 139:971–976, 1987

46. Kawase I, Komuta K, Hara H, Inoue T, Hosoe S, Ikeda T, Shirasaka T, Yokota S, Tanio Y, Masuno T, Kishimoto S: Combined therapy of mice bearing a lymphokine-activated killer-resistant tumor with recombinant interleukin-2 and an antitumor monoclonal antibody capable of inducing antibody-

dependent cellular cytotoxicity. Cancer Res 48:1173–1179, 1988

47. Gresser I, Bourali C: Antitumor effects of interferon preparations in mice. JNCI 45:365–376, 1970

48. Kataoka T, Matsuura N, Oh-hashi F, Suhara Y: Treatment regimen and host T-cell-dependent therapeutic effect of interferon in mouse solid tumors. Cancer Res 45:3548–3553, 1985

49. Quesada JR: Interferons in cancer research—An update. Cancer Bull 35:30–39, 1983

50. Imanishi J, Kishida T: Clinical trials with interferon in Japan. Tex Rep Biol Med 41:647–652, 1982

51. Matsumori A, Crumpacker CS, Abelmann WH: Prevention of viral myocarditis with recombinant human leukocyte interferon alpha A/D in a murine model. J Am Coll Cardiol 9: 1320–1325, 1987

52. Mora I, Porres JC, Bartolome J, Quiroga JA, Gutiez J, Hernandez GC, Bas C, Carreno V: Changes of hepatitis B virus (HBV) markers during prolonged recombinant interferon alpha-2A treatment of chronic HBV infection. J Hepatol 4:29–36, 1987

53. Cheson BD, Martin A: Clinical trials in hairy cell leukemia: current status and future directions. Ann Intern Med 106: 871–878, 1987

54. Spiegel RJ: Clinical overview of alpha interferon: Studies and future directions. Cancer 59(Suppl 3):626–631, 1987

55. Brosjo O, Bauer HCF, Brostrom L, Nilsson OS, Reinholt FP, Tribukait B: Growth inhibition of human osteosarcomas in nude mice by human interferon: Significance of dose and tumor differentiation. Cancer Res 47:258–262, 1987

56. Fidler IJ, Heicappell R, Saiki I, Grutter G, Horisberger MA, Nuesch J: Direct antiproliferative effects of recombinant human interferon-B/D hybrids on human tumor cell lines. Cancer Res 47:2020–2027, 1987

57. Hicks NJ, Morris AG, Burke DC: Partial reversion of the transformed phenotype of murine sarcoma virus-transformed cells in the presence of interferon: A possible mechanism for the antitumor effect of interferon. J Cell Sci 49:225–236, 1981

58. Samid D, Flessate DM, Friedman RM: Interferon-induced revertants of ras-transformed cells: Resistance to transformation by specific oncogenes and retransformation by 5-azacytidine. Mol Cell Biol 7:2196–2200, 1987

59. Kohlhepp EA, Condon ME, Hamburger AW: Recombinant human interferon alpha enhancement of retinoic-acid-induced differentiation of HL-60 cells. Exp Hematol 15:414–418, 1987

60. Wan YJ, Orrison BM, Lieberman R, Lazarovici P, Ozato K: Induction of major histocompatibility class 1 antigens by interferons in undifferentiated F9 cells. J Cell Physiol 130:276–283, 1987

61. Fertsch D, Schoenberg DR, Germain RN, Tou JYL, Vogel SN: Induction of macrophage Ia antigen expression by rIFN-gamma and down-regulation by IFN-alpha/beta and dexamethasone are mediated by changes in steady-state levels of Ia mRNA. J Immunol 139:244–249, 1987

62. Aguet M, Vignaux F, Fridman WH, Gresser I: Enhancement of Fc receptor expression in interferon-treated mice. Eur J Immunol 11:926–930, 1981

63. van den Berg HW, Leahey WJ, Lynch M, Clarke R, Nelson J: Recombinant human interferon alpha increases oestrogen receptor expression in human breast cancer cells (ZR-75-1) and sensitises them to the anti-proliferative effects of tamoxifen. Br J Cancer 55:255–257, 1987

64. Greiner JW, Guadagni F, Noguchi P, Pestka S, Colcher D, Fisher PB, Schlom J: Recombinant interferon enhances

monoclonal antibody-targeting of carcinoma lesions *in vivo*. Science 235:895–898, 1987

65. Heron I, Hokland M, Berg K: Enhanced expression of β-2-microglobulin and HLA antigens on human lymphoid cells by interferon. Proc Natl Acad Sci USA 75:6215–6219, 1978

66. Matsumoto S, Moriyama M, Imanishi H: Effects of recombinant human interferon-gamma (Met-Gin form) on expression of Fc receptor and Ia-like antigen on human peripheral monocytes and lymphocytes: A comparative study with natural human interferon-alpha and beta. Chem Pharm Bull (Tokyo) 35:335–343, 1987

67. Talmadge JE, Herberman RB, Chirigos MA, Maluish AE, Schneider MA, Adams JS, Phillips H, Thurman GB, Varesio L, Long CW, Oldham RK, Wiltrout RH: Hyporesponsiveness to augmentation of murine natural killer cell activity in different anatomical compartments by multiple injections of various immunomodulators including recombinant interferons and interleukin-2. J Immunol 135:2483–2488, 1985

68. Herberman RB, Ortaldo JR, Timonen T, Reynolds CW, Djeu JY, Pestka S, Stanton J: Interferon and natural killer (NK) cells. Tex Rep Biol Med 41:590–602, 1981

69. Evans SS, Ozer H: Enhancement of a human antibody response in vitro mediated by interaction of interferon-α with T lymphocytes. J Immunol 138:2451–2456, 1987

70. Goodman MG: Interaction between cytokines and 8-mercaptoguanosine in humoral immunity: Synergy with interferon. J Immunol 139:142–146, 1987

71. Knop J, Taborski B, DeMaeyer-Guignard J: Selective inhibition of the generation of T suppressor cells of contact sensitivity in vitro by interferon. J Immunol 138:3684–3687, 1987

72. Chen BD, Najor F: Macrophage activation by interferon α + β is associated with a loss of proliferative capacity: Role of interferon α + β in the regulation of macrophage proliferation and function. Cell Immunol 106:343–354, 1987

73. Jett JR, Mantovani A, Herberman RB: Augmentation of human monocyte-mediated cytolysis by interferon. Cell Immunol 54:425–434, 1980

74. Brunda MT, Bellantoni D, Sulich V: *In vivo* anti-tumor activity of combinations of interferon alpha and interleukin-2 in a murine model. Correlation of efficacy with the induction of cytotoxic cells resembling natural killer cells. Int J Cancer 40:365–371, 1987

75. Iigo M, Sakurai M, Tamura T, Saijo N, Hoshi A: In vivo antitumor activity of multiple injections of recombinant interleukin-2, alone and in combination with three different types of recombinant interferon, on various syngeneic murine tumors. Cancer Res 48:260–264, 1988

76. Silagi S, Dutkowski R, Schaefer A: Eradication of mouse melanoma by combined treatment with recombinant human interleukin-2 and recombinant murine interferon-gamma. Int J Cancer 41:315–322, 1988

77. Maeda S, McCandliss R, Gross M, Sloma A, Familletti PC, Tabor JM, Evinger M, Levy WP, Pestka S: Construction and identification of bacterial plasmids containing nucleotide sequence for human leukocyte interferon. Proc Natl Acad Sci 77:7010–7013, 1980

78. Rosenberg SA, Schwarz S, Spiess P: Combination immunotherapy of cancer: Synergistic anti-tumor interactions of interleukin-2, alpha-interferon and tumor infiltrating lymphocytes. Science JNCI 80:1393–1397, 1988

79. Prats I, Marino M, Rosenberg SA: Combined antitumor effect of interferon alpha and interleukin-2 in a murine subdermal tumor model. (Submitted for publication)

80. Rosenberg SA, Spiess P, Lafreniere R: A new approach to the adoptive immunotherapy of cancer with tumor-infiltrating lymphocytes. Science 223:1318–1321, 1986

81. Spiess PJ, Yang JC, Rosenberg SA: In vivo antitumor activity of tumor infiltrating lymphocytes expanded in recombinant interleukin-2. JNCI 79:1067–1075, 1987

82. Muul LM, Spiess PJ, Director EP, Rosenberg SA: Identification of specific cytolytic immune responses against autologous tumor in humans bearing malignant melanoma. J Immunol 138:989–995, 1987

83. Topalian SL, Muul LM, Solomon D, Rosenberg SA: Expansion of human tumor infiltrating lymphocytes for use in immunotherapy trials. J Immunol Meth 102:127–141, 1987

84. Belldegrun A, Muul LM, Rosenberg SA: Interleukin-2 expanded tumor infiltrating lymphocytes in human renal cell cancer: Isolation, characterization and antitumor activity. Cancer Res 48:206–214, 1988

85. Topalian S, Solomon D, Avis FP, Chang AE, Freerksen DL, Linehan WM, Lotze MT, Robertson CN, Seipp CA, Simon P, Simpson CG, Rosenberg SA: Immunotherapy of patients with advanced cancer using tumor infiltrating lymphocytes and recombinant interleukin-2: A pilot study. J Clin Oncol 6:839–853, 1988

86. Weber JS, Jay G, Rosenberg SA: Immunotherapy of a murine tumor with interleukin-2; increased sensitivity after MHC Class I gene transfection. J Exp Med 166:1716–1733, 1987

87. Topalian SL, Solomon D, Rosenberg SA: Tumor-specific cytolysis by lymphocytes infiltrating human melanomas. J Immunol (in press)

88. Rosenberg SA, Mulé JJ: Immunotherapy of cancer with lymphokine activated killer cells and recombinant interleukin-2. Surgery 98:437–443, 1985

89. Dailey MO, Pillemer E, Weissman IL: Protection against syngeneic lymphoma by a long-lived cytotoxic T-cell clone. Proc Natl Acad Sci USA 79:5384, 1982

90. Binz H, Fenner M, Engel R, Wigzell H: Studies on chemically induced rat tumors. II. Partial protection against syngeneic lethal tumors by cloned syngeneic cytotoxic T lymphocytes. Int J Cancer 32:491, 1983

91. Engers HD, Glasebrook AL, Sorenson GD: Allogeneic tumor rejection induced by the intravenous injection of Lyt-2+ cytolytic T lymphocyte clones. J Exp Med 156:1280, 1982

92. Rosenstein M, Rosenberg SA: Generation of lytic and proliferative lymphoid clones to syngeneic tumor: In vitro and in vivo studies. JNCI 72:1161, 1986

93. Matis LA, Shu S, Groves ES, Zinn S, Cho T, Kruisbeek AM, Rosenstein M, Rosenberg SA: Adoptive immunotherapy of a syngeneic murine leukemia with a tumor-specific cytotoxic T cell clone and recombinant human interleukin-2: Correlation with clonal IL-2 receptor expression. J Immunol 136:3496, 1986

94. Klarnet JP, Matis LA, Kern DE, Mizuno MT, Peace DJ, Thompson JA, Greenberg PD, Cheever MA: Antigen-driven T cell clones can proliferate in vivo, eradicate disseminated leukemia, and provide specific immunologic memory. J Immunol 138:4012, 1987

95. DeGraaf PW, Horak E, Bookman MA: Adoptive immunotherapy of syngeneic murine leukemia is enhanced by the combination of recombinant IFN-gamma and a tumor-specific cytotoxic T cell clone. J Immunol 140:2853–2857, 1988

96. Old LJ: Tumor necrosis factor (TNF). Science 230:630, 1985

97. Asher A, Mulé JJ, Reichert CM, Shiloni E, Rosenberg SA: Studies on the anti-tumor efficacy of systemically administered recombinant tumor necrosis factor against several murine tumors in vivo. J Immunol 138:963–974, 1987

98. Aggarwal BB, Kohr WJ, Hass PE, Moffat B, Spencer SA, Henzel WJ, Bringman TS, Nedwin GE, Goeddel DV, Harkins RN: Human tumor necrosis factor. J Biol Chem 260:2345, 1985

99. Pennica D, Hayflick JS, Bringman TS, Palladino MA, Goeddel DV: Cloning and expression in Escherichia coli of the cDNA for murine tumor necrosis factor. Proc Natl Acad Sci USA 82:6060, 1985

100. Carswell EA, Old LJ, Kassel RL, Green S, Fiore N, Williamson B: An endotoxin-induced serum factor that causes necrosis of tumors. Proc Natl Acad Sci USA 72:3666, 1975

101. Wang AM, Creasey AA, Ladner MB, Lin LS, Strickler JN, Van Arsdell R, Yamamoto R, Mark DF: Molecular cloning of the complementary DNA for human tumor necrosis factor. Science 228:149, 1985

102. Pennica D, Nedwin GE, Hayflick JS, Seeburg PH, Derynck R, Palladino MA, Kohr WJ, Aggarwal BB, Goeddel DV: Human tumour necrosis factor: Precursor structure, expression and homology to lymphotoxin. Nature 312:724, 1984

103. Sugarman BJ, Aggarval BB, Hass PE, Figari IS, Palladino MA, Shepard HM: Recombinant human tumor necrosis factor-alpha: Effects on proliferation of normal and transformed cells in vitro. Science 230:943–945, 1985

104. Creasy AA, Doyle LV, Reynolds MT, Jung T, Lin LS, Vitt CR: Biological effects of recombinant human tumor necrosis factor and its novel muteins on tumor and normal cell lines. Cancer Res 47:145–149, 1987

105. Haranaka K, Satomi N, Sakurai A: Antitumor activity of murine tumor necrosis factor against transplanted murine tumors and heterotransplanted human tumors in nude mice. Int J Cancer 34:263–267, 1984

106. Creasy AA, Reynolds TR, Laird W: Cures and partial regression of murine and human tumors by recombinant tumor necrosis factor. Cancer Res 46:5687–5690, 1986

107. Mulé JJ, Asher A, McIntosh J, Lafreniere R, Shiloni E, Lefor A, Reichert CM, Rosenberg SA: Anti-tumor effects of recombinant tumor necrosis factor-against murine sarcomas at visceral sites: Tumor size influences the response to therapy. Cancer Immunol Immunother 26:202–208, 1988

108. International conference on tumor necrosis factor and related cytokines. Immunobiology 175:1–143, 1987

109. Blick M, Sherwin SA, Rosenblum M, Gutterman J: Phase I study of recombinant tumor necrosis factor in cancer patients. Cancer Res 47:2986–2989, 1987

110. Schiller JH, Bittner G, Storer B, Wilson JKV: Synergistic antitumor effects of tumor necrosis factor and gamma-interferon on human colon carcinoma cell lines. Cancer Res 47:2809–2813, 1987

111. Naomoto Y, Tanaka N, Fuchimoto S, Orita K: In vitro synergistic effects of natural human tumor necrosis factor and natural human interferon-alpha. Jpn J Cancer Res 78:87–92, 1987

112. Brouckaert PGG, Leroux-Roels GG, Guisez Y, Tavernier J, Fiers W: In vivo antitumor activity of recombinant human and murine TNF, alone and in combination with murine IFN-gamma, on a syngeneic murine melanoma. Int J Cancer 38:763–769, 1986

113. Balkwill FR, Ward BG, Moodie E, Fiers W: Therapeutic potential of tumor necrosis factor-alpha and gamma-interferon in experimental human ovarian cancer. Cancer Res 47:4755–4758, 1987

114. Talmadge JE, Tribble HR, Pennington RW, Phillips H, Wiltrout RH: Immunomodulatory and immunotherapeutic properties of gamma-interferon and recombinant tumor necrosis factor in mice. Cancer Res 47:2563–2570, 1987

115. Nishimura T, Ohta S, Sato N, Togashi Y, Goto M, Hashimoto Y: Combination tumor-immunotherapy with recombinant tumor necrosis factor and recombinant interleukin-2 in mice. Int J Cancer 40:255–261, 1987

116. Winkelhake JL, Stampfl S, Zimmerman RJ: Synergistic effects of combination therapy with human recombinant interleukin-2 and tumor necrosis factor in murine tumor models. Cancer Res 47:3948–3953, 1987

117. McIntosh JK, Mulé JJ, Merino MJ, Rosenberg SA: Synergistic anti-tumor effects of immunotherapy with recombinant interleukin-2 and recombinant tumor necrosis factor-alpha. Cancer Res 48:4011–4017, 1988

118. McIntosh JK, Mulé JJ, Krosnick J, Rosenberg SA: Combination lymphokine therapy: Synergistic antitumor effects of tumor necrosis factor, interleukin-2, and interferon-alpha against established murine subdermal and hepatic tumors. Surg Forum 1988 (in press)

119. Alexander RB, Isaacs JD, Coffey DS: Tumor necrosis factor enhances the in vitro and in vivo efficacy of chemotherapeutic drugs targeted at DNA topoisomerase II in the treatment of murine bladder cancer. J Urol 138:427–429, 1987

120. Regenass U, Muller M, Curachellas E: Anti-tumor effects of tumor necrosis factor in combination with chemotherapeutic agents. Int J Cancer 39:266–273, 1987

121. Haranaka K, Sakurai A, Satomi N: Anti-tumor activity of recombinant human tumor necrosis factor in combination with hyperthermia, chemotherapy or immunotherapy. J Biol Response Modifiers 6:379–391, 1987

122. Krosnick JA, Mulé JJ, McIntosh JK, Rosenberg SA: Augmentation of anti-tumor efficacy by the combination of recombinant tumor necrosis factor and chemotherapeutic agents in vivo. Cancer Res (in press)

123. Dinarello CA: Biology of interleukin-2. FASEB J 2:108–115, 1988

124. Lotze MT, Rosenberg SA: Interleukin-2 as a pharmacologic reagent. In Smith K (ed): Lymphokines. Orlando, FL, Academic Press (in press)

125. Happel AJ, Lee JC, Farrar WF, Ihle JN: Establishment of continuous cultures of Thy 1-2+, Lyt 1+, 2− T cells using purified interleukin-3. Cell 25:179, 1981

126. Hattori M, Sudo T, Iizuka M, Kobayashi S, Nishio S, Kano S, Minato N: Generation of continuous large granular lymphocyte lines by interleukin-2 from the spleen cells of mice infected with Moloney leukemia virus: Involvement of interleukin-3. J Exp Med 166:833–849, 1987

127. Paul WE: Interleukin-4/B-cell stimulatory factor 1: One lymphokine, many functions. FASEB J 1:456, 1987

128. Yokota T, Arai N, DeVries J, Spits H, Banchereau J, Zlotnik A, Rennick D, Howard M, Takebe Y, Mujatake S, Lee F, Arai KI: Molecular biology of interleukin-4 and interleukin-5 genes and biology of their products that stimulate B cells, T cells, and hemopoietic cells. Immunol Rev 102:137–187, 1988

129. Loughnan MS, Sanderson CJ, Nossal GJV: Soluble interleukin-2 receptors are released from the cell surface of normal murine B lymphocytes stimulated with interleukin-5. Proc Natl Acad Sci USA 85:3115–3119, 1988

130. Lotz M, Jirik F, Kabouridis P, Tsoukas C, Hirano T, Kishimoto T, Carson D: B cell stimulating factor 2/interleukin-6 is a costimulant for human thymocytes and T lymphocytes. J Exp Med 167:1253–1258, 1988

131. Takai Y, Wong GG, Clark SC, Burakoff SJ, Herrmann SH: B-cell stimulatory factor-2 is involved in the differentiation of cytotoxic T lymphocytes. J Immunol 40:508, 1987

132. Namen AE, Lupton S, Hjerrild K, Wignall J, Mochizuki DY, Schmierer A, Mosley B, March CJ, Urdal D, Gillis S, Cosman D, Goodwin RG: Stimulation of B-cell progenetors by cloned murine interleukin-7. Nature 333:571–573, 1988

133. Kern DE, Peace DJ, Klarnet JP, Cheever MA, Greenberg PD: IL-4 is an endogenous T cell growth factor during the immune response to a syngeneic retrovirus-induced tumor. J Immunol 141:2824–2830, 1988

134. Mulé JJ, Smith CA, Rosenberg SA: Interleukin-4 (B-cell stimulatory factor-1) can mediate the induction of LAK activity directed against fresh tumor cells. J Exp Med 166:792–797, 1987

135. Peace DJ, Kern DE, Schultz KR, Greenberg PD, Cheever MA: IL-4 induced lymphokine-activated killer cells: Lytic activity is mediated by phenotypically distinct natural killer-like and T cell-like large granular lymphocytes. J Immunol 140:3679–3685, 1988

136. Mulé JJ, Krosnick JA, Rosenberg SA: Interleukin-4 regulation of murine lymphokine-activated killer (LAK) activity in vitro: Effects on the interleukin-2 induced expansion, cytotoxicity and phenotype of LAK effectors. J Immunol (in press)

137. Muul LM, Director EP, Hyatt CL, Rosenberg SA: Large scale production of human lymphokine activated killer cells for use in adoptive immunotherapy. J Immunol Meth 88:265–275, 1986

138. Kawakami Y, Custer M, Rosenberg SA, Lotze MT: Interleukin-4 regulates interleukin-2 induction of lymphokine activated killer activity from human lymphocytes. (Submitted for publication)

139. Widner MB, Acres RB, Sassenfeld HM, Grabstein KH: Regulation of cytolytic cell populations from human peripheral blood by B cell stimulatory factor 1 (interleukin-4). J Exp Med 166:1447, 1987

140. Fisher B, Packard BS, Read EJ, Carrasquillo JA, Carter CS, Topalian SL, Yang JC, Rosenberg SA: Tumor localization of adoptively transferred indium-111 labeled tumor infiltrating lymphocytes in patients with advanced cancer. J Clin Oncol (in press)

141. Kawakami Y, Rosenberg SA, Lotze MT: Interleukin-4 promotes the growth of tumor infiltrating lymphocytes specific for human autologous melanoma. J Exp Med (in press)

142. Tanaka K, Hayashi H, Hamada G, Khoury G, Jay G: Expression of major histocompatibility complex class I antigens as a strategy for the potentiation of immune recognition of tumor cells. Proc Natl Acad Sci USA 83:8723, 1986

143. De Baestelier P, Katsav S, Gorelik E, Feldman M, Segal S: Differential expression of H-2 gene products in tumor cells is associated with their metastatogenic properties. Nature 288:179, 1983

144. Wallich R, Bulbuc N, Halmmerling GJ, Katsav S, Segal S, Feldman M: Abrogation of metastatic properties of tumor cells by de novo expression of H-2K antigens following H-2 gene transfection. Nature 315:301, 1985

145. Hui K, Grosveld F, Festenstein H: Rejection of transplantable AKR leukemia cells following MHC DNA-mediated cell transformation. Nature 311:740, 1985

146. Tanaka K, Isselbacher KJ, Khoury G, Jay G: Reversal of oncogenesis by the expression of a major histocompatibility class I gene. Science 228:26, 1985

147. Weber JS, Jay G, Rosenberg SA: Immunotherapy of a murine tumor with interleukin-2; increased sensitivity after MHC class I gene transfection. J Exp Med 166:1716–1733, 1987

148. Weber JS, Rosenberg SA: Modulation of murine tumor major histocompatibility antigens by cytokines in vivo and in vitro. Cancer Res 48:5818–5824, 1988

149. Asher AL, Mulé JJ, Rosenberg SA: Recombinant human tumor necrosis factor mediates regression of a murine sarcoma in vivo via Lyt-2+ cells. Cancer Immunol Immunother (in press)

150. Scheurich P, Thoma B, Ucer U, Pfizenmaier K: Immunoregulatory activity of recombinant human tumor necrosis factor-alpha: Induction of TNF receptors on human T cells and TNF-alpha-mediated enhancement of T cell responses. J Immunol 138:1786, 1987

151. Ostensen ME, Thiele DL, Lipsky PE: Tumor necrosis factor-alpha enhances cytolytic activity of human natural killer cells. J Immunol 138:4185, 1987

152. Philip R, Epstein LB: Tumor necrosis factor as immunomodulator and mediator of monocyte cytotoxicity induced by itself, gamma-interferon, and interleukin-1. Nature 323: 86, 1986

153. Shalaby MR, Aggarwal BB, Rinderknecht E, Svedersky LP, Finkle BS, Palladino MA: Activation of human polymorphonuclear neutrophil functions by interferon-gamma and tumor necrosis factors. J Immunol 135:2069, 1985

154. Kehrl JH, Miller A, Fauci AS: Effect of tumor necrosis factor-alpha on mitogen-activated human B cells. J Exp Med 166: 786, 1987

155. Wiebke EA, Lotze MT, Rosenberg SA: Tumor cell susceptibility to lysis: Marked increase in lysis by tumor infiltrating lymphocytes following target stimulation with interferon-γ and tumor necrosis factor-α. Implication for immunotherapy. Surg Forum 38:436–438, 1987

156. Stotter H, Wiebke EA, Tomita S, Belldegrun A, Topalian S, Rosenberg SA, Lotze MT: Cytokines alter target cell susceptibility to lysis: II. Evaluation of tumor infiltrating lymphocytes. (Submitted for publication)

Part Two

Clinical Progress

Sandra Meta Swain

Marc E. Lippman

Treatment of Patients With Inflammatory Breast Cancer

7

Introduction ■

Early reports described inflammatory breast cancer by various names, including mastitis carcinomatosa, acute brawny cancer, acute scirrhous carcinoma, acute medullary cancer, acute mammary cancer, acute mammary carcinomatosis, lactation cancer, carcinoma mastitoides, inflamed cancer, acute cancer of the breast, acute encephaloid cancer, and lymphocytoma of the breast.[1-6] The term "inflammatory breast cancer" was first used by Lee and Tannenbaum in 1924.[1] They described the condition in detail to enhance its recognition by all physicians: "the breast of the affected side usually increases in size. . . . This enlargement is more often diffuse. . . . As the disease progresses the skin becomes deep red or reddish-purple and to the touch is brawny and infiltrated. The inflamed areas present a distinct raised periphery after the fashion of erysipelas."

Lee and Tannenbaum described 28 cases that had these characteristics.[1] They concluded that this was a distinct entity that was often mistaken for other diseases of the breast. In addition to the characteristic clinical signs, the pathology of the tumor varied and there was no specific histology; the one distinct pathologic feature was dermal lymphatic invasion.

Since that report, other investigators have described this disease and confirmed these findings. Haagensen followed one of the largest early series of patients with this disease.[7] His description of the clinical findings is used by many as the classic criteria for the diagnosis and will be described in the following sections.

This chapter discusses the incidence, patient characteristics, and symptoms and signs of the disease; its pathologic features, including the controversy over whether the diagnosis is clinical or pathologic; classification; and treatment. It concludes with a description of our experience treating patients with inflammatory breast cancer at the National Cancer Institute.

Incidence ■

Inflammatory carcinoma is uncommon, and accounts for 1% to 4% of all breast cancers.[1,7-17] Haagensen's cases[7] represented 1% of all of his breast cancer patients, whereas Taylor and Meltzer[17] reported a 4% incidence. However, they included what they called both primary and secondary inflammatory carcinoma. The Surveillance, Epidemiology, and End Results (SEER) program presented an analysis of data collected from 1975 to 1981.[18] Of the 60,479 cases of breast cancer reported, 153 patients had both the clinical and pathologic features of inflammatory cancer and 2937 had the clinical diagnosis only, for an overall incidence of 5.1%. There were also 81 cases with only the pathologic finding of dermal lymphatic invasion. These were considered "occult" inflammatory breast cancer and are not included in the incidence figures.

Patient Characteristics ■

The age at which inflammatory breast cancer is diagnosed is similar to that of the more common invasive breast carcinomas, with means in various series ranging from 45 to 54 years.[1,7-9,11,12,14,15,17] There was one recent case report of inflammatory breast cancer in a child.[19] A 12-year-old girl in Thailand presented with classical inflammatory features and was treated with radiation therapy, during which she developed bone metastases. Despite treatment with chemotherapy, she died within 8 months of her diagnosis.

Early reports by Klotz in 1869,[6] von Volkmann in 1875,[5] and Schumann in 1911[3] suggested that inflammatory breast cancer was associated in most cases with pregnancy and lactation. However, other reports have not substantiated this association. Lee and Tannenbaum's classic description of 28 patients did not include any women who were lactating.[1] Taylor and Meltzer's series of 38 patients included only one who developed inflammatory cancer during pregnancy.[17] However, in 1938 Meltzer reviewed the literature on the subject and found that of 205 cases of cancer associated with pregnancy, 85 occurred prior to pregnancy, 72 occurred during pregnancy and 48 during lactation. Of those cancers occurring during pregnancy, 24% were inflammatory; for those associated with lactation, the figure was 40%. Haagensen reported in his series of 89 cases only 4 that occurred during pregnancy or lactation.[7] The conclusion from these series is that inflammatory cancer can occur during pregnancy but is not more common in this setting.

The largest data base on patients with inflammatory breast cancer is from SEER.[18] The average age is not listed, but a majority of patients were over 55 years. This report also found that the incidence of inflammatory breast cancer in the black population (using the broadest definition, which included occult inflammatory cancer) was 10.1%. This incidence is substantially higher than that among white patients and other nonwhite patients.

Clinical Signs and Symptoms ■

The symptoms that bring inflammatory carcinoma to the patient's attention include heaviness of the breast, a slight burning sensation, aching, and an increase in the size, tenderness, firmness, and redness of the breast. There is usually no fever, which might indicate an infection. However, patients are often treated with a course of antibiotics for a presumed infection, thereby delaying the diagnosis.

The signs include those mentioned in the introduction. The breast is reddened and edematous, especially in the dependent part or inferior aspect. Coloration varies from reddish-purple or reddish-brown to faint pink which may be mottled. These changes can occur beyond the normal extent of the breast.

The breast is enlarged and frequently lacks an associated mass. At times, the breast may be warm and tender to the touch. Nipple retraction may be present later in the course of the disease. A classic presentation is shown in Figure 7–1.

Haagensen described the clinical features of inflammatory breast cancer in his series of 89 patients.[7] The diagnosis was not made unless redness was present over at least one-third of the breast. A tumor mass was present in 57% of patients, erythema in 57%, breast enlargement in 48%, edema of the skin in 13%, warmth of the skin in 8%, nipple retraction in 13%, and pain in 29%. Many investigators rely on these criteria for the diagnosis of inflammatory breast cancer.

Other reports include two types of inflammatory carcinoma, primary and secondary. Taylor and Meltzer described the primary type, with features listed above.[17] The secondary type occurred when a localized tumor had been present for some time and inflammatory signs appeared late in the course of the disease. This category also includes recurrences in the site of the mastectomy scar and recurrences in a previously irradiated breast.

Piera and colleagues[20] described locally advanced breast cancer (LABC) with an inflammatory component in 1986. There were 50 patients in their institution in Barcelona, Spain, with LABC and 30 with LABC and an inflammatory component (LAIC). Patients were treated with radiation therapy, and all but one had systemic therapy with either hormones or chemotherapeutic drug regimens such as cyclophosphamide/methotrexate/5-fluorouracil (CMF) or doxorubicin/cyclophosphamide (AC). Median overall survival was 25 months for the LAIC group and 70 months for the LABC group. These figures are similar

FIG. 7–1   Clinical presentation of inflammatory breast cancer in the left breast, revealing edema, erythema, and peau d'orange.

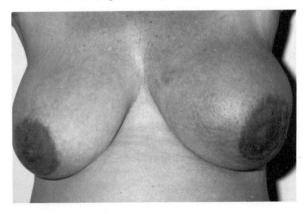

to those for the more classic cases of inflammatory carcinomas. Piera and colleagues suggest that patients who have inflammatory signs that are secondary or involve less than one-third of the breast should be considered as having inflammatory carcinoma because of their poor prognosis and should be treated accordingly.

Differential Diagnosis ■

The following diseases are often confused with inflammatory breast carcinoma, which can lead to a delay in diagnosis:

Bacterial infections of the breast: Mastitis and abscess are usually seen only in lactating breasts. Features that distinguish infections from inflammatory cancer are areas of localized tenderness, fever, and leukocytosis, which rarely occur in the latter.

Radiation dermatitis and fibrosis: Erythema after radiation therapy to the intact breast usually occurs 2 to 4 weeks after treatment has begun, and inflammation corresponds to the fields of treatment. However, radiation fibrosis, which occurs much later, can more closely mimic inflammatory cancer and may be difficult to distinguish from an aggressive recurrence of carcinoma. Physical examination in both fibrosis and carcinoma can reveal areas of thickening and mass-like lesions with skin edema.

Leukemia, lymphoma, or sarcoma: These can be indistinguishable clinically, and the correct diagnosis can be made only by biopsy.

In the past, tuberculosis, syphilis, and carcinoma en cuirasse were included in the differential diagnosis, but are now rarely considered in this country.

Pathology ■

There is no consistent microscopic type of breast carcinoma associated with the inflammatory subset. Histology ranges from infiltrating ductal to medullary. Haagensen's series of 40 patients included 19 (47%) with large cell, undifferentiated tumors.[21]

The initial observation of dermal lymphatic invasion by tumor in inflammatory carcinoma was made by Bryant in 1887.[22] This pathologic appearance was also reported by other investigators, and it became an integral part of the diagnosis.[1,2,17] Others have also reported involvement of subepidermal capillaries or venules, but most authors agree that the disease is primarily of the lymphatic vessels.[7,23] The edema and erythema seen clinically are thought to result from lymphatic blockage and subsequent capillary congestion.[17]

A controversy exists in the literature as to whether inflammatory carcinoma is a clinical or pathologic diagnosis. Several investigators have attempted to define the disease more specifically. Ellis and Teitelbaum[24] in 1974 proposed the name "dermal lymphatic carcinomatosis of the breast," making the presence of dermal lymphatic invasion mandatory for the diagnosis. They based this criterion on a review of the literature of all patients diagnosed with inflammatory cancer who were disease-free at 5 years. They found eight such patients, seven of whom had pathologic material available for review at the Mayo Clinic. Four of these had lymphatic invasion in the breast tumor, and six had axillary nodal involvement. Skin biopsy of four patients did not reveal dermal lymphatic invasion. Skin biopsies were not available for the other three patients, two of whom were still disease-free. Thus, six patients were disease-free, and four of these had negative skin biopsies. The two other patients either had no pathologic material available or no evidence of dermal lymphatic invasion. The authors concluded that disease-free status was related to the absence of dermal lymphatic invasion.

In 1974, Saltzstein[25] described four patients who had no clinical evidence of inflammatory carcinoma but had dermal lymphatic invasion pathologically; all died rapidly of their disease. He concluded that these patients had "clinically occult inflammatory carcinoma," and suggested that inflammatory carcinoma is a histologic rather than clinical diagnosis.

Lucas and Mesa-Perez[13] attempted to clarify this controversy in a retrospective review of inflammatory carcinoma at the Ellis Fischel State Cancer Hospital in Missouri. Of 79 initial cases, 21 were excluded because of inadequate material; thus, there were 58 patients with clinical inflammatory disease and an additional 15 with occult disease. They also included cases of secondary inflammatory carcinoma if there was an acute onset of inflammation in a breast with a longstanding tumor. Median survival was about 14 months for the 39 patients with clinical and pathologic evidence of inflammatory carcinoma and for those with clinical signs alone (N = 19); the 15 patients with pathologic evidence only had a longer median survival, about 40 months. The patients were treated with different modalities—radiation therapy, mastectomy, hormonal therapy, and chemotherapy were used alone or in combination. The authors concluded that patients with clinical evidence of inflammation, regardless of pathologic findings, had a prognosis as poor as that of patients with both clinical and pathologic evidence, and therefore should be included in the diagnosis of inflammatory carcinoma.

Levine and coworkers[18] presented the SEER data in an attempt to make criteria for diagnosis more uniform. There were 153 cases with both the clinical and pathologic diagnosis (3-year relative survival rate = 34%), 2937 with clinical features alone with a (3-year survival = 60%), and 81 with pathologic features alone (3-year survival = 52%). This suggests a better prognosis in those patients with a clinical diagnosis alone. Obviously, there are many shortcomings to this kind of analysis; the records come from abstracted charts provided by many different investigators. Several clinical characteristics may not have been noted, and skin biopsies were not done routinely. Also, patients were treated with different modalities of therapy. This issue can be resolved only by prospective studies.

Classification ■

Inflammatory breast carcinoma was a T_4 tumor by the standard tumor–node–metastasis (TNM) staging classification of the American Joint Committee (AJC) and the International Union Against Cancer (UICC) of 1983[26] and remains so in the 1987–1988 TNM staging.[27] It is considered Stage IIIb breast carcinoma (see Table 7–1).

The Columbia clinical classification proposed by Haagensen classifies inflammatory breast carcinoma as Stage D.[28] Stage C includes patients with any one of the following: edema of less than one-third of skin of the breast, ulceration of skin, chest wall fixation, axillary nodes >2.5 cm in diameter, and fixation of axillary nodes to deeper structures. If the patient has two or more of these "grave signs," the disease is considered Stage D.

Table 7–1
American Joint Committee TNM Breast Cancer Staging: Stage III[26]*

Stage	Tumor	Nodes	Metastasis
IIIa	T_0, T_1, T_2, T_3	N_2	M_0
	T_3	N_0, N_1, N_2	M_0
IIIb	Any T	N_3	M_0
	Any T_4	Any N	M_0

* N_2 = fixed ipsilateral axillary nodes; T_3 = tumors > 5 cm; N_3 = supraclavicular or infraclavicular nodes or arm edema; T_4 = tumor of any size with direct extension to chest wall or skin, edema of skin (peau d'orange), ulceration, or satellite skin nodules.

Investigators at the Institut Gustave-Roussy (Villejuif, France) have created a classification called *poussee evolutirie* (PEV) for breast cancer, which differs from the TNM staging.[29] This classification is descriptive, and takes into consideration recent tumor growth and inflammatory signs. The PEV categories are as follows: PEV 0—a tumor without recent increase in volume and without inflammatory signs; PEV 1—a tumor showing marked increase in volume during the last 2 months but without inflammatory signs; PEV 2—a tumor in which the overlying breast tissue, particularly the skin, is affected by subacute inflammation and edema involving less than half of the breast surface; and PEV 3—a tumor with acute or subacute inflammation and edema involving more than half of the breast surface. This classification is also used by investigators in Tunisia.[30]

Prognostic Factors ■

The most important prognostic factor in breast cancer is the presence and extent of axillary nodal involvement. Nodal disease is indicative of systemic microscopic metastatic disease. In inflammatory breast cancer, an overwhelming majority of patients have clinically evident involved nodes. Haagensen described axillary nodal involvement in 100% of his 30 patients treated by radical mastectomy.[7] In his larger series, 81 of 89 patients had positive nodes, with 50% of these being >2.5 cm.[7] Taylor and Meltzer's 25 patients with primary inflammatory cancer included 10 with supraclavicular nodal involvement.[17] Only 5 of these patients had disease localized to the breast and axilla, and 4 of these 5 had clinically evident nodal involvement.

Lee and Tannenbaum[1] stated that axillary nodes are involved early.[1] Of their 18 patients, 17 (98%) had gross axillary nodal involvement and many had clinically positive supraclavicular nodal disease. Knight and colleagues[31] described 18 patients treated with preoperative chemotherapy, of whom 14 (78%) had axillary nodal metastases at mastectomy. Meyer and coworkers[12] reported 61 cases of inflammatory carcinoma in which radical mastectomy was performed: of those cases in which nodes were examined, 86% contained carcinoma. Other reports substantiate this high incidence of axillary nodal involvement. Rogers and Fitts[14] reported a 95% incidence of clinical axillary nodal involvement in 46 patients and 43% supraclavicular nodal involvement. Droulias and associates[15] described an 89% evidence of clinically positive nodes in 67 patients. Finally, Barber and colleagues[8] found a 100% incidence of clinically positive nodes; many patients had supraclavicular nodal involvement.

Another prognostic factor in breast cancer is the presence of estrogen receptors (ER) or progesterone receptors (PR) in the tumor. DeLarue and coworkers[32] found that in 59 patients with inflammatory carcinoma, 28 cases were ER+ (48%) and 31 ER− (52%); 28 patients were ER− PR−; 3 were ER− PR+; 11 were ER+ PR−; 17 were ER+ PR+; and 1 was "status unknown." Kokal and colleagues[33] described 22 patients, of whom 7 had ER assays done; all were negative. Harvey and associates[34] reported 16 cases of inflammatory carcinoma, with 5 ER+ and 11 ER−. The Schäfer and colleagues series[35] included 5 cases that were ER+ PR+; 5 ER+ PR−; and 11 ER− PR−. Keiling and colleagues[36] reported that 57 of 78 patients (73%) with inflammatory breast cancer were ER− PR−; 8 ER+ PR−; 10 ER+ PR+; and 2 ER− PR+. The numbers are small, but the data suggest that the receptor content of this subset of patients does not differ from that of the more common breast carcinomas.

Distant metastatic disease at diagnosis is more frequent in inflammatory than other breast carcinomas. Taylor and Meltzer[17] found visceral or bone metastases in 9 (36%) of their patients with primary inflammatory disease. Haagensen[7] reported that 15 of his 89 patients (17%) had distant metastases (9 lung, 5 bone, and 1 brain). In the DeLarue and associates[32] series of 59 cases, 21 (36%) had metastases at diagnosis. There was an equal distribution of ER+ and ER− tumors. Bozzetti and colleagues,[37] of the National Cancer Institute of Milan, confirmed the presence of distant metastases in 20 of 114 patients (17%).[37] The SEER data[18] revealed metastatic disease in 24% of 3171 white patients with inflammatory carcinoma diagnosed from 1975 to 1981. This range of reported metastatic disease at diagnosis, from 17% to 36%, far exceeds that for other presentations of apparently localized breast cancer ($\approx$5%).[18]

The Tunisian Experience ■

Investigators at the Institut Salah Azaiz (ISA) in Tunis, Tunisia, described the clinical and prognostic features of a rapidly progressive breast cancer among women in their country.[30] The 581 patients diagnosed with breast cancer between 1969 and 1974 included a remarkably higher incidence of inflammatory carcinoma than is seen in the United States: 58.9% of patients were distributed in PEV Groups 1–3, with

6.5% PEV 2 and 48.7% PEV 3. Although this classification is different from that used by most authors, the PEV 3 group is similar to the inflammatory cancer reported in studies in the United States. In that group, there were 283 patients, of whom 116 (41%) had metastatic disease at diagnosis. Also, 98% had clinical N_1 (55 patients), N_2 (107 patients), or N_3 (116 patients) disease. Patients were treated with surgical castration (if they were premenopausal or within 3 years of menopause), followed by radiation therapy and mastectomy (if the tumor was operable and no distant metastases were present). The date of detection of metastases was considered the survival endpoint by the authors because follow-up was not possible in many patients. The median survival was 16 months in the nonmetastatic PEV 3 group (152 patients) compared to 26 months in 29 patients with PEV 2, 23 months in 21 patients with PEV 1, and 64 months in the 210 patients with PEV 0.

Examination of prognostic factors revealed that rural residence, blood type A, and recent pregnancy were risk factors in premenopausal women for the development of rapidly progressive carcinoma.[38] Older age, rural residence, blood type A, late menarche, and delay in diagnosis were risk factors for postmenopausal women.

A review of the histopathology of 94 cases of rapidly progressive breast carcinoma in Tunisia was done by Costa and colleagues.[39] There were 31 PEV 3 cases, 94% of which had nuclear grade 3 tumors. Skin biopsies were available for 24 patients, 12 of whom had tumor emboli in the dermal lymphatics compared to 3 of 24 patients without any PEV features. Although these numbers are small, the data suggest that the presence of clinical inflammatory signs is sufficient to make the diagnosis of PEV 3 or inflammatory breast cancer because the prognosis is much worse in this group compared to PEV 0 patients.

Natural History ■

In the literature of the 1800s, there are several vivid descriptions of untreated inflammatory breast cancer. The following case report[3] is one example:

"A married woman of fifty-three, who had borne 11 children, was seen June, 1857. She had an acute brawny infiltration of her right breast and the skin over it, with oedema of the right arm. She had been perfectly well until three months before, when she noticed a swelling in the breast, which rapidly increased and became complicated with pain down the right arm. When seen, the axillary and supraclavicular glands were much enlarged, the breast was like brawn, the skin over it oedematous, and evidently infiltrated with new elements. Death occurred in three months from toxaemia."

Surgery ■

Learmonth's 1916 review of 45 cases reported in the literature discussed the poor prognosis of the disease, with only 1 patient who was disease-free at 5 years.[4] Many of these cases had been treated as chronic mastitis for months; by the time the diagnosis was evident, the disease was too advanced for treatment. Therefore, the goal of many early reports was to ensure more rapid diagnosis and treatment. Learmonth suggested that "the most radical operation possible should be performed with thorough removal of the axillary glands and also the supraclavicular if deemed necessary."

In 1938, Taylor and Meltzer[17] treated six patients with primary inflammatory breast carcinoma with radical mastectomy. All of these patients developed either local, regional, or contralateral breast recurrences fairly rapidly. The average survival was 21 months, with a range of 11 to 34 months.

Haagensen and Stout[40] wrote a treatise on the criteria for operability in 1943. Those authors were convinced that radical mastectomy should not be done in patients with classic inflammatory breast carcinoma. They reported that 20 patients with inflammatory signs treated by radical mastectomy had a local recurrence rate of 50% and a mean survival of 15.5 months. Haagensen[7] then presented his data on 30 patients treated by radical mastectomy before the criteria for operability had been established. There

was a mean survival of 19 months, with only one 5-year survivor (her disease recurred and she died 68 months after surgery). He was therefore convinced that radical mastectomy should not be done in any patient with inflammatory disease.

Results described by several other physicians are summarized in Table 7–2. It is evident that survival is poor when patients are treated by surgery alone. Treves wrote an editorial in 1959 stating that radical mastectomy was contraindicated in this disease, based on six reports in the literature.[41] He believed that the disease was disseminated at the time of diagnosis in most patients. In his review of 114 cases in which radical mastectomy was performed, only 3.5% of the patients were alive at 5 years.

Radiation Therapy ■

It became obvious to many physicians in the 1800s and early 1900s that inflammatory breast cancer was often diagnosed at a point that precluded surgical treatment alone. Therefore, many patients who were considered inoperable were treated by radiation therapy alone. It is difficult to compare early results of radiation therapy to more recent outcomes because of differences in technique and in stages of the disease. For example, Taylor and Meltzer's series included many patients who had metastatic disease at diagnosis.[17]

Several reports of patients treated with radiation therapy as the primary modality of therapy are summarized in Table 7–3. In many of these series, patients underwent hormonal manipulation, a popular modality at one time.

Table 7–2
Surgical Treatment of Inflammatory Breast Cancer

Study	Treatment*	No. Patients	Survival
Taylor and Meltzer (1938)[17]	RM	6	Mean = 19 mo
Meyer et al (1948)[12]†	RM	61	6% 5-yr survival
	SM	2	
Chris (1950)[23]	RM	2	Mean = 14 mo
	SM	1	
Haagensen (1956)[7]	RM	30	Mean = 19 mo
Stocks and Patterson (1976)[11]	RM ±hormones	10	Mean = 32 mo
Bozzetti (1981)[37]	RM	8	Mean = 11.5 mo

* RM = radical mastectomy; SM = simple mastectomy.

† Follow-up available in 50 patients.

One series not included in the table is by Baclesse,[52] from the Foundation Curie in Paris. He described the treatment of 431 patients with breast cancer with 200 kV roentgen rays. Patients were staged by the Columbia system that Haagensen described (in which inflammatory breast cancer is stage D, as is breast cancer with two or more of Haagensen's grave signs). For 200 Stage D patients, radiation therapy resulted in a 13% 5-year survival and a 10% 5-year disease-free survival (DFS). Even though this group as a whole had a perhaps slightly better prognosis than a "pure" inflammatory group, the results are still poor.

Wang and Griscom[43] described 33 patients with inflammatory breast cancer (6 with metastatic disease) treated from 1944 to 1959.[43] Orthovoltage radiation was used for 23 of these patients and supervoltage radiation for 10. The average dose was 2600 cGy in 30 days for the orthovoltage-treated patients and 5200 cGy for the supervoltage group. Also, 16 of the patients were treated with hormonal manipulation. The orthovoltage-treated tumors were controlled locally for a mean of 9.8 months compared to 27.4 months for the supervoltage-treated patients. There was a local recurrence rate of 67% for all patients. Mean survival was 14.3 months for orthovoltage-treated patients and 30 months for supervoltage-treated patients. Overall

Table 7–3
Radiation Therapy for Inflammatory Breast Cancer*

Study	Treatment	No. Patients	Survival
Lee and Tannenbaum (1924)[1]	RT	13	Mean = 11 mo
Taylor and Meltzer (1938)[17]	RT	19	Mean = 9.2 mo
		(9/25 M_1)	
Meyer et al (1948)[12]	RT	10	0 3-yr OS
		(follow-up in 7)	
Chris (1950)[23]	RT	5	Mean = 9.2 mo
	RT + hormones	3	Mean = 16 mo
Rogers and Fitts (1956)[14]	RT	24	4% 5-yr OS
Dao and McCarthy (1957)[42]	RT	3	Mean = 4 mo
Wang and Griscom (1964)[43]	RT	17	
	RT + hormones	16	Mean = 20.5 mo
		(6/33 M_1)	
Haagensen (1971)[7]	RT ± hormones (Ox in 4)	38	Mean = 16.3 mo
Stocks and Patterson (1976)[11]	RT	5	Mean = 11 mo (for 3 pts.)
Zucali (1976)[44]	RT, x-ray	21	
	RT, cobalt	37	Mean = 14 mo
	Other	12	
Droulias (1976)[15]	RT	31	Mean = 23 mo
	RT + hormones	22	Mean = 22 mo
Nussbaum (1977)[45]	RT	15	Mean = 15 mo; median = 12 mo for 54 pts.
		(13/54 M_1)	
Bruckman (1979)[46]	RT ± hormones chemo	18	13% 5-yr RFS (actuarial)
Chu (1980)[47]	RT	28	Mean = 28.5 mo
		(± hormones ± chemo)	
Barker (1980)[48]	RT	80	19% 2-yr OS
Bozzetti (1981)[37]	RT, x-ray	20	Mean = 16.5 mo
	RT, cobalt	12	Mean = 12 mo
Rao (1982)[49]	RT (7 + surgery)	29	Median = 7 mo
		(36 total)	
Hagelberg (1984)[10]	RT (2 + surgery)	10	Mean = 21 mo
Rouësse (1986)[50]	RT + Ox	60	16% 4-yr RFS
			28% 4-yr OS
			Median RFS = 13 mo
			Median survival = 33 mo
Perez (1987)[51]	RT	28	Median RFS = 8 mo; median OS = 18 mo

* RT = radiation therapy; M_1 = metastatic disease; ox = oophorectomy; OS = overall survival; RFS = relapse free survival.

survival from the date of diagnosis averaged 20.5 months. Wang and Griscom concluded that supervoltage treatment was preferred because of better dose delivery to the tumor, which resulted in better local control.

Bruckman and colleagues,[46] at the Joint Center for Radiation Therapy, treated 116 patients with Stage III carcinoma of the breast with radiation therapy; 36% received adjuvant treatments (hormonal manipulation, 15 patients; hormonal and chemotherapy, 10 patients; and chemotherapy alone, 16 patients). Several patients also received an iridium implant. Among the 18 patients with inflammatory breast cancer, the 5-year actuarial local control rate was 65%. Local control was achieved in 11 of 13 patients who received doses >6000 cGy but only 1 of 5 who received <6000 cGy. These authors concluded that doses of 6000 cGy or more were needed for optimal local control.

Chu and coworkers,[47] at the Massachusetts General Hospital, treated 62 patients with inflammatory breast cancer by radical radiotherapy; 14 also received hormonal manipulation and 20 adjuvant chemotherapy (4 single agent; 16 CMF VP or CMF). Twenty-six patients were treated with megavoltage therapy, 29 with orthovoltage, and 7 with both. Patients were treated with different tumor doses. Time dose factors (TDFs) were calculated from the total dose, interfraction schedule, and dose per fraction to assess treatment efficacy based on the radiation dose actually delivered. TDFs from 30 to 131 are equivalent to 1800–8000 cGy tumor doses given at 200 cGy/day for 5 days. The local recurrence rate was 70% in patients who had a TDF of <30–70, 58% in those with a TDF of 71–110, and 55% in those with a TDF of 111–131; the overall local recurrence rate was 63%. When rate of local recurrence was analyzed by tumor size, it was shown that increasing the TDF in tumors <10 cm decreased local recurrences, but this was not true for tumors >10 cm. The mean duration of local control by TDF was as follows: <30–70, 3.9 months; 71–110, 5.6 months; and 111–131, 12.2 months. For tumors >10 cm, the time to local recurrence was longer. Mean survival was 28 months for the 28 patients treated by radiation therapy alone and 24 months for the whole group (median = 18 months). Chu and colleagues concluded that doses >6000 cGy were needed for optimal local control; in tumors larger than 10 cm, an increase in dose did not decrease the local recurrence rate but prolonged time to local recurrence. This study also included 6 patients treated with twice-daily fractionation; their local recurrence rate of 33% suggests that better local control may be achieved by using this schedule.

Barker and colleagues[48] described the experience at M. D. Anderson from July 1948 through July 1972 in treating 80 patients with inflammatory breast cancer. Once-daily fractionation was used in 69 patients (45 treated with 250 kV with a 4800 cGy air dose and a midaxillary tumor dose of 6000–6500 cGy, and 24 treated with cobalt at a 6000 cGy tumor dose with a boost of 2000–3000 cGy). Eleven patients were treated with twice-daily fractionation with a 5400 cGy tumor dose. There was a 46% local recurrence rate in the single-fractionation group compared to 27% in those given twice-daily fractionation. Two-year DFS was seen in 17% of patients treated with conventional once-daily radiation and 27% treated with twice-daily fractionation. It was concluded that a twice-daily fractionation may improve local control.

Perez and Fields[51] analyzed 95 patients with inflammatory breast cancer treated at Washington University, St. Louis. Among 28 patients treated with radiotherapy alone, the median DFS was 8 months and overall survival was 18 months. There were 19 local recurrences (68%), with 18 of these patients also having distant metastases.

From studies in which patients were treated with radiation therapy alone, we conclude that a tumor dose $\geq$6000 cGy is necessary for optimal local control. Also, the literature suggests that twice-daily fractionation may improve local control. However, radiation therapy alone has little impact on survival.

Surgery Plus Radiation Therapy ■

Several physicians have treated patients with inflammatory breast cancer with the combination of surgery and radiation therapy in an effort to improve local control (Table 7-4). The details of radiation therapy, especially in earlier series, are often unclear, and local recurrence rates are not always given.

Barker and colleagues[53] treated 17 patients with simple mastectomy followed by radiation therapy. The radiation dose was 5000 cGy in 5 weeks to the chest wall, axilla, supraclavicular nodes, and internal mammary nodes. There was a local recurrence rate of 53%, and none of these patients was alive at 5 years.

For 12 patients treated with radiation and mastectomy, Perez and Fields[51] reported a median DFS of 24 months and median survival of 42 months. The DFS was significantly better than that seen in a previous series of 28 patients from the same institute who were treated with radiation therapy alone (*p*

Table 7–4
Radiation Therapy and Surgery as Treatment of Inflammatory Breast Carcinoma

Study	Treatment	No. Patients	Survival
Lee and Tannenbaum (1924)[1]	M + RT	4	Mean = 24 mo
Chris (1950)[23]	SM (3 pre- and post-RT, 1 post)	4	Mean = 10.8 mo
Rogers and Fitts (1956)[14]	SM (10), RM (10); post-op RT (18) pre-op RT (6)	20	10% 3-yr OS
Dao and McCarthy (1957)[42]	RM + post-op RT (3) Pre-op RT + RM (2) Pre-op RT + hormone (1)	6	Mean = 11.5 mo
Barber (1961)[8]	RM and post-op RT	42 (53 total)	0% 5-yr OS (5/50)
Zucali (1976)[44]	x-ray + RM Cobalt + RM	3 9 (70 total)	Mean = 14 mo (entire sample)
Droulias (1976)[15]	M + RT	5	Mean = 29 mo
Barker (1976)[53]	SM + post-op RT	17	0 5-yr OS
Nussbaum (1977)[45]	SM + RT	7 (54 total)	Mean = 15 mo (entire sample); median = 12 mo
Rao (1982)[49]	M + RT	7 (36 total)	Mean = 7 mo (entire sample)
Bozzetti (1981)[37]	RM + post-op RT	24	Mean = 18 mo
Haagensen (1986)[21]	RM + post-op RT	2	Mean = 16 mo
Perez (1987)[51]	M + RT	12	Median RFS = 24 mo; median OS = 42 mo

= 0.01). The local recurrence rate of 33% was also less than that associated with radiation alone (68%).

The mean survival in several other series ranges from 7 to 29 months. Thus, overall survival is still very poor with the combination of radiation therapy and mastectomy and does not differ from rates in patients treated with either surgery or radiation therapy alone (see Tables 7–2 and 7–3).

Hormonal Manipulation ■

Hormonal therapy with testosterone or estrogen or by hormonal ablation (oophorectomy, adrenalectomy, or hypophysectomy) was not uncommon in the treatment of inflammatory breast cancer and other advanced cancers in earlier studies (see Table 7–3). There are two examples in the literature of large series of patients with advanced breast cancer treated with adrenalectomy.

Fracchia and colleagues[54] treated 500 patients by adrenalectomy. There were 27 patients with primary inoperable inflammatory carcinoma; 21 were treated with combined adrenalectomy and oophorectomy and 6 with adrenalectomy alone. There were 12 responses (57%) in the combined group and 2 (33%) in the adrenalectomy-only group. Because these re-

sponses are not rigorously defined, it is difficult to know how they would correspond to the objective response criteria now in use. Disease-free and overall survival are also not discussed.

Yonemoto and colleagues[55] treated 14 patients with inflammatory breast cancer (11 considered primary) from 1956 to 1966. Haagensen's criteria were used for diagnosis. A majority of the patients had other treatments in addition to adrenalectomy: 10 also had bilateral oophorectomy, and the other 4 had previously had ovarian ablation. Four of the primary cases received radiation, hormones, or chemotherapy before adrenalectomy. There was an objective response rate of 50% lasting 6 months. The median survival for the entire series was 12 months, with a mean of 22 months. Only one of the patients with primary disease was alive at 5 years.

These two reports suggest that patients with inflammatory breast carcinoma have an objective response to adrenalectomy. However, survival duration is not improved compared to that of patients treated with local therapy alone.

In two studies, tamoxifen has been used in LABC. Veronesi and colleagues[56] treated 46 postmenopausal women with inoperable T_{3-4} breast carcinoma ($\approx$50% of whom had metastatic disease) with tamoxifen, 10–20 mg/day for at least 6 weeks. Eight patients (17%) had an objective response after the first 6-week eval-

Table 7-5
Combination Chemotherapy Treatment of Inflammatory Breast Carcinoma*

Study	Chemotherapy Regimen	No. Patients	Percent Response (CR/PR)	Median Follow-up	DFS	Survival
Fastenberg et al (1985)[60]	FAC	63	68 (14/54)	60 mo	Median = 24 mo	Median = 43 mo
DeLena et al (1978)[58]	AV	36	67 (20/47)	NA	NA	Median = 25 mo
Schäfer (1987)[35]	Chlorambucil + MAF	21 (15 primary, 6 secondary)	NA	37 mo	NA	Median = 43 mo
Loprinzi et al (1984)[62]	CMFP ± T alt. AV ± T	9 (32 total)	NA	NA	Median = 29.5 mo (entire sample)	Median >25 mo
Burton et al (1987)[61]	CAFV	22	95 (22/73)	NA	Median = 16.4 mo	Median = 23.6 mo
Pawlicki (1983)[63]	CMVF	72 (total 87 LABC)	42 (1/41)	NA	10% 3-yr DFS	28% 3-yr OS
Zylberberg et al (1982)[64]	CAVF + mel + BCG	15	93 (20/73)	NA	66% NED	ND >56 mo
Israël et al (1986)[65]	High-dose CTX + 5-FU	25	96 (8/88)	35 mo	Median = 33 mo	ND
Keiling et al (1985)[36]	CAVF + mel	41	NA	30 mo	54% 58-mo DFS	63% 58-mo OS
	CEVF + mVindTt	18	NA	16 mo	86% 3-yr DFS	86% 3-yr OS
	CEVF	19	NA		58% 3-yr DFS	77% 3-yr OS
Schwartz et al (1987)[66]	CMF ± TAM + dox	17	71	27 mo	NA	>85% 5-yr OS
Knight et al (1986)[31]	CFP	18	NA	NA	NA	Median = 23 mo
Fowble et al (1986)[67]	CMFPT or CAF	16	88 (75/13)	22 mo	65% 3-yr DFS	84% 3-yr OS
Hagelberg et al (1984)[10]	CMF CAVFP Misc.	8 6 4 (19 total)	NA	28 mo	NA	Median = 38 mo
Jacquillat et al (1987)[68]	Vel, Tt + MFA + T	66 (+29 T₃N₁ᵦ)	NA	48 mo	73% 4-yr (Obs)	62% 4-yr OS
Perloff et al (1988)[69]	CAFVP	14	50	37 mo	Median = 17.5 mo	Median = 26.9 mo
Sherry et al (1985)[70]	CAF or CMF ± T	17 (6 M₁)	NA	NA	NA	Median = 18 mos (LABC ND)
Conte et al (1987)[71]	DES + FAC	14	NA	NA	Median = 15 mo	NA

Author	Regimen	No.	Response	Median DFS	Survival	Survival
Noguchi et al (1988)[9]	I_a FMmC (ITA) } +C FMmC (SCA) } I_a CT(ITA) teg (9) } • I_a AT(SCA) teg (5) } (premenopausal ox) (postmenopausal adrenalectomy) in 2 patients	14 14	89 (25/64)	111 mo	59% 5-yr 53% 10-yr	63% 5-yr 47% 10-yr
Wiseman et al (1982)[72]	FAC + BCG → CMF	13	NA	21 mo	ND	ND
Perez et al (1987)[51]	FAC + RT FAC + mastectomy + RT	23 32	NA NA	NA NA	18 mo 4-yr 41 mo 4-yr	25 mo 46 mo
Rouëssé (1986)[50]	AVM + VCF AVCMF + AVM + VCF	91 79	14 27	NA NA	Median = 20 mo; 28% 4-yr Median = 37 mo; 46% 4-yr	Median = 38 mo; 44% 4-yr Median = ND; 66% 4-yr
Chevallier (1987)[73]	CMF → AVCF	64	47	NA	Median = 19 mo	Median = 32 mo
Brun (1988)[74]	AVCF	26	23	NA	Median = 12 mo	Median = 31 mo
Swain and Lippman (in progress)	CAMF + T Pre	45	98 (55/43)	32 mo	Median = 23 mo	Median = 36 mo

* Drugs cited in combination regimens as follows: F = 5-FU; A = dox; C = CTX; V = VCR; M = MTX; P = prednisone; T = tamoxifen; mel = melphalan; E = epidorubicin; vind = vindesine; Tt = thiotepa; Vel = vinblastine. Other abbreviations as follows: DES = diethylstilbesterol; Mmc = mitomycin; teg = tegafur; pre = premarin; M_I = metastases; I_A = intra-arterial; ITA = internal thoracic artery; SCA = subclavian artery; ND = not determined; alt = alternately; NA = not available; Obs = observed.

uation, and a total of 14 (30%) had a response noted at subsequent evaluations. However, none of the 5 patients with inflammatory disease responded. The median survival for the whole series was 10 months.

Campbell and colleagues[57] treated 51 postmenopausal women with LABC using tamoxifen, 10–20 mg BID. Estrogen receptor values were assessed in 40 patients. There was an overall objective response rate of 45%, with 7 (17%) clinical complete responses (CRs) and 16 (31%) partial responses (PRs). Response was seen in 63% of ER+ patients versus 33% of ER− patients and 36% of those with unknown ER status. By extrapolation from the graph presented, the median overall survival was 48 months for the tamoxifen responders and 18 months for the nonresponders. It is not stated whether any patients with inflammatory disease were treated in this series. The data suggest that the response rate in LABC is low with tamoxifen alone.

Combination Chemotherapy Treatment ■

It is evident that inflammatory breast carcinoma is a systemic disease at diagnosis and that local therapy alone is therefore inadequate. Several earlier investigators treated this disease with a combination of different modalities, including hormonal manipulation and chemotherapy. However, this approach was not tested systematically until the early 1970s.

Table 7–5 includes most series in which patients were treated with combination chemotherapy, with radiation or surgical therapy as local therapy. Response rates range from 14% to 98%. Median DFS ranges from 12 to 41 months, with median overall survival of 23 to 46 months.

DeLena and coworkers,[58] at the National Cancer Institute in Milan, began a randomized trial in patients with LABC in 1973. They treated 110 patients with doxorubicin (dox) and vincristine (VCR) for four cycles, followed by radiation therapy in responders. Doses were as follows: dox, 75 mg/m² IV on day 1; and VCR, 1.4 mg/m² IV on days 1 and 8, every 3 weeks. Patients who were off study at any time for progressive disease or no response received CMF therapy. Patients older than 60 years were given lower doses (dox, 60 mg/m²; MTX, 30 mg/m²; and 5-FU, 400 mg/m²). After radiation therapy was complete, patients who had no evidence of disease were randomized to either maintenance chemotherapy with six more cycles or observation only. The six cycles consisted of dox + VCR (AV regimen) for patients achieving CR or PR during induction and CMF regimen for patients not achieving PR. The 36 patients with inflammatory disease achieved a 67% objective response to induction chemotherapy, with 7 CRs (20%) and 17 PRs (47%). The median survival for the inflammatory group overall was 25 months (including patients who received maintenance or observation only). Their 3-year survival was 25%, which was not different from these investigators' previous experience with radiation alone (28%). For the LABC patients as a whole, the median disease-free survival was 19 months for those who received maintenance chemotherapy and 11 months for those who did not ($p = 0.02$). The 3-year survival rate for the entire sample was 52%. This represents an improvement over local therapy alone. The study also suggested that maintenance chemotherapy increased disease-free survival overall. As noted previously, the older patients had a substantial dose reduction, and 16 of inflammatory patients were postmenopausal. Also, not all inflammatory patients received maintenance therapy. These data were therefore not conclusive, but stimulated other investigators to take a more aggressive approach to this disease.

Buzdar and colleagues[59] reported treatment results for 32 patients with inflammatory breast cancer seen at M. D. Anderson between 1973 and 1977. Results were compared to a historical control group of 32 patients treated with radiation alone at the same institution. The treatment regimen consisted of 5-FU, 500 mg/m^2 IV on days 1 and 8; dox, 50 mg/m^2 IV on day 1, CTX 500 mg/m^2 IV day 1, plus bacillus Calmette–Guerin (BCG) every 3 weeks for three or four cycles. Patients then received radiation therapy with twice-daily fractionation. The total dose was 5100 cGy to the breast and supraclavicular and internal mammary nodes, with a boost to the entire breast and skin. Patients were then scheduled to receive chemotherapy for 2 years. With a median follow-up of 62 months, the median disease-free interval was 22.8 months for the chemotherapy-treated group and 9 months for the controls. Median survival was 30.1 and 18 months, respectively. Locoregional failures were seen in 26% of chemotherapy-treated patients compared to 43% of historical controls treated with once-daily fractionation radiation. The difference in local control was thought to result from the twice-daily fractionation given to the chemotherapy patients. Also, when they evaluated the radiation-only group who received twice-daily fractionation Buzdar and colleagues found only 27% locoregional recurrences.

The group at M. D. Anderson has updated this series to include 63 patients treated from 1973 to 1981.[60] The patients received chemotherapy as described above plus radiation therapy. Fifty patients received 5-FU/dox/CTX (FAC) plus immunotherapy (BCG), 12 received other dox-containing regimens, and one received CMF. In addition, 21 had a simple mastectomy during their primary treatment; 7 of these patients did not receive consolidation radiation therapy. The median follow-up was 60 months. A median of three cycles of chemotherapy was given and, after there was no further improvement on physical examination, mastectomy was performed (in patients treated after the initial report described above). Fifty patients (87%) received maintenance chemotherapy, first with FAC and then with CMF, for 2 years. The response to induction therapy was 68% overall (14% CR, 54% PR). The median DFS was 24 months and the median survival was 43 months. Evaluation of patients by results of skin biopsy to assess dermal lymphatic invasion revealed a median DFS of 31 and 46 months for patients with positive (N = 16) and negative (N = 10) skin biopsies, respectively ($p = 0.45$). Evaluation by response to induction therapy revealed a DFS of 31 months in patients who achieved an objective response compared to 19 months in those who did not ($p = 0.01$). The conclusion was that disease-free and overall survival were improved with the use of combination chemotherapy. Also, it was thought that since there was no difference in DFS based on the presence of dermal lymphatic invasion, the clinical diagnosis of inflammatory breast cancer alone portends a poor prognosis.

Another large series of patients with inflammatory breast cancer was reported by Perez and Fields in 1987.[51] The authors compared the treatment outcomes of different combined-modality therapies in 95 patients treated at a single institution. They found a significant benefit in DFS and survival in patients receiving chemotherapy in their regimens. The details of the chemotherapy are not given, but it is stated that patients received two or three cycles of FAC prior to mastectomy. The median DFS for 28 patients receiving radiation alone was 8 months, compared to 41 months for 32 patients receiving chemotherapy, surgery, radiation, and more chemotherapy (CSRC; $p < 0.0001$). The median overall survival for radiation alone was 18 months versus 47 months for CSRC ($p = 0.0002$). There was also a significant increase in survival in patients who received CSRC versus radiation and chemotherapy alone (N = 23; $p = 0.02$). There was a decrease in local recurrences in patients treated with all three modalities. The local recurrence rate was 16% for CSRC, 57% for radiation plus chemotherapy, 33% for radiation plus mastectomy, and 68% for radiation alone.

The largest series of patients with inflammatory

breast carcinoma is that reported by Rouëssé and colleagues in 1986 from the Institut Gustave-Roussy.[50] They presented results of treatment of 230 cases of inflammatory breast carcinoma. The difficulty in comparing these findings to the North American literature is that these physicians use the PEV classification. However, it is stated that all patients would be classified as T_{4b} in the TNM classification (UICC). Three different protocols were used. Radiation alone was the treatment from 1973 to 1975 (group C). Group A, treated between 1976 and 1980, received three cycles of AVM—dox, 40 mg/m^2 IV on day 1; VCR, 1 mg/m^2 IV on day 2; and MTX 3 mg/m^2 SC for six doses every 12 hours beginning day 3, all repeated every 3 or 4 weeks before radiation for three courses, one cycle during radiation, and five cycles postirradiation. Group B, treated between 1980 and 1982, received three cycles of AVMCF—dox, 50 mg/m^2 IV on day 1; VCR, 0.6 mg/m^2 IV on day 2; CTX, 200 mg/m^2 IM on days 3–5; MTX, 10 mg/m^2 IM on days 3–5; and 5-FU, 300 mg/m^2 IM days 3–5 every 4 weeks for three courses, followed by radiation with one cycle of AVM, then five more cycles of AVM. Both groups A and B received maintenance with VCR 1 mg/m^2 IV on day 1, CTX, 200 mg/m^2 IM on days 2–4; and 5-FU, 300 mg/m^2 IM on days 2–4 every 4 weeks for 4 to 12 cycles. The median number of maintenance cycles was 9 for group A patients and 10 for group B. Maintenance was given only to patients who did not relapse. The radiation dosage was the same in all three groups: 4500 cGy to the breast and draining lymph nodes, with a 2000–3000 cGy boost to the tumor. All patients had hormonal manipulation, which took the form of radiocastration for pre- or perimenopausal women. Postmenopausal women treated after 1973 were given tamoxifen, 20 mg/day for 1 year.

Patient characteristics were equivalent across groups. The patients with PEV 2 or PEV 3 were equally distributed, with 68% and 32% in the control group, respectively, 69% and 31% in group A, and 73% and 27% in group B. There were 60 patients in group C, 91 in group A, and 79 in group B.

The objective response to induction chemotherapy was 14% in group A and 27% in group B ($p = 0.04$). The 4-year DFS and overall survival, respectively, were 16% and 28% for group C, 28% and 44% for group A, and 46% and 66% for group B (DFS, group C and A, $p < 0.005$; group C and B, $p < 0.00001$; and group A and B, $p < 0.01$). There was a survival difference between groups C and A ($p = 0.03$), groups A and B ($p < 0.001$), and groups C and B ($p = 0.0001$). The authors also analyzed DFS and survival in 91 patients who did not relapse during or

within 3 months after maintenance chemotherapy. There was no difference in DFS or survival in relation to the duration of chemotherapy. At 4 years, DFS for patients with PEV 2 and PEV 3 disease, respectively, within study groups were as follows: group C, 8% and 0 ($p = 0.0001$); group A, 35% and 11% ($p = 0.005$); group B, 52% and 30% ($p = 0.11$). There was an improvement in DFS in PEV 3 patients who received more intensive chemotherapy (group B and A, $p = 0.03$). However, when patients with N_2 or N_3 disease were analyzed, there was no difference in DFS in the group receiving more intensive chemotherapy (group C, 6%; group A, 18%; and group B, 15%; p = NS). There was a benefit in those patients with N_0 or N_1 disease: 4-year DFS was 6% in group C, 30% in group A, and 53% in group B (all ps = 0.00001). The majority of patients actually fall into the N_0 plus N_1 category: group C, 70%; group A, 76%; and group B, 82%.

The conclusions from this study are that the more aggressive chemotherapy prolonged DFS in patients with PEV 3 disease but not N_2 or N_3 disease. A more intensive induction may be needed for the latter patients.

Another interesting report, using a different approach, is that of Noguchi and colleagues.[9] The treatment regimen is shown in Table 7–5. Patients were all treated with intra-arterial (IA) infusional chemotherapy, surgical ablation, extended radical mastectomy, and adjuvant chemotherapy. The median follow-up was 111 months. There was complete necrosis of the tumor at mastectomy in 13 patients (46%). The local recurrence rate of 32% is not much different than that seen with radiation therapy and surgery. Leukopenia, with white blood cell (WBC) count <3000/mm^3, was seen in 75% of patients treated with IA therapy alone, indicating systemic distribution of the drugs. The median 10-year DFS was 53%, and overall survival was 47%.

The issue of whether dermal lymphatic invasion influences DFS was addressed in two other small studies. Burton and colleagues[61] treated patients with CAFV chemotherapy and found a median DFS for patients with lymphatic invasion (N = 12) of 17 months versus 15 months for those without dermal lymphatic invasion (N = 5). In 21 patients treated with chlorambucil, MTX, 5-FU, and dox, Schafer and colleagues found a median distant-disease-free survival of 22.5 and 12 months for patients with and without dermal lymphatic invasion, respectively (p = NS). From the evidence presented, it seems that when clinical inflammatory signs are present, dermal lymphatic invasion is not necessary to make the diagnosis.

National Cancer Institute Experience ■

We have treated 107 patients with LABC at the National Cancer Institute (NCI) from April 1980 to February 1988 using primary induction chemotherapy, including an attempted hormonal synchronization in 101 patients. There are 47 patients with Stage IIIa disease, 56 with Stage IIIb disease (45 with inflammatory disease; 11 with noninflammatory) and 4 with Stage IV disease. All patients were treated to best response, which included at least four cycles of induction chemotherapy, before local therapy was given. The following discussion includes only the 45 patients with inflammatory breast cancer. A preliminary report of results in patients with locally advanced disease has been published.[75] The chemotherapy regimen chosen was hormonal synchronization, based on work in the laboratory showing that tamoxifen causes an arrest of cells in G_1, and estrogen increases DNA synthesis.[76] The hypothesis is that more cells will be put into the cell cycle, therefore making them more sensitive to cell-cycle-specific chemotherapeutic agents such as 5-FU.

Patient Selection ■

Patients were included if they had clinical signs of inflammatory cancer, such as erythema and edema involving more than one-third of the breast. A skin biopsy was considered positive for inflammatory breast cancer if there was dermal lymphatic invasion. Patients were required to have locoregional disease, without evidence of metastasis. However, four patients who were entered in the study were later found to have had metastatic disease at the time of study entry. These patients are included in the analysis of all LABC patients but not in the following analysis of inflammatory breast cancer. Patients were required to have a leukocyte count greater than 4000/mm³, platelet count greater than 100,000/mm³, and normal hepatic and renal function. All patients gave written informed consent.

Initial and Follow-up Evaluations ■

Prior to treatment, all patients had a complete history and physical examination, complete blood cell count, chemistry profile, urinalysis, electrocardiogram, radionuclide scans of bone and liver, mammogram, chest radiograph, metastatic bone survey, and bone marrow biopsy. Rehabilitation therapy and radiation therapy consultation evaluations were also done. Beginning in 1987, all patients had a radionuclide ventriculogram at study entry, when 300 mg/m² of dox was given, and at the end of treatment. Blood counts were monitored on a weekly basis. With the institution of each new chemotherapy cycle, chemistry profiles were repeated, along with formal quantitation of any palpable tumor burden. Mammograms were performed at best response and annually thereafter. Patients eligible for bone marrow transplant were fully reevaluated at the end of local therapy with radionuclide scans, chest radiograph, metastatic bone survey, and bone marrow biopsy. All other patients were restaged at the end of treatment; radionuclide scans of bone and liver, chest and bone radiographs, and annual tests were done thereafter.

Induction and Maintenance Chemotherapy Regimens ■

The initial 9 patients with inflammatory breast cancer were part of a randomized study of advanced breast cancer comparing a chemotherapy regimen with or without attempted hormonal synchronization.[77] Therefore, 4 patients in the total sample did not undergo hormonal synchronization. The initial patients also received different drug doses: CTX, 750 mg/m² IV on day 1; dox, 30 mg/m² IV on day 1, with or without tamoxifen, 10 mg PO b.i.d. on days 2–6 and conjugated estrogens (Premarin), 0.625 mg PO every 12 hours in three doses on day 7; MTX, 40 mg/m² IV on day 8, and 5-FU, 500 mg/m² IV on day 8. This protocol was closed as a randomized study in June 1983. Subsequent patients were accrued to the hormonal arm of this study, with drug doses as follows: CTX, 500 mg/m² IV on day 1; dox, 30 mg/m² IV on day 1; tamoxifen, 40 mg PO on days 2–6; Premarin, 0.625 mg PO every 12 hours in three doses on day 7; MTX, 300 mg/m² IV on day 8, followed in 1 hour by 5-FU, 500 mg/m² IV; and leucovorin, 10 mg/m² PO every 6 hours in six doses on day 9. A 25% dose escalation of either MTX or 5-FU in alternate cycles was used to achieve maximum doses of these drugs.

All patients were treated with induction therapy to the point of maximum objective response. Maximum objective clinical response was formally scored when response parameters remained stable for two consecutive determinations separated by 6 weeks. Analyses of time to best response used the time when maximum objective clinical response was first observed. A CR was defined as disappearance of any palpable tumor mass in the breast and any axillary, infraclavicular, or supraclavicular nodes present initially. A PR was defined as a decrease ≥50% in the sum of the products of the greatest length and width of the mass in the breast and any involved nodes. A tumor reduction of <50% was rated as no change (NC). Progressive disease denoted when there was an increase ≥25% in the size of the breast mass. Dose reductions for this regimen have been described previously.[78]

Local Therapy With Mastectomy and Radiation Therapy ■

After patients achieved maximal objective clinical response to chemotherapy, they were evaluated for local therapy. This was done routinely by the authors (S.S. and M.L.) using pre- and postchemotherapy mammograms and physical examinations. Patients achieving a clinical CR underwent incisional biopsy at the site of the original lesion, with a biopsy of any surrounding suspicious areas seen at the time of the procedure. If skin involvement was present at diagnosis, a skin biopsy was obtained. If biopsies were negative, the patients received a course of radical radiotherapy to the previously involved breast and adjacent draining lymph node areas. No axillary surgery was performed. For patients with residual disease, and those achieving only a PR or NC after induction chemotherapy, a total mastectomy was performed, including removal of any gross axillary disease. This was followed by a course of radical radiotherapy. All patients continued to receive chemotherapy, with the exclusion of dox during radiotherapy. Randomized patients received maintenance chemotherapy for either 1 year or 6 months after local therapy was completed. All other patients received maintenance chemotherapy for 6 months, with dox included in every cycle (not to exceed 525 mg/m^2).

Patients achieving a CR received radiation to the previously involved breast and peripheral lymphatic areas; therapy included breast tangents (including the internal mammary nodes), a supraclavicular field, and a posterior axillary boost. Patients who had a PR, NC, or NC on restaging biopsy underwent mastectomy and removal of any grossly involved axillary lymph nodes. This was followed by chest wall tangent irradiation and similar treatment of peripheral lymphatics. Only the portion of the axilla that was not dissected received radiation. Bolus was used every other day for all chest wall tangents and for any intact breast that had inflammatory involvement at presentation. Dose (and dose per fraction) ranged from 4400 to 5400 cGy to the prescribed 150 dose for tangents and to the supraclavicular field at 3 cm. A boost (to 6000 cGy total dose) was given to the original tumor volume for intact breasts. Radiation boost was also used for areas of gross residual nodal disease and positive chest wall margins following mastectomy.

Autologous Bone Marrow Transplant and High-dose Melphalan ■

The early analysis of this study indicated that patients with inflammatory breast cancer had a much shorter disease-free survival than other patients with LABC. In the hope of increasing overall survival in this subset of patients, randomization to high-dose therapy was introduced in October 1984. The treatment options were autologous bone marrow transplant (BMT) and high-dose melphalan followed by maintenance chemotherapy versus maintenance chemotherapy alone. Patients were eligible for randomization if they had a diagnosis of inflammatory breast cancer and achieved a CR with induction chemotherapy or could be rendered free of disease surgically. After local therapy with radiation therapy alone or surgery in combination with radiation, both given concomitantly with chemotherapy, the patients were restaged. If they had no evidence of disease, they were offered randomization. The patients who were randomized to high-dose melphalan were admitted to the hospital and a bone marrow biopsy was done. If the result was negative for tumor, the patients' bone marrow was harvested. These patients then received melphalan, 60 mg/m^2 for 3 consecutive days, with return of their marrow on the following day. They remained hospitalized until their blood counts returned to normal and received maintenance chemotherapy at reduced doses (initially at 50% and then at the dose tolerated).

Statistical Analysis ■

Time to progression and survival time were estimated actuarially using the Kaplan–Meier procedure.[79] The significance of the difference between actuarial curves used to evaluate prognostic factors and outcomes of treatment modalities was determined by the Mantel–Haenszel method.[80]

Results ■

At the time of this analysis, 45 patients with inflammatory breast cancer had been entered on the study; and all but 1 were evaluable for response. Time to progression and survival analysis includes 45 patients,

Table 7–6
Clinical Characteristics of 45 Patients in NCI Study*

Characteristic	Number
Estrogen receptor status	
Positive	13
Negative	14
Unknown	18
Skin biopsy	
Positive	22
Negative	17
Not done	6
Menopausal status	
Premenopausal	15
Postmenopausal	30
Clinical nodal status	
N_0	11
N_1	21
N_2	9
N_3	4

* Mean age = 53 years; range, 33–73. Study in progress.

with 1 patient lost to follow-up 4 months after treatment began and after achieving a PR. All patients are evaluable for toxicity. The characteristics of the patients are listed in Table 7–6.

Response to Induction Chemotherapy ■

The overall objective response rate was 98%, with 24 (55%) clinical CRs, 19 (43%) PRs, and 1 NC (2%); no patients had progressive disease. The median number of cycles needed to achieve a CR was 5, with a range of 3 to 11. For PR, the median was 4, with a range of 2 to 9. The time course to best response to chemotherapy is shown in Figure 7–2.

Patients who achieved a clinical CR were evaluated by repeat biopsy: 58% (N = 14) had a negative biopsy and 38% (N = 9) were positive (1 patient did not have a repeat biopsy).

Local Therapy ■

There were 27 patients who had a mastectomy before receiving radiation therapy as local therapy. Of the 17 patients who did not undergo mastectomy, 14 had negative repeat biopsies and 13 received radiation therapy alone as local treatment. One patient who had a negative repeat biopsy refused any local therapy. A patient with a positive repeat biopsy was found to have residual microscopic disease, with a few scattered tumor cells that appeared to be nonviable; this patient proceeded to local therapy with radiation alone. One patient who did not have a repeat biopsy (because of a negative mammogram and the judgment of physicians involved early in the study) received radiation therapy alone. One patient was lost to follow-up at the time of best response. Thus, there were 15 patients who actually received radiation therapy alone as local therapy, with an additional patient who refused radiation. This patient is included in analyses of the group scheduled to receive radiation therapy.

Toxicity ■

The major toxicities in this study are listed in Table 7–7. The extent of hematologic toxicity was graded according to the World Health Organization (WHO) guidelines.[81] There were three episodes of neutropenia

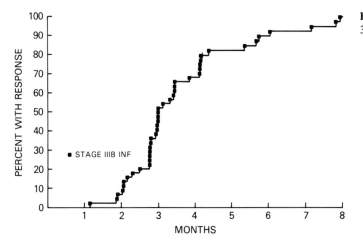

FIG. 7–2 Time to best response. The median time was 3.0 months.

Table 7–7
Toxicities Observed in NCI Study*

Toxicity	Severity†	No. (%)
Hematologic		
WBC	Grade 1	4 (9%)
	Grade 2	16 (36%)
	Grade 3	19 (42%)
	Grade 4	6 (13%)
Platelets	Grade 1	2 (4%)
	Grade 4	4 (9%)
Hepatic	SGOT, 1.1 to 2 × nml	18 (40%)
	SGOT, 2.1 to 5 × nml	7 (16%)
	SGOT, >5 × nml	1 (22%)
Gastrointestinal		
Nausea and vomiting	Grade 1	3 (7%)
	Grade 2	21 (47%)
	Grade 3	6 (13%)
Diarrhea	Grade 1	5 (11%)
	Grade 2	5 (11%)
	Grade 3	1 (2%)
Stomatitis	Grade 1	0 (0%)
	Grade 2	21 (47%)
	Grade 3	7 (16%)

* Study in progress.
†NML = normal.

and fever during induction or maintenance chemotherapy that required hospitalization. Five episodes of neutropenia and fever requiring antibiotics were seen in patients receiving high-dose melphalan and autologous BMT. There were six cases of cardiomyopathy: three with ejection fractions of 38%–40%, one with an ejection fraction of 23%, and two with ejection fractions <15%. One of these patients, who had received 513 mg/m² of dox, died of congestive heart failure, with no evidence of disease at death. Five of the six patients with cardiomyopathy had left-sided lesions and received radiation therapy along with dox therapy. In these patients, total dox doses ranged from 352 mg/m² to 518 mg/m².

Disease-free and Overall Survival ■

Relapses have occurred in 21 patients. The initial relapse was locoregional only in 7 patients, distant only in 10, and both locoregional and distant in 4. Locoregional recurrences included 4 on the chest wall, 2 in ipsilateral axillary nodes, and 5 breast recurrences. Three of the 5 patients with breast recurrences have died with metastatic disease, 1 patient currently is being treated with salvage chemotherapy for unresectable local disease, and 1 patient had a mastectomy and has been disease-free for 7 months.

The 2-year actuarial probability of local control was 67% (Fig. 7–3). At 1 year, the actuarial probability of not having a regional failure is 95% for patients treated with both mastectomy and radiation versus 93% for those treated with radiation alone; at 2 years, these figures are 59% and 77%, respectively. The life table curves for local recurrence by local treatment modality tend to overlap greatly, and there is no evidence of any significant differences ($p = 0.95$).

Relapses were also evaluated by response: 7 of 19 patients with PRs (37%) and 13 of 24 patients with CRs (54%) relapsed. The one patient rated NC also relapsed. Relapses by results of skin biopsies are as follows: 9 of 22 with positive biopsies (41%), 7 of 17 with negative biopsies (41%), and 5 of 6 (83%) with unknown biopsy results.

FIG. 7–3 Time to locoregional recurrence. The 2-year actuarial local control rate for patients with inflammatory breast cancer was 67%.

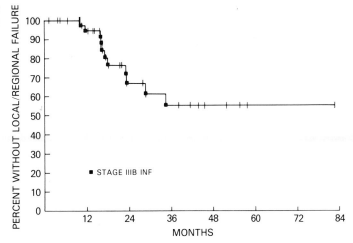

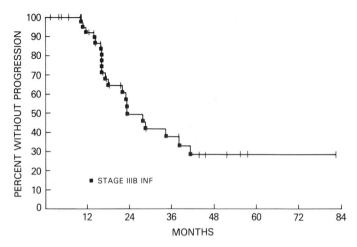

FIG. 7–4   Time to progression. The median was 23 months for patients with inflammatory cancer.

The median potential follow-up at the time of this analysis is 32 months. The median time to progression is 23 months (Fig. 7–4), and the median survival is 36 months (Fig. 7–5). Median time to progression and survival did not differ on the basis of skin biopsy results (presence or absence of dermal lymphatic invasion). The median time to progression was 23 months for patients with a positive skin biopsy, 24.8 months for those with a negative biopsy, and 16 months for those with unknown biopsy results (all ps = NS). Similarly, the median survival for the biopsy-positive group was 37.2 months; the negative-biopsy group has not reached median survival at the present time, and the median for the unknown-results group 35.3 months (all ps = NS). Patients were also analyzed by the type of local treatment received. Patients who had mastectomy and radiation had DFS identical to that of those who received radiation therapy alone (23.1 months, Fig. 7–6).

Results of BMT and High-dose Melphalan Versus Maintenance Chemotherapy ■

At the time of the February 1988 analysis, 16 patients with inflammatory disease had been randomized—7 to BMT and 9 to maintenance chemotherapy; ten patients refused randomization. Only 5 patients actually received BMT because 2 had positive bone marrow biopsies immediately prior to bone marrow storage.

The toxicities of high-dose melphalan in the five patients who received the treatment comprised grade 2 stomatitis in one patient and grade 3 stomatitis in one patient; grade 2 diarrhea in two patients and grade 4 in one patient; and grade 2 nausea and vomiting in three patients and grade 4 in one. The patient with grade 4 diarrhea was admitted to the intensive care unit for profound diarrhea, severe abdominal pain, and bowel edema on CT scan. All 5 patients had fevers

FIG. 7–5   Overall survival. The median was 36 months for patients with inflammatory cancer.

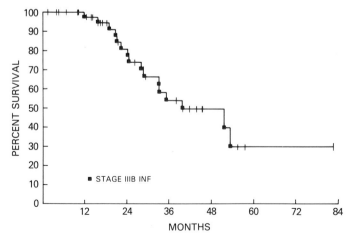

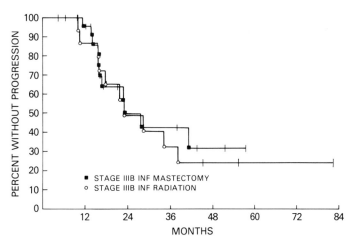

PERCENT WITHOUT PROGRESSION

■ STAGE IIIB INF MASTECTOMY
○ STAGE IIIB INF RADIATION

MONTHS

FIG. 7-6 Time to progression. The median was 23.1 months for patients treated by mastectomy followed by radiation (■) and 23.1 months for patients treated by radiation alone.

during neutropenia and required antibiotic treatment. The median length of WBC nadir was 10 days and platelet nadir was 6 days. The median hospital stay was 27 days.

There have been two relapses in the BMT arm and six in the maintenance arm, with one death on the BMT arm and two on maintenance arm. These numbers are too small to make any conclusions regarding the therapeutic efficacy of autologous BMT and high-dose melphalan.

The median number of maintenance cycles reduced $\leq 75\%$ was 1 for high-dose melphalan and BMT and 3 for maintenance ($p = .15$); medians for $\leq 50\%$ reductions were 1 for BMT and 3 for maintenance 3 ($p = 0.70$); overall, the median number of cycles reduced was 3.5 for BMT and 8 for maintenance therapy ($p = .51$). One patient who underwent BMT was hospitalized during maintenance chemotherapy for neutropenic sepsis; no patient receiving maintenance alone required hospitalization for this side-effect. The median nadir WBC for patients receiving BMT while on maintenance was $2100/\text{mm}^3$ and for those receiving only maintenance was $1800/\text{mm}^3$ ($p = .63$); median nadir platelet counts were $102,500/\text{mm}^3$ for BMT patients during maintenance $130,000/\text{mm}^3$ for maintenance ($p = 0.15$).

Conclusion ■

The median overall survival in the NCI study was 36 months, which is an improvement over treatment with local therapy alone. However, it is evident that more intensive, or altogether different, modalities of therapy must be undertaken to cure patients with this disease.

Future directions in the treatment of inflammatory breast cancer include the use of very-high-dose chemotherapy and autologous marrow transplant, as incorporated in our regimen. Patients with locally advanced inflammatory breast cancer are ideal for this modality of therapy because of their low disease burden at the time of best response.

One of the largest studies of high-dose chemotherapy in breast cancer was by Peters and colleagues.[82] They treated 21 patients with a combination of CTX, cisplatin, and carmustine. There were eight CRs, 3 of which were continuous (duration, 3 to 21 months), and 6 PRs. This represents an objective response rate of 67%. There were 3 deaths resulting from toxicity. The median duration of response for all patients was 7.5 months. Although the response rates are excellent in this study, this level of response can be achieved in untreated patients with conventional chemotherapy, and the duration of response has not been prolonged.

An excellent review of autologous BMT and high-dose therapy in breast cancer has been published by Antman and Gale.[83] They evaluated 27 trials of high-dose chemotherapy and autologous BMT in 172 breast cancer patients. There were 73 patients treated with single-agent chemotherapy with various drugs, such as melphalan, thiotepa, CTX, and mitomycin C. The overall CR rate was 5% (4 patients) and the PR rate was 26% (19 patients). There were 40 patients treated with high-dose combination chemotherapy or a single agent combined with radiation, with a 25% CR rate and 48% PR rate. The median duration of response ranged from 2 to >16 months. Finally, six studies were evaluated in which single agents or combination chemotherapy were given in high dose with autologous BMT to a total of 59 previously untreated patients with inflammatory or Stage IV breast cancer.

In three studies, high-dose therapy was the only treatment given and in the others, induction therapy was given before high-dose therapy. There was an objective response rate of 81%, with 64% CR and 17% PR. However, the median duration of response ranged from 3 to 8 months (one study had a median duration >5 months). Also, there were 6 (10%) early deaths. The authors concluded that single- or multiple-agent high-dose chemotherapy with or without radiation produced responses in a substantial number of patients resistant to conventional therapy. However, disease-free survival was not prolonged. They suggested that autologous transplant should be done earlier in the disease course but noted that the efficacy of this therapy can only be evaluated in prospective studies.

One of the largest problems with high-dose chemotherapy is severe and prolonged myelosuppression, with resultant infections and treatment-related deaths. As mentioned above, there was a 10% incidence of early deaths in patients treated with high-dose therapy and autologous BMT. There has been recent interest in using granulocyte-macrophage colony-stimulating factor (GM-CSF) to accelerate hematopoietic recovery in the setting of high-dose therapy, thereby reducing treatment-related toxicity. Recombinant human GM-CSF has been shown to promote proliferation of granulocyte-macrophage progenitor cells.[84]

Brandt and colleagues[85] published a Phase I study using recombinant human GM-CSF after high-dose chemotherapy with CTX, carmustine, and cisplatin in 19 patients with breast cancer or melanoma.[85] Results were compared with 24 historical controls. Patients were treated with doses ranging from 2 μg to 32 μg/day for 14 days, starting after bone marrow reinfusion. The mean granulocyte count at day 15 (the end of GM-CSF infusion) was significantly higher than that of controls (1160 ± 1030 versus 318 ± 314, $p = 0.0035$). There was no difference in platelet counts. After GM-CSF infusion was stopped, leukocyte counts fell within 3 to 4 days to control levels. There was considerable toxicity with this therapy, especially at the dose of 32 μg, including myalgia, weight gain, edema, pleural effusion, and hypotension. Although these results are preliminary, the study suggests that GM-CSF may be helpful in accelerating myeloid recovery, thereby decreasing treatment-related toxicity. This promising therapy will require extensive evaluation in well-designed prospective studies.

Other future directions in the treatment of breast cancer could involve the use of growth factors, such as transforming growth factor beta (TGF-β) or antibodies to growth factors or their receptors, such as TGF-α. TGF-β has been shown to inhibit the growth of breast cancer cells *in vitro*.[86] It is contained in and secreted by breast cancer cells in culture. TGF-β is increased by the antiestrogen tamoxifen and may be responsible for the inhibition of growth of breast cancer that is seen clinically with the use of tamoxifen. TGF-β also inhibits estrogen-independent cell lines *in vitro*. TGF-β may have effects on stromal proliferation[87] and bone resorption.[88] Thus, this growth factor may be used in the future in breast cancer treatment.

Two other growth factors that have been shown to be important in the biology of breast cancer are TGF-α[89] and insulin-like growth factor-I (IGF-I) activity.[90] These factors are stimulated by estrogen treatment *in vitro* in breast cancer cell lines. TGF-α may be an important autostimulatory component in the growth regulation of breast cancer. New therapies may be designed to interrupt TGF-α or enhance growth-inhibitory effects of TGF-β. Future chemotherapeutic approaches could use antireceptor molecules conjugated with toxins to tumor-specific agents. These approaches have produced encouraging results in animal model systems.[91,92]

Other goals of research programs for breast cancer treatment include development of monoclonal antibodies to tumor antigens for cytotoxic targeting against tumor cells, development of methods to change breast cancer kinetics *in vivo,* and increasing binding of drugs to certain enzymes important for tumor growth. Also, drug sensitivity assays are being developed to determine optimal drug combinations.

References ■

1. Lee BJ, Tannenbaum NE: Inflammatory carcinoma of the breast: A report of twenty-eight cases from the breast clinic of Memorial Hospital. Surg Gynecol Obstet 39:580–595, 1924
2. Leitch A: Peau d'orange in acute mammary carcinoma: Its cause and diagnostic value. Lancet 1:861–863, 1909
3. Schumann EA: A study of carcinoma mastitoides. Ann Surg 54:69–77, 1911
4. Learmonth GE: Acute mammary carcinoma. Can Med Assoc J 6:499–511, 1916
5. von Volkmann R: Brust Krebse. Beiträge zur Chirurgie, pp 319–334. Leipzig, Breitkopf und Härtel, 1875
6. Klotz ID: Über Mastitis Carcinomatosa Gravidarum et Lactantium. These, Halle, 1869
7. Haagensen CD: Diseases of the Breast, 2nd ed, pp 576–584. Philadelphia, WB Saunders, 1971
8. Barber KW, Dockerty MB, Clagett OT: Inflammatory carcinoma of the breast. Surg Gynecol Obstet 112:406–410, 1961
9. Noguchi S, Miyauchi K, Nishizawa Y et al: Management of inflammatory carcinoma of the breast with combined modality therapy including intraarterial infusion chemotherapy as induction therapy. Cancer 61:1483–1491, 1988

10. Hagelberg RS, Jolly PC, Anderson RP: Role of surgery in the treatment of inflammatory breast carcinoma. Am J Surg 148:125–131, 1984
11. Stock LH, Patterson MS: Inflammatory carcinoma of the breast. Surg Gynecol Obstet 143:885–889, 1976
12. Meyer AC, Dockerty MB, Harrington SW: Inflammatory carcinoma of the breast. Surg Gynecol Obstet 87:417–424, 1948
13. Lucas FV, Mesa-Perez C: Inflammatory carcinoma of the breast. Cancer 41:1595–1605, 1978
14. Rogers CS, Fitts WT: Inflammatory carcinoma of the breast: A critique of therapy. Surgery 39:367–370, 1956
15. Droulias CA, Sewell CW, McSweeney MB, Powell RW: Inflammatory carcinoma of the breast: A correlation of clinical, radiologic and pathologic findings. Ann Surg 184:217–222, 1976
16. Donnelly B: Primary "inflammatory" carcinoma of the breast: A report of five cases and a review of the literature. Ann Surg 128:918–930, 1948
17. Taylor GW, Meltzer A: Inflammatory carcinoma of the breast. Ann Surg 33:33–49, 1938
18. Levine PH, Steinhorn SC, Ries LE, Aaron JL: Inflammatory breast cancer: The experience of the Surveillance Epidemiology and End Results (SEER) Program. JNCI 74:291–297, 1985
19. Chamadol W, Pesie M, Puapairoj A: Inflammatory carcinoma of the breast in a 12-year-old Thai girl. J Med Assoc Thailand 70:543–547, 1987
20. Piera JM, Alonso MC, Ojeda MB, Biete A: Locally advanced breast cancer with inflammatory component: A clinical entity with a poor prognosis. Radiother Oncol 7:199–208, 1986
21. Haagensen CD: Diseases of the Breast, 3rd ed, pp 808–814. Philadelphia, WB Saunders, 1986
22. Bryant T: Diseases of the Breast, pp 171–194. London, Cassell & Co Ltd, 1987
23. Chris SM: Inflammatory carcinoma of the breast: A report of 20 cases and a review of the literature. Br J Surg 38:163–174, 1950
24. Ellis DL, Teitelbaum SL: Inflammatory carcinoma of the breast: A pathologic definition. Cancer 33:1045–1047, 1974
25. Saltzstein SL: Clinically occult inflammatory carcinoma of the breast. Cancer 34:382–388, 1974
26. Beahrs OH, Myers MH (eds): Manual for Staging of Cancer, 2nd ed, pp 127–135. Philadelphia, JB Lippincott, 1983
27. Hermanek P, Sobin LH (eds): TNM Classification of Malignant Tumors: UICC International Union Against Cancer, 4th ed, pp 93–99. Berlin, Springer-Verlag, 1987
28. Haagensen CD: Diseases of the Breast, p 858. Philadelphia, WB Saunders, 1986
29. Lacour J, Hourtoule FG: La place de la chirurgie dans le traitement des formes evolutives du cancer du sein. Mem Acad Chir 93:635–643, 1967
30. Tabbane F, Muenz L, Jaziri M et al: Clinical and prognostic features of a rapidly progressing breast cancer in Tunisia. Cancer 40:376–382, 1977
31. Knight CD, Martin JK, Welch JS: Surgical considerations after chemotherapy and radiation therapy for inflammatory breast cancer. Surgery 99:385–391, 1986
32. DeLarue JC, Levin F, Mouriesse H et al: Oestrogen and progesterone cytosolic receptors in clinically inflammatory tumors of the human breast. Br J Cancer 44:911–916, 1981
33. Kokal WA, Hill CR, Porudominsky D et al: Inflammatory breast carcinoma: A distinct entity? Surg Oncol 30:152–155, 1985
34. Harvey HA, Lipton A, Lawrence BV et al: Estrogen receptor in inflammatory breast carcinoma. J Surg Oncol 21:42–44, 1982
35. Schäfer P, Alberto P, Forni M et al: Surgery as part of a combined modality approach for inflammatory breast carcinoma. Cancer 59:1063–1067, 1987
36. Keiling R, Guiochet N, Calderoli H et al: Preoperative chemotherapy in the treatment of inflammatory breast cancer. In Primary Chemotherapy in Cancer Medicine, pp 95–104. New York, Alan R Liss, 1985
37. Bozzetti F, Saccozzi R, DeLena M, Salvadori B: Inflammatory cancer of the breast: Analysis of 114 cases. J Surg Oncol 18:355–361, 1981
38. Mourali N, Muenz LR, Tabbane F et al: Epidemiologic features of rapidly progressing breast cancer in Tunisia. Cancer 46:2741–2746, 1980
39. Costa J, Webber BL, Levine PL et al: Histopathological features of rapidly progressing breast carcinoma in Tunisia: A study of 94 cases. Int J Cancer 30:35–37, 1982
40. Haagensen CD, Stout AP: Carcinoma of the breast: II. Criteria of operability. Ann Surg 118:859–870, 1032–1051, 1943
41. Treves N: The inoperability of inflammatory carcinoma of the breast. Surg Gynecol Obstet 109:240–242, 1959
42. Dao TL, MacCarthy JD: Treatment of inflammatory carcinoma of the breast. Surg Gynecol Obstet 105:289–294, 1957
43. Wang CC, Griscom NT: Inflammatory carcinoma of the breast: Results following orthovoltage and supervoltage radiation therapy. Clin Radiol 15:168–174, 1964
44. Zucali R, Uslenghi C, Kenda R, BonaDonna G: Natural history and survival of inoperable breast cancer treated with radiotherapy and radiotherapy followed by radical mastectomy. Cancer 37:1422–1431, 1976
45. Nussbaum H, Kagan AR, Gilbert H et al: Management of inflammatory breast carcinoma. Breast 3:25–29, 1977
46. Bruckman JE, Harris JR, Levene MB et al: Results of treating stage III carcinoma of the breast by primary radiation therapy. Cancer 43:985–993, 1979
47. Chu AM, Wood WC, Doucette JA: Inflammatory breast carcinoma treated by radical radiotherapy. Cancer 45:2730–2737, 1980
48. Barker JL, Montague ED, Peters LJ: Clinical experience of irradiation of inflammatory carcinoma of the breast with and without elective chemotherapy. Cancer 45:625–629, 1980
49. Rao DV, Bedwineck J, Perez C et al: Prognostic indicators in stage III and localized stage IV breast cancer. Cancer 50:2037–2043, 1982
50. Rouësse S, Sarrazin D, Mouriesse H et al: Primary chemotherapy in the treatment of inflammatory breast carcinoma: A study of 230 cases from the Institut Gustave-Roussy. J Clin Oncol 4:1765–1771, 1986
51. Perez CA, Fields JN: Role of radiation therapy for locally advanced and inflammatory carcinoma of the breast. Oncology 1:81–93, 1987
52. Baclesse F: Five-year results in 431 breast cancers treated solely by roentgen rays. Ann Surg 161:103–104, 1965
53. Barker JL, Nelson AJ, Montague ED: Inflammatory carcinoma of the breast. Radiology 121:173–176, 1976
54. Fracchia AA, Randall HT, Farrow JH: The results of adrenalectomy in advanced breast cancer in 500 consecutive patients. Surg Gynecol Obstet 125:747–756, 1967
55. Yonemoto RH, Keating JL, Byron RL et al: Inflammatory carcinoma of the breast treated by bilateral adrenalectomy. Surgery 68:461–467, 1970
56. Veronesi A, Frustaci S, Tirelli U et al: Tamoxifen therapy in postmenopausal advanced breast cancer: Efficacy at the primary tumor site in 46 evaluable patients. Tumori 67:235–238, 1981
57. Campbell FC, Morgan AL, Bishop HM et al: The management of locally advanced carcinoma of the breast by Nolvadex (tamoxifen): A pilot study. Br Assoc Surg Oncol 10:111–115, 1984

58. DeLena M, Zucali R, Viganotti G et al: Combined chemotherapy-radiotherapy approach in locally advanced (T_{3b}-T_4) breast cancer. Cancer Chemother Pharmacol 1:53–59, 1978

59. Buzdar AU, Montague ED, Barker JL et al: Management of inflammatory carcinoma of breast with combined modality approach—An update. Cancer 47:2537–2542, 1981

60. Fastenberg NA, Buzdar AV, Montague ED et al: Management of inflammatory carcinoma of the breast. A combined modality approach. Am J Clin Oncol 8:134–141, 1985

61. Burton GV, Cox EB, Leight GS et al: Inflammatory breast carcinoma, effective multimodal approach. Arch Surg 122: 1329–1332, 1987

62. Loprinzi CL, Carbone PP, Tormey DC et al: Aggressive combined modality therapy for advanced local-regional breast carcinoma. J Clin Oncol 2:157–163, 1984

63. Pawlicki M, Skolyszewski J, Brandys A: Results of combined treatment of patients with locally advanced breast cancer. Tumori 69:249–253, 1983

64. Zylberberg B, Salat-Baroux J, Ravina JH et al: Initial chemoimmunotherapy in inflammatory carcinoma of the breast. Cancer 49:1537–1543, 1982

65. Israël L, Brew J-L, Morere J-F: Two years of high dose cyclophosphamide and 5-fluorouracil followed by surgery after 3 months for acute inflammatory breast carcinomas: A phase II study of 25 cases with a median follow-up of 35 months. Cancer 57:24–28, 1986

66. Schwartz GF, Cantor RI, Biermann WA: Neoadjuvant chemotherapy before definitive treatment for stage III carcinoma of the breast. Arch Surg 122:1430–1434, 1987

67. Fowble B, Glover D, Rosato EF, Goodman RL: Combined modality treatment of inflammatory breast cancer. Int J Radiat Oncol Biol Phys 12:11–12, 1986

68. Jacquillat C, Weil M, Auclerc G et al: Neo-adjuvant chemotherapy in the conservative management of breast cancer: A study of 205 patients. In Adjuvant Therapy of Cancer, vol 5, pp 403–409. New York, Grune & Stratton, 1987

69. Perloff M, Lesnick GJ, Korzun A et al: Chemotherapy with mastectomy or radiotherapy for stage III breast carcinoma: A Cancer and Leukemia Group B Study. J Clin Oncol 6:261–269, 1988

70. Sherry MM, Johnson DH, Page DL et al: Inflammatory carcinoma of the breast. Am J Med 79:355–364, 1985

71. Conte PF, Alama A, Bertelli G et al: Chemotherapy with estrogenic recruitment and surgery in locally advanced breast cancer: clinical and cytokinetic results. Int J Cancer 40:490–494, 1987

72. Wiseman C, Jessup JM, Smith TL et al: Inflammatory breast cancer treated with surgery, chemotherapy and allogenic tumor cell/BCG immunotherapy. Cancer 49:1266–1271, 1982

73. Chevallier B, Asselain B, Kunlin A et al: Inflammatory breast cancer—Determination of prognostic factors by univariate and multivariate analysis. Cancer 60:897–902, 1987

74. Brun B, Otmezguine Y, Feuilhade F et al: Treatment of inflammatory breast cancer with combination chemotherapy and mastectomy versus breast conservation. Cancer 61:1096–1103, 1988

75. Swain SM, Sorace RA, Bagley CS et al: Neoadjuvant chemotherapy in the combined modality approach of locally advanced nonmetastatic breast cancer. Cancer Res 47:3889–3894, 1987

76. Lippman ME, Bolan G, Huff K: The effects of estrogens and antiestrogens on hormone-responsive human breast cancer in long-term tissue culture. Cancer Res 36:4595–4601, 1976

77. Lippman ME, Cassidy J, Wesley M, Young RC: A randomized attempt to increase the efficacy of cytotoxic chemotherapy in metastatic breast cancer by hormonal synchronization. J Clin Oncol 2:28–36, 1984

78. Sorace RA, Bagley CS, Lichter AS et al: The management of nonmetastatic locally advanced breast cancer using primary induction chemotherapy with hormonal synchronization followed by radiation therapy with or without debulking surgery. World J Surg 9:775–785, 1985

79. Kaplan EL, Meier P: Nonparametric estimation from incomplete observations. J Am Stat Assoc 53:457–481, 1958

80. Mantel N: Evaluation of survival data and two new rank order statistics arising in its consideration. Cancer Chemo Rep 50: 163–170, 1966

81. Miller AB, Hoogstraten B, Staquet M et al: Reporting results of cancer treatment. Cancer 47:207–214, 1981

82. Peters WP, Jones RP, Shpall EJ et al: High dose combination alkylating agents with autologous bone marrow support as initial therapy for metastatic breast cancer. Proc Am Assoc Cancer Res 28:227, 1987

83. Antman K, Gale RP: Advanced breast cancer: High-dose chemotherapy and bone marrow autotransplant. Ann Intern Med 108:570–574, 1988

84. Metcalf D, Begley CG, Johnson GR et al: Biologic properties in vitro of a recombinant human granulocyte-macrophage colony-stimulating factor. Blood 67:37–45, 1986

85. Brandt SJ, Peters WP, Atwater SK et al: Effect of recombinant human granulocyte-macrophage colony-stimulating factor on hematopoietic reconstitution after high-dose chemotherapy and autologous bone marrow transplantation. N Engl J Med 318: 869–876, 1988

86. Knabbe C, Lippman ME, Wakefield L et al: Evidence that TGFβ is a hormonally regulated negative growth factor in human breast cancer. Cell 48:417–428, 1987

87. Derynck R, Goeddel DV, Ullrich A et al: Synthesis of messenger RNAs for transforming growth factors α and β and the epidermal growth factor receptor by human tumors. Cancer Res 47:707–712, 1987

88. Tasjian AH, Voelkel EF, Lazzaro M et al: α and β human transforming growth factors stimulate prostaglandin and bone resorption in cultured mouse calvaria. Proc Natl Acad Sci (USA) 82:4535–4538, 1985

89. Bates S, McManaway ME, Lippman ME, Dickson RB: Characterization of estrogen responsive transforming activity in human breast cancer cell lines. Cancer Res 46:1707–1713, 1986

90. Huff KK, Knabbe C, Lindsey R et al: Multihormonal regulation of insulin-like growth factor-1-related protein in MCF-7 human breast cancer cells. Molec Endocrinol 2:200–208, 1988

91. Vitella ES, Uhu JW: Immunotoxins: Redirecting nature's poisons. Cell 41:653–665, 1985

92. Pastan I, Willingham MC, Fitzgerald DP: Immunotoxins. Cell 47:641–648, 1986

Gianni Bonadonna

Pinuccia Valagussa

Role of Chemotherapy in Stage I Breast Cancer

8

Introduction ■

For many decades, the size of primary tumor and the status of regional lymph nodes have been the main prognostic indicators in primary breast cancer. These two variables have influenced surgical decisions about tumor resectability, as well as relapse-free and total survival rates. Since the initial reports of the National Surgical Adjuvant Breast Project (NSABP) in 1968,[1] surgeons have gradually become more aware of the prognostic significance of the histologic status of ipsilateral axillary nodes and, in particular, the inverse relationship between number of involved lymph nodes and treatment outcome.[2-9] In more recent years, randomized trials of adjuvant chemotherapy have used as stratification parameters two nodal subsets—1–3 and >3 positive lymph nodes.[10,11] A retrospective evaluation of the earlier trials confirmed that increasing numbers of involved nodes were associated with greater probability of failure to respond to treatment or death.[12-14] As a consequence of these observations, the National Institutes of Health (NIH) Consensus Development Conference[15,16] defined four lymph node categories: negative nodes, 1–3 positive nodes, 4–9 positive nodes, and ≥10 positive nodes.

For many years, surgeons have thought that a histologically negative nodal status was associated with a very favorable treatment outcome, particularly in the presence of a small tumor size. However, retrospective evaluations reported in the 1970s clearly documented that the overall recurrence rate within the first 10 years after mastectomy was about 25%, regardless of tumor size.[2,3]

Natural History of Node-Negative Tumors ■

This section briefly summarizes data on the natural history of node-negative breast cancer treated with surgery alone (Halsted radical mastectomy or modified radical mastectomy). Of women with resectable breast cancer who undergo axillary dissection, approximately half are classified as node-negative. It is well known that the overall error in clinical (versus histopathologic) assessment of axillary nodal status is about 33%. In the NSABP experience, based on 937 cases, 38.6% of patients judged to be clinically node-negative were found upon pathologic examination to have tumor-positive nodes.[17] The accuracy of physical examination in predicting histologic involvement of axillary nodes in other case series is reported in Table 8–1.

An important issue is the number of axillary lymph nodes that should be removed to ensure the accuracy of a node-negative assessment. The NSABP studies provide the most accurate information in this regard. Fisher and colleagues[17] stated that "when relatively few nodes are found and examined . . . the nodal status can be determined with accuracy. There is no evidence to indicate that the removal of more nodes increases the likelihood of determining the true nodal status. . . . To quantify accurately the degree of *positive* nodal involvement, a more complete axillary dissection is required." Also Veronesi and colleagues,[21] evaluating 539 cases, noted that the chances of finding metastatic nodes at the second and third axillary levels are negligible when the first level is clear.

Tumor Size ■

Conventional clinical–histopathologic evaluation has shown prognosis in node-negative tumors to be related to the primary tumor size (Table 8–2). Tumors <2 cm in largest diameter show a very good prognosis, with a 5-year relapse rate of approximately 10%. Comparable 5-year results were recently reported in T_1 tumors (≤2 cm) treated with conservative surgery and postoperative irradiation.[23] As detailed by Valagussa and associates[3] in 335 cases, 15% of node-negative patients relapse during the first 3 years after mastectomy; in the subsequent 7 years another 13% relapse. Also in this series, tumors measuring up to

Table 8–1
Accuracy of Physical Examination in Predicting Histologic Involvement of Axillary Nodes (Percentages)

Study	False Positive	False Negative
Butcher[18]	25	32
Haagensen[19]	31	28
Schottenfeld and Nash[5]	26	27
Bucalossi et al[20]	29	29
Fisher et al[17]	39	27

2 cm had a lower relapse rate compared to larger tumors (Table 8–3).

Tumor Grading ■

Tumor grading as prognostic factor in node-negative breast cancer has not been systematically reported in most series. In the evaluation of discriminants for 10-year treatment failure, Fisher and associates[24] examined 279 node-negative women and noticed an adverse effect on outcome in patients whose tumors were assessed as being most malignant (histologic grade III by the NSABP old and newer methods). The Memorial Hospital group[25] concluded that whether defined in terms of cytologic type (nuclear grade) or growth pattern (histologic grade), differentiation was significant with respect to recurrence and survival in node-negative tumors. The major criticism concerning the prognostic value of tumor grade is the degree of interobserver reproducibility.[26] As correctly stressed by Fisher,[27] a considerable degree of practice in large case series and a thorough review (at least 15 minutes) are necessary to eventually reach internal and external comparability >90%.

Steroid Receptors ■

During the past 15 years, innumerable reports have appeared on steroid receptor assays and their correlation with clinical response in various stages of breast

Table 8–2
Five-year Relapse Rate in Node-negative Patients by Primary Tumor Size (Percentages)

Study	Primary Tumor Size		
	<2 cm	2–5 cm	>5 cm
Fisher et al[2]	12	24	27
Nemoto et al[22]	13	19	25
Valagussa et al[3]	8	24	19

cancer. Not all reports have provided unambiguous and consistent information, probably reflecting different technical methods used in the receptor assay.[28,29] The San Antonio group[30] was the first to demonstrate that in node-negative women, treatment outcome—at least during the first 5 years postsurgery—was better in estrogen receptor-positive (ER+) tumors than ER-negative tumors. Most subsequent studies have confirmed this observation (Table 8–4). More recent findings have also indicated that in Stage II disease, progesterone (PgR) levels are more important than ER levels for predicting time to recurrence, and the addition of PgR data to ER findings significantly added to the predictive value of the latter.[39] The most recent data from the San Antonio group on Stage I disease (1647 patients)[40] revealed that ER and tumor size are the most important factors for predicting recurrence in node-negative tumors; in contrast, age and PgR status were not independent prognostic variables.

Tumor Cell Proliferative Activity ■

Pathologists have known for decades that the presence of numerous mitotic figures in a tumor specimen was often associated with an aggressive clinical course and with shortened relapse-free and total survival. During the past few years, quantitative measurements of the proliferative activity of tumor cells have been done by thymidine-labeling index[41–43] and flow cytometry.[44,45] Several studies have consistently concluded that the higher the percentage of tumor cells engaging in DNA synthesis, the more likely a patient is to have a breast cancer recurrence and shorter survival. Of particular importance, these studies on tumor cell kinetics have indicated that the proliferative rate is a prognostic indicator independent of tumor size, stage, and estrogen receptor content. Figures 8–1 and 8–2 illustrate the prognostic importance of the thymidine-labeling index in predicting both relapse-free and overall survival in a series of 215 node-negative breast cancer patients treated with mastectomy alone at the Milan Cancer Institute.[46] The regression analysis revealed superiority of the labeling index over the other factors.

Flow cytometry, using frozen pulverized breast tumors, to measure the proliferative rate (the percentage of cells in S phase) and to determine ploidy, was investigated by the San Antonio group.[44,45] Their analysis indicated that receptor-negative tumors are much more likely to be aneuploid and to have a high median S phase than receptor-positive tumors. The investigators concluded that in node-negative breast cancer,

Table 8–3
Progressive Increment of Relapse Rate in Node-negative Patients Treated with Surgery Alone (Percentages)

Stratification Variable	Relapse at 3 Years	Increment		Total at 10 Years
		3–5 Years	5–10 Years	
Primary size				
≤2 cm	1.9	5.8	12.2	19.9
2–5 cm	17.7	6.6	5.9	30.2
>5 cm	18.7	0	6.4	25.1
Menopause				
Pre	23.0	0.8	7.0	30.8
Post	14.0	5.4	7.0	26.4
Total series	15.0	6.0	6.9	27.9

Adapted from Valagussa et al, Cancer 41:1170–1178, 1978.

both percent S phase and ploidy are significant prognostic factors for relapse.

The monoclonal antibody Ki-67, which is expressed only in continuously cycling cells, was studied by Lellé and coworkers[47] to determine the growth fraction of breast tumors by immunostaining of fresh tissue. A correlation was found between growth fractions and histologic grading, and a significantly higher growth fraction was detected in node-positive than node-negative tumors. The results of this interesting study, however, do not show whether Ki-67 represents a potentially useful predictor of clinical course.

Other Prognostic Indicators ■

More recent investigations have called attention to the possible prognostic relevance of oncogene amplification. The San Antonio group has reported that overexpression of the HER-2/*neu* oncogene, a member of the *erb*B-like family, predicts short disease-free and overall survival in Stage II breast cancer.[48,49] No data are as yet available for Stage I patients. Proto-oncogene abnormalities were correlated with anatomic features and clinical course of human breast cancer by Cline and coworkers.[50] Briefly, the presence of altered proto-oncogenes correlated with clinical stage (67% in node-positive cancer versus 43% in node-negative cancer), and all but one of the cancers that recurred or progressed had detectably altered proto-oncogenes.

Monoclonal antibodies were used to detect micrometastases in the bone marrow of breast cancer patients who had local disease on staging by conventional methods.[51] The bone marrow of 307 women with primary breast cancer was examined for tumor cells by immunocytochemistry, using an antiserum to epithelial membrane antigen. Micrometastases were found in 26.4% of the patients, and their presence was related to various prognostic factors. In 152 node-negative women, bone marrow micrometastases were found in 19%. Analysis of the sites of relapse

Table 8–4
Relapse-free Survival as a Function of ER Status in Resectable Breast Cancer

Study	Stage	No. Pts.	Time of Analysis (yr)	RFS (%)		*p* Value
				ER+	ER−	
Knight et al[30]	I, II	145	1.6	86	66	0.01
Rich et al[31]	I, II	285	1.6	93	73	NR
Allegra et al[32]	I, II	292	2	91	62	<0.001
Cooke et al[33]	I, II	144	3	85	35	<0.001
Maynard et al[34]	I, II	232	3	71	63	<0.05
Adami et al[35]	I	94	5	83	73	<0.05
Butler et al[36]	I	556	6	83	86	NS
Crowe et al[37]	I	510	5	78	67	<0.034
Valagussa et al[38]	I	464	5	80	63	<0.001

* Minor local recurrences excluded from analysis.

NR = not reported.

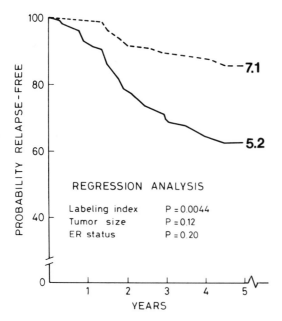

FIG. 8-1 Relapse-free survival of patients with node-negative breast cancer as a function of labeling index (---- slowly proliferating tumors; ——— highly proliferating tumors). Regression analysis is by the Cox model. (Adapted from Silvestrini R et al: Breast Cancer Res Treat 7:161–169, 1986)

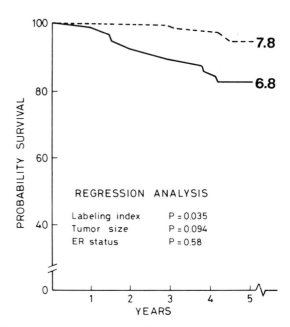

FIG. 8-2 Total survival of patients with node-negative breast cancer as a function of labeling index (---- slowly proliferating tumors; ——— highly proliferating tumors). Regression analysis is by the Cox model (Adapted from Silvestrini R *et al:* Breast Cancer Res Treat 7:161–169, 1986)

showed that this test predicts bone metastases only. Both relapse-free and total survival were significantly shorter for women with micrometastases. The authors concluded that the detection of micrometastases in primary breast cancer is a useful, albeit not independent, prognostic factor.

The Early Clinical Trials ■

The early adjuvant trials for node-negative breast cancer date back to 1958,[1] and the patients studied represent only a subgroup of larger studies concentrating on node-positive tumors. The essential results of trials started before 1980 are reported in Table 8-5 and described below.

NSABP Trial ■

The multicenter NSABP trial, started in April 1958,[1] included a total of 826 patients, 382 of whom were node-negative. Conventional Halsted radical mastectomy was followed by (randomly assigned) placebo or a short course of perioperative thiotepa (TPA). Initially, TPA patients received 0.8 mg/kg of body weight of this drug (0.4 mg/kg at the time of operation and

0.2 mg/kg on each of the first 2 postoperative days). Because of drug toxicity, the total amount of TPA administered was reduced to 0.6 mg/kg (0.2 mg/kg on the day of operation and on each of 2 subsequent days). The 10-year relapse-free survival (RFS) for all patients, regardless of menopausal or nodal status, was 50%.

Scandinavian Trial ■

This multicenter study, initiated in 1965,[61] included 1026 women, of whom 609 were classified as node-negative. Randomization was done by telephone from the operating room, with stratification by hospital only. In about 80% of the patients, surgery consisted of either Halsted radical mastectomy or modified radical mastectomy; the remaining patients underwent simple mastectomy without dissection of the axilla. The 507 patients in the treatment group received IV cyclophosphamide (5 mg/kg/day for 6 consecutive days), with the first injection immediately after closure of the surgical wound. The control group consisted of 509 patients. Both groups received postoperative irradiation. Primary oophorectomy or radiation castration was performed in 26% of the patients. The 20-year RFS for the entire series of patients was 39.5% in the control group and 52% in the treat-

Table 8–5
Synopsis of Published Results with Adjuvant Chemotherapy in Node-negative Breast Cancer*

Study	No. Pts.	Years of Follow-up	Trial Design	RFS (%)
Early Trials				
NSABP[52]	382	10	Placebo vs. short course perioperative thiotepa	76 vs. 73
Scandinavian[53]	609	20	Control vs. short course perioperative cyclophosphamide	55 vs. 63
Osako[54]	123	10	Control vs. LMF + BCG × 6	62 vs. 68
Midlands[55]	543	5	Control vs. LMF × 8	74 vs. 75
Mainz[56]	175	5	Radiotherapy vs. CMF × 12	72 vs. 82
Wien[57]	128	6	Control vs. CMFVP ± immuno-stimulants × 4 → 2 → 2 cycles	77 vs. 84
Recent Trials				
Milan[58]	90†	5	Control vs. IV CMF × 12	45 vs. 87
NSABP[59]	679†	4	Control vs. IV M → F × 12	71 vs. 80
Cardiff[60]	52†	3	Control vs. AVC × 6	71 vs. 83

* Abbreviations: L = leukeran; M = methotrexate; F = 5-fluorouracil; C = cyclophosphamide; V = vinblastine; A = Adriamycin.

† Receptor-negative tumors.

ment group, respectively. The number of relapses in the node-negative subgroup was considered too small for a meaningful testing of significance.[53]

OSAKO Trial ■

A multicenter randomized Swiss study, the OSAKO trial, was started in 1974[62] and included 240 evaluable patients (node-positive and node-negative). Patients were allocated to either surgery alone (modified radical mastectomy without postoperative radiotherapy) or the same type of surgery plus six cycles of oral LMF (Leukeran [chlorambucil], methotrexate, and 5-fluorouracil) followed by monthly skin scarification with bacillus Calmette–Guerin (BCG; Glaxo strain) up to relapse or 2 years. The dose schedule was as follows: Leukeran, 6–8 mg PO on days 1–14; methotrexate, 5–7.5 mg PO on days 1–3 and 8–10; and 5-fluorouracil, 500–750 mg PO on days 1 and 8. The 10-year RFS for the series was 40% in the control group and 51% for the chemoimmunotherapy group. Although node-negative women had an impressive RFS advantage during the first 3 to 4 years, this advantage began to vanish at 5 or more years of median follow-up.

West Midlands Trial ■

In a multicenter British trial, initiated in 1977,[55] all patients underwent simple mastectomy with axillary

node sampling after histologic confirmation of the diagnosis. Postoperative radiotherapy was not employed. After definition of axillary node status, patients were randomized to a surgery-only control group or surgery plus chemotherapy. Prospective stratification was done for menopausal status and tumor size. Of 574 node-negative women randomized, 543 were eligible for study. In this group, adjuvant chemotherapy consisted of an LMF-like regimen (Leukeran, 10 mg PO on days 1 and 2; methotrexate, 25 mg PO on day 1; 5-fluorouracil, 500 mg PO on days 1 and 2). Treatment has had no significant effect on 5-year RFS, either overall or when analyzed by subsets.

Mainz Trial ■

This German trial, started in 1977,[56] involved 175 patients treated by modified radical mastectomy or simple mastectomy with axillary node dissection. Only those patients whose axillary specimens contained at least four lymph nodes entered the study. Following surgery, patients were allocated randomly to receive postoperative irradiation (102 women) or adjuvant standard CMF (cyclophosphamide, methotrexate, 5-fluorouracil) chemotherapy for 12 monthly cycles (73 women). There were significantly more patients with T_2 tumors in the CMF group than the radiation group. With a median follow-up of 5 years, the RFS was 80% in the CMF group and 71% in the radiotherapy group.

Wien Trial ■

This single-institution trial was initiated in 1977.[57] All women who had a quadrantectomy plus axillary dissection or modified radical mastectomy for T_1 or T_2 breast cancer and who had no histologic evidence of axillary node metastases were eligible for study. A total of 128 patients were randomized into three groups: no adjuvant chemotherapy; chemotherapy; and chemotherapy plus the aspecific immunostimulant azimexon. Chemotherapy consisted of cyclophosphamide, 100 mg PO b.i.d. for 10 days; 5-fluorouracil, 750 mg IV on days 1 and 7; vinblastine, 5 mg IV on days 1 and 7; and methotrexate, 25 mg IV on days 1 and 7. Four treatment cycles were administered in the first year, and two cycles in the second and third year. No patient received postoperative irradiation. Because data for patients treated with chemotherapy and chemoimmunotherapy showed identical survival results, the authors grouped these patient subsets and compared them with the untreated controls. After a 6-year follow-up, the RFS was not significantly influenced by therapy.

Recent Clinical Trials ■

Four prospective randomized trials limited to node-negative and receptor-negative breast cancer have been designed and activated since December 1980.

Milan Trial ■

In December 1980, the Milan Cancer Institute started a prospective randomized trial in node-negative and ER− tumors.[58] Patient accrual was terminated in September 1985. The selection criteria were based on prior findings indicating the unfavorable prognosis of node-negative women whose ER assays were negative.[37,38] Study patients had T_{1-3a} disease. Within 1 month from locoregional therapy (modified radical mastectomy or quadrantectomy, full axillary dissection, and breast irradiation), patients were randomly allocated to receive no further treatment or intravenous CMF every 3 weeks for a total of 12 courses in about 9 months. Doses, in mg/m² of IV drug, were as follows: cyclophosphamide and 5-fluorouracil, 600; and methotrexate, 40. Adjuvant treatment was delivered at full dose whenever possible; in the presence of myelosuppression on day 21, the dose of CMF was delayed for 7 to 14 days rather than being reduced by 50%. A total of 90 patients were prospectively randomized (45 in each group). Stratification was limited to menopausal status. Eleven of 45 women allocated to receive CMF refused to complete the initial treatment program, and 4 patients dropped out after the first drug course. Figures 8–3 and 8–4 display the comparative treatment results. The actuarial 5-year RFS was 45% for the control group versus 87% for the treatment group ($p < 0.001$). Total survival was 65% versus 90% ($p = 0.02$). There were no remarkable differences in the treatment outcome between pre- and postmenopausal patients. Of the four relapses in the CMF group, one woman had received only a single dose of CMF because of treatment refusal. Many women in both treatment groups whose disease relapsed presented with new disease manifestations in visceral sites (11 of 25, or 44%) and, despite prompt institution of salvage therapies, 15 patients died of progressive disease within a median of 1 year (range, 4–19 months) from relapse.

NSABP Trial ■

In this study of node-negative and ER-negative tumors, started in August 1981,[59] 679 patients were randomized between locoregional therapy and the

FIG. 8–3 CMF adjuvant program in node-negative, ER-negative tumors: relapse-free survival compared to controls (CTR).

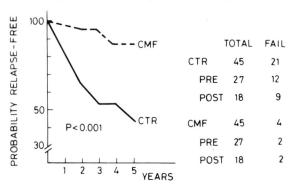

FIG. 8–4 CMF adjuvant program in node-negative, ER-negative tumors: total survival compared to controls (CTR).

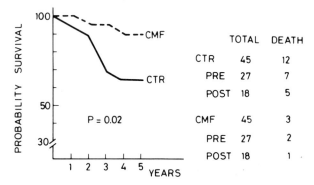

same treatment followed by sequential combination chemotherapy. Surgery consisted of total or segmental mastectomy plus postoperative irradiation; axillary dissection included at least complete removal of the lower two levels of the lymph nodes. M→F chemotherapy consisted of methotrexate, 100 mg/m^2 IV on days 1 and 8; 5-fluorouracil 600 mg/m^2 IV 1 hour after methotrexate; and leucovorin 10 mg/m^2 every 6 hours for 6 doses, started 24 hours after methotrexate. Treatment cycles were repeated every 4 weeks for 12 months.

The 4-year results revealed a highly significant difference ($p = 0.003$) in RFS favoring patients who received adjuvant M→F. The benefit was present during the entire period of observation, and the odds that a woman would remain free of disease after 4 years of follow-up were 1.81 (1.24–2.65) better for those who received the MF chemotherapy. When all patients were evaluated for overall survival, no significant difference was yet evident at 4 years.

Cardiff Trial ■

Between January 1981 and December 1985, 52 patients with T_1 or T_2 tumors treated with simple mastectomy and axillary clearance were randomly allocated to either no further treatment or to AVC chemotherapy.[60] The drug regimen was as follows: Adriamycin, 40 mg/m^2 IV on day 1; vincristine, 1.4 mg/m^2 IV (maximum dose = 2.0 mg) on day 1; and cyclophosphamide, 200 mg/m^2 PO on days 2–5. Six treatment cycles were administered at 3-week intervals. Of 28 patients randomized to receive adjuvant AVC, only 21 accepted the assigned therapy. The 3-year RFS was 83% for the 28 women randomized to receive chemotherapy compared to 71% for the control group. The authors stated that the analysis of the study was complicated by its small size and by the refusal of 25% of the patients to accept randomization to adjuvant chemotherapy.[60]

Eastern Cooperative and Southwest Oncology Group Trial ■

In May 1981 these American cooperative groups activated a comparative study to assess the impact of short-term intensive chemotherapy on disease recurrence and survival in node-negative patients with either ER-negative tumors of any size or ER-positive tumors ≥3 cm.[63] Initially, only women who had had total mastectomy plus either axillary dissection or low axillary sampling were admitted to the study. After surgery, patients were randomized to either no further treatment or to CMFP (cyclophosphamide, 100 mg/m^2 PO on days 1–14; methotrexate, 40 mg/m^2 IV on days 1 and 8; 5-fluorouracil, 600 mg/m^2 IV on days 1 and 8; prednisone 40 mg/m^2 PO on days 1–14) for 6 monthly cycles.

Data on 422 randomized patients with a median follow-up of 3 years indicated an improved relapse-free survival for women receiving adjuvant chemotherapy (84%) compared to the control group (67%, $p = 0.0001$). The efficacy of therapy was apparent for both ER-positive and negative tumors as well as for pre- and postmenopausal women. Data on total survival are not yet available.

Future Directions ■

The initial results of the first two adjuvant trials for node-positive women[10,11] provided the strategic principles and the driving force to expand the concept of a multidisciplinary approach to primary breast cancer. As result of many efforts carried out in scientific institutions all over the world, the NIH Consensus Development Conference on Adjuvant Chemotherapy and Endocrine Therapy for Breast Cancer formulated the guidelines for treatment of patients outside the context of clinical trial.[15,16] The most important statements concerning node-positive patients were the recognition that adjuvant combination chemotherapy should become standard medical care in premenopausal women, regardless of hormone receptor status, while tamoxifen represented the treatment of choice for postmenopausal women with receptor-positive tumors. The findings related to tumor mortality collected from over 30,000 study patients were thoroughly analyzed at the Oxford University and culminated in a milestone publication that reaffirmed the clinical usefulness of multimodal strategy.[64]

At the NIH Consensus Conference, not enough clinical data were available on node-negative tumors to allow meaningful conclusions in terms of guidelines for systemic adjuvant therapy. However, histopathologic,[65] cell kinetic,[66] and endocrine[67] findings as well as data from one clinical report,[68] led the panel to recognize that certain tumor characteristics (as summarized earlier in this chapter) represented important prognostic indicators, and thus could contribute to the selection of candidates for adjuvant chemotherapy.

The results from the recent Milan and NSABP prospective randomized trials[58,59] using negative ER status as the parameter for high-risk of recurrence are showing that systemic adjuvant chemotherapy can improve treatment outcome in this subset of patients. Although the two research groups are providing information based on studies that differ in terms of size of patient population and type of drug regimen, the similarity of the observed findings indicates that adjuvant chemotherapy can effectively alter the natural history of ER-negative tumors. Thus, the reported results strongly support the concept that systemic adjuvant therapy is also indicated in high-risk subsets of node-negative tumors. The failure to identify these subsets within the node-negative group is probably the reason why the early adjuvant trials, regardless of size of patient population and drug treatment, failed to detect significant benefit from adjuvant chemotherapy. The possible advantage from postoperative drug treatment may have been blurred by the mix of low- and high-risk subsets.

Drug selection and intensity of treatment during the first 6 months after operation can also represent another important variable. It is our own opinion that if the NSABP investigators had added an alkylating agent to the M→F regimen, the effect on treatment outcome would have been more pronounced. The fear of using cyclophosphamide in the adjuvant treatment of selected node-negative tumors now appears unjustified. Prior long-term experience with alkylating-agent-containing regimens for node-positive tumors should have largely dispelled the concern about the high risk of chemotherapy-induced carcinogenesis,[69,70] particularly if cytotoxic drugs are delivered for a relatively short period of time.

As previously mentioned, many prognostic indicators are now available to predict early relapse and short-term survival in node-negative breast cancer. In addition to negative hormone receptor status, cell proliferative activity—either expressed as high labeling index[43,46] or high percent of S-phase cells[44,45]—should now be taken into consideration. Histopathologic evidence of undifferentiated (grade III) neoplastic cells and aneuploidy can also be added to the list of unfavorable prognostic parameters to improve patient selection. It should be stressed that we do not yet know the precise interrelationship of the unfavorable prognostic discriminants, and thus cannot determine how many and which indicators will be necessary to more accurately define the best candidates for systemic adjuvant treatment. Each of the above mentioned prognostic factors requires further study to convince clinicians that the new biologic findings can further improve treatment selection.[71]

We suggest that clinicians seriously consider adjuvant chemotherapy in node-negative breast cancer when there are at least two unfavorable prognostic indicators, such as grade III tumor and negative hormone receptors—particularly when both ER and PgR

are absent. In hospitals where more sophisticated diagnostic facilities are available, the additional evidence of aneuploidy in the resected specimen or of increased tumor cell proliferative activity by either thymidine-labeling index or flow cytometry should further alert physicians that the patient is at high risk for micrometastatic disease, and adjuvant chemotherapy must be strongly advised. In pathologically node-negative breast cancer with ER-positive tumors, prognostic indicators following locoregional therapy alone are less well defined. At the time of present writing, three research groups[72–74] have consistently reported RFS advantage but not always significant total survival benefit[74] from the prolonged administration of adjuvant tamoxifen.

Conclusion ■

The results of recent trials indicate that the contribution of medicine to the primary treatment of breast cancer can be extended to a selected subset of node-negative women.[75] Current findings have not yet clearly established the contribution of prognostic discriminants that would permit unquestionable selection of high-risk patients, or development of a standard adjuvant systemic therapy. However, there are no biologic or clinical reasons to believe that the drug regimens effective in node-positive patients[64,75] should not be used in the treatment of high risk node-negative women. Clinicians should become aware that the prognosis of primary breast cancer is no longer based only on anatomic findings (histologically node-positive versus node-negative tumors). Rather, a new constellation of biologic indicators will be gradually, if not rapidly, introduced at the clinical level, that is, at the time of treatment decision making.

Supported in part by Contract N01-CM-07338 with DCT, NCI, NIH.

References ■

1. Fisher B, Ravdin RG, Ausman RK et al: Surgical adjuvant chemotherapy in cancer of the breast: Results of a decade of cooperative investigation. Ann Surg 168:337–356, 1968
2. Fisher B, Slack N, Katrych D, Wolmark N: Ten-year follow-up results of patients with carcinoma of the breast in a cooperative clinical trial evaluating surgical adjuvant chemotherapy. Surg Gynecol Obstet 140:528–534, 1975
3. Valagussa P, Bonadonna G, Veronesi U: Patterns of relapse and survival following radical mastectomy. Analysis of 716 consecutive patients. Cancer 41:1170–1178, 1978
4. Haagensen CD: Treatment of curable carcinoma of the breast. Int J Radiat Oncol Biol Phys 2:975–980, 1977
5. Schottenfeld D, Nash AG, Robbins GF et al: Ten-year results of the treatment of primary operable breast carcinoma. Cancer 38:1001–1007, 1976

6. Spratt JS, Donegan WL: Carcinoma of the Breast, p 136. Philadelphia, WB Saunders, 1971

7. Payne WS, Taylor WF, Khonsari S et al: Surgical treatment of breast cancer: Trends and factors affecting survival. Arch Surg 101:105–113, 1970

8. Wilson RE, Donegan WL, Mettlin C et al: The 1982 national survey of carcinoma of the breast in the United States by the American College of Surgeons. Surg Gynecol Obstet 159:309–318, 1984

9. Moon TE, Jones SE, Bonadonna G et al: Development and use of a natural history data base of breast cancer studies. Am J Clin Oncol (CCT) 10:396–403, 1987

10. Fisher B, Carbone P, Economou SG et al: L-phenylalanine mustard (L-PAM) in the management of primary breast cancer: A report of early findings. N Engl J Med 292:117–122, 1975

11. Bonadonna G, Brusamolino E, Valagussa P et al: Combination chemotherapy as an adjuvant treatment in operable breast cancer. N Engl J Med 294:405–410, 1976

12. Fisher B, Bauer M, Wickerham DL et al: Relation of number of positive axillary nodes to the prognosis of patients with primary breast cancer. An NSABP update. Cancer 52:1551–1557, 1983

13. Bonadonna G, Valagussa P: Adjuvant systemic therapy for resectable breast cancer. J Clin Oncol 3:259–275, 1985

14. Budzar A, Smith T, Blumenschein G et al: Adjuvant chemotherapy with fluorouracil, doxorubicin, and cyclophosphamide (FAC) for stage II or III breast cancer: 5-year results. In Salmon SE, Jones SE (eds): Adjuvant Therapy of Cancer III, pp 419–426. Orlando, FL, Grune & Stratton, 1981

15. Consensus Conference: Adjuvant chemotherapy for breast cancer. JAMA 254:3461–3463, 1985

16. Lippman ME (ed): Proceedings of the NIH Consensus Development Conference on adjuvant chemotherapy and endocrine therapy for breast cancer. Natl Cancer Inst Monogr 1:1–159, 1986

17. Fisher B, Wolmark N, Bauer M et al: The accuracy of clinical nodal staging and of limited axillary dissection as a determinant of histological nodal status in carcinoma of the breast. Surg Gynecol Obstet 152:765–772, 1981

18. Butcher HR: Radical mastectomy for mammary carcinoma. Ann Surg 170:833–884, 1969

19. Haagensen CD: Diseases of the Breast, 3rd ed, p 656. Philadelphia, WB Saunders, 1986

20. Bucalossi P, Veronesi U, Zingo L et al: Enlarged mastectomy for breast cancer: Review of 1213 cases. Am J Roentgenol Radium Ther Nuclear Med 111:119–122, 1971

21. Veronesi U, Rilke F, Luini A et al: Distribution of axillary node metastases by level of invasion. An analysis of 539 cases. Cancer 59:682–687, 1987

22. Nemoto T, Vana J, Bedwani RN et al: Management and survival of female breast cancer: Results of a national survey by the American College of Surgeons. Cancer 45:2917–2924, 1980

23. Veronesi U, Banfi A, Del Vecchio M et al: Comparison of Halsted mastectomy with quadrantectomy, axillary dissection, and radiotherapy in early breast cancer: Long-term results. Eur J Cancer Clin Oncol 22:1085–1089, 1986

24. Fisher ER, Sass R, Fisher B et al: Pathologic findings from the National Surgical Adjuvant Project for breast cancers (Protocol No. 4): X. Discriminants for the tenth year treatment failure. Cancer 53:712–723, 1984

25. Rosen PP, Kinne DW, Lesser M, Hellman S: Are prognostic factors for local control of breast cancer treated by primary radiotherapy significant for patients treated by mastectomy? Cancer 57:1415–1420, 1986

26. Gilchrist KW, Kalish L, Gould VE et al: Interobserver reproducibility of histopathological features in Stage II breast cancer. An ECOG study. Breast Cancer Res Treat 5:3–10, 1985

27. Fisher ER: Comment on "Interobserver reproducibility of histopathological features in Stage II breast cancer." Breast Cancer Res Treat 5:11–13, 1985

28. Borjesson BW, McGinley R, Foo TMS et al: Estrogen and progesterone receptor assays in human breast cancer: Sources of variation between laboratories. Eur J Cancer Clin Oncol 23:999–1004, 1987

29. Thorpe SM: Steroid receptors in breast cancer: Sources of interlaboratory variation in dextran-charcoal assays. Breast Cancer Res Treat 9:175–189, 1987

30. Knight WA III, Livingston RB, Gregory EJ, McGuire WL: Estrogen receptor as an independent prognostic factor for early recurrence in breast cancer. Cancer Res 37:4669–4671, 1977

31. Rich MA, Furmanski P, Brooks CS: Prognostic value of estrogen receptor determinations in patients with breast cancer. Cancer Res 38:4296–4298, 1978

32. Allegra J, Simon R, Lippman M: The association between steroid hormone receptor status and the disease-free interval in breast cancer. In Jones SE, Salmon SE (eds): Adjuvant Therapy of Cancer II, pp 47–54. Orlando, FL, Grune & Stratton, 1979

33. Cooke T, George D, Shields R et al: Oestrogen receptors and prognosis in early breast cancer. Lancet 1:995–997, 1979

34. Maynard PV, Blamey RW, Elston CW et al: Estrogen receptor assay in primary breast cancer and early recurrence of the disease. Cancer Res 38:4292–4295, 1978

35. Adami HO, Graffman S, Lindgren A, Sallstrom J: Prognostic implication of estrogen receptor content in breast cancer. Breast Cancer Res Treat 5:293–300, 1985

36. Butler JA, Bretsky S, Menendez-Botet C, Kinne DW: Estrogen receptor protein of breast cancer as a predictor of recurrence. Cancer 55:1178–1181, 1985

37. Crowe JP, Hubay CA, Pearson OH, et al: Estrogen receptor status as a prognostic indication for stage I breast cancer patients. Breast Cancer Res Treat 2:171–176, 1982

38. Valagussa P, Bignami P, Buzzoni R et al: Are estrogen receptors alone a reliable prognostic factor in node negative breast cancer? In Jones SE, Salmon SE (eds): Adjuvant Therapy of Cancer, Vol 4, pp 407–415. Orlando, FL, Grune & Stratton, 1984

39. Clark GM, McGuire WL, Hubay CA et al: Progesterone receptor as a prognostic factor in stage II breast cancer. N Engl J Med 309:1343–1347, 1983

40. McGuire WL: Prognostic factors for recurrence and survival in human breast cancer. Breast Cancer Res Treat 10:5–9, 1987

41. Meyer JS, Friedman E, McCrate MM, Bauer WC: Prediction of early course of breast carcinoma by thymidine labeling. Cancer 51:1879–1886, 1983

42. Tubiana M, Pejovic MH, Chavaudra N et al: The long-term prognostic significance of the thymidine labelling index in breast cancer. Int J Cancer 33:441–445, 1984

43. Silvestrini R, Daidone MG, Gasparini G: Cell kinetics as a persistent prognostic marker in node negative breast cancer. Cancer 56:1982–1987, 1985

44. Merkel DE, Dressler LG, McGuire WL: Flow cytometry, cellular DNA content, and prognosis in human malignancy. J Clin Oncol 5:1690–1703, 1987

45. Dressler LG, Seamer LC, Owens MA et al: DNA flow cytometry and prognostic factors in 1331 frozen breast cancer specimens. Cancer 61:420–427, 1988

46. Silvestrini R, Daidone MG, Di Fronzo G et al: Prognostic implication of labeling index versus estrogen receptors and tumor size in node-negative breast cancer. Breast Cancer Res Treat 7:161–169, 1986

47. Lellé RJ, Heidenreich W, Stauch G, Gerdes J: The correlation of growth fractions with histologic grading and lymph node status in human mammary carcinoma. Cancer 59:83–88, 1987

48. Slamon DJ, Clark GM, Wong SG et al: Amplification of the

HER-2/*neu* oncogene correlates with relapse and survival in human breast cancer. Science 235:177–182, 1987

49. Tandon A, Clark G, Ullrich A et al: Overexpression of the HER-2/*neu* oncogene predicts relapse and survival in Stage II human breast cancers. Proc Am Soc Clin Oncol (in press)

50. Cline MJ, Battifora H, Yokata J: Proto-oncogene abnormalities in human breast cancer: Correlation with anatomic features and clinical course of disease. J Clin Oncol 5:999–1006, 1987

51. Mansi JL, Berger U, Easton D et al: Micrometastases in bone marrow in patients with primary breast cancer: Evaluation as an early predictor of bone metastases. Br Med J 295:1093–1096, 1987

52. Fisher B, Redmond CK, Wolmark N et al: Long-term results from NSABP trials of adjuvant therapy for breast cancer. In Salmon SE (ed): Adjuvant Therapy of Cancer V, pp 283–295, Orlando, FL, Grune & Stratton, 1987

53. Nissen-Meyer R, Høst H, Kjellgren K et al: Treatment of node-negative breast cancer patients with short course of chemotherapy immediately after surgery. Natl Cancer Inst Monogr 1:125–128, 1986

54. Senn HJ, Barett-Mahler R, for the OSAKO and SAKK Groups: Update of Swiss adjuvant trials with LMF and CMF in operable breast cancer. In Salmon SE (ed): Adjuvant Therapy of Cancer, Vol 5, pp 243–252. Orlando, FL, Grune & Stratton, 1987

55. Morrison JM, Howell A, Grieve RJ et al: The West Midlands Oncology Association Trials of adjuvant chemotherapy for operable breast cancer. In Salmon SE (ed): Adjuvant Therapy of Cancer, Vol 5, pp 311–318. Orlando, FL, Grune & Stratton, 1987

56. Caffier H, Rotte K, Haeggqwist O: Adjuvant chemotherapy versus postoperative irradiation in node negative breast cancer. In Jones SE, Salmon SE (eds): Adjuvant Therapy of Cancer, Vol 4, pp 417–424. Orlando, FL, Grune & Stratton, 1984

57. Jackez R, Kolb R, Reiner G et al: Adjuvant chemotherapy in node-negative breast cancer patients. In Salmon SE (ed): Adjuvant Therapy of Cancer, Vol 5, pp 223–231. Orlando, FL, Grune & Stratton, 1987

58. Bonadonna G, Zambetti M, Valagussa P et al: Adjuvant CMF in node negative breast cancer. Proc Am Soc Clin Oncol 5:74, 1986

59. Fisher B, and NSABP investigators. N Engl J Med (in press).

60. Williams CJ, Buchanan RB, Hall H et al: Adjuvant chemotherapy for T1-2, N0, M0 estrogen receptor negative breast cancer: Preliminary results of a randomised trial. In Salmon SE (ed): Adjuvant Therapy of Cancer, Vol 5, pp 233–241. Orlando, FL, Grune & Stratton, 1987

61. Nissen-Meyer R, Kjellgren K, Malmio K et al: Surgical adjuvant chemotherapy. Results with one short course with cyclophosphamide after mastectomy for breast cancer. Cancer 41:2088–2098, 1978

62. Senn HJ, Jungi WF, Amgwerd R et al: Swiss adjuvant trial (OSAKO 06/74) with chlorambucil, methotrexate, and 5-fluorouracil plus BCG in node-negative breast cancer patients: Nine year results. Natl Cancer Inst Monogr 1:129–134, 1986

63. Friedman MA, Dorr FA, Perloff M: Adjuvant therapy for breast cancer patients with negative lymph nodes. NCI Clinical Alert, May 18, 1988

64. Early Breast Cancer Trialists Collaborative Group: The effects of adjuvant tamoxifen and of cytotoxic therapy on mortality in early breast cancer: An overview of 61 randomized trials among 28,896 women. N Engl J Med 1988 (in press)

65. Fisher ER: Prognostic and therapeutic significance of pathological features of breast cancer. Natl Cancer Inst Monogr 1: 29–34, 1986

66. Meyer JS: Cell kinetics in selection and stratification of patients for adjuvant therapy of breast carcinoma. Natl Cancer Inst Monogr 1:25–28, 1986

67. McGuire WL, Clark GM, Dressler LG, Owens MA: Role of steroid hormone receptors as prognostic factors in primary breast cancer. Natl Cancer Inst Monogr 1:19–23, 1986

68. Bonadonna G, Valagussa P, Tancini G et al: Current status of Milan adjuvant chemotherapy trials for node-positive and node-negative breast cancer. Natl Cancer Inst Monogr 1:65–69, 1986

69. Fisher B, Rockette H, Fisher ER et al: Leukemia in breast cancer patients following adjuvant chemotherapy or postoperative radiotherapy: The NSABP experience. J Clin Oncol 3: 1640–1658, 1985

70. Valagussa P, Tancini G, Bonadonna G: Second malignancies after CMF for resectable breast cancer. J Clin Oncol 5:1138–1142, 1987

71. Bonadonna G, Valagussa P: New prognostic variables in primary breast cancer: How useful to clinicians? Oncology Journal Club 1988

72. Nolvadex Adjuvant Trial Organization: Controlled trial of tamoxifen as single adjuvant agent in management of early breast cancer. Analysis at six years. Lancet 1:836–840, 1985

73. Breast Cancer Trials Committee: Adjuvant tamoxifen in the management of operable breast cancer: The Scottish trial. Lancet 2:171–175, 1987

74. Fisher B, and NSABP investigators. N Engl J Med (in press)

75. Bonadonna G, Valagussa P: The contribution of medicine to the primary treatment of breast cancer. Cancer Res 48:2316–2324, 1988

Norman D. Nigro

Vainutis K. Vaitkeviceus

Arnold M. Herskovic

Preservation of Function in the Treatment of Cancer of the Anus

9

Introduction ■

For years, abdominoperineal resection (APR) of the rectum, with the formation of a permanent colostomy, has been the treatment of choice for cancer of the rectum and anal canal. The operation, first described by Miles in 1908, was designed to remove the primary lesion, its extensions in the lymphatic tissue, and a wide margin of surrounding tissue.[1] This concept was first described by Halsted when he devised radical mastectomy for breast cancer, and Miles applied these principles in his operation for rectal cancer. The projected improvement in disease control was considered to be well worth the resultant loss of structure and function in both instances.

Cancers of the rectum and anal canal are so close physically that it was reasonable to treat both with the same operation. However, APR is not as effective in removing a malignant lesion in the anal canal as it is in the rectum. There are anatomic constraints in the anal area that prevent wide excision of tissue surrounding the primary lesion, and it is not possible to remove all of the lymphatic tissue leading to the pelvic wall and in the approaches to the inguinal area. In addition, cancers of the rectum are typically adenocarcinomas, whereas anal canal cancers are squamous cell tumors or their variants, and are more sensitive to radiation. This fact is in part responsible for the general interest in new approaches to the management of squamous cell cancers of the anal canal. Radiation, chemotherapy, and surgery, singly and in various combinations, are being investigated. Initial results using radiation and chemotherapy are so encouraging that an extensive review of the subject is justified.

Anatomy ■

The anal region is divided into an internal part called the anal canal and an external, perianal area, often called the anal margin (Fig. 9–1). Though the gross anatomy was first described several centuries ago, and the microscopic features have been studied for more than a hundred years, confusion still exists as to definitions, nomenclature, and boundaries. This is due to the dense, complex anatomic structures, individual variations, and lack of identifiable boundary lines. An important structure that can be identified on anoscopic examination is the dentate line, also called the pectinate line, anorectal line, or mucocutaneus junction. The dentate line, as it is most frequently termed today, is the site where the entoderm and ectoderm join during embryonic development. Anal papillae, numbering up to six or eight, are thought to be remnants of the proctodeal membrane. They are small, sawtooth-like triangular projections that encircle the area at the base of the longitudinal mucosal columns of Morgagni. These columns presumably result from the downsizing of the hindgut to meet the anal canal. The anal valves are a series of semilunar folds located between the base of the vertical columns. Behind each is a recess or anal crypt into which the anal glands empty. Together, these structures help to identify the dentate line. In addition, the tissue above resembles mucosa, whereas the distal surface is more like skin.

The anal margin refers to the perianal area extending 5 or 6 cm from the anal verge. The anal verge refers to the opening itself, and there is no gross or microscopic line to mark it. In fact, the precise level of the opening varies depending on the degree of

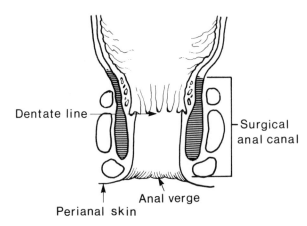

FIG. 9–1   Important anatomic landmarks in the anal area. The perianal skin area for about 6 cm in all directions from the anal verge is called the anal margin.

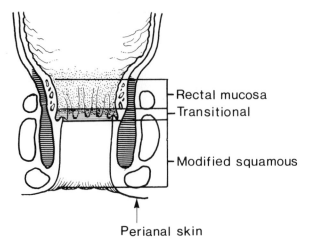

FIG. 9–2   The four surfaces covering the anal canal and the anal margin.

muscle contraction around it. Just inside the opening, the skin is lighter in color and lacks hair. Outside the anal verge, the skin appears more normal. Microscopically, there is a gradual change from skin containing hair follicles and sweat glands on the outside to modified skin without these structures on the inside.

The term anal canal is defined in two ways. The anatomic anal canal describes the ectodermal areas. It extends approximately 2 cm, from the dentate line to the anal verge. The surgical anal canal is the part of the channel within the grasp of the anorectal sphincter musculature, and extends from the pelvic floor to the anal verge. It is approximately 5 cm in length. Fenger, in an excellent review of the anatomy of the anal canal, defined it more simply as extending from the top to the bottom of the internal sphincter.[2] Thus, in its most proximal part, the canal is lined with normal rectal mucosa. Today, "surgical anal canal" is the term most frequently used.

The anal canal and the perianal area have a rich supply of blood vessels and lymphatics. The middle rectal blood vessels help supply the lower part of the rectum and the upper part of the anal canal. The inferior rectal vessels supply the lower part of the canal, as well as the surrounding muscles and skin. There is a profuse network of lymphatic vessels under the anal canal lining. The vessels above the dentate line drain into the internal iliac nodes and those below the line pass to the superficial inguinal nodes. Innervation is derived from the middle rectal plexuses and from the pudendal nerves by way of the inferior rectal nerves. The part of the canal above the dentate line (allowing for a little overlap) is insensitive to pain, whereas the area below is very sensitive.[3]

Histology ■

The tissues of the anal canal can be divided into three zones (Fig. 9–2). The most proximal is simply normal rectal mucosa. The middle zone is called the transitional zone, or the cloacogenic zone. It is a narrow strip that extends 1 to 2 cm above the dentate line, although Fenger has shown that it can involve any part of the area from 0.6 cm below to 2.0 cm above the dentate line.[2] This area contains a complex mixture of predominantly cuboidal or polygonal cells of varying size. Interspersed are islands of rectal mucosal cells that migrate into the area from above, and normal squamous cells from below. A few endocrine and some melanin-containing cells have been found in this area. Mucin histochemical studies suggest that the mucin pattern of cells in this zone differs from that which is secreted by colorectal mucosal cells. Fenger suggests that mucin histochemistry may be useful in classifying the numerous malignant epithelial tumors that occur in the anal canal. The surface covering the lower third is modified skin which has no hair follicles and no skin glands. (For a more detailed description of the histology of this area, see the recent review by Fenger.[2])

Incidence ■

Cancers of the anus are uncommon and are not listed separately in epidemiologic surveys of cancer incidence. However, some information regarding their frequency can be obtained from published reviews regarding institutions' experience with series of patients over a period of time. On average, anal cancers represent about 1% of colorectal cancers or about 4% of those in the rectum. At Memorial Hospital in New York, Stearns and coworkers saw 117 patients from 1950 to 1978, an average of nearly 4 per year.[4] At a special cancer clinic in France, Papillon and his colleagues saw 276 patients with anal canal cancer during the years 1971 to 1984.[5] In a 7-year period, Flam and colleagues[6] in California reported that their group had seen 30 patients, while Glimelius and coworkers in Sweden published a report of 44 patients seen during a 6-year period.[7]

Cancer of the anal canal is more common than that of the anal margin. Morson analyzed the experience at St. Marks Hospital in London.[8] Of 157 patients with cancers of the anal region, 103 had anal canal cancer, 38 had anal margin cancers, and 16 were not specified. Hintz and colleagues, in reviewing the literature, concluded that approximately 75% of cancers of the anus occur in the anal canal, with 25% in the anal margin.[9] On the other hand, McConnell, in a review of 96 patients, found a more equal distribution (55 versus 41).[10]

Distribution between cancers in the canal and those in the margin varies by sex. The former are more common in women while the latter are more frequent in men. In Papillon's series of 276 patients with anal canal cancers, 228 were women and 48 were men.[5] In Nigro's series of 104 patients, 76 were women and 28 were men.[11] In contrast, Morson indicated that of 38 patients with anal margin cancer, 31 were men and 7 were women.[8] The range and average of age of patients with anal cancer is similar to that in colorectal cancer.

Etiology ■

The cause of anal cancer is unknown, although its association with other conditions has led to speculation regarding predisposing conditions in at least some patients. There has long been an impression that anal margin cancer is due, in part, to constant irritation of the perianal skin from such conditions as anal fissure, fistulas, anal pruritus, and even poor anal hygiene. However, these problems are common and their association may be merely circumstantial. There is now somewhat better evidence to suggest significant association of squamous cell cancer with condylomata acuminata in genital and perianal areas. These soft, wart-like lesions are caused by human papilloma viruses. Early in this century, several papers suggested an association between vulval carcinoma and condylomata. In 1962, Siegal described their association with cancers in the perianal area, and other reports followed.[12] In a series of 35 patients with anal cancer, Brennan and Stewart found 5 associated with condylomata.[13]

Recent case reports of anal cancer in male homosexuals suggest an increased risk for the disease, and have initiated considerable interest.[17] Peters and Mack investigated the association of anal cancer and marital status in 970 patients in Los Angeles County.[15] They found that anal carcinomas are more common in women than men, and that single men and divorced persons of both sexes have a higher risk for this form of cancer. An increased risk for cervical cancer, thought to be associated with sexual behavior, has also been reported in divorced women. It seems reasonable from such information to theorize that the increased risk for anal cancer is due to atypical sexual behavior, specifically anal intercourse. Peters and Mack also suggest that the pattern of anal cancer in women is consistent with this hypothesis.

Among the possible mechanisms by which anal intercourse may promote cancer formation is infection with one or more viral agents. As already mentioned, the papilloma virus is found in condylomata acuminata tissue. Other possibilities include some of the herpes viruses that are associated with cervical cancer. Obviously, more evidence is needed to implicate viral infection due to sexual activity in the etiology of anal cancer. As Daling and colleagues pointed out, the practical consequences of finding such an association, while important on an individual basis, would not have a great impact on overall cancer incidence because of the generally low incidence of the disease.[16] It is also quite possible that there are several predisposing factors and that not all are sexually related.

Pathology ■

It is not surprising, considering the variation of epithelial surfaces in the anal region, that carcinomas here vary from well-differentiated, highly keratinized squamous cell cancer to very undifferentiated carcinoma. In discussions that deal primarily with therapy, it is most convenient to divide these cancers into anal canal and anal margin cancers (Fig. 9–3).

Most tumors of the anal canal develop from cells located in the anal transitional (cloacogenic) zone. Normal cells in the area vary considerably, as do the cancers that develop from them. Accordingly, pathologists classify these tumors as basaloid, transi-

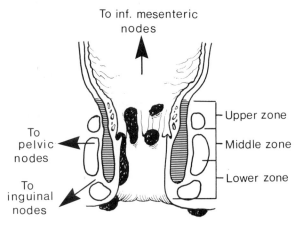

FIG. 9-3 Location of tumors, with the general direction of lymphatic spread, in the three zones of the canal and in the anal margin. Because interconnections exist, involvement may be in more than one direction.

tional, epidermoid, cloacogenic, squamous cell, and undifferentiated. Boman and associates, in a report from the Mayo Clinic, identified a highly lethal small cell type.[17] On rare occasions, adenocarcinomas develop in the anal canal, arising either from the rectal mucosa in the most proximal part of the canal or from the anal glands in the tissues at the level of the dentate line. Malignant melanoma may occur in the same location.

Anal margin cancers, which constitute only about a third of all cancers in the anal region, reflect the characteristics of the normal skin present in the perianal region.[8] Most are differentiated squamous cell cancers. Others that occur less frequently are basal cell cancer, Bowen's disease, and Paget's disease—the latter being an intradermal adenocarcinoma developing from apocrine glands in the perianal skin.[8]

Routes of Spread ■

Like most gastrointestinal cancer, anal cancer spreads by direct extension through the lymphatic system and via the blood stream. The tumors often spread directly to adjacent tissues, including the sphincter muscles, to the vagina or to the capsule of the prostate, and then to the urethra. Wolfe and Bussey found that tumors occasionally spread upward along tissue planes, particularly the submucosal space, for 5 or 6 cm before ulcerating into the rectum.[18]

Because there is an extensive lymphatic plexus in the area, spread through this system is the most common. It can occur in all directions: upward through the superior hemorrhoidal and inferior mesenteric vessels and nodes, laterally through the pelvic system, and downward to the inguinal nodes. In general, lesions in the upper third of the anal canal spread primarily to the mesenteric system. Those in the midportion spread to the pelvic nodes, and tumors in the lower part of the canal and in the anal margin spread to the inguinal nodes. Because there are extensive communications among the three lymphatic systems in the anal region, a lesion in any location may spread in more than one direction. Stearns and Quan studied the routes of lymphatic spread in 109 patients with cancer of the anus.[19] In 67 patients who had a routine APR, they found 16 (24%) with lymphatic spread to the superior hemorrhoidal and inferior mesentric nodal system. In 45 patients on whom they performed an abdominopelvic lymphadenectomy, 15 (33%) had cancer in the pelvic lymph nodes. Finally, in the 109 patients, they found that 44 (40%) developed inguinal lymph node metastases. Interestingly, they observed that the incidence of spread (regardless of direction) was not correlated with the location of the primary lesion.

Bloodstream metastases in patients with squamous cell cancer of the anus are not nearly as common as in patients with adenocarcinoma of the rectum or colon. In a review by Kuehn and colleagues, 13 of 189 patients had metastases to the liver while six had spread to the lungs.[20] The primary lesion in these 19 patients was located in the area above the dentate line. Stearns and coworkers found 4 patients with liver metastases out of 180 patients examined.[4] Three others developed liver metastases at a later date. Only two patients developed pulmonary metastases diagnosed before death.

Staging ■

The ability to objectively categorize the extent of disease in cancer patients permits an accurate assessment of prognosis and is extremely helpful in comparing the effect of different therapeutic measures. The classical method for staging cancer is Dukes' classification of colorectal cancer. Richards and associates at the Mayo Clinic applied this to cancer of the anal canal, but the anatomic features of this area do not lend themselves to the precise localization of extent of disease as they do in the rectum or colon.[21] The lining of the canal is not defined by separate layers as in the colon. In addition, the canal is surrounded by a thick ring of muscle consisting of the internal and external sphincters and part of the puborectalis muscle. Consequently, the degree of penetration is difficult to evaluate, making Dukes' classification difficult to apply. The tumor–node–metastasis (TNM) system is difficult to apply for the same reason, because it is based in part on the degree of infiltration of the external sphincter muscle. If preoperative therapy is given, the surgical specimen is not suitable for evaluation, and if operation is not a part of therapy, staging is based on a clinical appraisal. Variations have been proposed by Frost,[22] Boman and associates,[17] Singh and colleagues,[23] and Papillon.[5] All include the extent of local invasion, which we believe should not be used in a staging system for anal canal cancer because the extent is too difficult to determine.

According to Papillon, Russeau and associates were the first to suggest a staging system to include the size of the primary lesion. In 1971, Papillon and his associates adopted a system based on tumor size and gross invasion of surrounding organs, such as the vagina and genitourinary tract.[5] Most recent reports indicate that tumor size correlates well with prognosis. There is general agreement that lymph node involvement is a significant sign of disease progression in anal cancer (as in cancer in general). Particularly important in anal canal cancer is the involvement of the inguinal nodes, which are easily accessible to clinical evaluation. Cell type of the primary tumor does not appear to correlate well with survival potential, although an exception may be the small cell type described by Boman and associates.[17] From the foregoing, it appears that a staging system based on the size of the primary lesion, the condition of the inguinal nodes, and whether or not there are distant organ metastases would be the best approach for anal cancer. We propose a simplified clinical staging system for cancer of the anal canal based on the parameters listed in Table 9–1. This is similar to the one used by Papillon, but is simplified by removing extension features, which we do not think necessarily imply a poor diagnosis. Because the emphasis is on tumor size, the measurement should be made, under anesthesia, at the time of biopsy. These cancers occur in an extremely sensitive area, and an accurate appraisal of the features of the tumor and its surrounding area can only be made when the patient has been properly anesthetized. The staging of patients in our combined therapy series is also shown in Table 9–1.

Patterns of Treatment Failure ■

The establishment of objective criteria to estimate probable outcomes in anal cancer is hampered by relatively small patient numbers, marked variation in neoplasm cell type, difficulty in assessing the degree of invasion due to anatomic peculiarities, and by marked differences in malignant potential between lesions that occur inside the anus compared to those on the outside. Consequently, investigators vary in their analysis of patients, which has led to some confusion. However, some aspects of this problem have become clearer due to increased interest in the disease and dramatic changes in therapy.

All evidence indicates that anal canal cancer should be considered separately from anal margin cancer, as first suggested by Gabriel in 1941.[24] Anal canal cancer is an invasive cancer while the other generally is a localized skin tumor. Moreover, recent information suggests that squamous cell and cloacogenic anal canal cancer should not be considered as separate entities. Singh has shown that they act similarly in their ability to spread locally, to involve regional lymph nodes, and to metastasize to distant organs.[23] In addition, Schraut and coworkers found no differences between the two in the degree of cellular differentiation.[25] There is considerable agreement that size of the primary lesion correlates well with survival, and investigators therefore tend to base their staging systems, in part, on this characteristic. For many years, there has been consensus on the importance of regional lymph node metastases, with particular emphasis on inguinal nodes, whose involvement is often a bad prognostic sign.

Investigators from several institutions have analyzed their patients with anal cancer to determine the incidence of recurrence and to identify areas of disease progression after treatment. Frost and associates, at M. D. Anderson Hospital, reviewed the records of 192 patients treated between 1954 and 1979.[22] In a

Table 9–1
Suggested Clinical Staging System

Stage	Criteria	No. of Patients*
0	No gross lesion after local excision	0
Ia	Tumor < 2 cm	0
Ib	Tumor < 2 cm, positive inguinal lymph nodes	0
IIa	Tumor 2–5 cm	62
IIb	Tumor 2–5 cm, positive inguinal lymph nodes	3
IIIa	Tumor > 5 cm	38
IIIb	Tumor > 5 cm, positive inguinal lymph nodes	1
IV	Distant metastases	0

* Suggested staging of the 104 patients in combined-therapy series.

subgroup of 132 patients who underwent APR, they found that the survival rate was related to tumor size, extent of local invasion, and the status of regional lymph nodes. The 5-year survival rate for early lesions (1–2 cm with only superficial invasion) was 76%, whereas for late lesions (deep invasion or positive lymph node involvement) it was 29%. Survival rates by size are as follows: 1–2 cm, 78%; 3–5 cm, 55%; and 6 cm, 40%. Cell type was not a factor; in fact, survival for patients with squamous cell and cloacogenic cancer was virtually the same. Some patients had radiation therapy either before or after operation. The gross tumor disappeared in 11 patients who had preoperative radiation, but three of these patients were found to have positive lymph nodes in the operative specimen. For this group, the survival rate was 83%. Ten patients with fixed primary lesions were converted to operability by radiation therapy. Thirty-one patients who developed local recurrences were treated with surgery, radiation alone, or a combination of the two. Retreatment resulted in a 38% 5-year survival rate in that group. Twenty-nine patients had inguinal node involvement at the time of diagnosis of the primary lesion; of these, 29% survived 5 years after treatment. Eleven of 16 patients who underwent APR were found to have other positive lymph nodes in addition to those in the inguinal area. There were 20 patients who developed inguinal node metastases after the original therapy, but who still had a chance for cure. Eighteen had groin dissections, and 42% survived at least 5 years.

Recently, Boman and associates analyzed the Mayo Clinic experience.[17] The records of 188 patients with anal cancer were reviewed. Among 114 who had an APR and who were followed for at least 5 years, 71% were long-term survivors. They found that tumor size, depth of invasion, regional lymph node involvement, and histologic grading were predictive of survival. Forty percent of the entire series developed recurrences. Exact site of recurrence after APR was documented in 38 patients: 24 recurred locally (*i.e.,* in the pelvis or groin), 5 had both local and distant metastases, and 6 developed only distant metastatic disease. The incidence of failure by stage of the initial lesion were as follows: patients with extension of disease to but not beyond the external sphincter, 23%; extension beyond the sphincter, 48%; and lymph node involvement, 36%. Patients with recurrent disease were treated with surgery, radiation, or a combination of both. Only two of these patients survived more than 5 years after treatment of the recurrence. The authors described a highly aggressive small cell carcinoma of the anal canal, which they suggest is a separate entity. Of the 13 patients in this series, 5 had distant metastases at the time of diagnosis, and only 1 of 7 who could be treated surgically survived 5 years.

Papillon and associates recently updated their series of 272 patients with anal canal cancer who had a chance for cure; 159 were followed for at least 5 years after treatment.[5] The survival rate was 65.4%. Treatment failure occurred in 47 patients and the recurrence was either local, pelvic, inguinal, or distant. Some patients had recurrence in more than one area. However, there were 17 patients with only local recurrence, 19 with only pelvic recurrence, and 11 only in the inguinal area. Of the 47 patients who developed recurrence, 27 died of cancer. The authors concluded that tumor size and involvement of inguinal lymph nodes correlated best with survival.

Symptoms and Diagnosis ■

Unfortunately, early symptoms of anal canal cancer are minimal; usually there is only slight bleeding and discomfort following defecation. Patients assume they have hemorrhoids or a fissure, which leads to self-medication and a delay in seeking medical care. As the growth increases in size, the complaints, especially of pain, become severe enough to cause the patient to seek medical care. Loss of weight is not common but suggests advanced disease when present. Patients sometimes voluntarily reduce food intake because defecation is so painful. In rare situations, patients will notice a lump in the groin as the first indication of anal canal cancer.

The diagnosis is made on examination and biopsy. The long duration of continuous symptoms, plus the induration characteristic of cancer, suggests the possibility of malignancy and the need for biopsy. The lesion may extend proximally into the rectum or distally to and even outside the anal verge. The cancer is generally ulcerative and the size varies. Some are elongated, elliptical, fissure-like lesions, whereas others encircle the anal canal to varying degrees. Advanced cancers may completely encircle it and extend upward or distally to involve tissues beyond the anal canal. An important point, however, is that most—if not all—anal canal cancers, whatever their size, involve the area of the dentate line.

In general, appraisal of the location, measurement of the size, and estimate of the depth of invasion is best done with the patient under anesthesia (usually caudal or spinal); biopsy is done at the same time. If treatment with chemotherapy and radiation is a possibility, only a portion of the lesion should be removed for biopsy. Complete removal is unwise because it will not be possible to estimate the effect of the treatment, and decisions regarding further therapy may be more difficult.

Therapy ■

Surgery ■

For over a half-century, the accepted treatment for invasive cancer of the anal canal has been radical operation. This consists of APR of the rectum as described by Miles in 1908 and later expanded by others to include an extensive perineal phase. In women, the rectovaginal septum is often removed. Some surgeons added a pelvic lymph node dissection in selected patients;[26] there is some rationale for this, but it has not been adopted generally because of the excessive morbidity. Years ago, inguinal lymph node dissection was done prophylactically either during APR or shortly afterward. However, Stearns and colleagues showed this was not effective enough to warrant routine use.[26] Groin dissection is now indicated only when the lymph nodes are involved.

The group at the Mayo Clinic recently reported their results following APR in 118 patients with cancer of the anal canal.[17] The operative mortality rate was 2.5%, with a 71% long-term survival rate for the 114 patients followed for at least 5 years. Local excision was done on 13 patients with lesions less than 2 cm in diameter. All survived at least 5 years, although one patient had to have an APR done for a local recurrence.

Greenall and coworkers reported a 5-year survival rate of 55% in 103 patients treated by APR.[27] Another 11 patients were treated by local excision; 7 of these developed local recurrences. Of 11 patients who had inguinal node involvement at the time of diagnosis, only 2 (18%) survived 5 years. Sixteen others developed groin metastases during follow-up; 69% of these survived at least 5 years after management of the complication. Frost and associates, in a review of the M. D. Anderson Hospital experience, reported 76% long-term survival after APR for early lesions, and 29% survival for deeply invasive primary lesions.[22] Twenty patients with small lesions were treated by local excision, with a 5-year survival rate of 66%. Among 29 patients who had inguinal node metastases at the time of diagnosis (15.2%), 5-year survival after APR and groin dissection was 49%.

In summary, it appears that small, superficial lesions (<2 cm) in the anal canal can be excised locally with significant effectiveness. The 5-year survival rate in a small series reported by Frost and associates was 66%.[22] In the discussion, the authors collected a total of 111 such patients from the literature and calculated an overall 5-year survival rate of 68.5%. Over the years, APR for invasive cancers of the anal canal has been moderately successful. Five-year survival rates as high as 71% have been reported. Any other equally effective therapy would naturally be preferable to avoid the extensive operation and its associated morbidity and mortality risks. Perhaps more important, patients would avoid a permanent colostomy, thereby retaining normal structure and bowel function.

Radiation Therapy ■

Squamous cell carcinomas of the anus have radiosensitivity similar to that of squamous cell carcinomas in other sites. Radiation therapy, as the sole treatment technique, has been limited in the past because of the poor tolerance of the perineum and the limitations of orthovoltage equipment. From the 1920s to the early 1940s, anal cancers were treated with radiation therapy by the groups of Gordon-Watson[28] and Roux-Berger,[29] but their good results were not confirmed by their contemporaries. Despite encouraging results from radium implants, Gabriel recommended surgery for all patients because of some degree of unreliability of the radiation equipment and the complications of the radiation therapy.[24] Nevertheless, some investigators continued to use radiation therapy for anal cancer.

Currently, Papillon and Montbaron probably have the largest experience, with a series of 276 patients last described in 1987.[5] They emphasized interstitial treatment because of the limitations of the orthovoltage equipment and suggested that the high incidence of complications was due to faulty technique and overdosage. They reported a 68% 5-year survival rate in 88 patients, with a 5% rate of severe radiation necrosis with implants, whereas Dalby and Pointon described a higher incidence of radionecrosis, which they attributed to treatment of larger lesions.[30] In 59 patients, the latter authors found a 5-year survival rate of 59% in patients with moderately advanced cancers and 20% in those with advanced tumors. The necrosis rate was 10%. Papillon's radiation therapy was as follows: for T_1 to T_3 tumors (tumors <2 cm to >4 cm, not infiltrating vaginal mucosa), 3000 cGy was delivered at 5 cm depth, with direct 8 cm × 8 cm perineal field in 10 fractions over 19 days. A 7 cm × 12 cm presacral radiation portal was added with a cobalt-60 machine through the posterior arc. With the patient prone, 1800 cGy in six fractions was delivered, with the bottom of the field 7 cm above the anal verge. After a 2-month rest, 2000 cGy was delivered in 1 day using a single-plane template technique.

Papillon and Montbarbon reported excellent results in the 222 patients in whom sphincter conservation was attempted—80% of the patients had their cancer controlled; and 90% of these patients were able to retain normal anal function.[5] Twenty-nine patients developed local pelvic failure alone, almost all within the first year. Distant metastases occurred in 8 patients, associated with locoregional failure in 7. Pelvic failures, usually as presacral or side wall masses, occurred in 19 patients whose primary lesion disappeared. The incidence of pelvic failure was decreased significantly by the use of the presacral field. In European centers, homogeneous doses of 5000 cGy of pelvic radiation in 5–6 weeks with an anal boost of 1000 cGy were commonly used without chemotherapy, as reported by Salmon and colleagues.[31] This appeared to be adequate for lesions < 4 cm. At the Institute Curie, 195 patients were treated with radiation alone. Of 160 patients whose response was complete, 100 were alive with no evidence of disease and with normal anal function after 2 years. Half of the 42 patients with local recurrence had salvage surgery, and half of those survived 3 years. The actual overall survival rate was 68.5% at 3 years and 58% at 5 years. The size of the tumor and the presence of inguinal nodes were important prognostic factors. Neither histology nor grade correlated with the response to radiation or survival. Papillon and others believe that anal canal tumors are suitable for split-course regimens because of their slow regression rate, accessibility for clinical evaluation, and high risk of radiation necrosis.[5]

Eschwege and associates, from the Gustave-Roussy Institute, reported on 64 patients who received radiation therapy alone.[32] They noted a 5-year survival rate of 72% for T_1 and T_2 tumors, but 35% for T_3 and T_4 tumors. Their technique from 1970 to 1977 involved a 240° posterior arc with 60–80 cm source access distance (SAD) cobalt machines that delivered 60 Gy in 6 weeks in 30 fractions. From 1977 to 1980, patients with $T_{1-2}N_0$ tumors were given 45 Gy in 18 fractions in 4.5 weeks via arc treatment. Patients with T_{3-4} tumors were given the above treatment followed by a rest period of 4–5 weeks, and then received an additional 20 Gy in eight fractions over 2 weeks with the same technique. There were nine Grade III complications in 64 patients, most occurring within 2

years, and the rate of complications was related to the size of the tumor. Two of 33 patients with staged T_{1-2} tumors had Grade III complications compared to 3 of 25 with T_3 tumors and 4 of 6 with T_4 tumors. Cummings and coworkers reported in 1984 on 51 patients treated with radiation therapy alone; surgery was reserved for those who had residual tumors. The actual 5-year survival rate was 59%. Primary tumor was controlled with radiation in 29 of 51 patients, but 3 of 29 patients required surgical correction of radiation complications. More recently, Cummings has been using combination chemotherapy and radiation.[33] Glimelius and Pahlman treated T_{1-2} lesions with 65 Gy or 60 Gy plus bleomycin.[34] Of 32 patients, 21 were cleared of their tumors and did well. A few patients were salvaged by perineal resection. Kheir and colleagues reported on 30 cases of cloacogenic carcinomas treated mostly surgically (only 7 received radiation). Seventeen patients died of their disease, suggesting that operation alone is inadequate.

In California, Cantrill and colleagues described 39 patients treated for cure between 1966 and 1981.[36] Of these patients, 34 had anal canal lesions (5 anal margin tumors and 30 lesions < 5 cm in diameter). Five of the 39 patients underwent APR. The tumor and nodal area received 4500–5000 cGy in 180–200 cGy fractions, with a boost field of an additional 1500–2500 cGy. Twenty-eight patients (82%) maintained local control without further treatment. Four patients were salvaged with surgery, bringing control in the 39 patients to 94%. Anal continence was maintained in 28 of 34 patients. Severe anal stenosis requiring colostomy occurred in 2 patients, and persistent painful bleeding ulcers requiring APR occurred in 2 patients.

Radiation is effective as an adjunct in properly selected patients following APR. Generally, radiation treatment for squamous cell carcinomas at other sites (*e.g.,* head and neck) is equivalent whether given preoperatively or postoperatively. In this situation, if there is adequate preoperative response, APR may be avoided. Loygue and colleagues noted that patients with large lesions receiving preoperative radiotherapy and APR had a 50% better 3-year survival than patients who underwent treatment by other modes.[37] The authors suggested 4000 cGy in 4 weeks given before operation. Boman and colleagues used radiation therapy in an attempt to salvage 21 patients with local surgical failure.[17] Only one salvage patient (4000 cGy) was known to be free of disease after 5 years, whereas two patients with recurrence lived longer than 5 years. The remaining 17 patients died of recurrent or metastatic tumor after 3.5 to 57 months.

Chemotherapy ∎

Only anecdotal information is available about the use of systemic chemotherapy alone in the treatment of anal carcinomas. Transient tumor responses have been observed in patients treated with nitrosoureas, Adriamycin, cisplatin, and bleomycin.[38–41] At Wayne State University Oncology Service, two of four patients with metastatic anal cancer responded to 5-fluorouracil (5-FU) and one to mitomycin C. We then decided to explore the use of a combination of these two agents.

In 1975, Seifert and coworkers reported that 5-FU, when infused continuously over 5 days, produced virtually no hematologic effect but regularly produced ulceration of oral and anal mucosa.[42] The lack of hematologic toxicity made it attractive to combine infused 5-FU with bone-marrow-suppressing cytotoxic drugs. The severe toxicity occurring in gastrointestinal squamous epithelium led to the exploration of the combination of these drugs in the treatment of squamous cell carcinomas of the intestinal tract.[43,44] Although a rather large number of patients with locally incurable head and neck and esophageal cancers were available for these studies, there were only two patients with disseminated squamous cell cancer of the anus. They responded to 5-FU infusion (1000 mg/m^2 daily for 5 days repeated every 4 weeks) combined with mitomycin C (20 mg/m^2 repeated every 8 weeks). This anecdotal observation led to our decision to combine infused 5-FU and mitomycin C with radiotherapy, first for preoperative and later for definitive treatment of squamous cell carcinomas of the anus.

Combined Therapy ∎

The initial attempt of combining 5-FU with mitomycin C and radiation given preoperatively by the Wayne State University group was intended to increase surgical curability of these patients. Therefore, a rather modest dose of radiation (3000 cGy over 3 weeks) was selected. The duration of 5-FU infusion, originally 5 days, was reduced to 4 days to avoid severe proctitis prior to surgery. Because of the observation by Vietti and associates that 5-FU given in vitro prior to radiation might act as a radiation protector, and because the drug has a marked radioenhancing effect when given after radiation, the infusion was started concurrently with radiotherapy.[45] The infusion was repeated 4 weeks later, usually 1 week after radiation

was completed. Mitomycin C was selected from the many cytotoxic bone marrow suppressing drugs because our experience had shown it to be active against other squamous carcinomas.[46,47] In addition, it was observed in in vitro studies that mitomycin C is particularly effective in anoxic tissues.[48,49] Recently, the advantages of using mitomycin C with radiotherapy in the treatment of tumors with anoxic areas were reviewed by Sartorelli.[50]

When radiotherapy is limited to 3000 cGy in 3 weeks, this combined chemoradiation therapy is rather well-tolerated. However, Cummings used larger amounts of radiation in an attempt to avoid the need for surgery.[51] Under these circumstances, more bone marrow suppression can be expected, and the dose of mitomycin C has to be reduced, to perhaps 10 mg/m^2. In malnourished, frail, or elderly patients, a reduction of 5-FU infusion to 600 mg/m^2 per day may be advisable to avoid excessive stomatitis and proctitis.

Nigro reported a series of 104 patients with squamous cell cancer of the anal canal treated from January 1972 to July 1983.[11] All cancers involved the area of the dentate line and they included each of the various cell types commonly described as arising in the anal transitional zone. We treated 44 patients at Wayne State University, and the remaining 60 were managed by individual surgeons around the country. The information was obtained by questionnaire and follow-up reports. Patients with inguinal metastases but not those with known metastases to distant organs, were included in the study. The lesions were ulcerative, and all but six were moderately to poorly differentiated. Thirty-nine patients had small lesions (2–3 cm), 46 had moderate-sized growths (4–5 cm), and 19 had large lesions (6–8 cm). Four patients had inguinal node metastases (one bilateral) at the time of diagnosis. All patients but one were judged to be candidates for APR of the rectum.

Preoperative radiation and chemotherapy was administered to all patients. Radiation and drug therapy were begun jointly on day 1. 5-FU was given via a central venous catheter in a dosage of 1000 mg/m^2 per day for 4 days as a continuous infusion. This 96-hour infusion was repeated in 1 month. Mitomycin C was given as a single bolus intravenous injection of 15 mg/m^2. Radiation therapy was given as 3000 cGy, calculated at the central axis midplane of the pelvis, at 200 cGy/day, 5 days per week starting on day 1. The parallel-opposing anteroposterior portals included the primary lesion with margin, the true pelvis, and the inguinal lymphatics. Abdominoperineal resection was performed 4 to 6 weeks after completion of radiation therapy. Leukocyte and platelet counts were obtained until the time of operation.

The first 5 patients in our series received the higher doses of 5-FU and mitomycin C suggested in our initial report;[52] however, toxicity was excessive in 3 patients, so the drug amounts were reduced to those described here. Ninety-nine patients, therefore, received the reduced drug regimen. The protocol was changed again in 1975 when we found that 5 of the first 6 patients had no cancer in the operative specimen after APR of the rectum. Subsequently, we did not perform radical operations unless cancer remained following chemoradiation therapy. Some surgeons who submitted questionnaires continued to operate routinely for varying times after 1975. In most patients whose primary lesion disappeared grossly, the scar was excised for biopsy purposes 4 to 6 weeks after completion of radiation treatment (a few patients refused to have this done). Abdominoperineal resection was performed on 38 patients in this series either routinely, for residual cancer remaining after chemoradiation therapy, or for recurrent disease.

All 104 patients were evaluable for the efficacy of chemoradiation therapy. Six weeks after treatment no gross tumor remained in the anal canal in 97 patients, and visible cancer was present in 7. Twenty-four patients underwent radical operations routinely after chemotherapy, with 7 other operations performed because gross cancer remained after initial therapy. The specimens were free of tumor in 22, microscopic cancer was found in 2 specimens and gross cancer in 7. Of 62 patients who had excision of the scar following chemoradiation therapy, there was no tumor in 61. One patient had a small area of microscopic cancer that was excised locally; she has been cancer-free for 4 years. Eleven patients whose cancer disappeared grossly refused to have the scar excised for biopsy purposes following chemoradiation therapy. Two of the latter patients died of their disease while the other 9 are alive, without evidence of disease, after 5 to 9 years. There were 8 recurrences in the patients treated conservatively after chemoradiation therapy. The recurrences became apparent 5 months to nearly 3 years after a negative biopsy following chemoradiation treatment. Abdominoperineal resection of the rectum was performed on 7 of these 8 patients; thus, of 104 patients, 38 underwent radical surgery.

Inguinal node metastases were initially present in only four patients; one had bilateral involvement while three had one positive node on one side. The three patients with unilateral disease had radical surgery and groin dissection, and the patient with extensive bilateral inguinal disease associated with a small primary lesion was treated (conservatively) with more radiation (3000 cGy to the inguinal area). Two of the four patients died: the patient with bilateral involvement, and one patient who underwent APR and groin dissection. Both died of distant metastases. The two survivors are free of disease, one for 6 years and one for 5 years. Two other patients developed inguinal node metastases subsequent to the initial chemoradiation therapy without operation. One of these patients had a bilateral groin dissection and only one node was found to contain cancer. The patient is alive without evidence of disease 4 years after groin dissection. The other patient developed extensive bilateral involvement and was treated with more radiation; she died 2 years later.

Toxicity from the chemoradiation therapy was mild or moderate in 99 of 104 patients. Symptoms consisted of mild stomatitis, diarrhea, temporary loss of hair, and redness of perineal skin. Fifteen patients had moderate depression of the white blood cell count or platelet count but did not require hospitalization. Five patients developed severe toxicity requiring hospitalization and significant therapy, including transfusions, intestinal intubation, and hyperalimentation. All patients recovered, however, without long-term complications. Drug therapy was interrupted during the fourth day of the infusion in 11 patients, but radiation therapy did not have to be stopped in any patient.

Eighty-one patients are alive and apparently free of cancer 5 to 16 years after treatment. Two others are alive but have been treated aggressively for extensive recurrent cancer. One of these patients has been in clinical remission for nearly 5 years after treatment for the recurrence. The other patient, who underwent an APR in 1982 for a local recurrence, developed extensive pelvic cancer diagnosed in July 1987; at this writing, she is still receiving therapy for symptomatic cancer.

There were 21 deaths: 13 due to squamous cell cancer and eight due to other causes. Of those who died of their disease, 7 underwent APR following completion of chemoradiation therapy, and 3 had the operation later for recurrent disease. The other 3 patients had only chemoradiation therapy. It is of interest to note that, of the 7 patients who had delayed radical operation after negative biopsy following chemoradiation therapy, 3 died, 3 are alive without evidence of disease 4 to 6 years after operation, and one is alive with residual disease 6 years after APR. The study began 16 years ago, and the last patient was entered in July, 1983; thus, all the patients have been followed for at least 5 years. The actual 5-year survival rate, counting all 21 deaths, is slightly less than 80%.

At Highland Hospital, Rochester, New York, Sischy treated 33 patients with cancer of the anal canal between 1976 and 1983 with combined therapy.[53] The chemotherapy consisted of 5-FU and mitomycin C given as described by the Wayne State University group, except for a reduction in the dose of mitomycin C to 10 mg/m^2 started on day 2 and an increase in radiation to the pelvis (4500 cGy). If inguinal nodes were involved, more radiation was administered directly to the inguinal area. Three patients in this series had positive nodes at the time of diagnosis. The first 4 patients of the 33 had routine APR, but all operative specimens were free of cancer. Consequently, routine APR was discontinued. Of the 29 remaining patients, 26 had local control of the disease. Three patients died of their disease, one of whom had inguinal node disease at the time of diagnosis. The other two patients with initial inguinal node disease are long-term survivors. One other patient has distant metastases but is still undergoing therapy. Five patients died of other causes. The crude survival rate was 81% at a minimum of 12 months and a maximum of 8 years.

Cummings and colleagues at Princess Margaret Hospital in Toronto have had a special interest in the management of anal canal cancer. They recently compared a group of patients treated with radiation alone (1958 to 1978) with a group treated with a similar amount of radiation combined with chemotherapy (1978 to 1982).[54] The first group consisted of 25 patients, with 30 in the second group. All patients treated with radiation only received 4500 to 6000 cGy in 4 to 6 weeks. The combined-therapy group received 5000 cGy in 4 weeks plus 5-FU and mitomycin C given in the manner described by the Wayne State University group except that the dose of mitomycin C was reduced to 10 mg/m^2. Sixteen patients were treated in this manner, but toxicity was excessive, and a split-course regimen was started in an effort to reduce complications. In the new protocol, patients then were given 2500 cGy plus chemotherapy, with the combination repeated in 4 weeks. There were 14 patients in the split-therapy group.

The size of the lesions was not indicated in the charts in many of the patients treated with radiation only. In the group treated with combined therapy, 50% of the cancers were greater than 5 cm in size. Lymph node involvement—inguinal, pelvic, or both—was present at the time of diagnosis in 28% of the first group and 27% in the combined-therapy group.

Control of the primary lesion was achieved in 60% (15/25) of the radiation-only treatment group but was over 90% in both the continuous and split-therapy combined-treatment groups. Surgical therapy (APR)

successfully controlled the disease in 7 patients after failure of radiation therapy alone, and there were 3 other failures that could not undergo the operation. Surgical therapy salvaged enough patients to bring the radiation group long-term survivors to 88%, which is practically the same as in the combined-therapy groups. In the combined-therapy group, local excision successfully managed a small residual tumor. In one other failure, laparotomy confirmed the presence of liver metastases. No patients developed inguinal lymph node disease during follow-up.

Patients in all groups developed a mild degree of toxicity, and some had moderate to severe hematologic toxicity or enterocolitis. Three patients from the radiation group required operation for radiation-related complications, as did 5 of the 30 who received combined therapy. In conclusion, the combined therapy, in both the single- and the split-course versions, greatly improved local disease control compared to radiation alone. Long-term survival rates were similar, but the numbers are too small and the time frame too short to be statistically significant.

Recently, Enker and coworkers updated the Memorial Hospital series of patients treated with combined therapy between 1973 and 1983.[55] The treatment was similar to the protocol developed at Wayne State University except that radiation therapy was given after chemotherapy. Operations were carried out 3 to 5 weeks after the preoperative therapy. Of 44 patients, 31 had lesions ≤ 5 cm, one had a larger lesion, and 12 had lesions of unrecorded size. Two patients had inguinal lymph node involvement at the time of diagnosis. Twenty patients had the scar excised after preoperative therapy and 24 had an APR. There was no cancer in the operative specimen in 26 patients. Ten patients developed recurrences, either local or pelvic. When the paper was written, 32 patients were alive without evidence of disease, 4 were alive with disease, and 8 had died of cancer. The median follow-up was 39 months (range, 1–89).

Flam and associates recently published an update of their series, which included 30 patients treated from 1979 to 1986 by chemoradiation therapy without operation.[6] The treatment protocol was adapted from the one initiated by the Wayne State group and consisted of two cycles of 5-FU and mitomycin C concomitant with pelvic radiation therapy. It differed in that mitomycin C was given with the second infusion of 5-FU and the dose of radiation was increased to 4140–4500 cGy. Additional therapy (900 cGy) was given to the perineum in advanced local lesions or to the inguinal area if there was nodal involvement. Any failures were given additional chemoradiation (dosage varied) rather than APR. Seven patients had inguinal lymph node involvement. Of the 30 patients, 26 were free of cancer after the initial therapy, the other 4 had residual local disease and were rendered free of cancer by additional chemoradiation therapy. The salvage treatment varied, but 2 patients received a combination of 5-FU and cisplatin with five fractions of radiation therapy at 180 cGy. Another was treated with the original drug therapy plus low-dose radiation. The last patient received three chemotherapeutic drugs plus radiation (radiation was given to the perineum in each of the four patients). Acute toxicity was a problem, in that 4 patients required therapy in the hospital. However, all recovered. Late complications were minimal. After 9–76 months, 27 patients were alive and free of disease, and 3 died of unrelated causes.

Meeker and coworkers reported a series of 19 patients treated with the protocol used at Wayne State University.[56] Nine patients had APR but 7 had no cancer in the operative specimen. Seven patients had biopsies after therapy and all tissue was cancer-free, but one had a local recurrence 4 months later and underwent an APR. Three refused biopsy. One of the latter died of cancer, whereas 2 are long-term survivors. There were two other deaths in patients who had APR with no cancer in the specimen. Of these, one died of distant metastases and the other probably died of breast cancer. Three patients with inguinal lymph node disease underwent groin dissection after the chemoradiation therapy. All tissue removed from the groin was free of cancer. Finally, the actuarial disease-free survival at 40 months was 87.5% ± 8.8%.

Papillon and his group have treated patients with anal canal cancer for many years with radiation therapy alone. In 1977, they added chemotherapy consisting of 5-FU and mitomycin C (at a lower dose than in the Wayne State protocol) in the treatment of patients with lesions > 4 cm. The results improved significantly, and, since 1985, this group has included chemotherapy with radiation for all patients with carcinoma of the anal canal, regardless of the disease stage or lesion size. In comparing patients treated by radiation alone to those with combined therapy, the local failure rate was reduced from 26% to 13%.[5]

The Radiation Therapy Oncology Group (RTOG), under the direction of Sischy, initiated a protocol for the treatment of squamous cell cancer of the anal canal (Sischy B: personal communication). The therapy consisted of radiation (4080 cGy to the pelvis in 170 cGy fractions) plus chemotherapy, which included an infusion of 5-FU 1000 mg/m^2 per 24 hours for 4 days and mitomycin C 10 mg/m^2 as a single bolus injection on day 1. Seventy-nine patients were available for evaluation. Generally, the therapy caused minimal toxicity, although it was moderate in several patients; there were no long-term toxic effects. Local tumor control rate was 84% for patients with small tumors (≤3 cm) and 62% for those with tumors >3 cm. The 3-year survival rate was 85% for patients with small tumors and 67.5% for those with the larger lesions. It appears that neither the radiation dose used in this study nor the 3000 cGy used in the Wayne State University study was likely to have been solely responsible for the control of so high a percentage of these cancers. The chemotherapy no doubt sensitizes the tumor to the radiation, but it may also have a significant cytotoxic effect of its own on the cancer cells. At any rate, the two treatments have an additive effect when given simultaneously.

It is difficult to draw precise conclusions from the literature regarding the best therapy for patients with anal cancer, because there are too many variations in the combined therapy approach and because the number of patients in each study is too small. Radical surgery has been used most frequently, but even here the 5-year survival rate varies among series, from less than 30% to more than 71%. Long-term survival rates reported after radiotherapy alone are comparable to those after radical surgery. For example, Papillon and colleagues report a 5-year survival rate of 65% for patients with anal canal cancer.[5] However, radiation has not been widely accepted as the sole therapy for this disease, apparently because the complications of the therapy itself have been considered unacceptable. Finally, it is clear from reports of several investigators that a regimen consisting of pelvic radiation and two cycles of 5-FU infusion and one dose of mitomycin C is effective in eradicating the local lesion in cancer of the anal canal in 75% to 80% of patients. We believe that radical surgery has not been successful enough in the management of failures after chemoradiation therapy, and it would therefore be reasonable to use chemoradiation more often than APR for the failures. Preliminary evidence suggests this may be effective.[6]

Current Therapy ■

There is now sufficient evidence, from many investigators, to establish chemoradiation therapy as the primary treatment for all macroscopic squamous cell cancer of the anal canal (including its variants) and for invasive squamous cell cancers of the anal margin. This includes lesions less than 2 cm in size. Variations of the protocol initiated at Wayne State University School of Medicine have been reported, but the optimal regimen has not been established. Many investigators have questioned the wisdom of using mitomycin C in the therapy; it has prolonged and sometimes unpredictably severe bone-marrow-suppressing activity and is also known to produce a sometimes fatal hemolytic syndrome. Because of these properties, mitomycin C is not often used in the palliative care of cancer. In 1985, Salem and colleagues reported a favorable response to the use of cisplatin in patients with squamous cell carcinoma of the anus.[40] In 1986, Khater and associates successfully treated two patients with metastatic disease with a combination of a 5-FU infusion and cisplatin.[57] They used the same schedule that Weaver and associates advocated for the treatment of head and neck cancers.[43]

Cisplatin, however, is also capable of producing distressing and sometimes permanently disabling toxicity. Severe drug-induced nausea is probably the most undesirable effect. Nephrotoxicity generally can be managed by careful monitoring of hydration, by chloride administration, and by avoidance of potassium and magnesium depletion. Neurotoxicity (particularly eighth cranial nerve injury leading to deafness) is difficult to avoid, particularly in older patients requiring repeated administration of the drug.

A large-scale randomized study comparing combinations of mitomycin C or cisplatin with 5-FU infusion is needed to determine which of the two drugs is more active. Because of the relative rarity of anal carcinoma and because of the high response rate observed in mitomycin C-treated patients, such studies are not likely to be completed soon. Severe mitomycin C toxicity is usually not observed unless the drug is administered repeatedly. Therefore, mitomycin C is better tolerated than cisplatin for short-term use while the latter is better when multiple doses are required. We advise continued use of the following chemoradiation therapy as the initial therapy for all patients with this disease.

Chemotherapy and radiation therapy are begun jointly on day 1 of the treatment. Continuous infusion of 5-FU is given via a central venous catheter in a dosage of 1000 mg/m^2 per 24 hours for 4 days. This 96-hour infusion is repeated in 1 month, even in the presence of mild bone marrow depression, because 5-FU infusions have been shown to be nonmyelosuppressive. Mitomycin C is given as a single bolus intravenous injection of 15 mg/m^2. Radiation therapy is given as 3000 cGy, calculated at the midplane of the pelvis, at 1000 cGy/week starting on day one. The radiation portal includes the primary lesion with margin, the true pelvis, and the inguinal lymphatics (Fig. 9–4). The lower edge of the radiation field should include the ischial tuberosities and the perineum. A clinical evaluation is made 6 weeks after completion of radiation therapy. If the lesion disappears and if the tumor was less than 5 cm in size initially, the therapy is sufficient. Naturally, the patient is followed closely for signs of recurrence.

We continue with additional chemoradiation therapy for patients whose tumor does not disappear, and for all patients whose original lesion was 5 cm or larger, regardless of the effect of the first course of therapy. We suggest the latter because our experience indicates that all patients with large cancers are at high risk. Currently, we prefer to give the treatment 6 weeks after completion of the first course of radiation therapy. It consists of 2000 cGy in 2 weeks to the local lesion, together with an infusion of 5-FU, 1000 mg/m^2 for 4 days. On the first day of chemotherapy, after appropriate hydration, a single 100 mg/m^2 dose of cisplatin is given. Currently, we repeat the 5-FU infusion and the cisplatin twice more at 1-month intervals. Long-term evaluation of this second course of therapy is not yet available. If the local lesion persists 6 weeks after the second course of radiation therapy, we suggest the application of interstitial implants. The alternative, of course, is APR of the rectum. Finally, we are treating patients who develop metastatic disease or delayed recurrence after chemoradiation therapy with second-line chemotherapy. This consists of a combination of bleomycin, cisplatin, and VP-16, and more radiation if possible.

FIG. 9–4 Typical anteroposterior fields. The dotted lines represent typical electron field boost to the inguinal lymph nodal areas.

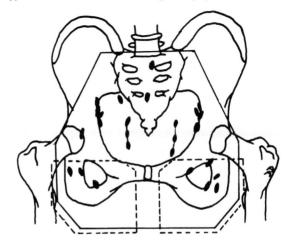

We have observed several remissions. Obviously, full doses of cisplatin can be given only to patients with normal renal function. Moreover, this drug combination needs more investigation for use for this purpose. Fortunately, patients requiring such therapy are not common, and its evaluation will long remain anecdotal. A schema representing all our recommendations for therapy is shown in Figure 9–5.

Inguinal Lymph Node Metastasis ■

Reports in the literature show that the incidence of lymph node metastasis varies significantly. For example, Wolfe and Bussey, in 1968, reported a 35% incidence of synchronous inguinal node involvement in a series of 170 patients, and Stearns and Quan, in 1970, found a 40% incidence in their patients.[18,58] However, more recent reports indicate that this incidence has decreased. Frost and coworkers found inguinal metastases in 29 of 192 patients (15.1%).[22] Papillon and coworkers found that only 13% of 276

FIG. 9–5 Chemoradiation therapy. All courses of therapy but the first are tentative, and experience is minimal. APR is an alternative to be considered in individual patients for residual or recurrent cancer. (See text for details of therapy.)

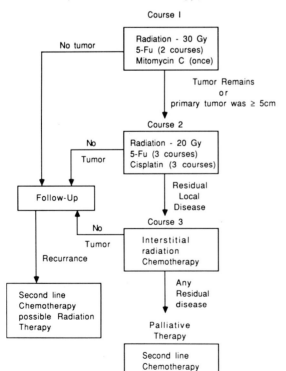

patients had inguinal node involvement at the time of diagnosis. In a series of 104 patients, Nigro found that only 4 patients had synchronous inguinal node metastases.[11] There is general agreement, however, that this is a grave prognostic sign. In 1980, Stearns and colleagues reported only 1 5-year survivor out of 11 patients.[4] In the series reported by Wolfe and Bussey, 21.3% survived at least 5 years.[18] More recent results are somewhat better because patients have been treated with a combination of surgery and radiotherapy. Papillon and colleagues, for example, report a survival rate of 57.8%.[5] The prognosis in patients with metachronous inguinal node involvement has been always better than when positive nodes are present at the time of diagnosis. Sugarbaker and associates consolidated patients from a number of major series, and found that 36 of 70 patients (51%) were long-term survivors.[59]

Treatment of metastatic inguinal lymph nodes has been surgical. In the past, groin dissection was done at the time of APR or shortly afterward. When positive nodes were found later, an operation was performed as soon as possible. At present, the role of radiation therapy in the management of this problem is not clearly defined. Although in the past it was believed that metastatic lymph nodes did not respond well to radiation therapy, Papillon and colleagues maintain that radiotherapy is effective in the management of nodal disease in patients with squamous cell cancer.[5] The trend now is to use a combination of operation and radiotherapy, and variations of this combination are no doubt being investigated. We treat all patients with squamous cell cancer of the anal canal, including those with inguinal node metastases, with the Wayne State University chemoradiation therapy protocol. As has been stated, the radiation field includes the inguinal areas. After 6 weeks, a superficial groin dissection is done on the affected side if the node is not clinically normal. Some surgeons operate in any event. It is quite clear, however, that patients with extensive, bilateral inguinal lymph node involvement should be treated only with additional radiation to the groin areas as soon as convenient after the first course of chemoradiation therapy. In our experience, this is only a palliative measure.

Treatment Prospects ■

It is reasonable to expect the development of more effective methods of radiation therapy and better cytotoxic drugs. Moreover, there are exciting prospects for new approaches to drug therapy. Experimental studies suggest the possibility of adding a biochemical modulator to the drug therapy. These chemicals do not kill cancer cells, but rather act to cause cell reversion to a more normal state.[60] A synergy of both destructive and reversion chemical mechanisms will perhaps be more effective than the current use of destructive agents alone. A representative biochemical modulator is difluoromethylornithine (DFMO), a specific inhibitor of polyamine biosynthesis undergoing clinical evaluation.[61] Singly, it does not appear to be effective in humans, but it may have some effect when combined with other drugs. Other chemicals closely related to DFMO have been synthesized and are being tested.[62] Hopefully, one of these will prove to be more effective clinically. They may retard tumor regrowth following exposure to a combination of cytotoxic agents and radiation therapy. Another class of drugs that may be found useful is the nonsteroidal anti-inflammatory agents. These drugs have an antitumor effect when given to animals undergoing intestinal carcinogenesis.[63] A preliminary study suggests that such therapy reduces the number of adenomas in patients with familial polyposis.[64] Another study showed that these drugs can prevent chemotherapy-induced deterioration of some aspects of immune function in cancer patients.[65] Investigators speculated that the drug acts by controlling excessive production of monocyte-synthesized prostaglandins.

Anal Margin Cancer ■

These tumors occur in the perianal skin and are similar to skin cancers elsewhere. Histologically, they include squamous cell carcinoma, basal cell cancer, Bowen's disease, and Paget's disease. Generally, these cancers are localized to the skin, and simple excision is curative. At times, a second or even third attempt is needed to completely remove the tumor if it involves a large area. Wounds may be left open because healing in the perianal skin is rapid and scarring minimal. Wounds may also be closed in any appropriate manner (including by skin graft).

Occasionally, anal margin tumors are invasive and require radical therapy. Since this problem is uncommon, individual experience is limited. However, we recommend these patients be treated with the chemoradiation therapy as described for anal canal cancer except that a part of the radiation may be given through a perineal portal. Abdominoperineal resection should be considered 8 weeks later on an individual basis, depending on the effect of chemoradiation therapy. If the lesion disappears, the patient should be followed at frequent intervals, at least initially. If it does not disappear, or if it recurs soon, a second course of chemoradiation should be given. If residual tumor still remains, surgery should be considered.

There is a group of miscellaneous lesions that occur outside the anus that must be treated aggressively. On rare occasions, anorectal fistulas contain malignant tissue, which may be either squamous cell or adenocarcinoma. The former occurs in a fistula that has been present for many years, whereas adenocarcinoma is present in fistulas of recent origin (the cancer is the cause of the fistula formation). Abdominoperineal resection with a wide excision of the affected area is the accepted treatment for the adenocarcinoma fistula. However, we suggest that chemoradiation therapy be given before the operation. We would speculate that the fistulas with squamous cell cancer would have a better prognosis, and radical operation may not be necessary.

Condyloma acuminatum, a common lesion of the perianal skin, occasionally is associated with squamous cell cancer. We have treated two such patients and, as mentioned above, Brennon and Stewart reported another five.[11,13] Radical surgery (APR) has been advocated for this lesion. We have, however, successfully treated two patients with chemoradiation therapy alone with no recurrence—one for 3 years and the other for 6 years. Recently Butler and colleagues published a report of a patient treated with chemoradiation therapy followed by APR.[66] There was no cancer in the operative specimen and there has been no recurrence in 3 years. Consequently, it appears that chemoradiation alone is an effective therapy for this lesion. We would suggest additional chemoradiation treatment be given if the lesion does not completely disappear after the first course of therapy. Radical surgery may not be required in most patients.

Conclusion ■

Abdominoperineal resection of the rectum, an extensive operation that results in the establishment of a permanent colostomy, is no longer the treatment of choice for invasive, squamous cell cancer of the anus. The preferred method of treatment is a combination of radiation and chemotherapy. There is sufficient evidence that this therapy is at least as effective as the radical operation, without the burden of a permanent colostomy. This development represents progress toward one objective of cancer therapy, namely, treatment with preservation of structure and function. In the early part of this century, Gordon-Watson had this objective in mind for the management of cancer of the anus, but the means were not available at the time. Now they are.

References ■

1. Miles EW: A method of performing abdominoperineal excision for carcinoma of the rectum and of the terminal portion of pelvic colon. Lancet 2:1812–1813, 1908
2. Fenger C: Histology of the anal canal. Am J Surg Pathol 12:41–55, 1988
3. Thorek P: Anatomy in Surgery, pp 477–490. Philadelphia, JB Lippincott, 1951
4. Stearns MW Jr, Urmacher C, Sternberg SS, Woodruff J, Attiyeh F: Cancer of the anal canal. Curr Probl Cancer 4:1–44, 1980
5. Papillon J, Montbarbon JF: Epidermoid carcinoma of the anal canal: A series of 276 cases. Dis Colon Rectum 30:324–333, 1987
6. Flam MS, Hohn MJ, Mowry PA, Lovalvo LJ, Ramalho LD, Wade J: Definitive combined modality therapy of carcinoma of the anus. Dis Colon Rectum 30:495–502, 1987
7. Glimelius B, Pahlman L: Radiation therapy of anal epidermoid carcinoma. Int J Radiation Oncology Biol Phys 13:305–312, 1987
8. Morson BC: The pathology and results of treatment of cancer of the anal region. Proc R Soc Med 52(Suppl):117–118, 1959
9. Hintz BL, Charyulu KKN, Sudarsanam A: Anal carcinoma: Basic concepts and management. J Surg Oncol 10:141–150, 1978
10. McConnell EM: Squamous cell carcinoma of the anus—A review of 96 cases. Br J Surg 57:89–92, 1970
11. Nigro ND: Multidisciplinary management of cancer of the anus. World J Surg 11:446–451, 1987
12. Siegel A: Malignant transformation of condyloma acuminatum. Am J Surg 103:613–617, 1962
13. Brennan JT, Stewart CF: Epidermoid carcinoma of the anus. Ann Surg 176:787–790, 1972
14. Wexner SD, Milsom JW, Dailey TH: The demographics of anal cancers are changing. Dis Colon Rectum 30:942–946, 1987
15. Peters RK, Mack TM: Patterns of anal carcinoma by gender and marital status in Los Angeles County. Br J Cancer 48:629–636, 1983
16. Daling JR, Weiss NS, Klopfenstein LL, Cochran LE, Chow WH, Daifuku R: Correlates of homosexual behavior and the incidence of anal cancer. JAMA 247:1988–1990, 1982
17. Boman BM, Moertez CG, O'Connez MJ: Carcinoma of the anal canal: A clinical and pathologic study of 188 cases. Cancer 54:114–125, 1984
18. Wolfe HRI, Bussey HJR: Squamous cell carcinoma of the anus. Br J Surg 55:295, 1968
19. Stearns MW Jr, Quan SHQ: Epidermoid carcinoma of the anorectum. Surg Gynecol Obstet 131:953–957, 1970
20. Kuehn PG, Eisenberg H, Reed JF: Epidermoid carcinoma of the perianal skin and anal canal. Cancer 22:932–938, 1968
21. Richards JC, Beahrs OH, Woolner LB: Squamous cell carcinoma of the anus, anal canal and rectum in 109 patients. Surg Gynecol Obstet 114:475–482, 1962
22. Frost D, Richards P, Montague E, Giaceo G, Martin R: Epidermoid cancer of the anorectum. Cancer 53:1285, 1984
23. Singh R, Nime F, Mittelman A: Malignant epithelial tumors of the anal canal. Cancer 48:411–415, 1981
24. Gabriel WB: Squamous-cell carcinoma of anus and anal canal: Analysis of 55 cases. Proc R Soc Med 34:139–157, 1941
25. Schraut WE, Wang C, Dawson PJ, Block GE: Depth of invasion, location, size of cancer of the anus dictate operative treatment. Cancer 51:1291–1296, 1983
26. Stearns MW Jr: Epidermoid carcinoma of the anal region. Am J Surg 90:727–733, 1955
27. Greenall MJ, Ivan SH, Urmacher C, Decosse JJ: Treatment of epidermoid carcinoma of the anal canal. Surg Gynecol Obstet 161:509–517, 1985
28. Gordon-Watson D, Dukes CE: The treatment of carcinoma of rectum with radium with introduction on spread of cancer of rectum. Br J Surg 17:643–672, 1930
29. Roux-Berger JL, Ennuyer A: Carcinoma of the anal canal. Am J Roentgenol 60:807–815, 1948
30. Dalby JE, Pointon RS: The treatment of anal carcinoma by interstitial irradiation. Am J Roentgenol 85:515–520, 1961
31. Salmon RJ, Zafrani B, Labib A, Asselain B, Girodet J, Durand JC, Fenton J, Mathieu G, Bataini P, Rousseau J: Cancer of the anal canal. Results of the treatment of a series of 195 cases. Gastro Clin Bio 9:911–917, 1984
32. Eschwege F, Lasser P, Chavy A, Wibault P, Kac J, Rougier P, Bognel C: Squamous cell carcinoma of the anal canal: Treatment by external beam irradiation. Radio Oncol 3:145–150, 1987
33. Cummings B, Keane T, Thomas G, Harwood A, Rider W: Results and toxicity of the treatment of anal canal carcinoma by radiation therapy or radiation therapy and chemotherapy. Cancer 54:2062–2068, 1984
34. Glimelius B, Pahlman L: Radiation therapy of anal epidermoid carcinoma. Int J Radiat Oncol Bio Phys 12:305–312, 1987
35. Kheir S, Hickey RC, Martin RG, MacKay B, Gallagher HS: Cloacogenic carcinoma of the anal canal. Arch Surg 104:407–416, 1972
36. Cantril ST, Green JP, Schall GL, Schaupp WC: Primary radiation therapy in the treatment of anal carcinoma. Int J Radiat Oncol Biol Phys 9:1271–1278, 1983
37. Loygue J, Langier A, Parc R, Weisberger G: Carcinoma epidermoids de l'anus a propos de 149 observations. Chirurgie 109:710–724, 1981
38. Moertel C: The anus. In Holland JF, Frei E III (eds): Cancer Medicine, pp 1859–1863. Philadelphia, Lea & Febiger, 1982
39. Fisher WB, Herbst KD, Sims JE, et al: Metastatic cloacogenic carcinoma of the anus: Sequential response to adriamycin and cis-dichlorodiamine-platinum (II). Cancer Treatment Rep 62:91–97, 1978
40. Salem PA, Habboubi N, Anaissie E, Brihi ER, Issa P, Abbas JS, Khalyl MF: Effectiveness of cisplatin in the treatment of anal squamous cell carcinoma. Cancer Treatment Rep 69:891–893, 1985
41. Glimelius B, Graffman S, Pahlman L, Wilander E: Radiation therapy of anal carcinoma. Acta Radiologica Oncol 22:273–279, 1983
42. Seifert P, Baker LH, Reed ML, Vaitkevicius VK: Comparison of continuously infused 5-fluorouracil with bolus injection in treatment of patients colorectal adenocarcinoma. Cancer 36:123–128, 1975
43. Weaver A, Fleming S, Ensley J, Kish JA, Jacobs J, Kinzie J, Crissman J, Al-Sarraf M: Superior complete clinical response and survival rates with initial bolus cis-platinum and 120 hour 5-FU infusion before definitive therapy in patients with locally advanced head and neck cancer. Am J Surg 148:525–529, 1984
44. Steiger Z, Franklin R, Wison RF, Leichman L, Asfaw I, Vaishanpayan G, Rosenberg JC, Loh JJK, Dindogru A, Seydel

HK, Hoschner J, Miller P, Knechtges T, Vaitkevicius VK: Complete eradication of squamous cell carcinoma of the esophagus with combined chemotherapy and radiotherapy. Am J Surg 47:95–98, 1981

45. Vietti T, Eggerding F, Valeriate F: Combined effect of x radiation and 5-fluorouracil on survival of transplanted leukemia cell. JNCI 47:865, 1971

46. Baker LH, Opipari M, Izbicki RM: Phase II study of mitomycin C, vincristine, and bleomycin in advanced squamous cell carcinoma of the uterine cervix. Cancer 38:2222–2224, 1976

47. Crooke ST, Brodner WT: Mitomycin C. Cancer Treat Rep 3: 121–139, 1976

48. Lin AJ, Cosby LA, Shansky CW, Sartorelli AC: Potential bioreproductive alkylating agents. I. Benzoquinone derivatives. J Med Chemo 15:1247–1252, 1972

49. Lin AJ, Pardini RS, Cosby LA, Lillis B, Shansky CW, Sartorelli AC: Potential bioreproductive alkylating agents. II. Antitumor effect and biochemical studies of naphtoquinone derivatives. J Med Chemo 16:1268–1271, 1973

50. Sartorelli AC: Therapeutic attack of hypoxic cells of solid tumors: Presidential address. Cancer Res 48:775–778, 1988

51. Cummings BJ: Current management of epidermoid carcinoma of the anal canal. Gastroenterol Clin North Am 16:125–142, 1987

52. Nigro ND, Vaitkevicius VK, Considine B Jr: Combined therapy for cancer of the anal canal. Dis Colon Rectum 17:354, 1974

53. Sischy B: The use of radiation therapy combined with chemotherapy in the management of squamous cell carcinoma of the anus and marginally resectable adenocarcinoma of the rectum. Int J Radiat Oncol Biol Phys 11:1587–1593, 1985

54. Cummings BJ, Keane T, Thomas G, Harwood A, Rider W: Results and toxicity of the treatment of anal canal carcinoma by radiation therapy or radiation therapy and chemotherapy. Cancer 54:2062, 1984

55. Enker WE, Heilwell M, Janov AJ, Quan SH, Magill G, Stearns MW Jr, Shank B, Leaming R, Sternberg SS: Improved survival in epidermoid carcinoma of the anus in association with preoperative multidisciplinary therapy. Arch Surg 121:1386–1390, 1986

56. Meeker WR, Sickle-Santanello BJ, Philpott G, Kenady D, Bland K, Hill GH, Popp MB: Combined chemotherapy, radiation, and surgery for epithelial cancer of the anal canal. Cancer 57:525–529, 1986

57. Khater R, Frenoy M, Bourry J, Milouo G, Namer M: Cisplatin plus 5-fluorouracil in the treatment of metastatic and squamous cell carcinoma: A report of 2 cases. Cancer Treat Rep 70:1345–1346, 1986

58. Stearns MW Jr, Quan SHQ: Epidermoid carcinoma of the anorectum. Surg Gynecol Obstet 131:953, 1970

59. Sugarbaker P, Gunderson L, Wittes R: Cancer of the anal region. In DeVita V, Hellman S, Rosenberg S (eds): Cancer: Principles and Practice of Oncology, pp 885–889. Philadelphia, JB Lippincott, 1985

60. Rifkind R: Differentiation inducers: Freeing cancer cells to mature. Adv Oncol 2:3, 1986

61. Porter CW, Janne J: Modulation of antineoplastic drug action by inhibitors of polyamine biosynthesis. In McCann PP, Pegg AE, Sjoerdsma A (eds): Inhibition of Polyamine Metabolism, pp 203–248. New York, Academic Press, 1987

62. Pegg AE: Polyamine metabolism and its importance in neoplastic growth and as a target for chemotherapy. Cancer Res 48:759–774, 1988

63. Pollard M, Luckert PH, Schmidt MA: The suppressive effect of piroxicam on autochthonous intestinal tumors in the rat. Cancer Letters 21:57–61, 1983

64. Waddell WR, Loughry RW: Sulindac for polyposis of the colon. J Surg Oncol 24:83–87, 1983

65. Braun DP, Harris JE: Modification of the effects of cytotoxic chemotherapy on the immune responses of cancer patients with a non-steroidal, anti-inflammatory drug, piroxicam (abstr). Proc Am Soc Clin Oncol 4:223, 1985

66. Butler TW, Gefter J, Kleto D, Shuck EH, Ruffner BW: Squamous-cell of the anus in condyloma acuminatum. Dis Colon Rectum 30:293–295, 1987

V. Craig Jordan

Long-term Tamoxifen Therapy for Breast Cancer

10

Introduction ■

Tamoxifen (ICI 46,474; Nolvadex) is a nonsteroidal antiestrogen[1,2] developed for the treatment of breast cancer.[3-6] Although the pharmacology of the antiestrogens is rather complex,[5,7] some general principles can be illustrated by a brief survey of the laboratory and clinical investigations with tamoxifen.[8]

Tamoxifen has a long biologic half-life (7 days); about 6 weeks of treatment at doses of 10 mg *b.i.d.* is necessary to reach a steady state plasma level. Tamoxifen is extensively metabolized; the principal metabolites found in serum are N-desmethyltamoxifen,[9] 4-hydroxytamoxifen,[10,11] and metabolite Y[12] (Fig. 10-1). These metabolites are antiestrogens in conventional laboratory assays,[12,13] so they probably contribute to the overall antitumor activity of tamoxifen.

There are very few reported side-effects with tamoxifen, which, along with its efficacy, has made it the front-line endocrine therapy in the treatment of advanced disease.[8] The changing approaches to the treatment of breast cancer including the concept of adjuvant therapy following mastectomy, resulted in the consideration of tamoxifen as a potential treatment agent.

This chapter describes the basic laboratory principles that led to the successful clinical testing of long-term adjuvant tamoxifen therapy. Future strategies to improve the encouraging early results from studies of long-term antiestrogen therapy are suggested.

The Biologic Basis of Long-term Antiestrogen Therapy ■

A variety of *in vivo* laboratory models have been used to support the development of clinical trials assessing the efficacy of long-term or indefinite tamoxifen ad-

juvant therapy in Stages I and II disease. Unfortunately, these models do not precisely replicate the clinical situation, but their results clearly demonstrate the advantages of extended therapy to suppress the appearance of palpable tumors. Tamoxifen can therefore be considered a chemosuppressive therapy.[14]

The laboratory evidence demonstrating the tumoristatic properties of tamoxifen is reviewed below, with examples from carcinogen-induced rat mammary tumor models, spontaneous mouse mammary tumors, and human breast tumors transplanted into athymic mice.[15]

Laboratory Models ■

DIMETHYLBENZANTHRACENE-INDUCED RAT MAMMARY CARCINOMA □

A single oral administration of dimethylbenzanthracene (DMBA; 20 mg in 2 ml peanut oil) to 50-day-old female Sprague Dawley rats results in the appearance of palpable mammary tumors after 50–150 days.[16] The biology and endocrinology of this animal model have been studied extensively.[17] Established tumors are hormone-dependent (predominantly prolactin) and respond to oophorectomy indirectly, by reducing estrogen-stimulated prolactin release (antiestrogens inhibit estrogen-stimulated prolactin release both *in vivo*[18] and *in vitro*[19]). Unfortunately, metastasis does not occur in this model, and a hormone-dependent model that precisely replicates adjuvant therapy is not available. Tamoxifen inhibits the initiation[20,21] and growth of DMBA-induced rat mammary tumors.[22-25] However, this design does not provide a model for the treatment of minimal disease. To create this situation, DMBA can produce microfoci of transformed cells in the mammary chains after several weeks of promotion by circulating hormones. Tamoxifen therapy (in different doses or different du-

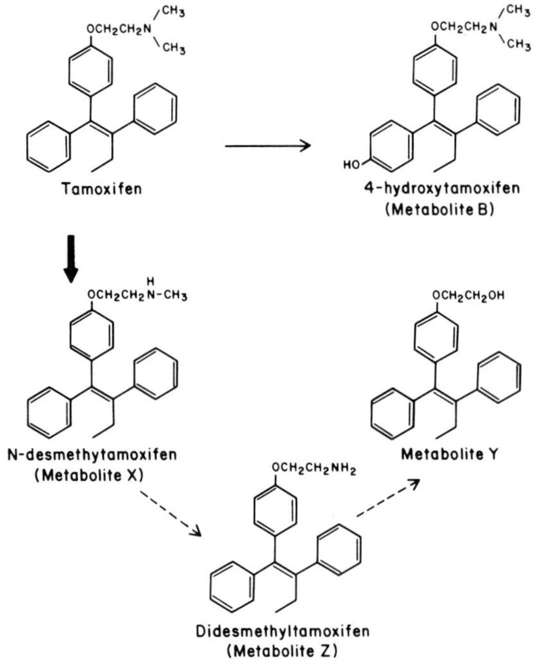

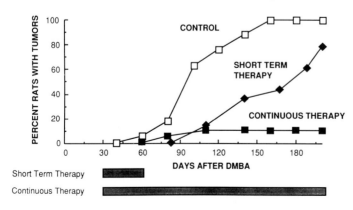

FIG. 10–1 The metabolism of tamoxifen in patients. N-Desmethyltamoxifen, the principal metabolite, is usually found at a serum concentration twice that of the parent. 4-Hydroxytamoxifen is a minor metabolite (usually <10% of the parent compound) but has a receptor binding affinity 25 times greater than tamoxifen's.

rations) can then be applied to determine whether the appearance of tumors can be prevented.[26–30]

Tamoxifen (12.5–800 μg/day), administered for a month (starting 1 month after DMBA), causes a dose-related decrease in the number of mammary tumors and a dose-related delay in the appearance of tumors.[27] However, all the animals eventually develop at least one tumor. In contrast, continuous treatment with tamoxifen prevents tumorigenesis,[28–30] although termination of therapy results in the appearance of

tumors.[31] Therefore, tamoxifen exhibits the properties of a tumoristatic agent in the DMBA-induced rat mammary carcinoma model. These principles are illustrated in Figure 10–2, where a short course of tamoxifen is compared with a continuous course of therapy.

N-NITROSOMETHYLUREA-INDUCED RAT MAMMARY CARCINOMA □

The N-nitrosomethylurea (NMU) model was originally believed to be metastatic,[32] but these reports have not been confirmed. Nevertheless, NMU-induced mammary tumors have been shown to be more directly dependent on estrogen for growth,[33] although a combination of pituitary and ovarian hormones is probably necessary to provide an optimal growth environment.

Administration of NMU to female rats, followed by the daily administration of tamoxifen for several weeks, results in a delay in the appearance of palpable mammary tumors.[34,35] In contrast, the continuous administration of tamoxifen completely suppresses the appearance of palpable tumors.[35,36] Cessation of therapy (even of large doses of tamoxifen) does, however, result in the appearance of mammary tumors in up to 50% of animals.[36]

SPONTANEOUS MOUSE MAMMARY TUMORS □

It has long been recognized that strains of mice can be bred that have a high incidence of mammary tumors. The tumor is transmitted via the mouse mammary tumor virus in the mother's milk, but development (or possibly promotion) of the tumors is regulated by the endocrine state of the host. Oophorectomy retards the development of tumors, whereas estrogen, pregnancy, or combinations of estrogen and progesterone cause an early development or increased

FIG. 10–2 Tumoristatic action of tamoxifen in the DMBA-induced rat mammary carcinoma model. The carcinogen (20 mg DMBA in 2 ml peanut oil) was administered orally to 50-day-old female Sprague Dawley rats. Short-term (50 μg/day SC for 1 month) or continuous (50 μg/day SC for the length of the experiment) tamoxifen therapy was started 30 days after DMBA. Control groups received injections of vehicle alone.

growth of tumors.[37–40] Short-term experiments have demonstrated the ability of tamoxifen to inhibit the steroid-hormone-stimulated growth of transplanted tumors[41,42]; however, long-term studies of tamoxifen's ability to prevent tumor development have not been reported. These experiments are currently under way in this laboratory. Early results in the model system show a decrease in the number of mammary tumors if tamoxifen is given continuously following a single pregnancy.

HETEROTRANSPLANTATION OF BREAST CANCER
CELL LINES INTO ATHYMIC MICE □

Primary breast tumors can be grown successfully in athymic (immune deficient) mice.[43] However, the "take rate" is often modest and hormone-dependent growth is difficult to demonstrate routinely, hindering efforts to establish a successful model for study in the laboratory.

In contrast, human breast cancer cell lines will grow into solid tumors following inoculation into the mammary fat in the axillary region of athymic mice. Estrogen receptor (ER)-negative lines grow without further treatment, whereas ER-positive lines only grow if the animals receive supplemental estrogen therapy.[44,45] Tamoxifen and its metabolites inhibit estrogen-stimulated growth of MCF-7 breast tumors.[46,47] However, tamoxifen does not appear to be tumoricidal; long-term treatment with tamoxifen alone does not destroy MCF-7 cells inoculated into athymic mice,[47,48] and therapy for up to 6 months does not prevent subsequent estrogen therapy from reactivating quiescent tumor cells (Fig. 10–3). Therefore, tamoxifen demonstrates the properties of a tumoristatic agent.

Summary of Laboratory Evidence for Tamoxifen as a Chemosuppressive Agent ■

Tamoxifen causes a reversible blockade in the G_1 phase of the breast cancer cell cycle.[49,50] The cumulative evidence from carcinogen-induced animal models *in vivo* suggests that continuous tamoxifen therapy is the best treatment strategy. However, there is recent evidence to demonstrate that ER-positive tumors grow in athymic mice despite long-term tamoxifen therapy.[51] Indeed, tamoxifen-dependent growth appears to occur with some tumors.[52–55] However, the facts that tamoxifen can exert estrogen-like effects in the mouse[56] and estrogens can reduce natural killer (NK) cell activity in mice suggest that these results should be viewed with caution. It is possible that the so-called antiestrogen can reduce the ability of athymic mice to mount any immunologic reaction to implanted cancer cells. We have recently reported that an ER-negative primary endometrial tumor can grow more rapidly in estrogen-treated athymic mice than in estrogen-deprived animals.[57] Perhaps future studies with human heterotransplants in athymic rats may show this to be a more effective model for human disease.

Adjuvant Monotherapy with Tamoxifen: Postmenopausal Patients ■

Several trials of tamoxifen monotherapy as an adjuvant to mastectomy were initiated toward the end of the 1970s. The major studies are summarized in Table 10–1. The study design compares tamoxifen therapy

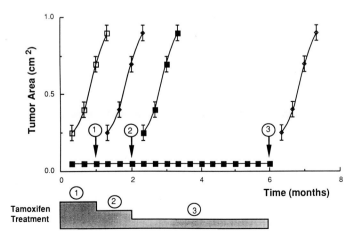

FIG. 10–3 The tumoristatic action of tamoxifen on MCF-7 breast cancer cells implanted into ovariectomized athymic mice (six per group). Sustained release preparations of tamoxifen (5 mg in cholesterol pellets; 4-week release) were implanted at monthly intervals to demonstrate tumoricidal action on breast cancer cells after various lengths of treatment. Estradiol therapy (1.7 mg in cholesterol pellets; 8-week release) was used to initiate tumor growth in remaining cells. Tumors grew after 1, 2, or 6 months of tamoxifen therapy. Each mouse was implanted with two MCF-7 tumors in the axillary region.

Table 10–1
Clinical Trials of Adjuvant Tamoxifen Therapy without Chemotherapy in Postmenopausal Patient Populations*

Group	Daily Dose (mg)	Duration (yr)	Increased DFS†	Increased Survival	Correlation with Receptor Status
Ludwig[58]	20	1	Yes	No	Yes
Christie[59,60]	20	1	Yes	No	Not done
NATO[61,62]	20	2	Yes	Yes	No
ECOG[63]	20	2	Yes	No	Not analyzed
Toronto[64]	30	2	Yes	No	Yes
Danish[65]	30	2	Yes	No	Yes
French[66]	40	3	Yes	Yes	Yes
Scottish[67]	20	≥5	Yes	Yes	Yes

* Some trials accepted premenopausal patients.

† Disease-free survival.

to a control arm, but only the Eastern Cooperative Oncology Group trial was designed as a double-blind placebo study. Most of the clinical trial experience is with postmenopausal patients with Stage II breast cancer. However, several trials include both premenopausal patients and patients with Stage I disease. This heterogeneity has the potential to dilute and confound analysis of the results.

Recently, Richard Peto of the University of Oxford has completed an overall analysis of the world literature on adjuvant therapy; such a review will not be attempted here. Two points, however, do merit mention in this short overview: duration of therapy, and the relationship of receptor status of the primary tumor to response to tamoxifen therapy.

Early trials with tamoxifen therapy were conservative, with only 1 year of therapy.[58,59] (Tamoxifen was then thought to be a tumoricidal agent.) The largest study of 2 years of tamoxifen therapy has been conducted by the Nolvadex Adjuvant Trial Organization (NATO) in Great Britain and New Zealand.[61,62] Only 46% of the entered patients (a mixture of pre- and postmenopausal patients with Stage I or II disease) had hormone receptor determinations, and these were assayed by different laboratories. This study is particularly important because it showed a survival advantage ($p = 0.0019$) for all patients receiving tamoxifen, regardless of receptor status. These data are substantially supported by the Scottish trial,[67] which also concluded that there is a steady improvement with tamoxifen treatment related to the receptor concentration of the primary tumor. The best disease-free survival is noted for those patients with ER values of over 100 fmol/mg cytosol protein. A controversial aspect of the Danish group's report[65] of 2-year tamoxifen adjuvant therapy is that, although patients with ER levels > 100 femtomol/mg cytosol protein

had an increased disease-free survival ($p < 0.01$), there was an apparent reversal of the effect when the assay showed levels of 10–99 fmol/mg cytosol protein.

All of the reported studies demonstrate an increase in disease-free interval for tamoxifen-treated women either overall or for some subgroup. Clearly, analyses of whether local versus distant recurrences are controlled by tamoxifen will mirror survival advantages. The available data are limited and also contradictory. The Christie[59,60] study reports (nonsignificantly) fewer distant recurrences, as does the ECOG study.[63] In contrast, the Ludwig group[58] found that the improvement was confined to a lower incidence of locoregional recurrences in the tamoxifen arm. The NATO[61] and Scottish[67] studies support both positions, with reductions in local and distant recurrences.

In conclusion, longer treatment regimens with adjuvant tamoxifen appear to provide more benefit than shorter (1 year) regimens. Not all trials support the position that ER-positive patients benefit from tamoxifen therapy. The NATO study does not provide a clear indication that receptor status is of relevance, although there has been criticism of these data based on the quality assurance of the assays and the fact that fewer than 50% of patients were evaluated.

Chemotherapy plus Tamoxifen: Extending Tamoxifen Therapy ■

In 1974, Hubay and coworkers[68] initiated a clinical trial of chemotherapy with cyclophosphamide, methotrexate, and 5-fluorouracil (CMF, low dose) versus chemotherapy plus tamoxifen (CMFT) versus CMFT plus Bacillus Calmette–Guerin (BCG) vaccinations. No control group could be justified in light of the encouraging data for the successful adjuvant therapy with CMF, so 312 Stage II pre- and postmenopausal patients were randomized to receive 1 year of treatment. Analysis of all the patients showed no benefit with the addition of tamoxifen. Nevertheless, subanalysis of the ER-positive patients approached significance ($p = 0.08$) for tamoxifen-treated groups and was significant in postmenopausal patients with four or more positive nodes ($p = 0.05$).

The Ludwig Breast Cancer Study Group[58] trial of 1 year of combination chemotherapy (CMF + prednisone) and tamoxifen in postmenopausal women showed a strong effect ($p < 0.0001$) for the adjuvant therapy on disease-free survival when compared to observation only.

The largest and most comprehensive analysis of adjuvant tamoxifen and chemotherapy has been conducted by the National Surgical Adjuvant Breast Project (NSABP),[70-72] in which 1890 patients with Stage II breast cancer (pre- and postmenopausal) have been randomized to combination chemotherapy with PF (L-phenylalanine mustard and 5-fluorouracil), with or without tamoxifen. The addition of tamoxifen to chemotherapy in premenopausal patients provides no additional benefit. This may not be too surprising, because chemotherapy is known to cause ovarian destruction,[73,74] so a maximal "endocrine" response may have already occurred. However, some patients appeared to show an adverse effect with the addition of tamoxifen. Patients with progesterone receptor (PgR)-negative tumors do less well ($p = 0.007$) when tamoxifen is added to chemotherapy. The reason for the ability of tamoxifen to negate the benefits of PF chemotherapy is unknown. A similar effect has not been observed with the CMF chemotherapy regimen.

An overall analysis of the NSABP trial (all entered patients) shows an increase in the disease-free survival for the tamoxifen-containing regimen ($p = 0.002$).

The benefit was observed entirely in the postmenopausal category. The response to tamoxifen is related to the nodal and steroid receptor status of the patients. Benefit with tamoxifen is noted in women over 50 years of age with steroid-receptor-positive tumors and four or more positive axillary nodes ($p < 0.001$).

The early laboratory data[29] indicate that long-term adjuvant tamoxifen therapy may provide additional benefit. There are indications from both the NATO and NSABP studies of 2-year tamoxifen therapy that benefit accrues only as long as tamoxifen is given. This raises the clinical question of how long tamoxifen should be given.

The first pilot clinical study of long-term tamoxifen therapy was initiated at the University of Wisconsin in 1977 by Tormey.[75] At the time this strategy was being considered, many patients with Stage II disease had already completed one year of adjuvant therapy with combination chemotherapy and tamoxifen. Because the data from the DMBA model showed tamoxifen to be tumoristatic, therapy with tamoxifen was continued initially for 5 years; subsequently, the decision was made to continue the drug indefinitely or until relapse.[76] The results of this study (Fig. 10–4) demonstrate the safety and potential efficacy of this treatment strategy.[75-78] Randomized trials are currently under way in the ECOG (EST 5181 and EST 4181) to test the efficacy of chemotherapy and tamoxifen adjuvant therapy followed by another 4 years of tamoxifen versus indefinite treatment (Fig. 10–5). The results are being prepared for publication.

The NSABP and the Stockholm trials group, have been persuaded by the laboratory evidence and developing clinical data to embark on long-term tamoxifen studies. The NSABP has recently reported[79] on a successive registration trial of Stage II breast cancer. Patients received chemotherapy (PF) and tamoxifen for 2 years, or the same regimen followed

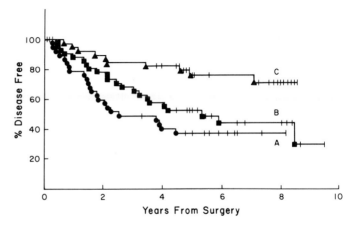

FIG. 10–4 Relapse-free survival for three adjuvant treatment groups: (A) combination chemotherapy only, 38 patients; (B) combination chemotherapy plus tamoxifen, 43 patients; (C) combination chemotherapy plus continuous tamoxifen therapy, 43 patients. Patients had a mean of 4 positive nodes; further patient information is contained in reference 75.

A

STRATIFICATION	STEP ONE	STEP TWO

Nodal Involvement

   1-3 postiive
   4-10 positive
   >10 positive

Estrogen Receptor Result

   Positive
   Negative

R A N D O M I Z E

R → CMFPT
   for 12 cycles

CMF(P)TH
   alternating with
   TˢAVᵇTH
   for 12 total cycles

R A N D O M I Z E

R → Observation

→ Continuous TAM
   to total of
   5 years

B

STRATIFICATION

Nodal Involvement

   1-3 postiive
   4-10 positive
   >10 positive

Estrogen Receptor Result

   Positive
   Negative

R A N D O M I Z E

→ CMFPT x 12 cycles +
   continuous TAM to a total of 5 years

→ CMFPT for 12 cycles + Observation

→ CMFPT x 4 cycles + Observation

FIG. 10-5 Schemas showing treatment in (*A*) ECOG study 5181 for premenopausal women, and (*B*) ECOG study 4181 for postmenopausal women. After completion of 5 years of tamoxifen therapy, there is subsequent randomization to stop tamoxifen or continue it indefinitely.

by an additional year of tamoxifen alone. The 3-year tamoxifen therapy seemed superior to 2 years. However, the study is not randomized, and only patients who have successfully completed 2 years of tamoxifen therapy are included for the third year.[80]

The Stockholm trial[81,82] is much more complex; a flow chart is presented in Figure 10-6. The postmenopausal patient population is a mixture of node-positive and node-negative patients. Node-positive patients receive either radiotherapy or chemotherapy, whereas the majority of node-negative patients received neither. All patients were subsequently randomized to 2 years of tamoxifen, 40 mg/day, or no endocrine therapy.

The interim analysis (53 months) is encouraging.[82] There is an increase in recurrence-free survival ($p < 0.01$), but not overall survival, for the tamoxifen-treated arm. Tamoxifen therapy was ineffective in ER-negative disease but very active in ER-positive disease.

A new extension trial was initiated in 1983 to randomize patients in the tamoxifen-treated arm who were disease-free at 2 years to either stop tamoxifen

or continue the drug for a further 3 years. Information concerning the efficacy of this strategy is not yet available.

Extended Tamoxifen Therapy Alone ■

In May 1978, Delozier and coworkers initiated a trial of tamoxifen (40 mg/day) for 3 years versus no further treatment.[66] The study population was 179 postmenopausal women. Overall survival at 5 years did not differ significantly, but in ER-positive patients, tamoxifen improved both disease-free and overall survival. Tamoxifen had no effect in ER-negative patients.

In April 1978, the Scottish Trials Office[67] (MRC) initiated a pilot clinical trial of tamoxifen versus no therapy in Stage I or II breast cancer. This successfully evolved to become a randomized trial with 1312 participants. A total of 1070 postmenopausal women were evaluated; almost half of these were Stage I (node negative) patients. Tamoxifen therapy (median = 5

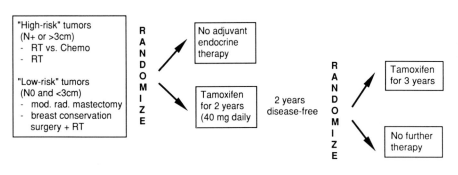

FIG. 10-6 Design of the Stockholm trial to determine the effectiveness of long-term tamoxifen therapy.

years) produced a survival advantage (hazard ratio = 0.61) for node-positive patients. This trial of adjuvant tamoxifen versus control and tamoxifen at first recurrence shows the benefit of early long-term adjuvant tamoxifen therapy alone. The fact that no chemotherapy was included in this evaluation brings into question the overall benefits of combined chemohormonal therapy. However, this direct comparison has not been undertaken in a randomized clinical trial.

Tamoxifen in Premenopausal Patients with Stage I Disease ■

The NATO[61] and Scottish Trials[67] groups both included significant numbers of Stage I patients, who were included in the overall analysis of the results. In the Scottish study, 242 premenopausal patients in the node-negative category were equally divided into tamoxifen versus observation. The encouraging result with tamoxifen (hazard ratio = 0.57) could not be reanalyzed by receptor status because of the small sample size.

In contrast, NSABP trial B14 has compared tamoxifen (for 5 or 10 years) versus placebo in women with Stage I disease and receptor-positive primary tumors. The trial has closed accrual and been found to favor the tamoxifen-treated arm. Publication of these data, and their subsequent examination, will obviously dictate future pattern of health care for breast cancer patients with Stage I disease.

Can We Improve the Effectiveness of Antiestrogen Therapy? ■

Tamoxifen can control the growth of Stage IV breast cancer in premenopausal patients,[83,84] and small clinical trials have demonstrated that tamoxifen and oophorectomy have similar efficacy.[85,86] However, patients who initially respond to tamoxifen therapy but later fail may subsequently respond to oophorectomy.[87–89] Although there is disagreement about the proportion of patients who subsequently respond to oophorectomy, there are clear indications that ovarian function can influence the disease.

Tamoxifen was initially used in premenopausal women to treat menometrorrhagia[90] and to induce ovulation in infertile women.[8] Subsequent evaluation of the endocrine effects of tamoxifen revealed an increase in ovarian estrogen production.[91] These findings have been confirmed by many groups of investigators.[83,92–97] Clearly, if tamoxifen is, as is believed,

a competitive inhibitor of estrogen action in the tumor cells, then removal of the ovaries may further enhance the effectiveness of the antiestrogen. Alternatively, the long-acting luteinizing-hormone-releasing-hormone (LHRH) agonist Zoladex could be used with tamoxifen to depress gonadotropin output and indirectly inhibit ovarian function.[98]

The nonsteroidal antiestrogens based on the triphenylethylene structure are not pure antagonists of estrogen action but weak estrogens in their own right. A spectrum of estrogen-like responses have been reported in animal systems[7] and in postmenopausal patients (see Table 10–2).[8] Indeed, tamoxifen and other antiestrogens, if used at low concentrations, can encourage breast cancer cell replication in vitro.[109,110] These data could argue for the use of higher doses of tamoxifen, but there are currently no consistent clinical data to support this position. However, higher daily doses of tamoxifen might avoid the serious fluctuation in tamoxifen serum levels that could occur with the sporadic or intermittent use of tamoxifen during long-term therapy.

Because tamoxifen is a known partial estrogen agonist, efforts are currently under way to develop additional nonestrogenic agents for clinical testing. A truly nonestrogenic agent might completely inhibit the production of stimulatory growth factors that could encourage cell replication through autocrine or paracrine mechanisms. Lippman's group[111] has developed the intriguing hypothesis that an antiestrogen can increase the induction of transforming growth factor beta, which could not only stop cell replication by an autocrine route but also regulate hormone-receptor-negative cells by a paracrine influence (Fig.

Table 10–2
Endocrine Effects of Tamoxifen in Postmenopausal Women

Effect	Change	Ref.
LH	Partial decrease	77, 99
FSH	Partial decrease	77, 99
Prolactin	Decrease	100
Vaginal cytology	Early estrogen-like stimulation	101, 102
Sex hormone binding globulin	Increase	78, 103, 104
Antithrombin III	Small decrease	78, 105
Estrogen-regulated serum protein	Increase	106
Uterine progesterone receptor	Early estrogen-like increase	107
Serum lipoproteins	Varied	108

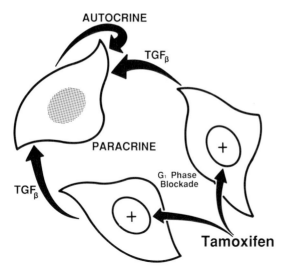

FIG. 10–7 A hypothetic model whereby ER-positive cells (+) can influence the replication of ER-negative cells. Tamoxifen may cause the release of TGF-β, which prevents cell replication by a paracrine mechanism.

10–7). Although no data have been offered from *in vivo* studies, a pure antiestrogen would seem to provide the best hope to validate the hypothesis.

The recent finding by Wakeling and Bowler[112] that the 7α substitution of estradiol with an amine-containing hydrocarbon side-chain can produce a pure antiestrogen (Fig. 10–8) has opened the door to the possibility of developing a clinically useful agent (perhaps a nonsteroidal compound, to avoid the problems of reduced oral activity often seen with steroids). We have successfully tested several compounds that inhibit tamoxifen-dependent breast and endometrial tumor growth in athymic mice.

FIG. 10–8 Formula of the nonestrogenic antiestrogen ICI 164,384.

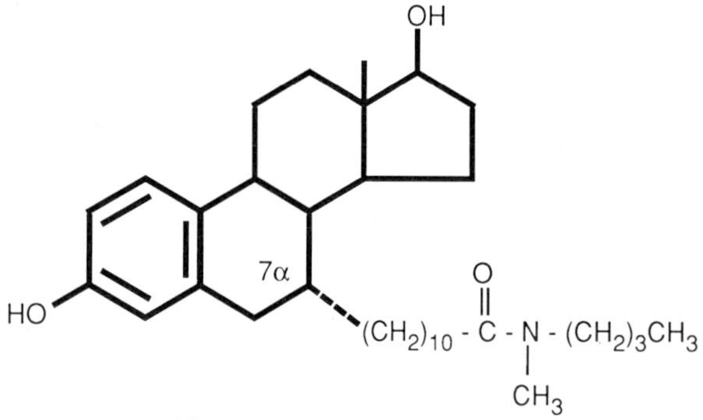

OH

HO

7α

$(CH_2)_{10} - \overset{\overset{\textstyle O}{\|}}{C} - \underset{\underset{\textstyle CH_3}{|}}{N} - (CH_2)_3CH_3$

ICI 164,384

Long-term Toxicology and Future Investigations ■

The clinical evaluation of long-term adjuvant tamoxifen therapy is nearing completion. The laboratory concept has been successfully transferred to the clinic, but several toxicologic questions need to be addressed. Obviously, the most important issue in the treatment of Stage II disease is efficacy; long-term toxicologic concerns are really secondary. However, there will be increasing numbers of women with Stage I disease (perhaps 50,000 women per year scheduled for at least 10 years of therapy) who are at a low risk for recurrence. This raises questions about the potential long-term side effects of decades of tamoxifen therapy for women in their late 20s and early 30s. In fact, there is currently an international debate about the wisdom of attempting to select women at high risk for breast cancer for efforts to prevent the appearance of the disease.[14,113] This idea is not new. Lacassagne[114] presented a paper entitled "Hormonal Pathogenesis of Adenocarcinoma of the Breast" to the American Association for Cancer Research on April 7, 1936. His work provided the link between hormones and the development of mouse mammary cancer. He concluded that if one concedes that breast cancer is the consequence of a special hereditary sensitivity to the proliferative action of estrone, then one might imagine the development of an antagonistic therapy. Fifty years later, tamoxifen is being considered as a candidate therapy.

The timing of the carcinogenic insult in breast cancer (unlike that in the DMBA-induced rat mammary carcinoma model[21]) is unknown, so a true preventive intervention strategy with tamoxifen seems impractical. Chemosuppression,[15] however, appears possible. With this approach, the carcinogenic insult would have occurred at some earlier time in the target population, but continuous tamoxifen therapy would suppress the development of the disease. In any event, whether Stage I breast cancer patients or "high-risk" women are to be treated, three major toxicologic issues should be addressed.

As mentioned previously, tamoxifen has a dramatic effect on the endocrine system in premenopausal women. There are elevations in circulating estradiol and follicle-stimulating hormone (FSH). The midcycle peak of luteinizing hormone (LH) indicates that ovulation occurs in menstruating patients during long-term tamoxifen therapy, and this is confirmed by the increase in circulating progesterone during the second half of the cycle. The circulating hormone profiles of women who continue to menstruate during tamoxifen therapy are shown in Figure 10–9.

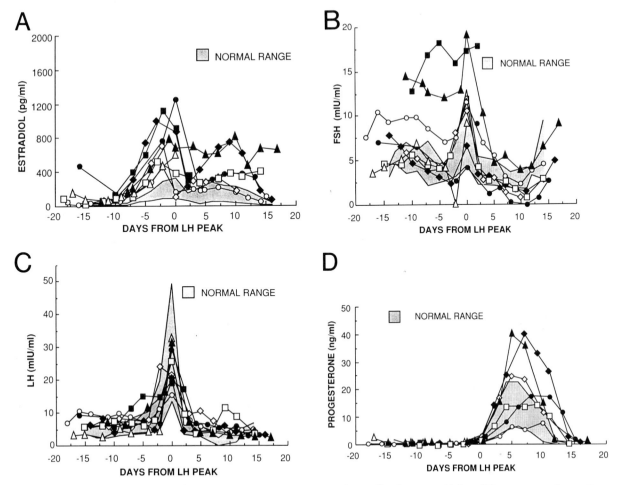

FIG. 10-9   The effect of adjuvant tamoxifen therapy (alone) on the endocrine profile of women with Stage II breast cancer who continue to menstruate. (*A*) Estradiol-17β (E$_2$). (*B*) Follicle-stimulating hormone (FSH). (*C*) Luteinizing hormone (LH). (*D*) Progesterone. *Shaded areas* are the limits of the hormone levels of 12 normal women. Blood was drawn three times weekly.

There is currently no information on the effects of long-term tamoxifen on the pathophysiology of the ovaries or on the drug's teratogenic potential in primates. Clearly, the participants in large long-term tamoxifen trials must be carefully counselled about contraception, or the physician and patient may be confronted with the moral issues of abortion.

These issues could be resolved if a large population of postmenopausal women were evaluated. However, estrogen appears to be physiologically important in maintaining bone density and preventing the development of atherosclerosis. One could therefore take the position that long-term antiestrogen therapy might not be beneficial.

We are currently studying these problems at the University of Wisconsin Clinical Cancer Center in the Wisconsin Tamoxifen Study (study coordinator,

Richard R. Love, M.D.). Postmenopausal patients with Stage I disease are being randomized to a two-arm study: tamoxifen, 10 mg *b.i.d.,* or placebo for 2 years (Fig. 10–10). Periodic bone density measurements and blood lipid analyses will determine the action of tamoxifen on these parameters. The study is double-blind, but the endocrine status of the postmenopausal women is being determined to study the effect of tamoxifen and to ensure that patients are truly postmenopausal. Compliance is established by the measurement of tamoxifen and metabolites.

We are optimistic that although tamoxifen is classified as an antiestrogen that controls estrogen-stimulated breast cancer growth, there may be sufficient estrogenic activity inherent in the molecule (see Table 10–2) to facilitate other estrogenic processes. Studies in intact rats demonstrate that antiestrogens do not

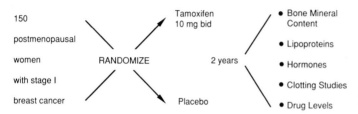

FIG. 10–10 Design of the Wisconsin study to evaluate the clinical toxicology of tamoxifen.

cause an oophorectomy-like decrease in bone density and that tamoxifen may in fact help to maintain bone density in oophorectomized rats.[115,116] As shown in Figure 10–11, tamoxifen plus estradiol produces an additive effect on bone density, but tamoxifen inhibits estradiol-stimulated uterine weight. This result reinforces the hypothesis that tamoxifen can produce a target-site-specific effect. Thus far, there are very few data concerning the effects of tamoxifen on bone density in patients. One preliminary report[117] of at least 2 years of adjuvant tamoxifen therapy in Stage II breast cancer has shown that patients receiving the antiestrogen do not suffer deleterious effects compared to those not receiving the drug.

Studies of the effects of tamoxifen on blood lipids have not been routinely reported. One report suggests that tamoxifen can produce an estrogen-like serum lipid profile.[108] This would obviously be beneficial during long-term tamoxifen therapy.

Conclusion ■

The successful evaluation of tamoxifen as an antiestrogenic therapy for advanced breast cancer in the 1970s has resulted in the drug's availability in more than 110 countries around the world. Currently, the drug development process is focusing attention on

long-term adjuvant therapy and the future prospect of chemosuppression in women at risk for the disease. Progress at this stage, however, must be cautious. Trials conducted in patients with Stage I disease will include a proportion of women who might never have a recurrence. At this point, the risk is justified because the toxicity of tamoxifen is low and disease recurrence is very difficult or impossible to control. Future studies in a high risk population must be carefully weighed to ensure that the toxicologic risks do not exceed the potential benefits.

The pharmacology of tamoxifen seems to be a balance of estrogenic and antiestrogenic effects. Long treatment regimens, even in postmenopausal women, must be carefully monitored. Uterine tissue should be examined to ensure that excessive stimulation does not occur. We have recently found that in mice, where short-term tamoxifen therapy produces estrogenic effects on the uterus, continuous therapy for several months produces a profound antiestrogenic effect. It is not yet known whether a similar effect occurs in the human uterus. This is particularly important in light of the recent report that a human uterine carcinoma transplanted into athymic mice grew rapidly during tamoxifen therapy.[55] Physicians should be vigilant to ensure that occult endometrial carcinoma growth does not occur during long-term tamoxifen adjuvant therapy for breast cancer.

The past two decades have witnessed the introduc-

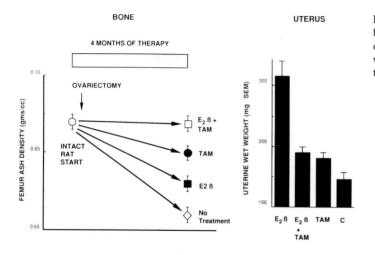

FIG. 10–11 The effect of oral tamoxifen, estradiol benzoate, or the combination on the bone density of ovariectomized rats after 4 months of therapy. Uterine wet weights were taken to illustrate the effectiveness of the respective agents.

tion and development of antiestrogens as a powerful new class of nontoxic drugs for the treatment of breast cancer. The close link between laboratory and clinical investigations has facilitated successful drug development. Tamoxifen is currently the agent of choice for the endocrine treatment of breast cancer. Future studies of long-term adjuvant therapy will seek to improve the efficacy of the drug in individual patients by optimizing a low-estrogen environment. The prospect of extensive chemosuppressive (preventive) trials would be facilitated by a precise study of tamoxifen's clinical toxicology. However, identification of target populations for chemosuppressive trials may be controversial, and the population selected may be too specific to have an overall impact on the incidence of breast cancer. As a final proposition, it may be that the ultimate focus of research should be shifted to consider use of tamoxifen-like molecules to treat osteoporosis or to alter blood lipids to protect from atherosclerosis. The general introduction of new therapeutic agents to treat these conditions in women may ultimately result in chemosuppression of occult breast cancer as a "side-effect" of the primary treatment.

The author thanks Douglass C. Tormey, M.D., Ph.D., and Richard R. Love, M.D., for collaborating in the clinical evaluation of tamoxifen, and Karen Blomstrom for typing the manuscript. Marco M. Gottardis performed the studies in athymic animals and Nancy F. Fritz conducted the radioimmunoassays on patient serum. Studies were supported by grants CA-14520 and CA-20432 from the National Institutes of Health.

References ∎

1. Harper MJK, Walpole AL: Contrasting endocrine activities of cis and trans isomers in a series of substituted triphenylethylenes. Nature 212:87, 1966
2. Harper MJK, Walpole AL: A new derivative of triphenylethylene: Effect on implantation and mode of action in rats. J Reprod Fertil 13:101–119, 1967
3. Cole MP, Jones CTA, Todd IDH: A new antioestrogenic agent in late breast cancer. An early clinical appraisal of ICI 46,474. Br J Cancer 25:270–275, 1971
4. Ward HWC: Antioestrogen therapy for breast cancer: A trial of tamoxifen at two dose levels. Br Med J 1:13–14, 1973
5. Jordan VC (ed): Estrogen/Antiestrogen Action and Breast Cancer Therapy. Madison, University of Wisconsin Press, 1986
6. Jordan VC: The development of tamoxifen for breast cancer therapy: A tribute to the late Arthur L. Walpole. Breast Cancer Res Treat 11:197–209, 1988
7. Jordan VC: Biochemical pharmacology of antiestrogen action. Pharmacol Rev 36:245–276, 1984
8. Furr BJA, Jordan VC: The pharmacology and clinical uses of tamoxifen. Pharmacol Ther 25:127–205, 1984
9. Adam HK, Douglas EJ, Kemp JV: The metabolism of tamoxifen in humans. Biochem Pharmacol 27:145–147, 1979
10. Daniel CP, Gaskell SJ, Bishop H, Nicholson RI: Determination of tamoxifen and an hydroxylated metabolite in plasma from patients with advanced breast cancer using gas chromatography-mass spectrometry. J Endocrinol 83:401–408, 1979
11. Jordan VC, Collins MM, Rowsby L, Prestwich G: A monohydroxylated metabolite of tamoxifen with potent antioestrogenic activity. J Endocrinol 75:305–316, 1977
12. Jordan VC, Bain RR, Brown RR, Gosden B, Santos MA: Determination and pharmacology of a new hydroxylated metabolite of tamoxifen observed in patient sera during therapy for advanced breast cancer. Cancer Res 43:1446–1450, 1983
13. Kemp JV, Adam HK, Wakeling AE, Slater R: Identification and biological activity of tamoxifen metabolites in human serum. Biochem Pharmacol 32:2045–2052, 1983
14. Jordan VC: Tamoxifen prophylaxis: Prevention is better than cure—Prevention is cure. In Cavalli F (ed): Endocrine Therapy of Breast Cancer: Strategies and Future Directions, pp 117–120. Heidelberg, Springer-Verlag, 1986
15. Jordan VC: Chemosuppression of breast cancer with tamoxifen—Laboratory evidence and future clinical investigation. Cancer Invest (in press)
16. Huggins C, Grand LC, Brillantes FB: Mammary cancer induced by a single feeding of polynuclear hydrocarbons and its suppression. Nature 189:204–207, 1961
17. Welsch CW: Host factors affecting the growth of carcinogen-induced rat mammary carcinomas: A review and tribute to Charles Brenton Huggins. Cancer Res 45:3415–3443, 1985
18. Jordan VC, Koerner S, Robison C: Inhibition of oestrogen-stimulated prolactin release by antioestrogens. J Endocrinol 65:151–152, 1975
19. Jordan VC, Koch R, Langan S, McCague R: Ligand interaction at the estrogen receptor to program antiestrogen action: A study with nonsteroidal compounds in vitro. Endocrinology 122:1449–1454, 1988
20. Jordan VC: Antitumour activity of the antioestrogen ICI 46,474 (tamoxifen) in the dimethylbenzanthracene (DMBA)-induced rat mammary carcinoma model. J Steroid Biochem 5:354, 1974
21. Jordan VC: Effect of tamoxifen (ICI 46,474) on initiation and growth of DMBA-induced rat mammary carcinoma. Eur J Cancer 12:419–424, 1976
22. Nicholson RI, Golder MP: The effect of synthetic antioestrogens on the growth and biochemistry of rat mammary tumours. Eur J Cancer 11:571–579, 1975
23. Jordan VC, Dowse LJ: Tamoxifen as an antitumour agent: Effect on oestrogen binding. J Endocrinol 68:297–303, 1976
24. Jordan VC, Koerner S: Tamoxifen as an antitumour agent: Role of oestradiol and prolactin. J Endocrinol 68:305–311, 1976
25. Jordan VC, Jaspan T: Tamoxifen as an antitumour agent: Oestrogen binding as a predictive test for tumour response. J Endocrinol 68:453–460, 1976
26. Jordan VC: Use of the DMBA-induced rat mammary carcinoma system for the evaluation of tamoxifen as a potential adjuvant therapy. In Reviews on Endocrine-Related Cancer, pp 49–55. Macclesfield, Cheshire, England, ICI Pharmaceuticals Division, 1978
27. Jordan VC, Dix CJ, Allen KE: The effectiveness of long-term tamoxifen treatment in a laboratory model for adjuvant hormone therapy of breast cancer. In Salmon SE, Jones SE (eds): Adjuvant Therapy of Cancer II, pp 19–26. New York, Grune & Stratton, 1979
28. Jordan VC, Allen KE, Dix CJ: The pharmacology of tamoxifen in laboratory animals. Cancer Treat Rep 64:745–759, 1980
29. Jordan VC, Allen KE: Evaluation of the antitumour activity of the nonsteroidal antiestrogen monohydroxytamoxifen in

the DMBA-induced rat mammary carcinoma model. Eur J Cancer 16:239–251, 1980

30. Jordan VC: Laboratory studies to develop general principles for the adjuvant treatment of breast cancer with antiestrogens: Problems and potential for future clinical applications. Breast Cancer Res Treat 3(Suppl):73–86, 1983

31. Robinson SP, Jordan VC: Reversal of the antitumor effects of tamoxifen by progesterone in the 7,12 dimethylbenzanthracene-induced rat mammary carcinoma model. Cancer Res 47:5386–5390, 1987

32. Gullino PM, Pettigrew HM, Grantham FH: N-Nitrosomethylurea as a mammary carcinogen in rats. JNCI 54:401–414, 1975

33. Arafah BM, Finegan HM, Roe J, Pearson OH: Hormone dependency in N-nitrosomethylurea induced rat mammary tumors. Endocrinology 101:666–671, 1982

34. Wilson AJ, Tehrani F, Baum M: Adjuvant tamoxifen therapy for early breast cancer: An experimental study with reference to oestrogen and progesterone receptors. Br J Surg 69:121–125, 1982

35. Jordan VC, Mirecki D, Gottardis MM: Continuous tamoxifen therapy prevents the appearance of mammary tumors in a laboratory model of adjuvant therapy. In Salmon SE, Jones SE (eds): Adjuvant Therapy of Cancer IV, pp 27–33. New York, Grune & Stratton, 1984

36. Gottardis MM, Jordan VC: The antitumor actions of keoxifene and tamoxifen in the N-nitrosomethylurea-induced rat mammary carcinoma model. Cancer Res 47:4020–4024, 1987

37. Lathrop AEC, Loeb L: Further investigations on the origin of tumors in mice III on the part played by internal secretion in the spontaneous development of tumors. J Cancer Res 1:1–19, 1916

38. Foulds L: Mammary tumours in hybrid mice: Growth and progression of spontaneous tumours. Br J Cancer 3:345–375, 1946

39. Van Nie R, Thung PJ: Responsiveness of mouse mammary tumors to pregnancy. Eur J Cancer 1:41–50, 1965

40. Matsuzawa A, Yamamoto T: Response of a pregnancy-dependent mouse mammary tumor to hormones. JNCI 55:447–453, 1975

41. Sluyser M, Evers SG, DeGoeij CCJ: Effect of monohydroxytamoxifen on mouse mammary tumors. Eur J Cancer 17:1063–1065, 1981

42. Matsuzawa A, Mizuno Y, Yamamoto T: Antitumor effect of the antiestrogen, tamoxifen, or a pregnancy dependent mouse mammary tumor (TPDMT-4). Cancer Res 41:316–324, 1981

43. Giovanella BC, Stehlin JS, Williams LJ, Lee S, Shepard R: Heterotransplantation of human cancer into "nude" mice: A model system for human cancer therapy. Cancer 42:2269–2281, 1978

44. Soule HD, McGrath CM: Estrogen responsive proliferation of clonal human breast carcinoma cells in athymic mice. Cancer Lett 10:177–189, 1980

45. Shafie SM, Grantham FH: Role of hormones in the growth and regression of human breast cancer cells (MCF-7) transplanted into athymic mice. JNCI 67:51–56, 1981

46. Osborne CK, Hobbs FK, Clark GM: Effect of estrogens and antiestrogens on growth of human breast cancer cells in athymic nude mice. Cancer Res 45:584–590, 1985

47. Gottardis MM, Robinson SP, Jordan VC: Estradiol-stimulated growth of MCF-7 tumors implanted in athymic mice: A model to study the tumoristatic action of tamoxifen. J Steroid Biochem 29:57–60, 1988

48. Gottardis MM, Martin MK, Jordan VC: Long-term tamoxifen therapy to control transplanted human breast tumor growth

in athymic mice. In Salmon SE (ed): Adjuvant Therapy of Cancer V, pp 447–454. New York, Grune & Stratton, 1987

49. Osborne CK, Boldt DH, Clark GM, Trent JM: Effects of tamoxifen on human breast cancer cell cycle kinetics: Accumulation of cells in early G_1 phase. Cancer Res 43:3583–3585, 1983

50. Sutherland RL, Reddel RR, Green MD: Effect of oestrogens on cell proliferation and cell cycle kinetics: A hypothesis on the cell cycle effects of antioestrogen. Eur J Cancer Clin Oncol 19:307–318, 1983

51. Osborne CK, Conarado EB, Robinson JP: Human breast cancer in the athymic nude mouse: Cytostatic effects of long-term antiestrogen therapy. Eur J Cancer Clin Oncol 23:1189–1196, 1987

52. Satyaswaroop PB, Zaino RJ, Mortel R: Estrogen-like effects of tamoxifen on human endometrial carcinoma transplanted into nude mice. Cancer Res 44:4006–4010, 1984

53. Gottardis MM, Jordan VC: Long-term tamoxifen treatment of athymic mice implanted with MCF-7 breast cancer cells: Critical importance of tumor burden. Breast Cancer Res Treat 10:85, 1987

54. Gottardis MM, Jordan VC: Development of tamoxifen-stimulated growth of MCF-7 tumors in athymic mice after long-term antiestrogen administration. Cancer Res 48:5183–5187, 1988

55. Gottardis MM, Robinson SP, Satyaswaroop PG, Jordan VC: Contrasting actions of tamoxifen on endometrial and breast tumor growth in the athymic mouse. Cancer Res 48:812–815, 1988

56. Jordan VC, Robinson SP: Species specific pharmacology of antiestrogens: Role of metabolism. Fed Proc 46:1870–1874, 1987

57. Friedl A, Gottardis MM, Buchler D, Jordan VC: Growth of estrogen receptor negative human endometrial adenocarcinoma in athymic mice—Stimulation by estradiol or tamoxifen. Proceedings of the Endocrinology Society, abstract 1317, 1988

58. Ludwig Breast Cancer Group: Randomized trial of chemo-endocrine therapy, endocrine therapy and mastectomy alone in postmenopausal patients with operable breast cancer and axillary node metastases. Lancet 1:1256–1260, 1984

59. Ribeiro G, Palmer MK: Adjuvant tamoxifen for operable carcinoma of the breast: Report of a clinical trial by the Christie Hospital and Holt Radium Institute. Br Med J 286:827–830, 1983

60. Ribeiro G, Swindell R: The Christie Hospital tamoxifen (Nolvadex) adjuvant trial for operable breast carcinoma—Seven year results. Eur J Cancer Clin Oncol 21:897–900, 1985

61. Baum M, and other members of the Nolvadex Adjuvant Trial Organization. Controlled trial of tamoxifen adjuvant agent in management of early breast cancer. Lancet 1:257–261, 1983

62. Baum M, and other members of the Nolvadex Adjuvant Trial Organization. Controlled trial of tamoxifen as single adjuvant agent in the management of early breast cancer. Lancet 1:836–840, 1985

63. Cummings FJ, Gray R, Davis TE, Tormey DC, Harris JE, Falkson G, Arsenau J: Adjuvant tamoxifen treatment of elderly women with stage II breast cancer. Ann Intern Med 103:324–329, 1985

64. Pritchard KI, Meakin JW, Boyd NF, Ambus K, DeBoer G, Dembo AJ, Paterson AHG, Sutherland DJA, Wilkinson RH, Bassett AA, Evan WK, Beale FA, Clark RM, Keane TJ: A randomized trial of adjuvant tamoxifen in postmenopausal women with axillary node positive breast cancer. In Jones SE, Salmon SE (eds): Adjuvant Therapy of Breast Cancer IV, pp 339–348. New York, Grune & Stratton, 1984

65. Rose C, Thorpe SM, Anderson KW, Pedersen BV, Mouridsen HT, Blicher-Toft M, Rasmussens BB: Beneficial effect of adjuvant tamoxifen therapy in primary breast cancer patients with high oestrogen receptor values. Lancet 1:16–19, 1985

66. Delozier T, Julien J-P, Juret P, Veynet C, Couette J-E, Grai Y, Olliver J-M, deRanieri E: Adjuvant tamoxifen in postmenopausal breast cancer: Preliminary results of a randomized trial. Breast Cancer Res Treat 7:105–110, 1986

67. Breast Cancer Trials Committee, Scottish Cancer Trials Office. Adjuvant tamoxifen in the management of operable breast cancer: The Scottish trial. Lancet 2:171–175, 1987

68. Hubay CA, Gordon NH, Crowe JP, Gayton SP, Pearson OH, Marshall JS, Mansour EG, Herman RE, Jones JC, Flynn WJ, Eckert C, Sparzo RW, McGuire WL, Evans D, and twenty-four participating investigators: Antiestrogen cytotoxic chemotherapy and bacillus Calmet-Guerin vaccination in stage II breast cancer: Seventy-two month follow-up. Surgery 96:61–72, 1984

69. Bonadonna G, Brusamolino E, Valagussa P, Rossi A, Brugnatelli L, Brombilla C, DeLena M, Tancini G, Bajetta E, Musumerci R, Veronesi U: Combination chemotherapy as an adjuvant treatment in operative breast cancer. N Engl J Med 294:405–410, 1976

70. Fisher B, Redmond C, Brown A, Wolmark N, Wittliff JL, Fisher ER, Plotkin D, Sachs S, Wolter J, Frelick R, Desser R, LiCalzi N, Geggie P, Campbell T, Elias EG, Prager D, Koontz P, Volk H, Dimitrov N, Gardner B, Lerner H, Shibata H, and other NSABP investigators: Treatment of primary breast cancer with chemotherapy and tamoxifen. N Engl J Med 305:1–6, 1981

71. Fisher B, Redmond C, Brown A, Wickerham DL, Wolmark N, Allegra J, Escher G, Lippman ME, Savlov E, Wittliff JL, Fisher ER, and other NSABP investigators: Influences of tumor estrogen and progesterone receptor levels on the responses to tamoxifen and chemotherapy in primary breast cancer. J Clin Oncol 1:227–241, 1983

72. Fisher B, Redmond C, Brown A, Fisher ER, Wolmark N, Bowman D, Plotkin D, Wolter J, Bornstein R, Legault-Poisson S, Saffer EA, and other NSABP investigators: Adjuvant chemotherapy with and without tamoxifen in the treatment of primary breast cancer: 5 year results from the National Surgical Adjuvant Breast and Bowel Project Trial. J Clin Oncol 4:459–471, 1986

73. Rose DP, Davis TE: Ovarian function in patients receiving adjuvant chemotherapy for breast cancer. Lancet 1:1174–1176, 1977

74. Samaan NA, deAsis DN, Buzdar AU, Blumenschein GR: Pituitary ovarian function in breast cancer patients on adjuvant chemoimmunotherapy. Cancer 41:2084–2087, 1978

75. Tormey DC, Jordan VC: Long-term tamoxifen adjuvant therapy is node-positive breast cancer: A metabolic and pilot clinical study. Breast Cancer Res Treat 4:297–302, 1984

76. Tormey DC, Rasmussen P, Jordan VC: Long-term adjuvant tamoxifen study: clinical update. Breast Cancer Res Treat 9:157–158, 1987

77. Jordan VC, Fritz NF, Tormey DC: Endocrine effects of adjuvant chemotherapy and long-term tamoxifen administration on node positive patients with breast cancer. Cancer Res 47:624–630, 1987

78. Jordan VC, Fritz NF, Tormey DC: Long-term adjuvant therapy with tamoxifen: effects on sex hormone binding globulin and antithrombin III. Cancer Res 47:4517–4519, 1987

79. Fisher B, Brown A, Wolmark N, Redmond C, Wickerman DL, Wittliff JL, Dimitrov N, Legault-Poisson S, Schipper H, Prager D, and other NSABP investigators: Prolonging tamoxifen therapy for primary breast cancer. Ann Intern Med 106:649–654, 1987

80. Tormey DC: Long-term adjuvant therapy with tamoxifen in breast cancer: How long is long? Ann Intern Med 106:762–764, 1987

81. Wallgren A, Baral E, Carstensen J, Friberg S, Glas U, Hjalmar M-L, Kaigas M, Nordenskjöld B, Skoog L, Theve N-O, Wilking N: Should adjuvant tamoxifen be given for several years in breast cancer? In Jones SE, Salmon SE (eds): Adjuvant Therapy of Cancer IV, pp 331–337. New York, Grune & Stratton, 1984

82. Rutqvist LE, Cedermark B, Glas U, Johansson H, Nordenskjöld B, Skoog L, Somell A, Theve T, Friberg S, Askergrekn J: The Stockholm trial on adjuvant tamoxifen in early breast cancer. Breast Cancer Res Treat 10:255–266, 1987

83. Manni A, Trujillo JE, Marshall JS, Brodskey J, Pearson OH: Antihormone treatment of stage IV breast cancer. Cancer 43:444–450, 1979

84. Pritchard KI, Thomson DM, Meyers RE, Sutherland DJA, Mobbs BG, Meakin JW: Tamoxifen therapy in premenopausal patients with metastatic breast cancer. Cancer Treat Rep 64:787–796, 1980

85. Ingle JN, Krook JE, Green SJ, Kubista TP, Everson LK, Ahman DL, Chang MN, Bisel HF, Windschild HE, Twito DI, Pfeifle DM: Randomized trial of bilateral oophorectomy versus tamoxifen in premenopausal women with metastatic breast cancer. J Clin Oncol 4:178–185, 1986

86. Buchanan RB, Blamey RW, Durrant KR, Howell A, Paterson AG, Preece PE, Smith DC, Williams CJ, Wilson RG: A randomized comparison of tamoxifen with surgical oophorectomy in premenopausal patients with advanced breast cancer. J Clin Oncol 4:1326–1330, 1986

87. Kalman AM, Thompson T, Vogel CL: Response to oophorectomy after tamoxifen failure in a premenopausal patient. Cancer Treat Rep 66:1867–1868, 1982

88. Planting AST, Alexiera-Figusch J, Blank-Wijst J, VanPatten WLJ: Tamoxifen therapy in premenopausal women with metastatic breast cancer. Cancer Treat Rep 69:363–368, 1985

89. Sawka CA, Pritchard KI, Paterson DJA, Thomson DB, Skelley WE, Myers RE, Mobbs BG, Malkin A, Meakin JW: Role and mechanism of action of tamoxifen in premenopausal women with metastatic breast cancer. Cancer Res 46:3152–3156, 1986

90. El-Sheikha Z, Klopper A, Beck JS: Treatment of menometrorrhagia with an antioestrogen. Clin Endocrinol 1:275–282, 1972

91. Groom GV, Griffiths K: Effect of the antioestrogen tamoxifen on plasma levels of luteinizing hormone, follicle-stimulating hormone, prolactin, oestradiol and progesterone in normal premenopausal women. J Endocrinol 70:421–428, 1976

92. Senior BE, Cawood ML, Oakey RE, McKiddie JM, Siddle DR: A comparison of the effects of clomiphene and tamoxifen treatment on the concentrations of oestradiol and progesterone in the peripheral plasma of infertile women. Clin Endocrinol 8:381–389, 1978

93. Sherman BM, Chapler FK, Crickard K, Wycoff D: Endocrine consequences of continuous antioestrogen therapy with tamoxifen in premenopausal women. J Clin Invest 64:398–404, 1979

94. Rose DP, Davis TE: Effects of adjuvant chemohormonal therapy on the ovarian and adrenal function of breast cancer patients. Cancer Res 40:4043–4047, 1980

95. Tajuma C, Fukushima T: Endocrine profiles in tamoxifen-induced ovulatory cycles. Fertil Steril 40:23–27, 1983

96. Dristrian AM, Greenberg EJ, Dillan HJ, Hakes TB, Fracchia AA, Schwartz MK: Chemohormonal therapy and endocrine function in breast cancer patients. Cancer 56:63–70, 1985

97. Ravdin PM, Fritz NF, Tormey DC, Jordan VC: Endocrine status of premenopausal node-positive breast cancer patients following adjuvant chemotherapy and long-term tamoxifen. Cancer Res 48:1026–1029, 1988

98. Nicholson RI, Walker KJ, Turkes AD, Dyas J, Blamey RW, Cambell FC, Robinson MRG, Griffiths K: Therapeutic significance and the mechanism of action of the LH-RH agonist, ICI 118, 630, in breast cancer and prostate cancer. J Steroid Biochem 20:129–135, 1984

99. Golder MP, Philips EA, Fahmy DR, Preece PE, Jones V, Henk JM, Griffiths K: Plasma hormones in patients with advanced breast cancer treated with tamoxifen. Eur J Cancer 12:719–723, 1976

100. Helgason S, Wilking N, Carlstrom K, Damber MG, van Schoultz B: A comparative study of the estrogenic effects of tamoxifen and 17 beta estradiol in postmenopausal women. J Clin Endocrinol Metab 54:404–408, 1982

101. Boccardo F, Bruzzi P, Rubagotti A, Nicolas G, Rosso R: Oestrogen-like action of tamoxifen on vaginal epithelium in breast cancer patients. Rev Endocrine-Related Cancer 9(Suppl):242–250, 1981

102. Ferrazzi E, Cartei G, Matarazzo R, Fiorentino M: Oestrogen-like effect of tamoxifen on vaginal epithelium. Br Med J 1: 1351–1352, 1977

103. Sakai F, Cheix F, Clavel M, Cohen J, Mayer M, Pannata E, Saez S: Increase in steroid binding globulins induced by tamoxifen in patients with carcinoma of the breast. J Endocrinol 76:219–226, 1978

104. Szamel I, Vincz B, Hindy I, Herman I, Borvendeg J, Eckhardt S: Hormonal changes during a prolonged tamoxifen treatment in patients with advanced breast cancer. Oncology 43:7–11, 1986

105. Enck RE, Rios CN: Tamoxifen treatment of metastatic breast cancer and antithrombin III levels. Cancer 53:2607–2609, 1984

106. Fex G, Adielson G, Mattson W: Oestrogen-like effects of tamoxifen on the concentration of proteins in plasma. Acta Endocrinol 97:109–113, 1981

107. Robel P, Mortel R, Levy C, Namer M, Baulieu EE: Steroid receptors and response to an antioestrogen in postmenopausal endometrial carcinoma and metastatic breast cancer. In Sutherland RL, Jordan VC (eds): Nonsteroidal Antioestrogens, pp 413–433. Sydney, Australia, Academic Press, 1981

108. Kossner S, Wallgren A: Serum lipoproteins and proteins after breast cancer surgery and effects of tamoxifen. Atherosclerosis 52:339–349, 1984

109. Reddel RR, Sutherland RL: Tamoxifen stimulation of human breast cancer cell proliferation in vitro: A possible model for tamoxifen tumour flare. Eur J Cancer Clin Oncol 20:1419–1424, 1984

110. Darbre PD, Curtis S, King RJB: Effects of estradiol and tamoxifen on human breast cancer cells in serum free culture. Cancer Res 44:2790–2793, 1984

111. Knabbe C, Lippman ME, Wakefield LM, Flanders KC, Kasid A, Derynck R, Dickson BB: Evidence that transforming growth factor β is a hormonally regulated negative growth factor in human breast cancer cells. Cell 48:417–428, 1987

112. Wakeling AE, Bowler J: Steroidal pure antioestrogens. J Endocrinol 112:R7–R10, 1987

113. Cuzik J, Wang DY, Bulbrook RD: The prevention of breast cancer. Lancet 1:83–86, 1986

114. Lacassagne A: Hormonal pathogenesis of adenocarcinoma of the breast. Am J Cancer 14:217–228, 1936

115. Turner RT, Wakeley GK, Hannon KS, Bell NH: Tamoxifen prevents the skeletal effects of ovarian hormone deficiency in rats. J Bone Min Res 2:449–456, 1987

116. Jordan VC, Phelps E, Lingren JU: Effects of antioestrogen on bone in castrated and intact female rats. Breast Cancer Res Treat 10:31–35, 1987

117. Love RR, Mazess RB, Tormey DC, Rasmussen P, Jordan VC: Bone mineral density in women with breast cancer treated with tamoxifen for two years (abstr). Breast Cancer Res Treat 10:112, 1987

Tom F. Lue

Peter R. Carroll

Connie Moore

Treatment of Impotence in Cancer Patients

11

Male sexual dysfunction is a relatively common problem. It has been estimated that 8% of men age 50 years suffer from impotence, and that this rate increases to 20% and 80% at ages 60 and 80 years, respectively. Changes in sexual function are even more common in men with cancer, and may occur as a result of anatomic damage to the penis or its neurovascular supply, changes in sex hormone levels, or alterations in mood, body image, and interpersonal communication. Although cancer cure or control is the major objective of oncologists, efforts to preserve the patient's quality of life are also very important. A better understanding of the physiologic mechanisms of normal sexual function, along with refinements in the diagnosis and treatment of impotence, allows for the preservation of sexual function in a large percentage of men treated for cancer. This chapter outlines the physiology of penile erection and the causes of impotence and presents an orderly approach to the diagnosis and management of this disorder.

Physiology of Penile Erection ∎

Functional Anatomy of the Penis ∎

The penis is composed of three cylindric bodies: the paired corpora cavernosa and the corpus spongiosum (Fig. 11–1). The corpus spongiosum, which includes the glans penis, lies inferiorly and contains the penile urethra. The arterial supply of the penis is mostly derived from the paired internal pudendal artery, a branch of the hypogastric artery, although accessory arteries from the obturator or inferior vesical arteries may contribute to the blood supply of the corpora cavernosa to some degree. Generally, the paired cavernous artery supplies the corpora cavernosa and is responsible for erection; the paired dorsal artery contributes to the engorgement of the glans penis; and the bulbar and urethral arteries supply the corpus spongiosum.

Penile venous drainage is more complex and comprises four major divisions: the superficial dorsal vein, which drains the penile skin and subcutaneous tissues and joins the saphenous vein; the deep dorsal vein, which drains the glans penis and the distal corpora cavernosa and joins the periprostatic plexus below the pubis; the urethral veins, which drain the corpus spongiosum; and the cavernous veins, which drain the proximal portion of the corpora cavernosa and join the urethral branches to form the internal pudendal veins. Communications exist among these systems.

Autonomic nerve contributions from the thoracolumbar (sympathetic) and sacral (parasympathetic) regions of the spinal cord converge in the pelvic nerve plexus, which lies along the lateral aspect of the rectum at the level of the seminal vesicles. This plexus innervates the bladder, rectum, and seminal vesicles. In addition, branches continue toward the perineum along the posterolateral surface of the prostate as the cavernous nerves.[1-2] These enter the corpus spongiosum and corpora cavernosa with accompanying arteries and veins. The pudendal nerve and its two major branches, the dorsal nerve (sensory) and the nerve to the bulbocavernosus and ischiocavernosus muscles (motor), provide somatic innervation of the penis.

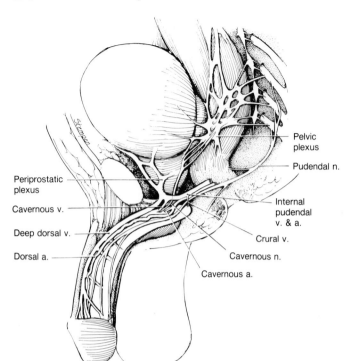

Periprostatic plexus

Cavernous v.

Deep dorsal v.

Dorsal a.

Pelvic plexus

Pudendal n.

Internal pudendal v. & a.

Crural v.

Cavernous n.

Cavernous a.

FIG. 11–1   Penile innervation, arterial supply, and venous drainage.

Mechanism of Penile Erection ■

Penile erection is a neurovascular phenomenon[3–6] that involves arterial dilation, sinusoidal relaxation, and venous outflow restriction. When the penis is flaccid, the smooth muscles of the arterioles and the sinusoidal walls are contracted. This exerts maximal resistance to the incoming blood flow. The venules draining the sinusoidal spaces are unimpeded. With stimulation of the cavernous nerves and subsequent release of neurotransmitters, the smooth muscles of the sinusoids and arterioles relax, resulting in increased sinusoidal compliance and decreased arteriolar resistance. Arterial inflow increases and sinusoidal engorgement occurs. The small venules between the sinusoids are compressed, as are the intermediary venules between the tunica and the sinusoidal walls. The overall decrease in venous outflow allows for maintenance of erection without a constant high arterial inflow.

Pharmacology of Erection and Detumescence ■

Although the neurotransmitters responsible for penile erection and detumescence are still under investigation, recent animal and human research has revealed several groups of agents that are able to induce or abolish erection when injected directly into the corpora cavernosa.[4] Among those which can induce erection (Table 11–1), papaverine hydrochloride has been extensively tested in both animal and human studies. When injected intracavernously, its action is similar to that of electrostimulation of the cavernous nerve: arterial dilatation, venous compression, and sinusoidal relaxation. Therefore, papaverine or other smooth muscle relaxants can be used to induce erection for studying penile arterial and venous function. Intracavernous injection can also be used to assist men with impotence resulting from neural dysfunction or mild arterial or venous impairment to achieve and maintain erection. These new discoveries have

Table 11–1
Erection-Inducing Agents

Drug Class	Agent
Smooth muscle relaxants	Papaverine, nitroglycerine
Alpha-adrenergic blockers	Phenoxybenzamine, phentolamine
Beta-adrenergic agonist	Isoxsuprine
Antidepressants	Chlorpromazine, trazodone
Calcium channel blocker	Verapamil
Peptide	Vasoactive intestinal polypeptide
Prostaglandin	PGE$_1$

revolutionized our diagnosis and treatment of impotence in the past 5 years.

Alpha-adrenergic agonists have been found to induce detumescence by contracting the cavernous and arteriolar smooth muscles, and can be used to treat abnormally prolonged erections (priapism) due to a variety of causes.[4] These agents include epinephrine, norepinephrine, dopamine, phenylephrine, metarominol, and ephedrine.

Etiology ■

Erection is a neurovascular phenomenon precipitated by physical or psychologic stimuli. Normal sexual function should be considered to encompass more than the ability to have and maintain erection; biologic, psychologic and social determinants of sexual behavior act in concert.[7] Thus, impotence may have more than one cause, and all these factors must be considered in treating male sexual dysfunction.

Normal penile tumescence occurs as a result of increased arterial perfusion, sinusoidal relaxation, and decreased venous drainage. Therefore, damage to the penis or its neurovascular supply caused by surgical management of male pelvic and penile cancers often leads to impotence. The neurovascular supply to the penis travels anterolaterally to the rectum and along the posterior surface of the bladder and prostate. Surgical extirpation of rectal, prostatic, and bladder malignancies commonly results in damage to either the penile nerves or arteries. The impotence rate after abdominoperineal resection for rectal carcinoma reportedly ranges from 33% to 100%; rates are much lower after proctocolectomy for benign disease.[8-11] This difference results from removal of the surrounding fibroareolar tissue, including the neurovascular structures, in the former procedure. Although impotence was once common after radical prostatectomy and cystectomy, a better understanding of the neurovascular supply has prompted refinements in technique that can avoid this outcome in selected patients.[12-14] Even preservation of only one neurovascular bundle will allow retention of erectile function in a large percentage of men undergoing pelvic surgery.[15] However, it should be remembered that preservation of sexual function is a product not only of surgical technique but also of the patient's preoperative level of sexual function, his age, and the anatomic extent of the malignancy. A review of pertinent surgical series reveals that older patients with higher stage malignancies are more likely to suffer from postoperative impotence.[14] Detailed vascular and neurologic evaluation of patients who have undergone either radical prostatectomy or cystectomy reveals that injury to the penile vasculature is a common cause of impotence.[16]

Radiation therapy for pelvic malignancies also may result in erectile dysfunction. Impotence has been reported to occur in 22% to 84% of patients receiving external beam radiotherapy for localized prostatic carcinoma and in approximately 10% of patients treated with interstitial radiotherapy.[17-19] Goldstein and colleagues[20] performed a detailed neurologic, vascular, and endocrinologic evaluation of patients who received external beam radiotherapy and found that radiation-induced occlusive disease of the penile arteries was the most common cause of impotence, rather than damage to penile nerves or to Leydig cell function. However, Mittal,[21] using somewhat different techniques, was unable to show a statistically significant difference between penile blood flow levels before and after radiation therapy.

Impotence may occur without injury to the penile neurovascular supply. The diagnosis of cancer, along with the financial, social, and physical sequelae of its treatment, represents a tremendous psychologic burden to the patient and his immediate family.[22] Impotence may be a result of depression, change in body image, or debilitation. Patients who require either urinary or fecal ostomy appliances frequently report a decrease in sexual activity and social interaction.[23-25] Medications prescribed to treat the malignancy or its sequelae may also produce impotence. Single-agent and combination-agent chemotherapy can both lead to sexual dysfunction, usually due to the morbidity of treatment itself. Cytotoxic chemotherapy may damage the germinal epithelium and lead to at least transitory changes in fertility but not in potency.[26,27] Although an elevation in serum luteinizing hormone (LH) is not uncommon after chemotherapy, serum testosterone determinations are usually within normal limits, reflecting compensatory Leydig cell function. In fact, men with Hodgkin's disease and testicular tumors frequently have abnormal gonadal endocrine and exocrine profiles before treatment.[28] Although impotence is rare, sexual dysfunction, as manifested by reduced orgasmic intensity and reduced libido, may occur in these patients.[29] Narcotics, barbiturates, and antidepressants all influence sexual function. Some medications or surgical procedures influence the hormonal axis responsible for libido and normal sexual function. Endocrine treatment of prostatic cancer at the level of the pituitary (*e.g.,* LH-releasing hormone agonists, estrogens), the adrenal gland (*e.g.,* ketoconazole, aminoglutethamide), or the testes (*e.g.,* orchiectomy) depresses plasma testosterone. The exact incidence of impotence in these patients has not been adequately studied, but some evidence suggests that a small percentage of men will maintain sexual potency despite low levels of serum testosterone.[30,31] A change in libido, rather than neurovascular compromise, seems responsible for impotence in these patients.

Finally, it should be remembered that impotence may be unrelated to the cancer or its method of treatment. As noted above, erectile dysfunction is a relatively common condition in the general male population. Patients with cancer may have associated conditions that predispose them to the development of impotence. Peripheral vascular disease induced by atherosclerosis, injury, or diabetes mellitus and managed by vascular bypass surgery may result in impotence. Similarly, neurologic impairment due to cerebrovascular disease, multiple sclerosis, diabetes mellitus, or direct nerve injury should be considered, as should disorders of the endocrine axis, including pituitary tumors and thyroid or adrenal disease. A variety of drugs cause sexual dysfunction. Some of the more common ones include cimetidine, several antihypertensive agents, antipsychotic medications,[32] and recreational drugs, including alcohol.

Evaluation ■

Ideally, sexual function should be addressed near the initial cancer diagnosis. Although it may be of little concern to some patients, for others it may represent an important means of displaying affection and a source of much pleasure. Early discussion regarding the impact of cancer diagnosis and treatment on sexual function serves two purposes: it allows the patient to feel comfortable discussing a variety of concerns, either initially or as they may develop, and it communicates interest not only in treating the patient's malignancy but in preserving his quality of life and dignity. Such discussions should be undertaken in an open and nonprejudicial manner.[22] A patient's cultural, religious, and educational background and sexual preference must be taken into account. The evaluation should be complete, and it should not be assumed that sexual dysfunction is due only to one cause. The initial evaluation should include the pertinent history, physical examination, and radiologic and laboratory tests necessary to determine the state of the patient's cancer.

Medical and Sexual History ■

Sexual dysfunction may be due to impotence, diminished libido, or ejaculatory disorder, and the precise cause must be determined. If impotence is identified

as the primary problem, it should be characterized further, noting its extent (*i.e.,* partial versus total inability to achieve erection, and whether erection is sufficient for vaginal intromission), its onset (*i.e.,* time of onset and whether it was abrupt or gradual), and its frequency (constant or intermittent). The patient's degree of sexual activity should be assessed, including whether he is sexually active, experiences normal orgasm or ejaculation, and has a regular sexual partner. It may be helpful to have the patient's sexual partner present at the initial interview.

Because impotence can result from a single cause or a combination of vascular, endocrine, neurologic, or psychologic causes, a thorough history and system review should be performed. A present or past history of coronary or peripheral vascular disease, hypertension, or hypercholesterolemia is often associated with erectile dysfunction resulting from atherosclerosis and decreased internal iliac or penile arterial flow.[33,34] Cigarette smoking is also associated with a greater likelihood of impotence, probably due to arterial occlusive disease.[35]

The incidence of impotence in patients with diabetes mellitus increases gradually with age, due to neurologic or vascular causes.[36] Neurologic disorders should be noted (*e.g.,* cerebrovascular disease, multiple sclerosis, or injury to the central or peripheral nervous system). A history of previous pelvic or retroperitoneal trauma or surgery should be recorded. For malignant disease, this description should include the tumor type, location, and the surgical technique used for biopsy or resection. Review of the operative report may be especially helpful in determining the extent of possible damage to the penile neurovascular supply. A history of radiation therapy should include the method (interstitial or external; electrons or neutrons), the total dose, and field size. Similarly, a history of chemotherapy or hormonal therapy should include a listing of all agents used, the total dose, and the frequency and number of doses. The relationship, if any, between the time of tumor diagnosis and its treatment should be noted.

A list of all medications and their doses, including recreational, prescription, and nonprescription drugs, as well as alcohol, should be recorded.

Physical and Neurologic Examination ■

A complete and careful physical examination should be performed on all patients. The assessment of tumor presence and extent depends on the malignancy, and might include careful rectal examination, stool guaiac determination, bimanual examination, and urinary cytology. The physical examination should assess the extent of previous treatment, noting the presence and extent of scars, stomas (including the fit of appliances), induration or fibrosis, and any other functional abnormalities that might interfere with normal sexual activity.

Physical examination should also include an assessment of body habitus, noting hair distribution, penile and testicular development, and the presence of gynecomastia. The penis should be examined for the presence of any surgical or congenital abnormalities, phimosis, or inflammation. The tunica albuginea of the corpora cavernosa should be palpated carefully to uncover any plaques that might result in curvature with erection (Peyronie's disease). Examination of the scrotum should include an assessment of the testicles and adnexal structures, noting testicular size and consistency and the presence of any inflammation. Assessment of the vascular system should include an examination of all peripheral pulses; transmission and the presence of bruits should be noted.

Neurologic examination should include sensory examination of the penis, scrotum, and perianal region. Biothesiometry can be used to quantify the sensory function of the penile skin.[35] Rectal examination should include an assessment of sphincter tone and the bulbocavernosus reflex. Careful motor and sensory examination of the extremities and all the deep tendon reflexes completes the neurologic examination. Further specialized tests, such as sacral evoked potential, dorsal penile nerve conduction velocity, and genitocerebral evoked-potential studies, can be used to confirm the diagnosis of sensory deficit.[35] However, a confirmatory test for penile autonomic neuropathy is still not available.

Laboratory Examination ■

Laboratory examination should include complete blood count, liver function tests, and determination of serum electrolytes, creatinine, and fasting glucose. Additional laboratory testing to assess disease presence or extent should also be performed as indicated.

The endocrine axis responsible for normal sexual function is complex and not completely understood.[37] A complete endocrine evaluation would include measurement of the gonadotropins, LH and follicle-stimulating hormone (FSH), serum testosterone, and prolactin. However, serum testosterone can be measured first and, if abnormal levels are identified or if major endocrinologic abnormalities are suspected, additional testing can then be undertaken. If low testosterone levels are noted, measurement of LH and FSH will differentiate hypergonadotropic hypogonadism (elevated LH and FSH, low testosterone) from hypogonadotropic hypogonadism (low LH, FSH, and testosterone).

Hypergonadotropic hypogonadism suggests primary testicular failure, which may be detected on physical examination as the absence of testicular tissue or presence of testicular atrophy due to age, radiation, chemotherapy, or surgery. Hypogonadotropic hypogonadism may be due to hyperprolactinemia, excess exogenous or endogenous hormones (i.e., estrogens, glucocorticoids, thyroid hormone), primary pituitary disorders, and certain rare congenital abnormalities. Additional endocrine testing is warranted in this group of patients to uncover disorders of prolactin secretion or thyroid, pituitary, and adrenal disease.[38] Hyperprolactinemia should be suspected in a patient who presents with both a decrease in libido and evidence of hypogonadism.[39]

Pharmacologic Evaluation of Impotence ■

Intracavernous injection of vasoactive substances (e.g., papaverine with or without phentolamine, prostaglandin E_1) can be substituted for neural stimulation and can effectively differentiate vasculogenic from nonvasculogenic impotence.[40]

For the patient with a normal-sized penis, pharmacologic testing is performed by placing a rubber band at the base and then injecting papaverine (30–60 mg) or prostaglandin E_1 (PGE_1; 5–15 μg) into one corpus cavernosum with a 28-gauge needle. The needle puncture site is manually compressed and the rubber band is kept in place for approximately 2 minutes. The patient is asked to stand and the response is assessed. A full erection is one that is firm to palpation and has an angle $\geq 90°$. If full erection develops within 15 minutes and lasts longer than 30 minutes, significant vasculogenic impotence is unlikely.

Pharmacologic testing does not differentiate among psychogenic, neurogenic, and hormonal impotence, as patients with these disorders usually respond normally to intracavernous injection. Nocturnal penile tumescence (NPT) testing may distinguish psychogenic from neurogenic impotence. Patients with psychogenic impotence usually have normal penile tumescence during REM sleep.[41] Although most patients who lose sexual function after radical pelvic surgery will be found to have suffered injury to either the cavernous nerves or arteries, selected patients may benefit from NPT testing. In addition, it may be helpful in documenting the return of potency after radical pelvic surgery. A recently introduced rigidity monitoring device, Rigiscan, has markedly improved our ability to document the duration, frequency, and degree of penile rigidity during sleep.

FUNCTIONAL EVALUATION OF CAVERNOUS ARTERIES □

The penile arteries can be evaluated with a variety of techniques including the penile–brachial pressure index (PBI), pudendal arteriography, and ultrasound and pulsed Doppler studies. The PBI is calculated by comparing the systolic pressure in the penile arteries with that of the brachial artery. Penile blood pressure is recorded by Doppler ultrasonography. An index above 0.8 is considered normal. Although the PBI may be a useful screening method for arterial insufficiency, it suffers from several limitations:[4] sclerotic vessels may give high pressure recordings, although flow may be minimal; the dorsal rather than the cavernous artery may be scanned; and the measurement of penile arterial pressure in the flaccid state gives no information regarding arterial dilatation and blood flow during erection. For these reasons, dynamic evaluation of the cavernous arteries with intracavernous papaverine or PGE₁ and duplex ultrasonography may be preferable for assessing penile arterial flow.

A real-time mechanical-sector duplex scanner (Diasonics DRF 400V; Milpitas, CA) is used in our institution.[42] The duplex probe allows simultaneous imaging and Doppler wave-form analysis. Anatomic evaluation is performed first in the flaccid state and then after injection of papaverine (45–60 mg) or PGE₁ (10–15 μg). Ultrasound evaluation (10 MHz) can depict the cavernous arteries, dorsal veins, tunica albuginea, corpus spongiosum, and corpora cavernosa. The diameter and thickness of the arterial lumina are recorded. A thick-walled, poorly dilated artery suggests sclerosis. A pulsed Doppler (4.5 MHz) study of each cavernous artery is then performed to determine flow. An increase in arterial diameter of more than 75% and a flow velocity of more than 30 cm/sec with a sharp upstroke wave-form constitute a normal arterial response.

Pharmacologic pudendal arteriography[43] is probably best reserved for patients with proximal occlusive disease of the larger arteries after blunt perineal or pelvic trauma, in preparation for surgical repair. Patients who become impotent after radiation or pelvic surgery are not good candidates for arterial revascularization because they are more likely to have suffered injury to small distal (penile) arteries, which do not respond well to these procedures. Because minimal arterial flow enters the cavernous arteries when the penis is in the flaccid state, arteriography performed without intracavernous injection of papaverine or PGE₁ is not adequate for functional evaluation of penile arteries.

FUNCTIONAL EVALUATION OF PENILE VEINS □

Venogenic impotence may be caused by poor relaxation of the cavernous smooth muscle cells as a result of cavernous nerve damage and impaired neurotransmitter release, atrophy of the cavernous smooth muscles, or cavernous fibrosis. Invasive testing should be reserved for the rare patient who fails to achieve an erection after papaverine injection yet is found to have a normal increase in arterial flow and diameter on ultrasonography.

The diagnosis of venogenic impotence is made with cavernosometry and cavernosography.[44–45] These are performed by inserting a 21-gauge scalp-vein needle into one corpus and connecting it to an arterial pressure monitor. A second 21-gauge needle is inserted into the opposite corpus and connected to an infusion pump. A papaverine/phentolamine (45 mg/1 mg) combination or PGE₁ (15 μg) is then injected into either corpus. The maximal intracavernous pressure and the time to achieve an erection are recorded. A good response is one in which the pressure reaches 90 mm Hg or more and the patient achieves a full erection. If the pressure is less than 90 mm Hg, an infusion of normal saline is begun (up to a maximal rate of 60–75 ml/min) and the response is assessed. The infusion rates that are required to achieve and maintain an intracavernous pressure of 90 mm Hg and the rate of pressure drop after infusion is stopped are recorded. Cavernosography is performed by infusing 60–150 ml of dilute contrast medium (1:1 with saline), with the patient in the supine and both oblique positions. Cavernosometry is the procedure of choice in diagnosing venogenic impotence. Cavernosography, although not as accurate, is essential in demonstrating the site of venous leakage for surgical repair.

Treatment Options for Impotence in Cancer Patients ■

Psychotherapy ■

Psychotherapy of the cancer patient and his sexual partner involves three phases: before surgery, after surgical recovery, and at about 1 year after surgery. The type of therapy and pertinent issues change with each phase.

Discussions about sexual function should begin after the diagnosis and before surgical intervention or radiation therapy. The patient will likely have many questions about capability for erection, ejaculation, and orgasm, but he may be hesitant to ask or may be overwhelmed by the idea of cancer and surgery. The possibilities of death and debility are utmost in his mind. Further, a feeling of loss of body integrity and control results from repeated examination, palpation, irradiation, and endoscopy. These stresses may provoke feelings of demasculinization and regression.

During this phase, the focus should first be on helping the patient cope with these issues and on encouraging the couple to express their grief, anger about their fate, and fears about the future. Addressing these feelings first often brings the couple closer together and sets the stage for a healthier adjustment later, sexually and generally. Education about sexual expectations can then begin.

During the second phase, the patient begins to think more realistically about his future and may be ready to resume sexual activity. Repeated education about sexual potentials and limitations is important. Visits to a sex therapist can help the couple make necessary attitude changes, which include a lessening of focus on coitus as sex and a broadening of sensuality and intimacy. For those patients who can achieve partial erections, practical diagrams about the most satisfactory positions for intercourse are useful. Many times the spouse has been nurse and caretaker of the patient during his recovery. This can be an asexual role. Discussion of the impact of role changes (his increased passivity and her increased activity) can help them to work out a comfortable sexual relationship. The couple may also want to explore erection-enhancing treatments (such as intracavernous injections) at this time.

In the last phase, about a year after surgery, the patient's erectile capabilities are usually clear. For the impotent patient, sexual psychotherapy now focuses on the decision regarding treatment options. The chief task becomes aiding the couple to choose the best means of intervention and for long-term sexual adjustment through behavioral, supportive, and exploratory psychotherapeutic techniques.

Hormonal Therapy ■

Patients with cancer of the pituitary, thyroid, adrenal, or testis who have a hormonal deficiency may benefit from hormone replacement therapy. For primary testicular failure, intramuscular injection of testosterone enanthate (200–300 mg every 2–3 weeks) can be effective. However, androgen therapy is contraindicated in patients with cancer of the prostate. If decreased libido is the major complaint, a trial of yohimbine, an alpha-2 blocker (5 mg *t.i.d.*), may be helpful in some patients.

Intracavernous Injection of Vasoactive Agents ■

Successful management of impotence with intracavernous injection of vasoactive agents has been well-documented.[40,46–48] In the United States, the most commonly used agent is papaverine hydrochloride, administered either alone or in combination with phentolamine mesylate. Recently, we have switched from papaverine to PGE_1 in all diagnostic and therapeutic procedures.

Intracavernous injection of pharmacologic agents provides an alternative to a penile prosthesis in neurogenic impotence, in selected cases of impotence due to arterial, venous, or sinusoidal disease, and in patients with combined disorders. Candidates should be advised of the treatment's investigational nature, the possibility of acute complications such as priapism, and the uncertainty about long-term side-effects such as cavernous fibrosis. Informed consent must be obtained.

Testing for the appropriate dosage should be done in the physician's office. The test and usual doses of PGE_1 and papaverine with or without phentolamine are summarized in Table 11–2. Medication is injected with a tuberculin or insulin syringe with a 28- or 30-gauge, 1- or 1.5-inch needle. The medication is injected along the lateral aspect of the penile shaft, avoiding the neurovascular bundle dorsally and the urethra ventrally. Only one side is injected and no tourniquet is used. Pressure is applied to the injection site for 5 minutes. The response is assessed as outlined above. If the patient fails to achieve a functional erection, the dose of medication can be increased, as outlined in Table 11–2. The injection site should be ro-

Table 11–2
Doses for Intracavernous Injection of Vasoactive Agents

Drugs	Test Dose*	Usual Dose
Papaverine hydrochloride	15–30 mg	15–60 mg
Papaverine and phentolamine†	0.1–0.3 ml	0.1–1 ml
PGE_1	5–10 μg	1–15 μg

* Lower doses should be used for patients with neurogenic impotence.

† (30 mg:1 mg)/ml.

tated. The auto-injection technique should be monitored by the physician until the appropriate dose is determined. Instruction of patient and partner should continue until the physician is confident that both understand the nature of the treatment and have mastered the injection technique.

Patients should be given a limited supply of medication (enough for 1 or 2 months) and injections should be limited to twice a week or less. Patients should be monitored monthly, and the penis should be carefully examined to determine if any fibrosis has resulted. Liver function tests should be performed every 1 to 3 months if papaverine is used for treatment.

Most patients with impotence can achieve a functional erection with intracavernous vasoactive agents. Patients with neurogenic impotence have a higher response rate and generally require lower doses; their erections tend to occur more rapidly, to be more rigid, and to last longer. Complications are few, although follow-up is as yet relatively short. The most common complications encountered with papaverine include pain or hematoma at the injection site, elevated results on liver function tests (in 4.5%), dizziness (1%–3%), intracavernous fibrosis, (0%–5%), and priapism (1%–3%).[47,48] The development of fibrosis is particularly disturbing. It may be the result of improper or too frequent injection or hematoma formation, or it may represent a tissue reaction to the medication itself, as papaverine is quite acidic.

Prolonged erection lasting more than 6 hours should be treated initially with aspiration. A 21-gauge scalp-vein needle is inserted into a corpus cavernosum, and both cavernous bodies are milked to facilitate drainage. Saline irrigation is not necessary. If aspiration is unsuccessful, instillation of an adrenergic agent will facilitate detumescence. Various agents have been used, including adrenaline, phenylephrine hydrochloride, metaraminol, and ephedrine.[4,47,48] Appropriate doses are listed in Table 11–3. These agents should be administered carefully, as systemic side-effects can occur. If necessary, administration can be repeated every 5 minutes until detumescence occurs.

Table 11–3
Intracavernous Medications for the Management of Priapism

Drug	Usual Dose
Epinephrine	10–20 μg
Phenylephrine	100–200 μg
Ephedrine	50–100 mg
Norepinephrine	10–20 μg

Arterial Revascularization ■

Anatomically, penile arterial insufficiency can be classified as extratunical and intratunical. The former includes disease of the terminal aorta and hypogastric, internal pudendal, and common penile arteries. Surgical correction or intraluminal balloon dilatation of these larger vessels reportedly yields good results in isolated lesions demonstrable on arteriography.[49,50] Intratunical arterial disease signifies not only terminal arterial disease but also end-organ failure. If the problem is minor, intracavernous injection can be the treatment of choice. In more advanced disease, surgical procedures have been advocated. These include epigastric–dorsal or epigastric–cavernous arterial bypass and an epigastric–deep dorsal vein shunt.[51–53] The results of arterial surgery are much poorer in patients with systemic atherosclerosis than in those with traumatic arterial disease.[54] Because cavernous smooth muscle atrophy may occur in patients with severe arterial insufficiency or tissue damage from radiation therapy, a penile prosthesis may be the only effective treatment.

Penile Vein Excision and Ligation ■

The incidence and cause of venous leakage in cancer patients is unknown. We recommend excision and ligation only for younger patients without diabetes or chronic hypertension who, despite good arterial flow, cannot achieve or maintain full erection after intracavernous injection of papaverine or PGE_1. In carefully selected patients, a 75% success rate can be achieved.[55,56] However, this procedure is new, and long-term follow up is not available.

Vacuum Suction Devices ■

These consist of a vacuum suction element and a tight constrictive elastic band. The suction on the penis induces tumescence and the tight constriction at the penile base retains blood in the corpora. With this device, a high percentage of patients can achieve an erection distal to the constrictive band that is sufficiently firm for sexual intercourse. If the patient does not elect the other treatment options, this is certainly a viable alternative, especially in cancer patients for whom a short life expectancy or poor general health precludes surgical intervention. Although some patients find this device unsatisfactory because the base of the penis remains flaccid, the majority find the partially erect penis adequate for sexual activity.

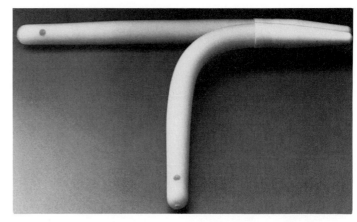

FIG. 11–2 A malleable (semirigid) penile prosthesis: AMS Malleable 600. (Courtesy of American Medical Systems, Minnetonka, MN)

Complications include numbness of the penis and ecchymosis of the penile skin, especially if the constrictive band is left in place too long.[57]

Penile Prostheses ■

A wide variety of penile prostheses are now available for the management of organic erectile dysfunction. Broad experience has been gained with the rigid, malleable, hinged, and inflatable prostheses (Figs. 11–2 and 11–3). All are manufactured in a variety of diameters and lengths to allow for accurate placement. A series of design changes in recent years has resulted

in excellent patient and partner satisfaction and a low complication rate. The semirigid and rigid prostheses have a lower complication rate than the inflatable models, but the latter allow the patient to control the timing and rigidity of his erections. Revision rates due to mechanical failure (fluid loss, pump migration, connector separation, or tubing kink) were high with earlier models of the inflatable prosthesis, but have declined to an acceptable level with the newer designs.[58]

Recently, a new generation of penile prostheses has been introduced. These single-component inflatable or articulated prostheses were designed to fill the gap between the more physiologic, but more mechanically complex, inflatable models and the simpler, but less cosmetically acceptable, rod prostheses. The Flexi-Flate and Hydroflex (Fig. 11–4) penile prostheses (Surgitek Corporation, Racine, Wisconsin; American Medical Systems, Minnetonka, Minnesota) are single-unit inflatable prostheses that, when activated, trans-

FIG. 11–3 A three-component inflatable prosthesis: AMS 700CX. (Courtesy of American Medical Systems, Minnetonka, MN)

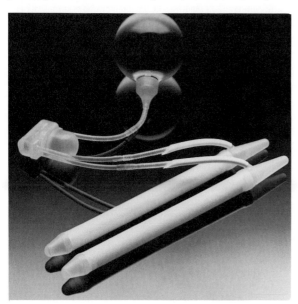

FIG. 11–4 A single-component inflatable prosthesis: AMS Hydroflex. (Courtesy of American Medical Systems, Minnetonka, MN)

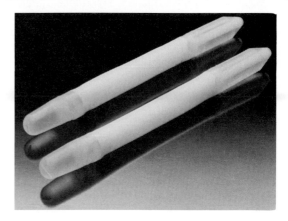

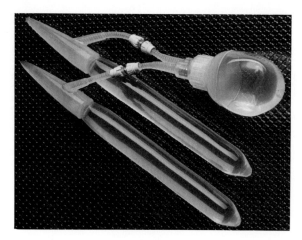

FIG. 11–5 A two-component inflatable prosthesis: Mentor Resi-pump. (Courtesy of Mentor Corporation, Goleta, CA)

fer fluid from an outer chamber to a nondistensible inner chamber until complete pressurization occurs. Rigidity is comparable to that obtained with most rod prostheses. The OmniPhase (Dacomed Corporation, Minneapolis, MN) is an articulated, nonhydraulic prosthesis. It consists of a proximal and rear tip, an anterior activator mechanism, and a central zone comprising a stack of interlocking polysulphone segments strung along a central cable. The prosthesis is activated by bending a spring within the activator mechanism. This shortens the central cable, pulls the interlocking segments together, and causes the prosthesis to become rigid. The most recent modification of the inflatable prosthesis consolidates the reservoir and pump into a single unit for easier implantation (Resipump; Mentor Corporation, Goleta, California [Fig. 11–5] and Uni-Flate 1000; Surgitek Corporation, Racine, Wisconsin). Experience with these new devices is still limited. The choice of design depends on the patient's preference, anatomy, and any associated illness, as well as the surgeon's experience.[59] Penile prostheses can be inserted through penile, suprapubic, scrotal, or perineal incisions.[60] Patient and partner satisfaction rates are generally reported to be quite high.[61]

References ■

1. Lue TF, Zeineh SJ, Schmidt RA, Tanagho EA: Neuroanatomy of penile erection: Its relevance to iatrogenic impotence. J Urol 131:273, 1984
2. Walsh PC, Donker PJ: Impotence following radical prostatectomy: Insight into etiology and prevention. J Urol 128:492, 1982
3. Lue TF, Takamura T, Schmidt RA, Palubinskas AJ, Tanagho EA: Hemodynamics of erection in the monkey. J Urol 130: 1237, 1983
4. Lue TF, Tanagho EA: Physiology of erection and pharmacological management of impotence. J Urol 137:829, 1987
5. Shirai M, Ishii N, Mitsukawa S, Matsuka S, Nakamura M: Hemodynamic mechanism of erection in the human penis. Arch Androl 1:345, 1978
6. Wagner G: Erection physiology and endocrinology. In Wagner G, Green R (eds): Impotence: Physiological, Psychological, and Surgical Diagnosis and Treatment, pp 25–36. New York, Plenum Press, 1981
7. Katchadourian HA, Lunde DT: Fundamentals of Human Sexuality. New York, Holt, Rinehart and Winston, 1975
8. Yeagher ES, Van Heerden JA: Sexual function following proctocolectomy and abdominoperineal resection. Ann Surg 191: 169, 1980
9. Weinstein M, Roberts M: Sexual potency following surgery for rectal carcinoma. Ann Surg 185:295, 1977
10. Jones TE: Complications of one stage abdominoperineal resection of rectum. JAMA 120:104, 1942
11. Davis LP, Jelenko C: Sexual function after abdominoperineal resection. South Med J 68:422, 1975
12. Walsh PC: Radical prostatectomy, preservation of sexual function, cancer control. Urol Clin North Am 14:663, 1987
13. Catalona WJ, Dresner SM: Nerve sparing radical prostatectomy: Extraprostatic tumor extension and preservation of erectile function. J Urol 134:1149, 1985
14. Schlegel PN, Walsh PC: Neuroanatomical approach to radical cystoprostatectomy with preservation of sexual function. J Urol 138:1402, 1987
15. Walsh PC, Epstein JI, Lowe FC: Potency following radical prostatectomy with wide unilateral excision of the neurovascular bundle. J Urol 138:823, 1987
16. Bergman B, Sivertsson R, Suurkula M: Penile blood pressure in erectile impotence following cystectomy. Scand J Urol Nephrol 16:81, 1982
17. Bagshaw MA, Ray RG, Pistenna DA, et al: External beam radiation therapy of primary carcinoma of the prostate. Cancer 36:723, 1975
18. McGowen DG: The value of extended field radiation therapy in carcinoma of the prostate. J Radiat Oncol Biol Phys 7:1332, 1981
19. Fowler JE, Barzell W, Hilaris BS, Whitmore WF: Complications of [125]iodine implantation and pelvic lymphadenectomy in treatment of prostatic cancer. J Urol 121:447, 1979
20. Goldstein I, Feldman MI, Deckers PJ, et al: Radiation-associated impotence: A clinical study of its mechanism. JAMA 251:903, 1984
21. Mittal B: Study of penile circulation before and after radiation in patients with prostate cancer and its effect on impotence. Int J Radiat Oncol Biol Phys 11:1121, 1985
22. Glasgow M, Halfin V, Althausen AF: Sexual response and cancer. CA 37:322, 1987
23. Fossa SD, Reitan JB, Ous S, Kaalhus O: Life with an ileal conduit in cystectomized bladder cancer patients: Expectations and experience. Scand J Urol Nephrol 21:97, 1987
24. Jones MA, Breckman B, Hendry WF: Life with an ileal conduit: Results of a questionnaire survey of patients and urological surgeons. Br J Urol 52:21, 1980
25. Gloekner MR: Perceptions of sexual attractiveness following ostomy surgery. Res Nurs Health 7:87, 1984
26. Thackil J, Jewet MAS, Rider WD: The effects of cancer and cancer therapy on male fertility. J Urol 126:141, 1981
27. Paoletti M, Straus FH: Effects of systemic chemotherapy on testicular morphology and fertility. In Talerman A, Roth LM

(eds): Pathology of the Testis and Its Adnexa. New York, Churchill Livingstone, 1986

28. Carroll PR, Whitmore WF, Herr HW, et al: Endocrine and exocrine profiles of men with testis tumors before orchiectomy. J Urol 137:420, 1987

29. Schover LR: Sexuality and infertility in urological cancer patients. Cancer 60:553, 1987

30. Bergman B, Damber JE, Littbrand B, Sjogren K, Tomic R: Sexual function in prostatic cancer patients treated with radiotherapy, orchiectomy or oestrogens. Br J Urol 56:64, 1984

31. Ellis WJ, Grayhack JT: Sexual function in aging males after orchiectomy and estrogen therapy. J Urol 89:895, 1963

32. Abramowizc M: Drugs that cause sexual dysfunction. Med Lett 25:73, 1983

33. Michal V: Arterial disease as a cause of impotence. Clin Endocrinol Metab 11:725, 1982

34. Tuttle WB, Cook WL, Fitch E: Sexual behavior in postmyocardial infarction patients. Am J Cardiol 13:140, 1964

35. Padma-Nathan H, Goldstein I, Krane RJ: Evaluation of the impotent patient. Semin Urol 4:225, 1986

36. Ellenberg M: Impotence in diabetes: The neurologic factor. Ann Int Med 75:213, 1971

37. McClure D: Endocrine evaluation and therapy of erectile dysfunction. Urol Clin North Am 15:53, 1988

38. Bardin CW, Paulsen CA: The testes. In Williams RH (ed): Textbook of Endocrinology. Philadelphia, WB Saunders, 1981

39. Perryman RL, Thorner MO: The effects of hyperprolactinemia on sexual and reproductive function. J Androl 5:233, 1981

40. Virag R, Frydman D, Legman M, Virag H: Intracavernous injection of papaverine as a diagnostic and therapeutic method in erectile failure. Angiology 35:79, 1984

41. Karacan I, Salis PJ, Williams RL: The role of the sleep laboratory in the diagnosis and treatment of impotence. In Williams RL, Karacan I, Frazier SH (eds): Sleep Disorders, Diagnosis and Treatment. New York, Wiley, 1978

42. Lue TF, Hricak H, Marich KW, Tanagho EA: Vasculogenic impotence evaluated by high resolution ultrasonography and pulsed Doppler spectrum analysis. Radiology 155:777, 1985

43. Zorgniotti AW, Lefleur RS: Auto-injection of the corpus cavernosum with a vasoactive drug combination for vasculogenic impotence. J Urol 133:39, 1985

44. Lue TF, Hricak H, Schmidt RA, Tanagho EA: Functional evaluation of penile veins by cavernosography in papaverine-induced erection. J Urol 135:479, 1986

45. Puyau FA, Lewis RW, Balkin P, Kaack MB, Hirsch A: Dynamic corpus cavernosography: Effect of papaverine injection. Radiology 164:179, 1987

46. Padma-Nathan H, Goldstein I, Payton T, Krane RJ: Intracavernosal pharmacotherapy: The pharmacologic erection program. World J Urol 5:160, 1987

47. Sidi AA, Chen KK: Clinical experience with vasoactive intracavernous pharmacotherapy for treatment of impotence. World J Urol 5:156, 1987

48. Zorgniotti AW: Pharmacologic injection therapy. Semin Urol 4:233, 1986

49. Metz P, Frimodt-Moller C, Mathiesen FR: Erectile function before and after arterial reconstructive surgery in men with occlusive arterial leg disease. Scand J Thorac Cardiovasc Surg 17:45, 1983

50. Castaneda-Zuniga WR, Smith A, Kaye K, et al: Transluminal angioplasty for treatment of vasculogenic impotence. AJR 139:371, 1982

51. Michal V, Kramar R, Hejhal L: Revascularization procedures of the cavernous bodies. In Zorgniotti AW, Rossi G (eds): Vasculogenic Impotence, pp 239–255. Springfield, IL, Charles C Thomas, 1980

52. Crespo E, Soltanik E, Bove D, et al: Treatment of vasculogenic impotence by revascularizing cavernous and/or dorsal arteries using microvascular techniques. Urology 20:271, 1982

53. Virag R: Revascularization of the penis. In Bennett AH (ed): Management of Male Impotence, pp 219–233. Baltimore, Williams & Wilkins, 1982

54. Goldstein I: Arterial revascularization procedures. Semin Urol 4:252, 1986

55. Wespes E, Schulman CC: Venous leakage: Surgical treatment of a curable cause of impotence. J Urol 133:796, 1985

56. Abber JC, Lue TF: Surgery for venogenic impotence: Early results. J Urol 139:297A, 1988

57. Nadig PW, Ware JC, Blumoff R: Noninvasive device to produce and maintain an erection-like state. Urology 27:126, 1986

58. Furlow WL, Barrett DM: Inflatable penile prosthesis: New device design and patient-partner satisfaction. Urology 24:559, 1984

59. Schlamowitz KE, Beulter LE, Scott FB, et al: Reactions to the implantation of an inflatable penile prosthesis among psychogenically and organically impotent men. J Urol 129:295, 1983

60. Benson RC, Pattereson DE, Barrett DM: Long term results with the Jonas malleable penile prosthesis. J Urol 134:899, 1985

61. Pedersen B, Tiefer L, Ruiz M, et al: Evaluation of patients and partners one to four years after penile prosthesis surgery. J Urol 139:956, 1988

Raymond P. Warrell, Jr.

Richard S. Bockman

Gallium in the Treatment of Hypercalcemia and Bone Metastasis

12

Introduction ■

The incidental observations that pharmacologic doses of gallium cause hypocalcemia and that this metal interacts with bone have led to an important research advance in bone metabolism. In this chapter, we review developments that led to this discovery and detail the extensive clinical and laboratory investigations that indicate gallium is an important new treatment for diseases characterized by accelerated calcium loss from bone.

Historical Development ■

Elemental gallium, originally predicted by Mendeleev as "ekaaluminum," was discovered spectroscopically by Lecoq de Boisbaudran in 1875 and named for France (*Gallia*). Gallium is classed as a Group IIIa metal along with aluminum, indium, and thallium. Each of the Group IIIa metals has been used medically—aluminum as a nonabsorbable antacid, and indium and thallium as radiopharmaceuticals for external scintiscanning. Trace amounts of gallium are found in bauxite and coal, and the pure metal exists as a liquid at temperatures above 29.8°C. In addition to its pharmaceutical uses, gallium also has major applications in electronic semiconductors. Gallium arsenide is extremely electroconductive and capable of converting electricity into highly coherent light.

Gallium as a Medical Radionuclide ■

The first report of radioactive gallium localization in proliferating tissues was by Dudley and colleagues in 1950.[1] Edwards and Hayes[2] first reported external

scintiscanning of human tumors using [67]Gallium in 1969, and this agent was subsequently shown to be useful for evaluating certain infectious processes.[3] As a radiopharmaceutical, ^{67}Ga citrate is now widely used for preoperative staging of lung cancer and for diagnostic staging of malignant lymphoma, although its utility in both diseases continues to be controversial.[4-6] The gallium scan has proven to be a highly sensitive (although nonspecific) diagnostic tool for evaluation of patients with acquired immunodeficiency syndrome (AIDS) and *Pneumocystis carinii* pneumonia.[7]

Gallium as an Anticancer Agent ■

Gallium nitrate was originally developed through work performed at the National Cancer Institute. After the antitumor activity of platinum-based compounds was recognized by Rosenberg,[8] a variety of metal-based compounds were screened as potential anticancer drugs. The Group IIIa elements were all shown to have cytotoxic activity against experimental tumors.[9,10] Gallium had the most activity and caused the least toxicity.[11] After completion of preclinical toxicologic testing, the drug entered clinical trials as an anticancer agent in 1976.

Results of the initial clinical studies generally showed a pattern of side-effects similar to those of cisplatin. High-dose intravenous injections were associated with considerable nausea, and nephrotoxicity was dose-limiting. The maximally tolerable dose proposed for broad Phase II testing was 700–900 mg/m,^{2} administered by brief infusion every 2 to 3 weeks.[12-14] A separate Phase I study using a continuous intravenous infusion over a 7-day period was started in 1982.[15] In that study, doses up to 400 mg/m^2 per day were administered. The intent of that study was to establish a satisfactory outpatient regimen, so dose escalation was halted when subjects developed nausea, which would preclude satisfactory oral hydration.

Reports from Phase II studies failed to confirm the preclinical results. Negative results were reported in studies of breast cancer,[16] non-small cell lung cancer,[13] head and neck cancer,[17] prostate cancer,[18] melanoma,[19] and sarcoma.[20] Despite its favorable activity in malignant lymphoma,[15,21,22] interest in high-dose gallium nitrate as an anticancer agent has waned.

Pharmacology ■

In clinical studies, gallium nitrate has been supplied as a clear solution in concentrations of 10 or 25 mg/ml (the former is most widely used). The medical formulation contains a small amount of sodium citrate, which enhances solubility and stability. The final mixture is extremely stable, with a shelf-life in excess of 1 year.

Variability in plasma half-life after injection has been reported and is dependent on the duration of the initial injection.[14,23,24] The initial half-life in plasma ($T_{1/2}$ alpha) is approximately 1 hour; the $T_{1/2}$ beta is approximately 24 hours. The terminal half-life is highly dependent on the method of administration. When administered by prolonged IV infusion, the plasma half-life dramatically lengthens to 72–115 hours.[25] This change undoubtedly reflects reversible binding and slow release from a deep tissue compartment (presumably bone). The volume of distribution (VD_{ss}) is also quite large for similar reasons. The major route of excretion is by the kidneys. Renal clearance of the drug is not affected by hydration and diuresis, although these maneuvers clearly reduce nephrotoxicity by lowering drug concentration in renal tubules.[14,26,27]

Observation of the Hypocalcemic Effect ■

In the study of prolonged IV infusion,[15] hypocalcemia was a particularly common side-effect. A previous report suggested that gallium nitrate induced hypocalcemia by increasing urinary calcium excretion,[27] a so-called "washout" effect. Over the long term, such an effect would clearly be deleterious because it would deplete calcium from bone and decrease bone strength. In unselected patients, it was observed that urinary calcium values were routinely quite low in the presence of low serum values. This apparent discrepancy prompted a reevaluation of the metabolic effects of gallium in patients who received the drug as anticancer therapy.

In contrast to previous reports, we found that gallium nitrate was associated with a major decrease in urinary calcium excretion.[28] This key finding suggested that significant effects on serum calcium could be induced only by two mechanisms—a decrease in gastrointestinal absorption or a decrease in calcium resorption from bone. The former possibility was excluded by the finding that there was no consistent change in fecal calcium excretion.[28]

These findings have stimulated an extensive series of laboratory-based investigations which show that gallium reduces bone resorption and may increase bone formation. As such, the drug might be broadly useful for diseases that are characterized by accelerated loss of bone mineral. In the following sections, the data from these experiments are summarized and clinical studies which showed that gallium nitrate is highly effective therapy for diseases such as cancer-related hypercalcemia are reviewed.

Laboratory Studies of Gallium ■

Gallium has certain physicochemical properties that are relevant to bone physiology. Elemental gallium precipitates in the presence of phosphate at pH $\geq$ 5.0, forming various metal/cation complexes of gallium-phosphate. Gallium also readily adsorbs to hydroxyapatite, the predominant calcium-phosphate species in mineralized and mineralizing bone.

Early studies indicated that gallium was a useful tool with which to study bone metabolism, as it was rapidly incorporated into osteogenic foci within bone.[29] Anghileri[30] first suggested that gallium could interact with "insoluble calcium" within cells, and also proposed a mechanism by which gallium might localize in metabolically active tissues. A variety of experiments have now been completed that elucidate the various effects of gallium on bone. These effects are as follows:

- Increases content of calcium and phosphorus.
- Increases hydroxyapatite crystallite size and/or perfection.
- Decreases solubility of bone mineral.
- Increases bone content of osteocalcin.
- Increases bone collagen synthesis.

Incorporation and Anatomic Localization in Bone ■

Preliminary experiments were done to determine whether gallium was normally found as a trace element in the skeleton and whether it was incorporated into bone after *in vivo* exposure. In these studies, young Sprague-Dawley rats were injected with gallium nitrate intraperitoneally (IP) at a dose of 25 mg/kg every other day for 14 days (total of 7 injections).[3] Although this dose is several times that given to human subjects, the rats showed no ill effects from the treatment, and they ate and gained weight normally. The animals were then killed and the long bones, including the diaphysis (shaft) and metaphysis (end-portions containing the growth plate), were separated. The gallium and calcium content of dried bone powder from these portions was measured by atomic absorption spectroscopy.

In the control animals, no detectable gallium was measured in the bones, even when large quantities of bone powder were tested. These data indicate that in rats gallium is not normally found in bone tissue, even in trace quantities. By contrast, in the gallium-treated rats, bone gallium content was directly correlated with the injected dose (Fig. 12-1).

In studies of long bones, a higher amount of gallium has been consistently measured in the metaphyseal compartment. This observation has now been verified by the technique of x-ray fluorescence microscopy. Using synchrotron-generated x-rays, the microscopic localization of several trace elements including gallium has been quantitatively determined. By this method, contour maps of gallium distribution have been constructed and its distribution patterns relative to calcium and other elements have been compared.

A typical contour plot of gallium in the tibia of a treated rat is shown in Figure 12-2. From such maps, the highest gallium content was measured in the metaphysis, notably in the region of the growth plate.[32] By contrast, extremely low levels of gallium were measured in mid-cortical regions. It is known that cortical bone is remodeled slowly[33] and that the mid-cortical region has the slowest turnover of skeletal calcium. Therefore, as in studies of other proliferating tissues, gallium preferentially localizes to metabolically active regions of bone.

Density separation has been used to differentiate newly formed bone particles from older, more mineralized bone. Normally, density fractionation of metaphyseal bone reveals a wide distribution of particle densities, with a mean density that is significantly less than particles from the diaphysis.[34] These differ-

FIG. 12-1 Gallium content in bones of rats receiving different total doses of gallium nitrate. Higher concentrations of gallium are consistently observed in the metaphyseal regions (*i.e.,* end portions containing the growth plate). *Solid bars* represent the diaphysis (shaft portion), *hatched bars* represent metaphysis. Data are expressed as mean ± SD for six animals. (Reprinted with permission from Bockman RS et al, in Sayre D, Howell M, Kirz J, Rayback H (eds): X-Ray Microscopy II. Springer Series in Optical Sciences. New York, Springer-Verlag, vol. 56, pp 391-394, 1988.)

FIG. 12-2 Contour plots for gallium (Ga) and calcium (Ca) distribution in tibial cross-sections taken from adult rats treated *in vivo* with gallium nitrate. Adjacent 100×100 μm^2 areas were sequentially scanned using the National Synchrotron Light Source, Brookhaven National Laboratory. (Reprinted with permission from Bockman RS et al, in Sayre D, Howell M, Kirz J, Rayback H (eds): X-Ray Microscopy II. Springer Series in Optical Sciences. New York, Springer-Verlag, vol. 56, pp 391-394, 1988.)

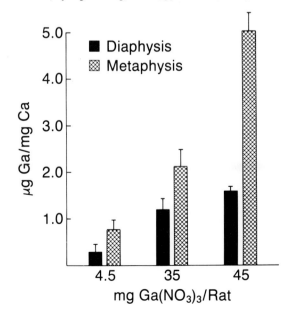

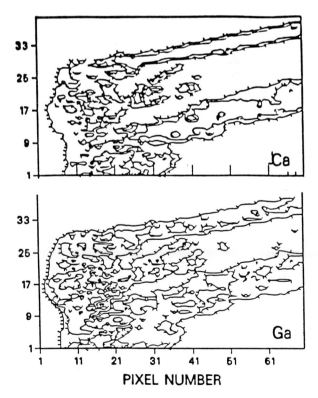

ences in particle density reflect the lower calcium content in the newly formed and maturing bone particles that are found in the growth plate region of the metaphysis. In these studies, rats were treated with gallium nitrate for 2 weeks. During this period, longitudinal bone growth continued and resulted in the formation of an entirely new metaphysis. Thus, all mineralizing components of the metaphyses would have been exposed to gallium.

Atomic absorptiometry showed that gallium was evenly distributed throughout bone particles of varying density derived from the growth plate. Less gallium was found in the older, more mineralized bone particles from diaphyseal bone. This suggests that newly formed as well as growing bone particles accumulated gallium. Thus, both the density fractionation studies and x-ray microscopy findings indicate that gallium accumulates in the growth plate and the endosteal and periosteal surfaces of cortical bone. Each of these regions is an active area of bone remodeling and new bone formation.

Gallium Effects on Bone Mineral ■

Short-term treatment with gallium exerts profound effects on the physical properties of bone mineral. Dissolution studies show that gallium treatment is associated with a significant decrease in the solubility of bone mineral. In one study, rats were injected with gallium nitrate over a period of 2 weeks. Bone powder obtained from treated and control animals was sus-

pended in an acid buffer. The subsequent dissolution of bone powder hydroxyapatite and calcium release into the media was measured over time (Fig. 12–3). Relative to untreated controls, the release of bone calcium was significantly slower for gallium-treated animals,[31] indicating that this treatment caused a significant decrease in the solubility of hydroxyapatite.

Gallium has also been found to increase calcium uptake into bone. To assess this effect, a series of young rats whose bones were undergoing active mineralization (i.e., growth and remodeling) were treated with gallium nitrate and injected with $^{45}CaCl_2$. The bones from gallium-treated rats showed a significantly higher specific activity of newly incorporated ^{45}Ca when compared to controls.[34] Because the ^{45}Ca-labeling period was relatively brief, this difference presumably reflects an increase in calcium uptake into newly formed (or newly remodeled) bone mineral. Atomic absorption measurements also showed an increase in calcium and phosphorus content in gallium-treated bone.[31]

The specific density of bone particles from the metaphyses of gallium-treated animals was evaluated using density fractionation studies. Relative to bones from control animals, a shift to denser bone was observed in the samples from the gallium-treated rats. This indicates that gallium treatment caused an increase in the growth of existing hydroxyapatite crystallites, with an increase in calcium/phosphate content.[31,34]

Finally, wide-angle x-ray diffraction and infrared measurements on bone samples from treated animals

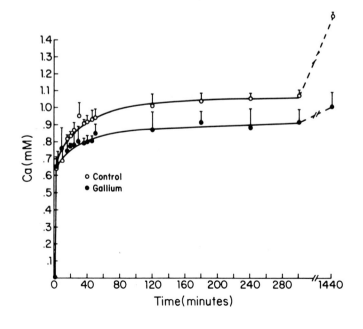

FIG. 12–3 Decreased solubility of bone powder taken from metaphyseal bone of rats treated *in vivo* with gallium nitrate. The release of calcium from bone into acid buffer was measured over time. Both the rate and total amount of calcium released were significantly higher for untreated controls than to gallium-treated samples ($p < 0.001$). (Reprinted with permission from Repo MA, et al: Calcif Tissue Int, 43:300–306, 1988)

were performed to characterize the physical properties of treated bone. In the x-ray diffraction studies, results showed that gallium treatment caused an increase in crystallite size or perfection, possibly reflecting a reduced level of contaminant substances.[31,35] The decreased solubility of hydroxyapatite mineral previously described is probably a reflection of this change in crystalline composition and structure.

Gallium Effects on Bone Cell Function ■

One possible explanation for the observed changes in bone mineral is that gallium alters the function of bone cells, leading to stabilization of crystal structure and yielding a matrix with more crystalline hydroxyapatite that has a higher calcium and phosphate content and lower carbonate content. To look more closely at the effects of gallium on bone cell function, bone resorption was studied *in vitro* using explants of fetal rat bones. In these studies, $^{45}CaCl_2$ was injected into pregnant rats to allow *in utero* mineralization of fetal rat bones with radiolabeled calcium. After 48 hours, the long bones from the fetal rats were excised and dissected. The bones were placed into media that contained various substances known to stimulate bone resorption, such as parathyroid hormone (PTH) or cytokines. The release of ^{45}Ca into the media is thus a measure of the rate of bone resorption.

Calcium release from bone was actively stimulated by the addition of bovine PTH or a lymphokine preparation containing interleukin-1 (IL-1) and cachectin/tumor necrosis factor (TNF). To test its effect, gallium nitrate was added to the culture media at concentrations ranging from 2.5 to 25 μM, either simultaneously with the addition of the bone-resorbing factors or 18 to 48 hours preceding their addition.

The inhibitory effect of gallium nitrate on PTH- and cytokine-induced bone resorption was found to be both time- and dose-dependent.[36] These results are shown in Figure 12–4. The addition of gallium nitrate simultaneously with—or 18 hours preceding—the addition of PTH or lymphokine caused only a slight decrease in ^{45}Ca release relative to controls. However, exposure of bones to gallium nitrate 24–48 hours preceding the addition of these resorbing substances caused a highly significant reduction in ^{45}Ca release.[38] In the absence of a resorbing factor, gallium nitrate had no effect on calcium release from bone. These experiments have since been repeated using highly purified recombinant human TNF, an agent which by itself dramatically increases bone resorption *in vitro*.[37] At concentrations that are readily achieved *in vivo*, gallium nitrate significantly abrogated the resorptive activity of human TNF.[38]

These inhibitory effects of gallium were clearly dose-dependent. After preincubation for 48 hours, 2.5 μM (1 μg/mL) of gallium nitrate did not inhibit ^{45}Ca release induced by either PTH or lymphokine. However, significant dose-related reductions in ^{45}Ca release were observed at concentrations of 12.5 and 25 μM (5 and 10 μg/mL) (Fig. 12–4).

Although the nitrate salt of gallium has been used predominantly, it is quite clear that elemental gallium is the biologically active substance, and that its potent activities on bone resorption are not dependent on the anion. Detailed dose-dependency studies with various salts of gallium have been conducted (*e.g.,*

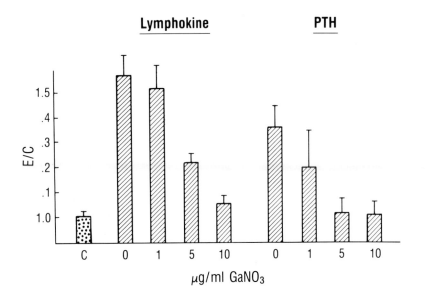

FIG. 12–4 Dose-dependent inhibition of bone resorption by gallium nitrate. Exposure of fetal rat bones to gallium nitrate *in vitro* inhibits resorption induced by both lymphokine and parathyroid hormone (PTH). (Reprinted with permission from Warrell RP Jr et al: J Clin Invest 73:1487–1490, 1984)

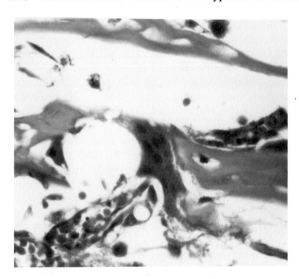

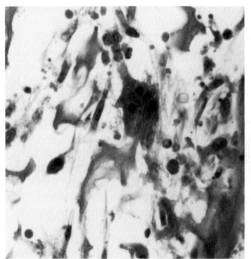

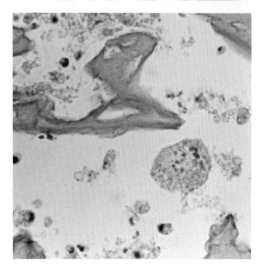

FIG. 12-5   Histologic section of fetal rat bones after drug exposure. (*Top*) Normal bone is shown with a multinucleated osteoclast apposed to a bone spicule after 48 hours in culture. (*Middle*) A bone explant exposed to gallium nitrate (50 μM) for 48 hours; no histologic abnormalities are noted and a normal appearing osteoclast is attached to a bone spicule. (*Bottom*) A bone sample cultured for 24 hours with mithramycin. Marked cellular destruction, with the remains of a pyknotic osteoclast, is evident. All micrographs shown at approximately 400$\times$.

gallium chloride, gallium acetate). All gallium salts tested at concentrations $\geq$ 2.5 μM have been found to inhibit bone resorption.

These effects of gallium on bone are not caused by toxic actions, as has been seen with mithramycin[39] and with other cytotoxic drugs, such as cisplatin.[40] Gallium has not been found to induce any change in bone cell morphology. In the fetal bone explant system described above, both the number and size of osteoclasts were similar in the treated and untreated explants.[41] These histologic results are in striking contrast to the results obtained with platinum- and germanium-containing drugs. Doses of cisplatinum, carboplatinum, and spirogermanium that block bone resorption are clearly cytotoxic, and no viable bone cells are evident after 24 to 48 hours of culture with these drugs (Fig. 12–5).[40] These important observations clearly distinguish gallium from cytotoxic agents.

Effects of Gallium on Bone Protein ■

Since bone is composed of hydroxyapatite mineral deposited in an organic, protein-containing matrix, it is essential to know whether drugs that affect bone cause deleterious effects on the synthesis of skeletal proteins. Osteocalcin is a bone-specific protein, and absolute levels of osteocalcin are thought to reflect bone turnover. Recent experiments have shown that gallium treatment results in substantial differences in bone osteocalcin content. Samples from both the metaphyseal and diaphyseal portions of bone from gallium-treated animals were found to contain significantly higher amounts of osteocalcin relative to untreated control animals.

The synthesis of bone collagen has also been measured using explanted rat calvaria. With this technique, the uptake of tritiated proline (^{3}H-Pro) and its subsequent conversion to hydroxyproline (^{3}H-OHP) was measured. Insulin, which is known to stimulate collagen synthesis, caused a 2-fold increase in ^{3}H-Pro incorporation into collagenase-digestible protein (CDP). Conversely, recombinant human TNF (in the absence of insulin) caused a decrease of approximately one-third in the ^{3}H-Pro and ^{3}H-OHP content of CDP. The addition of gallium alone caused a dose-dependent increase in ^{3}H-Pro uptake into CDP that was associated with increased conversion of ^{3}H-Pro to ^{3}H-OHP. The effects of gallium and insulin were additive. These data show that treatment with gallium increases osteocalcin content as well as proline and hydroxyproline incorporation into newly synthesized bone collagen, suggesting that gallium acts to enhance protein synthesis.[42] Because gallium also increases incorporation of calcium and phosphorus into growing or remodeling bone, it appears that gallium acts to enhance bone formation.

Clinical Studies in Cancer-Related Hypercalcemia ■

From the preceding laboratory investigations, compelling evidence has been assembled to indicate that gallium is a potent inhibitor of bone resorption and may also act to maintain or restore calcium content in bone. These effects suggested that gallium would be a useful treatment for a variety of diseases characterized by accelerated bone loss. Such conditions span a spectrum of disorders ranging from cancer-related hypercalcemia to senile osteoporosis.

In the first study of patients with cancer-related hypercalcemia, gallium nitrate was given as a continuous IV infusion at a daily dose of 200 mg/m² for periods ranging from 5 to 7 days. The first 10 patients

all responded with a reduction in serum calcium to normal (and occasionally below normal) levels.[36]

Several of these patients were treated with other hypocalcemic medications, either immediately before receiving gallium or after developing recurrent hypercalcemia. In these patients, a preliminary comparison could be made of the potency of gallium relative to other drugs. Results for two such patients are shown in Figure 12-6. The left panel illustrates results for a patient who received very large doses of salmon calcitonin (4800 IU/day) by continuous IV infusion. Serum calcium declined only slightly and never reached a normal level. The same patient then had an excellent response to treatment with gallium nitrate. Another patient with epidermoid carcinoma of the lung initially received an infusion of gallium nitrate and achieved normocalcemia. Because the protocol did not allow retreatment at that time, this patient received four injections of mithramycin (plicamycin) at a dose of 25 μg/kg when he developed recurrent hypercalcemia. As noted in Figure 12-6 (*right*), he had a minimal response to mithramycin and ultimately expired of hypercalcemia.

On the basis of these results, a broad Phase II study was initiated to evaluate a fixed dose and schedule of gallium nitrate for the treatment of moderate to severe hypercalcemia. The fixed dose schedule was employed to permit a clear evaluation of dose–response in many patients, rather than attempting to individualize these parameters for particular patients. Two principal dose levels were examined: 100 mg/m² and 200 mg/m², given daily for 5 days. As shown in Table 12-1, the results of the study indicated that both dose levels were highly effective. At the lower dose, 9 of 15 patients achieved normocalcemia, while 18 of 21 pa-

FIG. 12-6 Comparison of hypocalcemic activity of gallium nitrate compared to high doses of calcitonin (*left panel*) and serial injections of mithramycin, 25 μg/kg (*right panel*). (Right panel reprinted with permission from Warrell RP Jr et al: J Clin Invest 73:1487–1490, 1984)

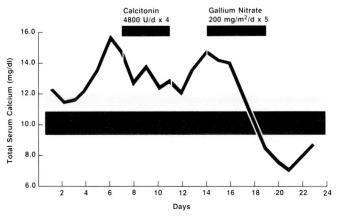

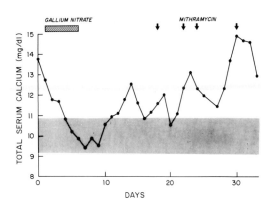

Table 12–1

Dose-related Changes in Mean Total Serum Calcium Concentration (±SD) and Percentage of Patients Achieving Normocalcemia in Response to Gallium Nitrate for Acute Control of Cancer-related Hypercalcemia

Dose (mg/m²)	No. of Infusions	Percent of Control	Serum Calcium (mg/100 ml)	
			Initial	Nadir
200	21	86*	14.6 ± 1.5	9.2 ± 1.5‡
100	15	60†	14.7 ± 1.2	10.5 ± 1.6§

* vs. †: No significant difference; ‡ vs. §: $p < 0.001$.

tients achieved normocalcemia at the high dose.[43] Both levels showed clear evidence of activity. However, the higher dose (200 mg/m² per day) caused a significantly greater reduction in total serum calcium (*i.e.*, a lower nadir value).

Controlled Studies in Hypercalcemia ■

A review of the clinical literature on cancer-related hypercalcemia can be quite dismaying. Almost all clinical studies consist of uncontrolled observations in patients receiving a variety of confounding medications, with inconsistent definitions of "response," extremely variable criteria for patient entry, and a variety of statistical manipulations, such as exclusion of early deaths.[44] When the Phase I and II studies with gallium nitrate had been completed, no study had been undertaken to compare active treatments in a double-blind randomized clinical trial.

In 1985, the first Phase III randomized double-blind study of hypercalcemia treatment was initiated. This study compared gallium nitrate to calcitonin for acute treatment of cancer-related hypercalcemia. The de-

sign of the study is shown in Figure 12–7. The study protocol required that all patients be hospitalized for at least 2 days, during which time they received intravenous hydration with or without diuretics. Exclusion criteria included (among other factors) recent treatment with chemotherapy, radiation, or mithramycin, and renal insufficiency (serum creatinine ≥ 2.5 mg/dl). Patients with hypercalcemia due to parathyroid carcinoma were also excluded because calcitonin was not believed to be effective for such patients. (These patients received gallium nitrate in a separate study, as discussed below.)

In this study, all patients who were admitted to Memorial Sloan–Kettering Cancer Center with a serum calcium ≥ 12.0 mg/dL were screened for eligibility. Patients with resistant hypercalcemia who met the eligibility criteria were then randomized to receive gallium nitrate (200 mg/m² per day) or maximally approved doses of salmon calcitonin (8 IU/kg IM every 6 hours). Both drugs were administered daily for 5 days.

Results from this study showed overwhelming superiority for treatment with gallium nitrate.[45] Overall, 18 of 24 patients (75%) who were randomized to receive gallium nitrate achieved a normal serum calcium, compared to 7 of 26 patients (27%) who received calcitonin ($p = 0.0006$). These statistics were calculated with conservative methods that allowed no exclusion for early deaths and used values of serum calcium that were adjusted for serum albumin. By more conventional (but less conservative) analyses (*i.e.*, early deaths excluded, uncorrected calcium values), 100% of patients treated with gallium nitrate achieved normal values. The response to calcitonin also improved (to 69%) using these criteria, but the treatment difference remained highly significant ($p < 0.001$).

Prior to the study, patients with hypercalcemia due to epidermoid (squamous) carcinomas were believed more likely to have a "humorally mediated" hyper-

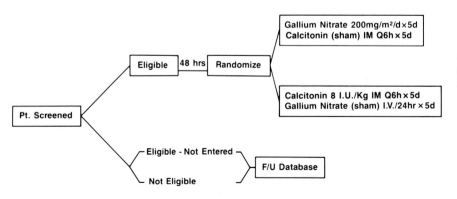

FIG. 12–7 Design of a randomized, double-blind study of gallium nitrate versus maximally approved doses of salmon calcitonin for acute treatment of cancer-related hypercalcemia.

calcemia that would be substantially more resistant to treatment. Therefore, patients were stratified according to histology (*i.e.,* epidermoid or nonepidermoid tumors). Patients with epidermoid carcinoma who received calcitonin in this study fared especially poorly. Only 1 of 10 such patients achieved a normal serum calcium when treated with calcitonin. The response to gallium nitrate was independent of histology, and equal proportions (75%) of patients in both the epidermoid and nonepidermoid groups responded with a normal serum calcium level.

The change in mean serum calcium in response to treatment in this study is shown in Figure 12–8. The initial response to both drugs was favorable; however, the mean serum calcium for patients treated with calcitonin began to increase after only 48 hours. By contrast, serum calcium continued to decrease in patients who received gallium nitrate, and the hypocalcemic response continued after the drug infusion was discontinued.

Duration of normocalcemia is exceptionally difficult to assess, given the multitude of confounding factors in these patients, particularly the subsequent use of hypocalcemic or cytotoxic drugs. If time to recurrence is censored at the time the serum calcium was first above the normal range or other treatment was administered (a very conservative method of analysis), the mean duration of normocalcemia was 6 days for patients treated with gallium nitrate and 1 day for patients treated with calcitonin ($p < 0.001$). If the effects of intercurrent treatment are ignored, the duration of normocalcemia was 11+ days for pa-

tients treated with gallium nitrate and 2 days for patients treated with calcitonin ($p < 0.01$).

An important advantage of double-blind studies is the ability to objectively assess adverse reactions. This factor is especially critical in disorders in which the natural history is characterized by frequent complications. In this study, all adverse reactions were assessed without knowledge of assignment to treatment. The incidence of toxic reactions is shown in Table 12-2. The incidence of serious renal damage was equally distributed between the two treatment groups. Two patients with multiple myeloma developed acute renal failure—one treated with gallium nitrate and one treated with calcitonin. A second patient treated with gallium nitrate who had previously undergone a nephrectomy developed renal failure after receiving a "loading dose" of an aminoglycoside antibiotic. Although hypercalcemia is frequently associated with nausea and vomiting, almost twice as many calcitonin-treated patients experienced this reaction compared to those treated with gallium.

Studies in Parathyroid Carcinoma ■

Patients with carcinoma of the parathyroid develop exceptionally virulent hypercalcemia due to grossly elevated levels of serum PTH. The metabolic disorder is highly resistant to treatment with standard agents. Metastatic parathyroid cancer is an uncommon neoplasm; thus far, three patients with parathyroid cancer

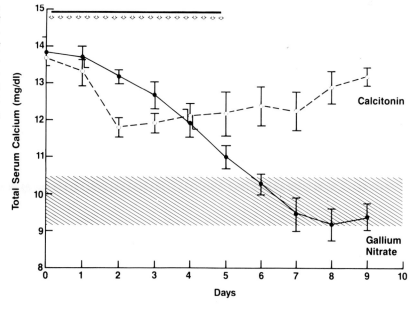

FIG. 12–8 Change in mean serum calcium concentration (±SE) after 5 days of treatment with gallium nitrate (— ● —) or calcitonin (– – – ○ – – –). The duration of treatment with gallium nitrate (—) and calcitonin (♢) is indicated at top left. The normal range for serum calcium is indicated by the shaded area. (Redrawn and reprinted with permission from Warrell RJ Jr: Ann Intern Med 108:669–674, 1988)

Table 12–2
Comparison of Adverse Reactions (in Percentages) in Patients with Hypercalcemia Treated with Gallium Nitrate or Calcitonin

Reaction	Gallium Nitrate (N = 24)	Calcitonin (N = 26)	p Value
Nausea/vomiting	14	35	0.094
Renal failure	8	4	NS
Hypophosphatemia			
Baseline	29	31	NS
Day 4–6	91	45	0.001
Pain at injection site	41*	62	0.15

* Placebo injection.

have received gallium nitrate. Each of these patients had an excellent initial response to this therapy.[25] As with other drugs, maintenance of normocalcemia after acute control remains a substantial problem. Although gallium nitrate can be safely administered subcutaneously (in daily doses up to 30 mg/m^2), studies of chronic treatment have not yet been carried out in these patients.

An important observation in these patients was the clear dissociation of the renal and skeletal effects of gallium and PTH. PTH classically stimulates calcium release from bone, decreases renal tubular resorption of phosphorus (causing hypophosphatemia and phosphaturia), increases conversion of 25-OH-vitamin D$_3$ to 1,25(OH)$_2$-vitamin D$_3$ through stimulation of the kidney enzyme 1-α-hydroxylase, and increases "nephrogenous" cyclic adenosine monophosphate. In these patients, gallium was found to exclusively inhibit the skeletal effects of PTH, without antagonizing the normal renal responses to the hormone.[25] In addition to decreasing serum calcium, administration of gallium caused a substantial decrease in urinary excretion of calcium and hydroxyproline (Fig. 12–9). Both of these parameters are indices of bone resorption.

Summary of Clinical Studies in Hypercalcemia ■

The clinical studies confirmed *in vitro* observations that gallium antagonizes bone resorption associated with all histologic types of cancer. The data show that gallium is effective irrespective of the presumed mechanism that induces hypercalcemia. Further studies comparing the effects of gallium to other forms of therapy, particularly the newer diphosphonates, are under way. At present, it appears that gallium nitrate is the most effective drug in clinical use for the acute treatment of cancer-related hypercalcemia.

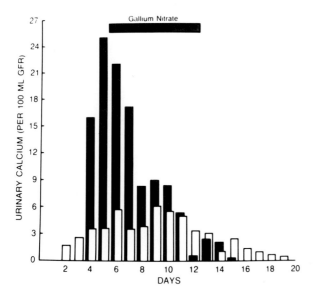
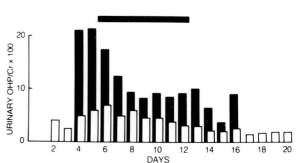

FIG. 12–9 Change in urinary excretion of calcium (*left*) and hydroxyproline (*right*) in two patients with accelerated bone resorption and severe hypercalcemia due to parathyroid carcinoma. (Reprinted with permission from Warrell RP Jr et al: Ann Intern Med 107:683–686, 1987)

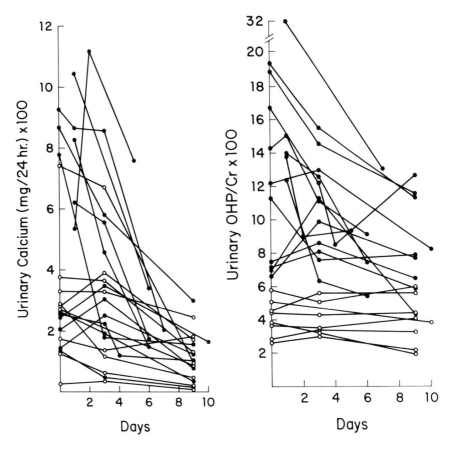

FIG. 12–10 Change in urinary excretion of calcium (*left*) and hydroxyproline (*right*) after short-term treatment with gallium nitrate in 22 patients with osteolytic bone metastases. (Reprinted with permission from Warrell RP Jr: J Clin Oncol 5: 292–298, 1987)

Osteolytic Bone Metastasis ■

The potent *in vitro* effects previously described suggested that gallium may be useful for a variety of diseases characterized by accelerated bone loss. Malignant osteolysis is the loss of bone mass due to local effects of bone metastases or the humoral release of bone-resorbing substances from tumors. The consequences of osteolytic bone disease (pain and pathologic fractures) are major sources of morbidity for patients with many prevalent types of cancer, such as carcinomas of the breast, lung, and prostate. Local radiation is commonly used for analgesic palliation, and various orthopedic surgical procedures are used for fractures.

The use of medical treatment to strengthen bone tissue against further erosion is becoming increasingly popular. Ideally, such therapy should not only minimize further bone loss but also restore bone that has been previously eroded. Preliminary reports using diphosphonates suggest that this form of treatment can be highly beneficial.[45-47] Because laboratory studies demonstrated that gallium nitrate reduces bone resorption and enhances bone formation, clinical trials have been initiated to evaluate the potential usefulness of this agent for the treatment of malignant osteolysis.

Gallium in Accelerated Bone Turnover ■

Diseases associated with accelerated breakdown of bone tissue are usually characterized by elevated serum levels of alkaline phosphatase and increased urinary excretion of calcium and hydroxyproline (an amino acid released during degradation of bone collagen). In a preliminary study, gallium nitrate was administered by IV infusion for 5 to 7 days to 22 patients with bone metastases. Pre- and posttreatment measurements of urinary calcium and hydroxyproline were determined.

Findings in this study confirmed the preliminary observations of reduced bone turnover seen in patients with hypercalcemia and parathyroid cancer.[25] The change in urinary calcium is shown in Figure 12–10. In 21 of 22 patients, urinary calcium was significantly reduced. The single exception was a patient who received an injection of furosemide—a known calciuretic drug—on the final day of collection. As had been seen in previous studies, this treatment was associated with a significant decline in serum phosphorus, perhaps suggesting that both calcium and phosphorous were being driven back into bone tissue.

Figure 12–10 also shows the change in urinary hydroxyproline excretion. Although urinary hydroxyproline excretion decreased significantly, overall, the decrease was most pronounced for those patients whose basal level of excretion was elevated (≥6.0). The values in patients with normal excretion did not change significantly.[49]

These data have since been confirmed in a study of patients with prostatic cancer and bone metastases,[18] which also found a significant decrease in urinary calcium and hydroxyproline excretion. Together, these results strongly indicate that gallium acutely lowers biochemical parameters associated with accelerated bone turnover. The important outstanding question is whether prolonged treatment can maintain these beneficial effects and whether such treatment will be associated with clinical improvement, as other studies have suggested.[46–48]

Studies in Malignant Osteolysis ■

One of the major issues in this general area of research is deciding on appropriate endpoints for study. For example, any treatment that does not result in a decrease of bone pain is unlikely to be very useful. Thus, pain assessment must be an integral component of any drug study used for treatment of this condition. However, analgesia can be provided by many drugs that have no direct effect on bone. An effective drug should also reduce the incidence of pathologic fractures. However, this endpoint requires large numbers of patients who would be treated in various stages of disease, each of whom would be receiving disparate forms of antitumor treatment that could significantly affect the outcome. Medical treatment must be also rapidly effective because, with few exceptions, bone metastases indicate systemic and incurable disease. Radiographic improvement of osteolytic foci could be used as a measurement of outcome. The disadvantage of this approach is its lack of precise quantitation and substantial interobserver variability.[50] The most useful, unbiased assessment would be a measurement of either regional or global changes in bone mineral. Fortunately, research technology derived from studies of patients with osteoporosis provides several methods that are suitable for such an analysis.

The technique that appears to be most sensitive to changes in total skeletal mineral and least subject to interpretive error is the analysis of total body calcium using neutron activation analysis.[51] The major disadvantage of this method is the requirement for reliable sources of neutrons and whole body scanners, which limits its applicability to a few, highly specialized research laboratories. A somewhat less precise assessment of total body bone mineral can be achieved using dual photon absorptiometry. This technique has the advantage of wider availability and is now in place at a number of hospitals. Regional changes in bone mass can be quantified by single and dual photon absorptiometry using the femur, forearm, and spine. With new developments in dual photon methodology, the precision of these measurements may soon be close to that achieved by neutron activation analysis. Theoretically, quantitative computed tomographic scanning could be used to measure serial changes in osteolytic foci; however, unless precise geometric realignment is ensured, minor changes in body position can result in very large measurement differences without any change in actual bone mineral content.

In clinical studies with gallium, a combination of tests that measure global and regional changes in bone mineral have been utilized. The major outcome determinant will be an increase in total body calcium (as measured by neutron activation analysis) or an

**Gallium Nitrate for Myeloma
Randomized Study Design**

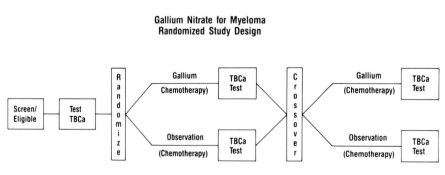

FIG. 12–11 Study design of patients with osteolysis due to multiple myeloma undergoing therapy with gallium nitrate. Pretreatment and posttreatment measurements of total body calcium are assessed by neutron activation analysis and dual photon absorptiometry to determine the increase in bone mass induced by treatment with gallium.

Table 12–3
Comparison of Certain Renal and Metabolic Effects of Cisplatin and Gallium

Effect	Drug	
	Cisplatin	Gallium Nitrate
Magnesium wasting	Common	Rare
Hypocalcemia	Uncommon	Common
Hypophosphatemia	Uncommon	Common
Sodium wasting	Occasional	Not observed
Renal insufficiency (characteristics)	Tubular necrosis, acute/ cumulative, occa- sionally reversible	Tubular plugging, acute/ noncumulative, gen- erally reversible

increase in total body bone mineral (as measured by dual photon absorptiometry). Serial changes in conventional radiographs will be blindly compared before and after treatment; however, these latter comparisons are subordinate outcome measurements.

A simplified study design for this disorder has been formulated, with the outline shown in Figure 12–11. Targets for the drug include breast cancer and multiple myeloma, relatively common diseases that are characterized by extensive osteolysis. In the myeloma study, total body calcium will be measured using both neutron activation analysis and dual photon absorptiometry. Patients will then be randomized to receive gallium nitrate or observation only for 6 months, followed by the other treatment for the succeeding 6 months. The initial period of no therapy with measurements is essential since the rate of bone loss has not previously been quantified in patients with myeloma (or any other malignant bone disease). It is quite likely that rates of osteolysis will vary substantially; thus, each patient will need to serve as his or her own control.

Side-effects ■

Renal Effects ■

Like many metal-based compounds (*e.g.*, gold, platinum), the principal serious side-effect of gallium nitrate is nephrotoxicity. Mechanisms of the renal injury differ considerably among these drugs. For example, gold is commonly associated with glomerular damage that is cumulative and probably irreversible. Platinum (particularly cisplatin) causes cumulative damage to renal tubular cells that is occasionally reversible. Nephrotoxicity due to gallium nitrate is not cumulative, is usually preventable by ensuring adequate urinary output during treatment, and is usually reversible when it occurs.

The pathology of the renal lesion also appears to be entirely different. For example, platinum is a highly reactive compound that can cause substantial toxicity to tubular "brush border" cells.[52–54] Conversely, gallium is an inert substance that can physically "plug" the lumen of renal tubule. Renal biopsies from animals and patients with gallium-induced toxicity show deposition of an amorphous eosinophilic material composed of gallium, calcium, and phosphorus.[14,27] Since nephrotoxicity is avoidable by ensuring large urine flow, it is surmised that this material can be dissolved and the renal lesion reversed by maintaining adequate urinary volume during treatment. It is recommended that patients maintain a urinary output of at least 2000 ml/day while receiving gallium nitrate during acute treatment for hypercalcemia. Because the drug does not cause nausea, hydration can be accomplished using either oral or parenteral fluids.

Cisplatin nephrotoxicity differs from that associated with gallium by other characteristics. A comparison of these effects is presented in Table 12–3. Platinum causes a cumulative renal injury that increases with the total cumulative dose. This injury is reflected in sensitive measurements of tubular damage, such as urinary excretion of β_2-microglobulin and "leakage" of enzymes such as N-acetyl glucosaminidase and leucine aminopeptidase.[55] Urinary excretion of both of these materials was shown to increase with increasing cumulative doses of cisplatin.[56] Conversely, chronic administration of gallium nitrate is not associated with cumulative renal damage. Large doses of gallium appear to be associated with an initial increase in β_2-microglobulinuria and enzymuria, which rapidly reverts to baseline levels, and which does not increase despite continued administration of the drug.[57]

Concurrent use of aminoglycosides has been reported to increase the likelihood of nephrotoxicity in patients who receive cisplatin,[58] and clinical experience suggests a similar additive role for gallium nitrate. It is recommended that aminoglycosides not be used concomitantly with gallium nitrate. It is recommended that aminoglycosides not be used concomitantly with gallium nitrate. If empiric antibiotic coverage is needed for gram-negative organisms, a third-generation cephalosporin should be used. Loading doses of aminoglycosides should be avoided.

Hematologic Effects ■

In large clinical trials, myelosuppression has not been a significant factor, and leukopenia and thrombocytopenia generally have not been observed as toxic reactions to gallium nitrate.[12-24] Anemia was observed in several clinical trials; however, since most patients had advanced cancer, the relationship of this condition to the drug was not clearly established. Anemia has not been observed in studies of short-term treatment for hypercalcemia.

The anemia that has been occasionally observed during chronic, low-dose therapy is usually mild in degree (a decrease of 1–2 g/dl in hemoglobin) and has not required transfusion. Red cell indices are characterized by hypochromia and microcytosis, similar to that seen in iron deficiency. Serum iron concentrations are generally normal, with little decrease in iron-binding capacity. Serum levels of transferrin and ferritin are also usually within the normal range.

Accumulation of gallium into cells was long thought to be mediated by transferrin. However, it is now clear that gallium enters cells by several different mechanisms, some of which are mediated by binding of a gallium–transferrin complex to the transferrin receptor, and others of which may involve active transport as well as passive diffusion.[59-66] While uptake of ^{67}Ga into tumor cells may be mediated by a transferrin receptor, recent studies have shown that the favorable effects of gallium on bone tissue *in vitro* are independent of transferrin, since they are also observed in transferrin-free media.[67] Theoretically, administration of iron supplements should increase the amount of transferrin that is saturated with iron (displacing gallium), thus preventing anemia without altering salutary effects on bone tissue.

Anemia has also been observed following administration of cisplatin. Although the mechanism of cisplatin-induced anemia is unclear, increased deposition of iron in hepatic tissue has been observed, suggesting some interference with iron reutilization.[68]

Metabolic Effects ■

A variety of metabolic effects have been observed in patients who receive gallium nitrate. One of the most common is a mild respiratory alkalosis, characterized by hyperchloremia and reduction in bicarbonate and P_{CO_2}.[15] Reasons for this phenomenon are unclear. The alkalosis does not cause symptoms and resolves shortly after discontinuance of the drug.

Hypophosphatemia is common when gallium is used for the treatment of hypercalcemia.[45] Since gallium can enhance bone formation, the drug may promote the incorporation of both calcium and phosphorus within bone.

In patients who develop hypocalcemia, an increase in serum levels of parathyroid hormone has been observed. Occasionally, an increase in serum PTH has occurred in the absence of any significant change in serum calcium or renal function.[28] This finding may reflect variability in the radioimmunoassay for PTH or a secondary effect on PTH secretion, possibly due to antagonism at the skeletal level.

Hypomagnesemia has been commonly observed after administration of cisplatin.[69-72] However, this effect is distinctly uncommon with the use of gallium nitrate, perhaps reflecting previously described differences in the action of the two drugs on the kidney.

Conclusion ■

Although gallium has been in clinical trials since 1976, its use as a treatment for osteolytic diseases has only recently been examined. It is fortuitous that a drug originally conceived as a cytotoxic agent should eventually be found to be a highly effective therapy for a metabolic disease. However, other drugs initially developed for anticancer use have proven useful for metabolic disorders. Allopurinol, originally synthesized as a cancer therapy, has become the leading treatment for hyperuricemic disorders. Further, many drugs useful in treating benign metabolic diseases are also used to treat cancer-related hypercalcemia. Examples include etidronate and mithramycin for Paget's disease, and calcitonin for osteoporosis.

Each of these diseases comprises a spectrum of conditions whose common theme is the accelerated loss of bone mass. The ideal therapy for each of these conditions will surely be a drug with characteristics similar to those described for gallium, namely, an agent that not only retards bone resorption but also enhances bone formation. Gallium has exceptional promise as an innovative medical therapy for hypercalcemia and osteolysis in patients with cancer, as well as other diseases associated with accelerated loss of bone.

This work was supported in part by US Department of Health and Human Services grants CA-37768, CA-42445, CA-38645, and CA-29502 from the National Cancer Institute, and by grant PDT-60 from the American Cancer Society.

References ■

1. Dudley HC, Imirie GW, Istock JT: Deposition of radiogallium (Ga-72) in proliferating tissues. Radiology 55:571–578, 1950
2. Edwards CL, Hayes RL: Tumor scanning with ^{67}Ga-citrate. J Nucl Med 10:103–105, 1969
3. Blair DC, Carroll M, Carr EA, Fekety FR: ^{67}Ga-citrate for scanning of experimental staphylococcal abscesses. J Nucl Med 14:99–101, 1973
4. Hoffer P: Status of gallium-67 in tumor detection. J Nucl Med 21:394–398, 1980
5. Longo DL, Schilsky RL, Beli L, Cano R, Johnston GS, Young RC: Gallium-67 scanning: Limited usefulness in staging patients with non-Hodgkin's lymphoma. Am J Med 68:695–700, 1980
6. Johnston GS, Go MF, Benua RS et al: Gallium-67 citrate imaging in Hodgkin's disease: Final report of cooperative group. J Nucl Med 18:692–698, 1977
7. Murray JF, Felton CP, Garay SM et al: Pulmonary complications of the acquired immune deficiency syndrome: Report of the National Heart, Lung, and Blood Institute Workshop. N Engl J Med 310:1682, 1984
8. Rosenberg B, Vancamp L, Trosko JE et al: Platinum compounds: A new class of potent antitumor compounds. Nature 222:385–386, 1969
9. Hart MM, Smith CF, Yancey ST et al: Toxicity and antitumor activity of gallium nitrate and periodically related metal salts. JNCI 47:1121–1127, 1971
10. Hart MM, Adamson RH: Antitumor activity and toxicity of salts of inorganic group IIIa metals: Aluminum, gallium, indium, and thallium. Proc Natl Acad Sci USA 68:1623–1626, 1971
11. Adamson RH, Cannellos GP, Sieber SM: Studies on the antitumor activity of gallium nitrate (NSC-15200) and other group IIIa metal salts. Cancer Chemother Rep 59:599–610, 1975
12. Bedikian AY, Valdivieso M, Bodey GP et al: Phase I clinical studies of gallium nitrate. Cancer Treat Rep 62:1449–1453, 1978
13. Samson MK, Fraile RJ, Baker LH et al: Phase I-II clinical trial of gallium nitrate (NSC-15200). Cancer Clin Trials 3:131–136, 1980
14. Krakoff IH, Newman RA, Goldberg RS: Clinical toxicologic and pharmacologic studies of gallium nitrate. Cancer 44:1722–1727, 1979
15. Warrell RP Jr, Coonley CJ, Straus DJ, Young CW: Treatment of advanced malignant lymphoma using gallium nitrate administered as a seven day continuous infusion. Cancer 51:1982–1987, 1983
16. Fabian CJ, Baker LH, Vaughn CB et al: Phase II evaluation of gallium nitrate in breast cancer: A Southwest Oncology Group study. Cancer Treat Rep 66:1591, 1982
17. Decker DA, Costanzi JJ, McCracken JD et al: Evaluation of gallium nitrate in metastatic or locally recurrent squamous cell carcinoma of the head and neck: A Southwest Oncology Group study. Cancer Treat Rep 68:1047–1048, 1984
18. Scher HI, Curley T, Geller N et al: Gallium nitrate in prostatic cancer: Evaluation of antitumor activity and effects on bone turnover. Cancer Treat Rep 71:887–893, 1987
19. Casper ES, Stanton GF, Sordillo PP et al: Phase II trial of gallium nitrate in patients with advanced malignant melanoma. Cancer Treat Rep 69:1019–1020, 1985
20. Saiki JH, Baker LH, Stephens RL et al: Gallium nitrate in advanced soft tissue and bone sarcomas: A Southwest Oncology Group study. Cancer Treat Rep 66:1673–1674, 1982
21. Weick JK, Stephens RL, Baker LH et al: Gallium nitrate in malignant lymphoma: A Southwest Oncology Group study. Cancer Treat Rep 67:823–825, 1983
22. Keller JW, Johnson L, Raney M et al: Phase II study of gallium nitrate (GaNO$_3$) (NSC-15200) in refractory lymphoproliferative diseases. Proc Am Soc Clin Oncol 3:247, 1984
23. Hall SW, Yeung K, Benjamin RS et al: Kinetics of gallium nitrate, a new anticancer agent. Clin Pharmacol Ther 25:82–87, 1979
24. Kelsen DP, Alcock N, Yeh S et al: Pharmacokinetics of gallium nitrate in man. Cancer 46:2009–2013, 1980
25. Warrell RP Jr, Isaacs M, Alcock NW, Bockman RS: Gallium nitrate for treatment of refractory hypercalcemia from parathyroid carcinoma. Ann Intern Med 107:683–686, 1987
26. Foster BJ, Clagett-Carr K, Hoth D, Leyland-Jones B: Gallium nitrate: The second metal with clinical activity. Cancer Treat Rep 70:1311–1319, 1986
27. Newman RA, Brody AR, Krakoff IH: Gallium nitrate (NSC-15200) induced toxicity in the rat: A pharmacologic, histopathologic and microanalytical investigation. Cancer 44:1728–1740, 1979
28. Warrell RP Jr, Isaacs M, Coonley CJ, Alcock NW, Bockman RS: Metabolic effects of gallium nitrate administered by prolonged intravenous infusion. Cancer Treat Rep 69:653–655, 1985
29. Dudley HC, Maddox GE: Deposition of radio gallium (Ga^{72}) in skeletal tissues. J Pharmacol Exp Ther 96:224–227, 1949
30. Anghileri L: Studies on the accumulation mechanisms of radioisotopes used in tumor diagnostic. Strahlentherapie 142:456–462, 1971
31. Bockman RS, Boskey AL, Blumenthal NC, Alcock NW, Warrell RP Jr: Gallium increases bone calcium and crystallite perfection of hydroxyapatite. Calcif Tissue Int 39:376–381, 1986
32. Bockman RS, Repo MA, Warrell RP Jr et al: X-ray microscopy studies on the pharmaco-dynamics of therapeutic gallium in rat bones. In Sayre D, Howell M, Kirz J, Rayback H (eds): X-Ray Microscopy II. Springer Series in Optical Sciences. New York, Springer-Verlag, vol 56, pp 391–394, 1988
33. Kimmel DB, Jee WSS: A quantitative histologic analysis of the growing long bone metaphysis. Calcif Tissue Int 32:113–122, 1980
34. Repo MA, Bockman RS, Betts F, Boskey AL, Warrell RP Jr: Effect of gallium on bone mineral properties. Calcif Tissue Int 43:300–306, 1988
35. Boskey AL, Bockman RS, Alcock N, Repo MA, Betts F, Blumenthal NC, Bansal M, Warrell RP Jr: Gallium nitrate alters bone mineral properties in the growing rat. Transactions of the 33rd Annual Meeting of the Orthopedic Research Society, Vol 12, p 170, 1987
36. Warrell RP Jr, Bockman RS, Coonley CJ, Isaacs M, Staszewski

H: Gallium nitrate inhibits calcium resorption from bone and is effective treatment for cancer-related hypercalcemia. J Clin Invest 73:1487–1490, 1984

37. Bertolini DR, Nedwin GE, Bringman TS, Smith DD, Mundy GR: Stimulation of bone resorption and inhibition of bone formation *in vitro* by human tumor necrosis factor. Nature 319:516–518, 1986

38. Bockman RS, Repo MA, Warrell RP Jr, Israel R, Gabrilove J: Gallium nitrate inhibits bone resorption induced by recombinant human tumor necrosis factor (TNF). Proc Am Assoc Cancer Res 28:449, 1987

39. Minkin C: Inhibition of parathyroid hormone stimulated bone resorption *in vitro* by the antibiotic mithramycin. Calcif Tissue Res 13:249–257, 1973

40. Bockman RS, Bohnsack R, Warrell RP, Jr: Effect of metal-based compounds on bone resorption. Clin Res 34:690A, 1986

41. Cournot-Witmer G, Bourdeau A, Lieberherr M et al: Bone modeling in gallium-nitrate-treated rats. Calcif Tissue Int 40: 270–275, 1987

42. Bockman RS, Israel R, Alcock NW, Ferguson R, Warrell RP Jr: Gallium nitrate stimulates bone collagen synthesis. Clin Res 35:620, 1987

43. Warrell RP Jr, Skelos A, Alcock NW, Bockman RS: Gallium nitrate for acute treatment of cancer-related hypercalcemia: Clinicopharmacological and dose-response analysis. Cancer Res 46:4208–4212, 1986

44. Warrell RP Jr: Editorial: Questions about clinical studies in hypercalcemia. J Clin Oncol (in press)

45. Warrell RP Jr, Israel R, Frisone M, Snyder T, Gaynor JJ, Bockman RS: Gallium nitrate for acute treatment of cancer-related hypercalcemia: A randomized double-blind comparison to calcitonin. Ann Intern Med (in press)

46. Siris ES, Hyman G, Canfield RE: Effects of dichloromethylene diphosphonate in woman with breast carcinoma metastatic to the skeleton. Am J Med 74:401–406, 1983

47. Elomaa I, Blomquist C, Grohn P et al: Long-term controlled trial with diphosphonate in patients with osteolytic bone metastases. Lancet 1:146–148, 1983

48. van Holten-Verzantvoort A Th, Bijvoet OLM, Cleton FJ et al: Reduced morbidity from skeletal metastases in breast cancer patients during long-term bisphosphonate (APD) treatment. Lancet 2:983–985, 1987

49. Warrell RP Jr, Alcock NW, Bockman RS: Gallium nitrate inhibits accelerated bone turnover in patients with bone metastases. J Clin Oncol 5:292–298, 1987

50. Powles TJ: Criteria for assessment of response of bone metastases to systemic therapy. In Garattini S (ed): Bone Resorption, Metastasis, and Diphosphonates, pp 93–98. New York, Raven Press, 1985

51. Cohn SH: Intercomparison of techniques for the non-invasive measurement of bone mass. In Dequeker JV, Johnston CC Jr (eds): Non-Invasive Bone Measurements: Methodological Problems, pp 17–26. Oxford, IRL Press, 1981

52. Madias NE, Harrington JT: Platinum nephrotoxicity. Am J Med 65:307–314, 1978

53. Goldstein RS, Mayor GH: Minireview: The nephrotoxicity of cisplatin. Life Sci 32:685–690, 1983

54. Doryan DC, Levi J, Jacobs C et al: Mechanism of cis-platinum

nephrotoxicity. II. Morphologic observations. J Pharmacol Ther 213:551–556, 1980

55. Sherman RI, Drayer DE, Leyland-Jones B et al: N-acetyl-beta-glucosaminidase and beta-2-microglobulin: Their urinary excretion in patients with renal parenchymal disease. Arch Intern Med 143:1183–1185, 1983

56. Jones BR, Bhalla RB, Mladek J et al: Comparison of methods of evaluating nephrotoxicity of cis-platinum. Clin Pharmacol Ther 27:557–562, 1980

57. Leyland-Jones B, Bhalla RB, Farag F et al: Administration of gallium nitrate by continuous infusion: Lack of chronic nephrotoxicity confirmed by studies of enzymuria and beta-2-microglobulinuria. Cancer Treat Rep 67:941–942, 1983

58. Pearson ADJ, Kohli M, Scott GW, Craft AW: Toxicity of high-dose cisplatinum (HDCP) in children—The additive role of aminoglycosides. Proc Am Assoc Cancer Res 28:221, 1987

59. Clausen J, Edeling CJ, Fogh I: ^{67}Ga binding to human serum proteins and tumor components. Cancer Res 34:1931–1937, 1974

60. Rasey JS, Nelson NJ, Larson SM: Relationship of iron metabolism to tumor cell toxicity of stable gallium salts. Int J Nucl Med Biol 8:303–313, 1981

61. Rasey JS, Nelson NJ, Larson SM: Tumor cell toxicity of stable gallium nitrate: Enhancement by transferrin and protection by iron. Eur J Cancer Clin Oncol 18:661–668, 1982

62. Larson SM, Rasey JS, Allan DR et al: Common pathway for tumor cell uptake of gallium-67 and iron-59 via a transferrin receptor. JNCI 64:41–53, 1980

63. Chitamber CR, Zivkovic Z: Uptake of gallium-67 by human leukemic cells: Demonstration of transferrin receptor-dependent and transferrin-independent mechanisms. Cancer Res 47:3929–3924, 1987

64. Chitamber CR, Massey EJ, Seligman PA: Regulation of transferrin receptor expression on human leukemic cells during proliferation and induction of differentiation: effects of gallium and dimethylsulfoxide. J Clin Invest 72:1314–1325, 1983

65. Chitamber CR, Seligman PA: Effects of different transferrin forms on transferrin receptor expression, iron uptake, and cellular proliferation of human leukemic HL60 cells. Mechanisms responsible for the specific cytotoxicity of transferrin-gallium. J Clin Invest 78:1538–1546, 1986

66. Chitamber CR, Zivkovic Z: Inhibition of hemoglobin production by transferrin-gallium. Blood 69:144–149, 1987

67. Bockman RS, Barcia M, Ferguson R, Warrell Jr RP: Gallium-induced inhibition of bone resorption is not mediated by iron-transferrin. Blood (Suppl) (in press)

68. McVie JG, Gordon M, ten Bokkel Huinink WW, Dubbelman R, Dikhoff T: Cisplatin and anaemia-protection by sodium thiosulfate (STS). Proc Am Assoc Cancer Res 27:172, 1986

69. Blachley JD, Hill JB: Renal and electrolyte disturbances associated with cisplatin. Ann Intern Med 95:628–632, 1981

70. Zumkley H, Bertram HP, Preusser P, Kellinghaus H, Straub C, Vetter H: Renal excretion of magnesium and trace elements during cisplatin treatment. Clin Nephrol 17:254–257, 1982

71. Hutchison FN, Perez EA, Gandara DR, Lawrence J, Kaysen GA: Renal salt wasting in patients treated with cisplatin. Ann Intern Med 108:21–25, 1988

72. Schilsky RL, Anderson T: Hypomagnesemia and renal magnesium wasting in patients receiving cis-platinum. Ann Intern Med 90:929–931, 1979

Thomas W. Griffin

Status of Clinical Trials With Neutron Irradiation

13

Introduction ∎

Fast neutrons are a type of high linear energy transfer (LET) radiation, and as such offer several specific advantages over conventional photon or electron radiation in the treatment of certain types of tumors. In brief, there are three main advantages to the use of fast neutrons in the treatment of various malignancies:

1. Fast neutrons are better able to kill hypoxic cells. The oxygen enhancement ratio (OER) is approximately 1.6 compared to 2.5–3.0 for conventional radiation.
2. Damage inflicted by fast neutrons is less readily repaired by the cells. This is true for both sublethal damage and potentially lethal damage.
3. There is less variation in radiosensitivity across the cell cycle as a function of the physical dose that is delivered.

Whether these properties have relevance to any given clinical situation depends on the cycling properties of the tumor compared to the cycling properties of the dose-limiting normal tissues in the treatment volume.

Investigations into the use of neutrons as a potential treatment for cancer date back to the 1930s, when R. S. Stone and coworkers used a neutron beam generated by the Berkeley cyclotron to treat patients with various advanced malignancies.[1] Although initial tumor responses were dramatic, almost all of the long-term survivors had severe late radiation sequelae in the normal tissues surrounding tumor sites. This effect, initially interpreted as being due to an increased relative biological effect (RBE) for late effects as compared to acute effects, deterred further clinical investigations of neutron radiation therapy for approximately 20 years. In the 1950s, when mammalian cell culture techniques were developed, it became apparent that the shapes of postirradiation cell survival curves following neutron irradiation were strikingly different from those following photon irradiation. The shoulder region of the cell survival curve following photon irradiation was greatly reduced on the neutron-irradiated cell survival curves. This difference demonstrated that the clinically used neutron fraction sizes corresponded to much higher RBEs than were extrapolated from the large-dose-increment animal model studies that preceded Stone's clinical work. Hence, nearly all of Stone's patients with serious radiation sequelae had inadvertently received extremely high radiation doses.

Clinical trials were first resumed at Hammersmith Hospital, London, in the 1960s. After several hundred patients with extensive cancers were treated, it was concluded that fast neutron radiation therapy was well tolerated and that many advanced malignancies responded amazingly well.[2,3] On the basis of these very encouraging results, various centers throughout the world again began clinical trials with fast neutrons.[4] In the United States, treatment was started in 1972 at the M. D. Anderson Hospital, using the Texas A&M University variable energy cyclotron (50 MeV d → Be reaction). Clinical trials were next instituted at the University of Washington in 1973, using a fixed-energy cyclotron (22 MeV d → Be reaction). Additional patients were treated using physics-laboratory-based machines at the MANTA facility (35 MeV d → Be reaction), centered at George Washington University, Washington D.C., the GLANTA facility (25 MeV d → Be reaction) in Cleveland, Ohio, and the Fermi Laboratory (66 MeV p → Be reaction) in Batavia, Illinois. Initially, Phase I clinical trials were carried out with patients who had advanced tumors and were estimated to have less than a 10% 5-year survival with conventional forms of treatment. This work yielded considerable information about the RBEs for different tissues and the variation of the neutron RBEs from facility to facility. More recently, patients receiving fast neutron radiation therapy have been entered into randomized, prospective clinical trials designed to compare neutron irradiation with the best available photon therapy as the control arm for a given tumor histology and site. Approximately 8000 patients have been treated worldwide, resulting in a fairly extensive patient data base.

Salivary Gland Tumors ■

Neutron irradiation was first used to treat advanced salivary gland tumors by Stone and colleagues, using a physics-laboratory-based cyclotron in Berkeley, California.[5] More recently, the results of fast neutron clinical trials have been reported from other treatment centers in Great Britain, Europe, the United States, and Japan.[6-15] Although treatment has been instituted on a more or less empiric basis, the results have been consistently encouraging, and it has been suggested that salivary gland tumors are much more responsive to neutrons than to photons.[7] The radiobiologic results strongly support this conclusion.

The first radiobiologic evidence that neutrons should be particularly effective in the treatment of salivary gland tumors came from Batterman and co-workers.[16] These investigators measured the RBE of neutrons produced by a d → T reaction relative to cobalt-60 radiation for human tumors metastatic to the lung. They determined the RBE for growth delay in terms of the time required for tumor mass to return to its preirradiation volume, as evaluated on serial radiographs. For patients with two or more metastases, lesions were simultaneously treated with the two types of radiation. The RBE for adenoidcystic carcinoma was 5.7 for a single radiation dose and 8.0 for fractionated radiation that would correspond to clinical treatment schemes. The RBEs for most other tumors were in the range of 2.5 to 4.0.

On the basis of encouraging results from earlier nonrandom clinical trials and the strong supporting evidence from Batterman's radiobiology studies, the Radiation Therapy Oncology Group (RTOG) in the United States and the Medical Research Council (MRC) in Great Britain sponsored a prospective randomized study comparing fast neutron irradiation with low-LET photon and/or electron treatment of inoperable malignant salivary gland tumors.

A total of 32 patients were entered on this study (25 from the United States and 7 from Scotland). Patients were randomized to receive irradiation with neutrons ($N = 17$) or standard photon and/or electron radiation therapy ($N = 15$). Inoperable or unresectable primary tumors were present in 61% of neutron-treated and 75% of photon-treated patients; the remaining patients had unresectable recurrent disease.

The minimum follow-up at the time of this analysis is 2 years.

Complete tumor clearance rates at the primary site were 85% for neutrons and 33% for photons following protocol treatment ($p = 0.01$). Complete clearance rates in the cervical lymph nodes were 86% for neutrons and 25% for photons. The overall locoregional complete tumor response rates were 85% and 33% for neutrons and photons, respectively (Fig. 13–1). The locoregional control rates at 2 years (Fig. 13–2) are 67% for neutron-treated and 17% for photon-treated patients ($p < 0.005$). The 2-year survival rates (Fig. 13–3) are 62% and 25% for these two groups, respectively ($p = 0.10$). There was no significant difference in the normal tissue complication rates between the two groups.

The results of neutron treatment of 289 patients with inoperable salivary gland tumors have been reported previously.[6-15] This number excludes patients who were treated for presumed residual disease following surgery. Some of these patients were treated with "mixed beam" treatment (2/5 neutrons, 3/5 photons); others were treated with neutrons alone. Treatment was delivered in 12 to 38 fractions over 4 to 7 weeks. In spite of this variability, the results are remarkably consistent. Table 13–1 summarizes the reported experience with neutron treatment in this

FIG. 13–1 Locoregional complete tumor response rates for neutron-treated and photon-treated patients. The difference is statistically significant, $p = 0.01$.

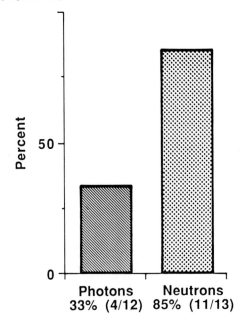

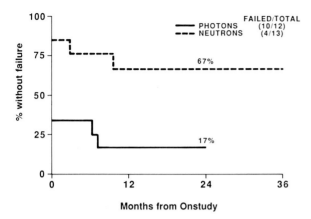

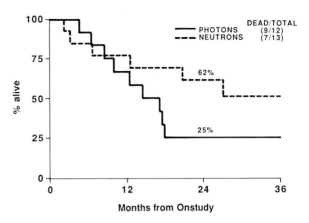

FIG. 13-2 Locoregional tumor control rates for neutron-treated and photon-treated patients. The difference is statistically significant, $p < 0.005$.

FIG. 13-3 Survival rates for neutron-treated and photon-treated patients. The trend is significant at the $p = 0.10$ level.

tumor system. The composite local control rate is 67% (194/289).

Local tumor control rates following low-LET photon and/or electron irradiation for inoperable salivary gland carcinomas are less satisfactory.[10,17–26] Table 13-2 lists the photon treatment results in this clinical situation. The composite local control rate in these series is 24% (61/254).

Table 13-3 presents a comparison of the randomized study results with historical results. As a whole, the data from the radiobiologic studies, the nonrandom clinical studies, and the prospective randomized clinical trial overwhelmingly support the contention that fast neutron radiotherapy represents a significant advance in the treatment of inoperable and unresectable primary and recurrent malignant salivary

gland tumors. There was no observable difference in tumor response to neutron therapy in relation to histology.

Prostate Tumors ■

Clinical investigations of neutron therapy in prostate cancer have been reported from the United States,[27,28] Europe,[29–32] and Japan.[33] The largest group of patients has been treated in the United States, under the auspices of RTOG. This trial, RTOG 77-04, is also the only randomized prospective trial that has compared neutron therapy directly to conventional megavoltage photon therapy. Details of the study design and ex-

Table 13-1
Neutron Locoregional Tumor Control Rates for Malignant Salivary Gland Tumors

Study	No. of Patients	Locoregional Control
Saroja et al[25]	113	71 (63%)
Catterall[3]	65	50 (77%)
Batterman et al[6]	32	21 (66%)
Griffin et al[12]	32	26 (81%)
Duncan et al[9]	22	12 (55%)
Maor et al[22]	9	6 (67%)
Ornitz et al[23]	8	3 (38%)
Eichhorn[10]	5	3 (60%)
Skolyszewski et al[26]	3	2 (67%)
Total	289	194 (67%)

Table 13-2
Low-LET (Photon/Electron) Locoregional Tumor Control Rates for Malignant Salivary Gland Tumors

Study	No. of Patients	Locoregional Control
Fitzpatrick and Theriault[20]	50	6 (12%)
Vikram[75]	49	2 (4%)
Borthne et al[7]	35	8 (23%)
Rafla[14]	25	9 (36%)
Fu et al[11]	19	6 (32%)
Stewart[76]	19	9 (47%)
Dobrowsky et al[8]	17	7 (41%)
Shidnia[77]	16	6 (38%)
Elkon et al[19]	13	2 (15%)
Rossman[15]	11	6 (54%)
Total	254	61 (24%)

Table 13–3
Comparison of the RTOG and MRC Study Results with Historical Results

Treatment	No. of Patients	Locoregional Control
Low LET		
Low-LET historical experience	254	24%
RTOG/MRC photon controls	12	17%
Neutron		
Historical neutron experience	289	67%
RTOG/MRC neutron results	13	67%

ecution have been fully reported,[27,28] and are reviewed briefly below.

In this study, patients with Clinical Stage C and D1 disease were randomized to receive treatment with either photon radiation or a combination of neutrons and photons (mixed-beam treatment). At the initiation of the study, several of the participating facilities had neutron beams similar to orthovoltage radiation in their penetrating properties. A major reservation regarding the use of the lower energy neutron beams stemmed from the lack of skin sparing with such units relative to that achievable with higher energy cyclotron beams or megavoltage photon irradiation. This lack of skin sparing, and the poor penetration of these beams, raised the possibility of unacceptably high rates of normal tissue complications, similar to those one might expect from orthovoltage-era photon units, if neutrons alone were used to treat the large treatment volumes required to incorporate pelvic lymph node chains. Therefore, the mixed-beam approach, which involved twice-weekly treatment with neutrons and thrice-weekly treatment with photons, was used. Because the RBE of neutrons varied with the facility, the daily neutron dose was adjusted (neutron dose + % of cyclotron output containing photon contamination × individual institutional RBE), so that equivalent biologic doses of neutrons or photons were given at each treatment.

Between 1977 and 1983, 91 patients were enrolled on the study, with a purposely skewed randomization leading to assignment of 55 patients to the mixed-beam arm and 36 to the conventional photon arm. Disease stage was C in 74 patients and D1 in 17. Prior hormonal treatment had been given to 25% of the patients randomized to receive photons and 11% of those randomized to mixed-beam therapy. The majority of patients had been staged by clinical and radiographic criteria (involving physical examination, serum acid phosphatase determination, pelvic CT scanning, lymphography, and radionuclide bone scans) alone; only 3 photon arm patients and 5 mixed-beam patients had undergone surgical sampling of pelvic lymph nodes. Chi-square analysis indicated that the two groups were balanced relative to all major prognostic factors.

Patients randomized to photon treatment received 5000 cGy in 180–200 cGy fractions, with treatment portals encompassing the prostate and regional pelvic lymph nodes. A subsequent boost of 2000 cGy was given to the prostate and areas of tumor extension beyond the prostate. Patients treated with mixed-beam irradiation received a dose of 5000 cGy "photon equivalent," followed by a similar 2000 cGy photon-equivalent boost, using the alternating schedule of neutrons and photons outlined above.

At the time of this analysis, with a median follow-up of 6.7 years, 81% of the neutron-treated patients remain clinically free of local tumor recurrence, compared to 61% of the patients treated with photons alone (Fig. 13–4). This difference is statistically significant ($p < 0.01$). Although no standard approach to routine posttreatment biopsy was mandated in this study, 11 patients had second biopsies a minimum of 2 years after treatment, while they were in clinical remission. Combining the pathologic criterion of a positive biopsy with the clinical criteria, 77% of the neutron-treated patients versus 31% of the photon-treated patients remained free of local disease. These differences remain statistically significant ($p < 0.01$),

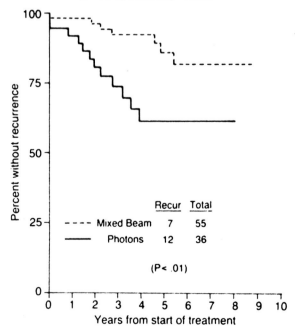

FIG. 13–4 Freedom from locoregional tumor recurrence. The two curves are significantly different, $p < 0.01$.

and the positive biopsy rate for photon-treated patients is consistent with other reports in the literature.

Survival data (Fig. 13–5) show that 63% of the neutron-treated group are alive at 8 years as opposed to 13% of the photon-only cohort ($p = 0.01$). There were many intercurrent deaths on this study, presumably due to the advanced average age of the patients entered. The disease-specific survival data, excluding intercurrent deaths from causes other than prostate cancer, are summarized in Figure 13–6. The rate for the neutron-treated group at 8 years is 82% compared to 54% for the photon-only group. The difference remains statistically significant ($p = 0.02$).

A stepwise Cox analysis has been used to identify the factors associated with overall survival in this study. The most significant factor was type of treatment (mixed beam versus photons, $p < 0.01$), followed by patient age ($p < 0.05$). No significant differences were noted for either acute or late normal tissue toxicity.

In Europe, clinical trials involving fast neutron irradiation of prostate cancer have been carried out primarily in the cyclotron facilities at Louvain-la-Neuve, Belgium, and Hamburg, Germany. In the Belgian experience, a neutron regimen similar to the RTOG mixed-beam approach has been employed, but photons were combined with high-energy 65 MeV

p → Be neutrons to allow better delivery of neutron dose to greater tissue depths. Accordingly, three treatments a week (or 60% of the total treatment) were composed of neutrons, as opposed to the 40% neutron contribution in the RTOG mixed-beam treatment. Treatment to the pelvis was carried to a total dose of 5000 cGy photon equivalent, and the prostate received an additional 1600 cGy photon-equivalent boost. Patients were treated in a Phase II setting without any attempt at randomization. At the time of last analysis, there were 50 treated patients, with a stage distribution of 14 Stage A, 30 Stage C, and 6 Stage D2. Of the 30 Stage C patients, 28 had been followed a minimum of 1 year.

Tumor local control rates of 93% and 90% were reported at 1 and 3 years, respectively, in the Stage C patients, with 28 and 10 patients available for analysis at these time points. Seven of the 10 patients followed for 3 years are alive and with no evidence of disease (NED). Complications in this group of patients have been minimal; only 1 patient had a urethral stricture requiring surgical attention.[29,30]

The group in Hamburg has reported similarly encouraging results. Originally, a mixed-beam schedule was employed, combining 14 MeV (deuterium-tri-

FIG. 13–5 Patient survival as a function of treatment. The two curves are significantly different, $p = 0.01$.

FIG. 13–6 Patient survival as a function of treatment using active cancer (local or distant) at the time of death as the endpoint. Deaths due to intercurrent disease with no evidence of cancer present are treated as censored observations. The two curves are different at the $p = 0.02$ level.

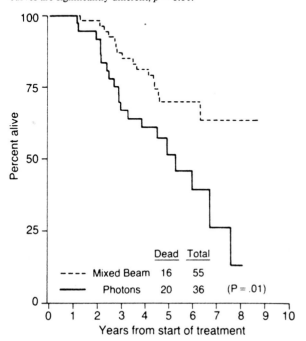

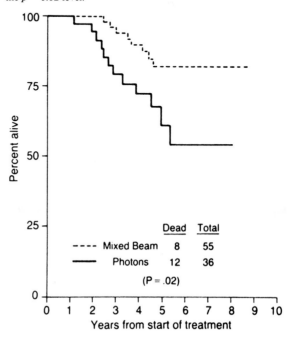

tium) neutrons and megavoltage photons. Pelvic nodes were treated with photons alone, to a total of 3000 to 4500 cGy over 3 to 4.5 weeks at conventional 200 cGy/day fractions. The boost dose to the prostate was carried out with neutrons alone, treating eight isocentrically centered fields a day, three treatments a week, for a total boost of 390 to 840 neutron cGy (approximately 1200–2600 photon cGy equivalent). The treatment of 13 Stage C (UICC Stage $T_3N_{X-2}M_{X-0}$ and $T_4N_{X-2}M_{X-0}$) tumors was well-tolerated; all patients obtained complete tumor regression with no adverse long-term reactions.[31] A recent update of this experience reported 5-year survival figures for the 12 evaluable patients; 7 of those with T_3 tumors (85%) and 5 of those with T_4 tumors (20%) are alive. No adverse sequelae of neutron treatment were observed in these patients with regard to bowel, bladder, or intestinal complications.

At Chiba University in Japan, 26 patients received primary radiotherapy consisting of either fast neutrons alone (15 patients) or mixed-beam radiation (11 patients). Treatment fields either encompassed the pelvic nodes, with a subsequent boost to the prostate (16 patients), or were limited to the prostate alone. A number of radiation doses were employed, reported as time-dose-fractionation (TDF) values,[34] ranging from 98 to 124. For the 14 patients with Stage C tumors, a 77% 3-year survival was reported.[33]

The results of the United States, European, and Japanese trials are summarized in Table 13–4. Survival results are tabulated for patients with locally advanced tumors, who constitute the majority of the patients treated to date and for whom the most complete published data are available.

The great majority of patients treated with fast neutrons for prostate cancer have been treated with mixed-beam schedules, for the reasons cited earlier. The implementation of a new generation of high-energy hospital-based cyclotrons capable of delivering neutrons to deep-seated tumors, with dose distributions comparable to those obtained from megavoltage linear accelerators, has presented the opportunity to advance clinical research efforts beyond what has been achieved to date with mixed-beam schedules and to treat patients with neutrons alone.

A successor study to RTOG 77-04 was recently initiated. Eligible patients include those with Stages B2 (Gleason pattern score > 6), C, and D1 adenocarcinomas of the prostate. Surgical staging of pelvic lymph nodes is encouraged, and patients are subjected to routine 2-year posttreatment biopsies. The patient randomization is between photon and neutron radiation. Patients randomized to neutron radiation receive treatments thrice weekly, 10 neutron cGy per fraction, for a total of 1360 neutron cGy to the pelvis and 2040 neutron cGy to the prostate. These were chosen as maximally tolerated safe doses based on data collected in an RTOG Phase I dose-searching protocol investigating tolerance of pelvic tissues to fast neutrons. Neutron treatments are therefore completed in 12 fractions over 4 weeks, compared to the 35 fractions over 7 weeks required to complete photon irradiation.

As of April 1988, 111 patients have been entered into this collaborative trial. To date, acute reactions among the patients treated with high-energy neutrons have been acceptable, and patient acceptance of the rapid treatment course has been high. It is expected that this study will provide definitive data to assess whether fast neutron irradiation of prostatic carcinoma provides the incremental improvement over photon irradiation suggested by earlier experiences.

Table 13–4
Fast Neutron Irradiation for Locally Advanced Prostate Cancer

Trial	No. of Patients	Treatment	Stage	Survival	Years of Follow-up*
RTOG[27]	55	Mixed beam	C/D₁	63%	8
RTOG[27]	36	Photons	C/D₁	13%	8
RTOG[28]	55	Mixed beam	C/D₁	82%*	8
RTOG[28]	36	Photons	C/D₁	54%*	8
Louvain-la-Neuve[29,30]	50	Mixed beam	A = 14	90% local control;	3
			C = 30	7/10 followed	
			D = 6	3 years = NED	
Hamburg[31]	13†	Mixed beam	T₃ = 7	85%	5
			T₄ = 5	20%	5
Chiba University[33]	25	Mixed beam = 11 Neutrons only = 15	C = 14	77%	3

* Adjusted to exclude intercurrent noncancer deaths.

† One of these patients was not evaluable.

Head and Neck Tumors ■

The use of fast neutron radiation therapy to treat patients with squamous cell head and neck cancer has been studied intermittently for four decades. Following Stone's early work, Catterall and coworkers conducted a randomized study in the 1960s at Hammersmith Hospital in London, reporting a significant advantage for neutrons over conventional photon treatment.[35] Using the low-energy MRC cyclotron, they observed a 76% (53/70) local control rate for neutrons compared to 19% (12/63) for photons in a group of patients with advanced disease. The survival rates were poor in both treatment groups. This early work led to many follow-up studies in Europe, Japan, and the United States.[36-38]

A second randomized study of fast neutrons in patients with earlier stage head and neck cancer has been reported by Duncan and colleagues.[39] This was a randomized cooperative study conducted at the Antoni van Leeuwenhoek Ziekenhuis in Amsterdam, the Department of Clinical Oncology in Edinburgh, and Universitatsklinikun in Essen. No significant advantage for neutrons over photons was demonstrated. Complete response rates were 70% for neutrons (70/100) and 66% for photons (63/95). The ultimate local control rates were 44% (44/100) for neutrons and 40% (38/95) for photons. There was no significant difference in the overall survival rates between the two groups. These results stand in contrast to those obtained at Hammersmith Hospital.

A third major study was carried out in the United States by the RTOG.[40,41] Patients with inoperable squamous cell carcinomas of the head and neck region were randomized to receive either photon radiation therapy or mixed-beam radiation therapy, as described in the previous section. Patients with previously untreated, histologically proven inoperable squamous cell carcinomas of T-stage T_2, T_3, or T_4 and any N-stage originating in the oral cavity, oropharynx, supraglottic larynx, or hypopharynx were eligible. Exclusion criteria were distant metastases, a Karnofsky performance score less than 60, and prior treatment for head and neck cancer. Of the 322 patients randomized, 297 were eligible for analysis.

Patients randomized to photons received 66 to 74 Gy in 1.8 to 2.0 Gy fractions, five fractions per week over 7 to 8 weeks. The uninvolved neck and supraclavicular regions received 46 to 50 Gy. Patients randomized to neutrons received equivalent doses, derived from the formula described previously, over 7 to 8 weeks. The minimum follow-up on this study is 5 years.

The complete tumor clearance rates at the primary site were 63% for mixed-beam treatment and 64% for photon treatment (p = NS). The primary site tumor control rates at 5 years were 34% for mixed-beam and 42% for photon treatment (p = NS). Figure 13–7 graphically displays the primary tumor control obtained in this study. Although no advantage was demonstrable for mixed-beam radiation therapy at the primary site, mixed-beam treatment was significantly better than photon treatment of the nodes (Fig. 13–8). The initial complete tumor clearance rates in patients with positive lymph nodes were 68% for mixed beam and 55% for photons. The nodal control rates at 5 years were 36% for mixed beam and 23% for photons (p = 0.007). The overall survival was equivalent at 5 years (17% for mixed beam, 23% for photons, p = 0.32), as was the overall complication rate.

The results of studies to date in this tumor system have been inconclusive and somewhat contradictory. The patient populations in these three randomized studies were distinctly different, as evidenced by differences in local control rates with photon therapy and the percentage of patients with neck node involvement (83% for the RTOG study; 66% in the Hammersmith study; approximately 50% in the Edinburgh study).[35,40-42] Currently, patients are being accrued to what promises to be a definitive study of fast neutrons in squamous cell carcinomas of the head and neck using the newer hospital-based, high-energy, isocentric neutron beams. Patients with T_3 or T_4 inoperable squamous cell carcinomas of the oral cavity, oropharynx, or supraglottic larynx are randomized to receive either 20.4 Gy neutron irradiation in 12 fractions over 4 weeks or 70 Gy photon irradiation in 35 fractions over 7 weeks. As of April 1988, 63 patients have been entered in this study, which is projected to be completed in 1991.

Soft Tissue Sarcomas ■

Soft tissue sarcomas historically have been considered radioresistant tumors because of poor results achieved with conventional photon irradiation. Current wisdom regards surgery as the main form of treatment, with radiotherapy and chemotherapy relegated to adjuvant status. The local recurrence rate following conservation surgery alone is about 50%;[43] the use of radiation therapy either preoperatively[44] or postoperatively[43] reduces this rate to about 10%. The effectiveness of chemotherapy in either preventing or eradicating distant metastases is less clear. For adjuvant photon or electron irradiation to be effective, it is generally thought that all gross tumor must be excised. The problem with this approach is that most types of soft tissue sarcoma tend to infiltrate along

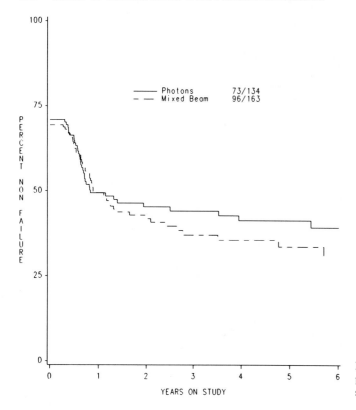

FIG. 13-7 Local control at the primary site following protocol treatment in RTOG 7610. The difference is not statistically significant ($p = 0.43$).

FIG. 13-8 Local control in the involved cervical lymph nodes following protocol treatment in RTOG 7610. The difference is statistically significant, $p = 0.007$.

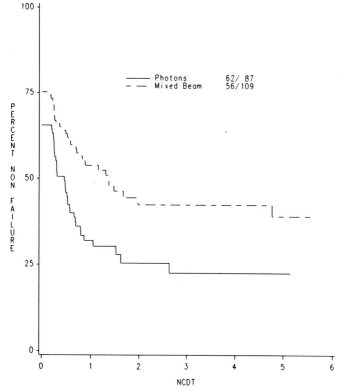

tissue planes or beyond obvious tumor margins, and thus may become quite extensive before they are discovered. This is especially true for lesions of the trunk, retroperitoneum, or proximal thigh.

Reported series of inoperable tumors treated definitively with radiotherapy tend to be rather small and contain many histologic subtypes, grades, and stages. Patients also may have been treated for local control rather than cure, as distant metastases may have been present when the patient first sought medical attention and may have ultimately been the main cause of death. Hence, it is not possible to directly compare the results of the various retrospective studies. Here, the focus will be on local control rather than survival. The results of definitive radiotherapy with neutrons[46-57] or photons/electrons[58-62] for soft tissue sarcomas are summarized in Table 13-5.

The experience with photon irradiation dates back to the work of Windeyer and colleagues[59] in 1966. They treated 11 patients *de novo* and 11 after a postsurgical recurrence (using high-dose radiation). All patients had fibrosarcomas. The overall control rate was 59%. McNeer and associates[58] treated 25 patients with mixed histologies and found an overall local control rate of 56%. The selection criteria for these patients were not well defined, but the authors concluded that a small (albeit unpredictable) group of patients with these lesions are curable by radiotherapy. Duncan and Dewar[60] reported on 25 patients with very extensive tumors treated with low-LET radiotherapy in whom the overall local control rate was 20%. They noted that amputation was the only alternative form of treatment. The most recent report is by Tepper and Suit,[61] who found a 33% local control rate at 5 years in a group of 51 patients treated with radiation alone. For patients receiving doses > 6400 cGy, the local control rate was 43.5%. The local control rate varied as a function of the lesion size: 87.5% for lesions < 5 cm, 53% for lesions between 5 and 10 cm, and 30% for lesions > 10 cm. This underscores both the importance of adequate radiation doses and the difficulty of comparing series dealing with different patient populations. The summed local control rate for all the series was 38% (49/128).

Paradoxically, although fast neutron radiotherapy is a newer form of radiotherapy practiced at a relatively small number of centers throughout the world, the number of definitively treated patients reported in the literature is about 2.5 times that of patients treated with photons and/or electrons. The treatment facilities and philosophies vary considerably; most facilities have used a horizontal neutron beam with relatively poor penetration, and some patients elected to be treated with a combination of neutrons and photons (rather than neutrons alone) in an attempt to reduce morbidity. For specific details of therapy, the reader is referred to the cited references. However, all patients were treated in what the attending physicians regarded as a definitive rather than strictly palliative manner. When neutrons alone were used, doses ranged from 15.6 to 26 Gy and fields were generally designed to cover the tumor volume plus a reasonable margin. The time for which the local control rate was quoted also varies from series to series, but in general exceeded 2 years posttreatment. (Reports that give only response rates after treatment are not included in the review.)

The most recently published series, from Hammersmith Hospital,[46] shows a local control rate of 52% (26/50). This is less than the rate of 77% (17/22) quoted in a previous work.[63] In this study, 20 patients were treated for recurrent tumors after previous surgery, radiotherapy, or both, and 62% of the tumors were > 10 cm in diameter. The main cause of death was metastatic disease, and the median survival was strongly related to tumor grade: 63 months for Grade I, 7 months for Grade II, and 9 months for Grade III. The two largest series are from Germany.[52-54] The Hamburg/Eppendorf group used a dT generator,[52] the Essen group used a low-energy cyclotron with a mean neutron energy of 5.8 MeV,[53,54]

Table 13–5
Local Control Rates for Soft Tissue Sarcomas Treated Definitively with Radiation Therapy*

Study	Local Control	Percent
Neutrons		
Hammersmith[46]	26/50	52
NIRS[47]	7/12	58
Fermi Laboratory[48]	13/26	50
MANTA[49]	4/10	40
TAMVEC[50]	18/29	62
Edinburgh[51]	5/12	42
Hamberg/Eppendorf[52]	27/45	60
Heidelberg/Essen[53]	31/60	52
Louvain[53,54]	4/19	21
Amsterdam[55]	8/13	61
Seattle†[57]	15/21	71
Total	158/297	53
Photons/Electrons		
McNeer et al[58]	14/25	56
Windeyer et al[59]	13/22	59
Duncan and Dewar[60]	5/25	20
Tepper and Suit[61]	17/51	33
Liebel et al[62]	0/5	—
Total	49/128	38

* Patients treated *de novo* or for gross disease after surgery are included, but not patients treated postoperatively for microscopic residual disease or for limited macroscopic residual disease.

† Two-year actuarial data.

and the Heidelberg group used a dT generator.[53,54] The beams from these systems were suboptimal in the treatment of large tumors; nevertheless, the two series summed together show a local control rate of 55% (58/105). The highest energy neutron beam was used at the Fermi Laboratory,[48] with a local control rate of 50% (13/26). The lowest local control rate was from Louvain (21%), for a study that excluded intraabdominal or intrathoracic tumors.[55] The results of the other series shown in Table 13–5 are remarkably similar; the overall local control rate was 53% (158/297). There are also some published data from Eichhorn and colleagues,[64] showing a complete response rate of 48% (39/82) in a group of patients treated by a Soviet-made 4120 cyclotron (mean neutron energy-6.1 MeV), but these patients are not included in Table 13–5) because follow-up times are not documented.

It was not possible to assess the complication rates from some of the published papers, but rates that are described tend to be remarkably similar, ranging between 25% and 40% for Grades III and above (using the combined RTOG/EORTC scoring scheme). Late effects often compromised motion around a joint, but again, the alternative form of treatment would have been amputation in many cases.

Although they are not sarcomas *per se,* cordomas are soft tissue tumors, which arise from remnants of the notochord (primarily in the clivus or sacrum). Lesions of the clivus generally are not amenable to fast neutron radiotherapy because the radiation dose that can be safely given is limited by the tolerance of the central nervous system. Lesions in this area are best referred for charged-particle radiotherapy. Sacral lesions, on the other hand, are readily irradiated. Three cases have been treated at Hammersmith Hospital[65] and five in Seattle. Local control rates were 2/3 and 3/5, respectively, a summed value of 63% (5/8). In our experience, these lesions regress quite slowly, over a period of months to years, but the overall locoregional response is similar to that of soft tissue sarcomas.

Osteogenic Sarcoma ■

Traditionally, osteogenic sarcomas have been treated with radical surgery—often by amputation. When this is feasible (and acceptable to the patient), local control can generally be achieved, and distant metastases constitute the primary failure mode. Chemotherapy is currently being used in an attempt to forestall distant dissemination. However, for tumors arising in the axial skeleton, radical surgery may not be possible.

In other patients, distant metastases may be present when the primary lesion is discovered, raising questions about the use of radical surgery. In such cases, radical radiotherapy would be an acceptable alternate form of treatment if local control could be achieved with acceptable morbidity.

Unfortunately, conventional radiotherapy for these lesions requires quite high radiation doses. DeMoor[66] described a series of 43 patients treated with 6600 to 7700 cGy over 6 to 8 weeks. All patients with lower extremity lesions who were followed for more than 1 year had pronounced subcutaneous fibrosis and partial flexion ankylosis of the knee. Eleven patients required amputation; in 3 cases, no tumor was present in the operative specimen. In another 3 cases, there was significant radiation change, and tumor cells of questionable viability were noted on pathologic examination. The net local control rate was 33% (9/43). Beck and colleagues[67] reported on a series of 21 patients treated at the University of California, San Francisco. There was only one long-term survivor with persisting local control. This patient had a lesion of the mandible and received 5200 cGy external beam radiation and an additional 5600 cGy via an implant. Tudway[68] reported on 9 patients treated with orthovoltage radiation to doses between 5500 and 8000 cGy. Local control was achieved in 5 of 9 patients (56%) but 3 patients had sequelae that restricted motion of the involved extremity. The photon data are summarized in Table 13–6. The overall local control rate in the photon-treated patients was 21% (15/73).

A total of 73 patients have received high-dose neutron radiation for osteogenic sarcomas (see Table 13–6).[47–51,56,69,70] The largest series is from the NIRS facility in Japan,[47,69,70] where patients received chemotherapy (doxorubicin, vincristine sulfate, and high-dose methotrexate) along with radiation treatments. Seventeen patients subsequently underwent either an amputation or a second-look incisional biopsy. A remarkably high proportion—15/17, or 88%—were found to be histologically free of viable tumor. The three failures in the Amsterdam series[56] and the four failures in the Edinburgh series[51] were classified as such because of persistent mass and calcification. Because it is doubtful that the osteoid matrix left behind would resolve even if the tumor cells were sterilized, these articles may have underestimated the local control rates. The one treatment "success" in the Edinburgh series died of metastatic disease; autopsy confirmed tumor control in the two treated regions. An updated report from Japan does not discuss local control at all but focuses instead on survival.[71] The 48 patients treated with fast neutrons had a 5-year survival of 67% compared to 19% for 17 patients

Table 13–6
Local Control Rates for Osteogenic Sarcomas Treated Definitively with Radiation Therapy*

Study	Local Control	Percent
Neutrons		
MANTA[49]	1/1	100
TAMVEC[50]	0/1	—
Fermi Laboratory[48]	2/9	22
Amsterdam[56]	0/3	—†
Edinburgh[51]	1/5	20†
NIRS[47,69,70]	33/41	80
Seattle‡	3/13	23
Total	40/73	55
Photons		
DeMoor[66]	9/43	33
Beck et al[67]	1/21	5
Tudway[68]	5/9	56
Total	15/73	21

* Patients treated postoperatively for microscopic residual disease or for limited macroscopic residual disease are not included.

† Persistent mass and calcification are treated as failures; hence, local control rates may be underestimated.

‡ Two-year actuarial data.

Table 13–7
Local Control Rates for Chondrosarcomas Treated Definitively with Radiation Therapy*

Study	Local Control	Percent
Neutrons		
MANTA[49]	7/9	78
TAMVEC[50]	4/4	100
Fermi Laboratory[48]	9/16	56
Amsterdam[56]	0/6	—†
Edinburgh[51]	0/5	—†
NIRS[47]	1/2	50
Seattle[57]†	4/9	44
Total	25/51	49
Photons		
McNaney et al[72]	3/10	30
Harwood et al[73]	7/20	35
Total	10/30	33

* Patients treated postoperatively for microscopic residual disease or for limited macroscopic residual disease are not included.

† Persistent mass and calcification are treated as failures; hence, local control rates may be underestimated.

‡ Two-year actuarial data.

treated with photon irradiation. However, this was not a randomized trial. The incidence of late skin reactions was found to be equivalent in the two groups. The overall local control rate for the summed series of patients is 55% (40/73). The complication rate is often difficult to determine; many authors tend to group the osteogenic sarcomas with the soft tissue sarcomas in reporting complications. Hence, it is reasonable to assume that, as a first approximation, complications would be site-dependent rather than histology-dependent, and thus would be in the range of 25% to 40%.

Chondrosarcoma ■

Chondrosarcomas occur at about half the frequency of osteogenic sarcomas, and reported patient series tend to be rather small. Like other types of sarcomas, they are generally thought of as radioresistant; therefore, surgery is the mainstay of treatment. However, unlike osteosarcoma, this tumor tends to arise in the axial skeleton rather than the extremities, and radical surgery may not be an option in many cases.

The literature on the results of radical photon irradiation for chondrosarcomas is rather sparse (Table 13–7). McNaney and associates[72] described 10 patients who were definitively treated at M. D. Ander-

son. They defined treatment failure as progression of symptoms and/or increase in the size of the mass lesion. The local control rate was 30% (3/10). The same group noted a local control rate of 100% in 4 patients treated with fast neutrons at the TAMVEC facility.[50] Of particular note is the fact that 3 of the failures in photon-treated patients occurred at long intervals after treatment (42 months, 132 months, and 156 months). The neutron-treated patients have not been at risk for these time periods. Harwood and colleagues[73] found a control rate of 35% (7/20) in patients who were treated definitively at Princess Margaret Hospital. They noted that the clinical response of the tumors was slow, requiring several months. Radiographically, the affected bone never returned to normal.[74] The authors concluded that chondrosarcomas should not be classified as radioresistant and that radical radiotherapy has a definite role in selected cases. The overall local control rate with photon irradiation for chondrosarcoma is 33% (10/30).

The experience with neutron irradiation for this lesion is summarized in Table 13–7.[47–51,56,69] The overall local control rate is 49% (25/51), despite the fact that two series[51,56] showed no local control in any of their patients. Both of these groups counted persistent mass and calcification as failures when, in reality, this may not be the case. The chondroid matrix elaborated by these tumors is left behind after

Table 13–8
Results of Fast Neutron Clinical Trials*

Site/Histology	No. of Patients	Results
Salivary gland	280	Positive (++++)
Prostate cancer	285	Positive (+++)
Bone sarcomas	75	Positive (++)
Soft tissue sarcomas	350	Positive (++)
Squamous cell head and neck cancer	>2000	Equivocal
Lung	425	Equivocal
Bladder	160	Equivocal
Cervix	260	Equivocal
Brain	>600	Negative
Esophagus	120	Negative
Pancreas	>100	Negative

* Patients were treated with physics-laboratory-based fixed beam machines.

radiotherapy, regardless of whether or not the tumor cells are sterilized. This matrix shows increasing calcification over time. There is initially some regression of the soft tissue component of the mass, but this is by no means complete. What is important is that the mass stabilizes and symptoms resolve. These are the criteria used by the other authors; therefore, the overall figure of 49% likely is an underestimate of the effectiveness of fast neutron radiotherapy for this class of tumor.

Other Tumor Sites ■

Neutron studies have been carried out in malignancies of the central nervous system, esophagus, lung, breast, pancreas, bladder, and cervix. Although some of the early results from these studies look promising, no definitive advantages have yet been demonstrated for neutron irradiation in these sites.

Conclusion ■

The biologic advantages of high- versus low-LET radiation can be summarized in terms of a decreased OER, a diminished capacity for cellular sublethal and potentially lethal damage repair, and diminished variability of radiosensitivity of cells in different stages of the cell cycle. These potential biologic advantages led to the neutron clinical trials outlined in the preceding pages. A summary of these and other trials is given in Table 12–8.

Until recently, heavy particle radiation research has been limited by equipment availability and versatility. Reliance on laboratory-based fixed horizontal beam machines severely handicaps the development of neutron radiotherapy. The installation of hospital-based high-energy cyclotrons capable of isocentric neutron beam delivery has greatly improved this situation. However, cost and size considerations still make these machines impractical for most hospital settings. New developments in superconductor technology hold a promise for the development of small, relatively inexpensive (at least comparatively) particle accelerators suitable for heavy particle radiation therapy. If this promise is realized, fast neutron radiation therapy may indeed become practical for a large number of treatment centers.

References ■

1. Stone RS: Neutron therapy and specific ionization. Am J Roentgenol 59:771, 1940
2. Catterall M, Bewley DK: Fast Neutrons in the Treatment of Cancer, pp 14–27. London, Academic Press, 1973
3. Catterall M: The treatment of advanced cancer by fast neutrons from the Medical Research Council's cyclotron at Hammersmith Hospital, London. Eur J Cancer 10:343, 1974
4. Eichhorn HJ: Results of a pilot study on neutron therapy with 600 patients. Int J Radiat Oncol Biol Phys 8:1561, 1982
5. Fowler PH, Perkins DH: The possibility of therapeutic applications of beams of negative pi mesons. Nature 189:524, 1981
6. Batterman JJ, Breur K, Hart GAM, van Peperzeel HA: Observations on pulmonary metastases in patients after single doses and multiple fractions of fast neutrons and cobalt-60 gamma rays. Eur J Cancer 17:539–548, 1981
7. Borthne A, Kjellevold K, Kaalhus O, Vermund H: Salivary gland malignant neoplasms: Treatment and prognosis. Int J Radiat Oncol Biol Phys 12:747–754, 1986
8. Dobrowsky W, Schlappack O, Karcher KH, Pavelka R, Kmet G: Electron beam therapy in treatment of parotid neoplasm. Radiother Oncol 6:293–299, 1986
9. Duncan W, Orr JA, Arnott SJ, Jack WJC: Neutron therapy for malignant tumors of the salivary glands. A report of the Edinburgh experience. Radiother Oncol 8:97–104, 1987
10. Eichhorn HJ: Pilot study on the applicability of neutron radiotherapy. Radiobiol Radiother 3:262–292, 1981
11. Fu KK, Leibel SA, Levine ML, Friedlander LM, Boles R, Phillips TL: Carcinoma of the major and minor salivary glands: Analysis of treatment results and sites and causes of failures. Cancer 40:2882–2890, 1977
12. Griffin BR, Laramore GE, Russell KJ, Griffin TW, Eenmaa J: Fast neutron radiotherapy for advanced malignant salivary gland tumors. Radiother Oncol 12:105–111, 1988
13. Kaplan EL, Meier P: Non-parametric estimation from incomplete observations. J Am Statist Assoc 53:457–481, 1958
14. Rafla S: Malignant parotid tumors: Natural history and treatment. Cancer 40:136, 1977
15. Rossman KJ: The role of radiation therapy in the treatment of parotid carcinomas. Am J Radiol 123:492–499, 1975

16. Armitage P: Statistical Methods in Medical Research, pp 135–136. New York, John Wiley & Sons, 1973

17. Batterman JJ, Mijnheer BJ: The Amsterdam fast neutron radiotherapy project: A final report. Int J Radiat Oncol Biol Phys 12:2093–2099, 1986

18. Conley J, Baker DG: Cancer of the salivary glands. In Cancer of the Head and Neck, pp 524–556. New York, Churchill Livingstone, 1981

19. Elkon D, Colman J, Hendrickson FR: Radiation therapy in the treatment of malignant salivary gland tumors. Cancer 41:502–506, 1978

20. Fitzpatrick PJ, Theriault C: Malignant salivary gland tumors. Int J Radiat Oncol Biol Phys 12:1743–1747, 1986

21. Mantel N: Evaluation of survival data and two new rank order statistics arising in its consideration. Cancer Chem Rep 5:163–170, 1966

22. Maor MH, Hussey DH, Fletcher GH, Jesse RH: Fast neutron radiotherapy for locally advanced head and neck tumors. Int J Radiat Oncol Biol Phys 7:155–163, 1981

23. Ornitz R, Herskovic A, Bradley E, Deyeand JA, Rogers CC: Clinical observations of early and late normal tissue injury and tumor control in patients receiving fast neutron irradiation. In Barendsen GW, Broerse J, Breur K (eds). High LET Radiations in Clinical Radiotherapy, pp 43–50. New York, Pergamon Press, 1979

24. Reddy EK, Mansfield CW, Hartman GV, Rouby E: Malignant salivary gland tumors: Role of radiation therapy. JAMA 71:959–961, 1979

25. Saroja KR, Mansell J, Hendrickson FR, Cohen L, Lennox A: An update on malignant salivary gland tumors treated with neutrons at Fermilab. Int J Radiat Oncol Biol Phys (in press)

26. Skolyszewski J, Byrski E, Chrzanowska A, Gasinka A, Reinfuss M, Huczkowski J, Lazarska B, Michalowski A, Meder J: A preliminary report on the clinical application of fast neutrons in Krakow. Int J Radiat Oncol Biol Phys 8:1781–1786, 1982

27. Laramore GE, Krall JM, Thomas FJ, Griffin TW, Maor MH, Hendrickson FR: Fast neutron radiotherapy for locally advanced prostate cancer: Results of an RTOG randomized study. Int J Radiat Oncol Biol Phys 11:1621–1627, 1985

28. Russell KJ, Laramore GE, Krall JM, Thomas FJ, Maor MH, Hendrickson FR, Krieger JN, Griffin TW: Eight years' experience with neutron radiotherapy in the treatment of Stages C and D prostate cancer: Updated results of the RTOG 7704 randomized clinical trial. Prostate 11:183–193, 1987

29. Wambersie A, Battermann JJ: Review and evolution of clinical results in the EORTC Heavy Particle Therapy Group. Strahlentherapie 161:746–755, 1985

30. Richard F, Renard L, Wambersie A: Current results of neutron therapy at the UCL, for soft tissue sarcomas and prostatic adenocarcinomas. Bull Cancer (Paris) 73:562–568, 1986

31. Franke HD, HeB A, Langendorff G, Borchers HD: The combined treatment of prostate cancer (Stage C) with definitive megavoltage irradiation and fast neutrons (DT, 14 MeV). Urologe A 19:341–349, 1980

32. Franke HD, Schmidt R: Clinical results with fast neutrons (DT, 14 MeV). Radiat Med 3(3):151–160, 1985

33. Maruoka M, Ando K, Nozumi K, Ito H, Shimazaki J, Matsuzaki O, Morita S, Tsunemoto H: Fast neutron therapy of prostatic cancer. Nippon Hinyokika Gakkai Zasshi 74:409–417, 1983

34. Orton CG, Ellis F: A simplification in the use of the NSD concept in practical radiotherapy. Br J Radiol 46:529–537, 1973

35. Catterall M, Bewley DK, Sutherland I: Second report on a randomized clinical trial of fast neutrons with X or gamma rays in the treatment of advanced cancers of the head and neck. Br Med J 1:1942, 1977

36. Laramore GE, Griffin TW, Tesh DW, Wong HH, Parker RG: Phase I pilot study on fast neutron teletherapy for advanced carcinoma of the head and neck region: Final report on local control rate and survival. Cancer 51:192–199, 1983

37. Maor MH, Hussey DH, Fletcher GH et al: Fast neutron therapy for locally advanced head and neck tumors. Int J Radiat Oncol Biol Phys 7:155–173, 1981 (also private communication)

38. Morita S, Tsunemoto H, Kurisu A et al: Results of fast neutron therapy at NIRS. Presented at Fourth High LET Radiotherapy Seminar, sponsored by the United States-Japan Cooperative Cancer Research Program. Philadelphia, PA, June 1978

39. Duncan W, Arnott SJ, Batterman JJ et al: Fast neutrons in the treatment of advanced head and neck cancers: The results of a multicentre randomly controlled trial. Radiother Oncol 2:293–305, 1984

40. Griffin TW, Davis R, Laramore GE, Hussey DH, Hendrickson FR, Rodriguez-Antunez A: Fast neutron irradiation of metastatic cervical adenopathy: the results of a randomized RTOG study. Int J Radiat Oncol Biol Phys 9:1267–1270, 1983

41. Griffin TW, Davis R, Hendrickson FR: Fast neutron therapy for unresectable squamous cell carcinomas of the head and neck: the results of a randomized RTOG study. Int J Radiat Oncol Biol Phys 10:2217–2221, 1984

42. Duncan W, Arnott SJ, Orr JA et al: The Edinburgh experience of fast neutron therapy. Int J Radiat Oncol Biol Phys 8:2155–2164, 1982

43. Lindberg RD: The role of radiation therapy in the treatment of soft-tissue sarcomas in adults. Semin Oncol 16:883–888, 1976

44. Suit H, Proppe K, Mankin H, Wood WC: Preoperative radiation therapy for sarcoma of soft tissue. Cancer 47:2269–2274, 1981

45. Lindberg RD, Martin RG, Romsdahl MM, Barkley HT: Conservative surgery and postoperative radiotherapy in 300 adults with soft tissue sarcoma. Cancer 47:2391–2397, 1981

46. Pickering DG, Stewart JS, Rampling DG, Errington RD, Stamp G, Chia V: Fast neutron therapy for soft tissue sarcoma. Int J Radiat Oncol Biol Phys 13:1489–1495, 1987

47. Tsunemoto H, Shinroku S, Arai T, Kutsutani Y, Kurisu A, Umegaki Y: Results of clinical trial with 30 MeV d → Be neutrons at NIRS. In Abey M, Sakamoto K, Phillips TL (eds). Treatment of Radioresistant Cancers, pp 115–126. Amsterdam, Elsevier North Holland, 1979

48. Cohen L, Hendrickson F, Mansell J, Kurup PD, Awschalom M, Rosenberg I, Tan Haken RK: Response of sarcomas of bone and of soft tissue to neutron beam therapy. Int J Radiat Oncol Biol Phys 10:821–824, 1984

49. Ornitz R, Herskovic A, Schell M, Fender F, Rogers CC: Treatment experience: Locally advanced sarcomas with 15 MeV fast neutrons. Cancer 45:2712–2716, 1980

50. Salinas R, Hussey DH, Fletcher G, Lindberg R, Martin R, Peters L, Sinkovics J: Experience with fast neutrons for locally advanced sarcomas. Int J Radiat Oncol Biol Phys 6:267–272, 1980

51. Duncan W, Arnott SJ, Jack WJL: The Edinburgh experience of treating sarcomas of soft tissue and bone with neutron irradiation. Clin Radiol 37:317–320, 1986

52. Franke HD: Clinical experiences with treatment of more than 50 patients with fast neutrons (DT, 14 MeV) since 1976 in Hamberg-Eppendorf. In Lopis, Eckhart (eds): Lectures and Symposia 14th International Cancer Congress, Budapest, 1986, Vol 8, pp 93–106. Basel, S Karger/Budapest, Akademiai Kiado, 1987

53. Schmitt G, Rassow J, Schnabel K, Borman R, Bamberg M, Scherer E, Streffer C: Radiotherapy of soft tissue sarcomas with neutrons or a neutron boost. Br J Radiol 57:247–250, 1984

54. Schmitt G, Schnabel K, Sauerwein W, Scherer E: Neutron and neutron-boost irradiation of soft-tissue sarcomas: A 4.5 year analysis of 139 patients. Radiother Oncol 1:23–29, 1983

55. Wambersie A: The European experience in neutron radiotherapy at the end of 1981. Int J Radiat Oncol Biol Phys 8:2145–2152, 1982

56. Batterman JJ, Breur K: Fast neutron radiotherapy for locally advanced sarcomas. Int J Radiat Oncol Biol Phys 7:1051–1053, 1981

57. Pelton JG, Del Rowe JD, Bolen JW, Russell AH, Laramore GE, Griffin TW, Griffin BR: Fast neutron radiotherapy for soft tissue sarcomas: University of Washington experience and review of the world's literature. Am J Clin Oncol 9:397–400, 1986 (and unpublished update)

58. McNeer GP, Cantin J, Chu F, Nickson JJ: Effectiveness of radiation therapy in the management of sarcoma of the soft somatic tissues. Cancer 22:391–397, 1968

59. Windeyer W, Dische S, Mansfield CM: The place of radiotherapy in the management of fibrosarcoma of the soft tissues. Clin Radiol 17:32–40, 1966

60. Duncan W, Dewar JA: A retrospective study of the role of radiotherapy in the treatment of soft tissue sarcoma. Clin Radiol 36:629–632, 1986

61. Tepper JE, Suit HD: Radiation therapy alone for sarcoma of soft tissue. Cancer 56:475–479, 1985

62. Leibel SA, Tranbaugh RF, Wara WM, Beckstead JH, Bovill EG, Phillips TL: Soft tissue sarcomas of the extremities: Survival and patterns of failure with conservative surgery with postoperative irradiation compared to surgery alone. Cancer 50:1076–1083, 1982

63. Batterman JJ, Breur K, Hart GAM, Van Peperzeel HA: Observations on pulmonary metastases in patients after single doses and multiple fractions of fast neutrons and cobalt-60 gamma rays. Eur J Cancer Clin Oncol 17:539–548, 1981

64. Eichhorn HJ, Dallage KH: Results of neutron therapy of soft tissue sarcomas. Strahlentherapie 61:801–803, 1985

65. Catterall M, Bewley D: Fast Neutrons in the Treatment of Cancer, Chap. 11. London, Academic Press, 1979

66. DeMoor NG: Osteosarcoma: A review of 72 cases treated by megavoltage radiation therapy with or without surgery. S Afr J Surg 13:137–146, 1975

67. Beck JC, Wara WM, Bovill EG, Phillips TL: The role of radiation therapy in the treatment of osteosarcoma. Radiology 120:163–165, 1976

68. Tudway RC: Radiotherapy for osteogenic sarcoma. J Bone Joint Surg 43B:61–67, 1961

69. Hodaka E, Maruyama K, Takada N, Tatezaki S: Multimodality treatment including fast neutron radiotherapy for osteosarcoma. Cancer Bull 31:216–219, 1979

70. Tsunemoto H, Arai T, Morita S, Ishikawa T, Aoki Y, Takada N, Kamata S: Japanese experience with clinical trials of fast neutrons. Int J Radiat Oncol Biol Phys 8:2169–2171, 1982

71. Tsunemoto H, Morita S, Sato S, Jino V, Yoo SY: Present status of fast neutron therapy in Asian countries. Strahlentherapie (in press)

72. McNaney D, Lindberg RD, Ayala AG, Barkley HT, Hussey DH: Fifteen-year radiotherapy experience with chondrosarcoma of bone. Int J Radiat Oncol Biol Phys 8:187–190, 1982

73. Harwood AR, Krajbich JI, Fornasier VL: Radiotherapy of chondrosarcoma of bone. Cancer 45:2769–2777, 1980

74. Krochak R, Harwood AR, Cummings BJ, Quirt IC: Results of radical radiation for chondrosarcoma of bone. Radiother Oncol 109–115, 1983

75. Vikram B, Strong EW, Shah JP, Spiro RH: Radiation therapy in adenoid-cystic carcinoma. Int J Radiat Oncol Biol Phys 10:221–223, 1984

76. Stewart JG, Jackson A, Chew M: The role of radiation therapy in the management of malignant tumors of the salivary glands. Am J Roentgenol Radium Ther Nucl Med 102:100–108, 1968

77. Shidnia H, Hornbeck N, Hamaker R, Lingeman R: Carcinoma of major salivary glands. Cancer 45:693–697, 1980

Part Three

Controversies
in Oncology

Bruce N. Ames

What Are the Major Carcinogens in the Etiology of Human Cancer?

Environmental Pollution, Natural Carcinogens, and the Causes of Human Cancer: Six Errors

14a

Introduction ■

Arguments that industrial pollutants are present in significant amounts or contribute substantially to cancer rates share several mistaken assumptions. These are discussed in the following sections, as is the danger inherent in diverting our attention away from tobacco and dietary, hormonal, occupational, and viral carcinogens to industrial pollutants.

Error 1: Cancer Rates Are Soaring ■

Overall, US cancer death rates are staying at the same levels or decreasing, the major exception being smoking-related cancer. A recent update from the National Cancer Institute (February 1988)[1] indicates that "the age adjusted mortality rate for all cancers combined except lung cancer has been declining since 1950 for all individual age groups except 85 and above" (13% decrease overall, 44,000 deaths below expected; 0.1% increase in the over-85 group). The types of cancer deaths that have been decreasing during this period are primarily those of the stomach (by 75%, 37,000 deaths below expected), cervix (73%, 11,000 deaths below expected), uterus (60%, 9,000 deaths below expected), and rectum (65%, 13,000 deaths below expected). The types of cancer deaths that are increasing

are primarily lung cancer (by 247%, 91,000 deaths above expected), which is caused by smoking (as is 30% of U.S. cancer) and non-Hodgkin's lymphoma (by 100%, 8,000 deaths above expected). The overall cancer mortality trends can be seen in the latest plot from the American Cancer Society (Fig. 14a–1).

Clearly, changes in survival rates and incidence rates are also relevant in interpreting those changes.[1,2] Incidence rates have been increasing for some types of cancer. Doll and Peto,[2] in their definitive study on cancer trends, pointed out that although incidence rates are of interest, they should not be taken in isolation because of the substantial extent to which trends in recorded incidence rates are biased by improvements in the level of registration and diagnosis, as appears to be the case with breast cancer. Even if particular types of cancer are shown to increase or decrease, establishing a causal relation among the many changing aspects of our lives remains difficult.[3-14] There is no convincing evidence that there is a general increase in cancer related to the conditions of the modern industrial world.[2,9,12]

Life expectancy is steadily increasing in the United States and other industrial countries; infant mortality is decreasing; and, although the statistics are not good, there is no evidence that birth defects are increasing. Thus, the conclusion is that Americans are healthier than they have ever been.

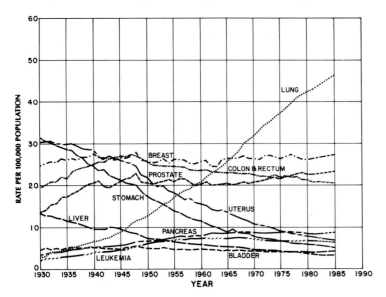

FIG. 14a–1   Cancer death rates by site, United States, 1930–1985. All figures are age-adjusted. Rate for the population standardized for age on the 1970 U.S. population. Sources of data: National Center for Health Statistics and Bureau of the Census, United States. Rates are for both sexes combined except breast and uterus, female population only, and prostate, male population only. (Reprinted with permission from Cancer Facts and Figures—1988, New York, American Cancer Society, 1988)

Error 2: Only a Small Number of Chemicals Are Carcinogenic or Teratogenic, and We Can Eliminate Them ■

More than 50% of the chemicals tested to date in rats and mice have been found to be carcinogens at the high doses administered,[3,15] the maximum tolerated dose (MTD). The exhaustive database of animal cancer tests developed by me and my colleagues[16,17] listed 392 chemicals tested in both rats and mice at the MTD. Of these, 58% of the synthetic chemicals and 45% of the natural chemicals were carcinogens in at least one species.[3,15] We concluded that the proportion of chemicals found to be carcinogens is strikingly high, a conclusion reached by others on the basis of smaller compilations. The earlier Innes and colleagues study[18] is sometimes cited to support the conclusion that the proportion of carcinogens is low. However, that study used a much smaller dataset (120 chemicals, 11 positive), and the tests, although appropriate for their time, used only one species and were less thorough than modern tests.[15]

Even when one considers that some chemicals are selected for testing based on a high index of suspicion, the large proportion of positive findings is disturbing. From considerations of carcinogenesis mechanisms, it is plausible that a large proportion of all chemicals we test in the future, both natural and man-made, will prove to be carcinogens (see "Error 4" below).[3]

Large proportions of positives are also reported for teratogenesis tests. Fully one-third of the 2800 chemicals tested in laboratory animals have been shown to induce birth defects at the MTD.[19] Thus, it seems likely that a sizable percentage of both natural and man-made chemicals will be reproductive toxins when tested at these doses. The world is full of carcinogens and reproductive toxins, and it always has been. The important issue is the human exposure dose, and, fortunately, this is almost always miniscule.

The major preventable risk factors for cancer causation, such as tobacco, dietary imbalances,[11,13,14,20–23] hormones,[10] and viruses,[24,25] have been discussed by us[3–8,26] and others.[2,9–12]

Error 3: Man-made Chemical Pollutants Are Present in Significant Amounts ■

We have attempted to address the issue of priority setting among possible carcinogenic hazards.[3] Carcinogens differ enormously in potency in rodent tests, and comparisons of possible hazards from various carcinogens ingested by humans must take this into account. Our analysis makes use of an exhaustive database of carcinogenic potency (currently 3500 experiments on 975 chemicals)[16,17] that analyzes animal cancer tests and calculates the TD_{50}, essentially the dose of the carcinogen sufficient to cause cancer in half of the animals. The TD_{50} is close to the high dose (MTD) actually given, and thus involves a minimal extrapolation. To calculate our index of possible hazard, we express each human exposure (daily lifetime dose, in mg/kg) as a percentage of the rodent TD_{50} dose (mg/kg) for each carcinogen. We call this percentage HERP (human exposure dose/rodent potency dose). Because rodent data are all calculated on the basis of lifetime exposure at the indicated daily dose rate,[16,17] the human exposure data are similarly

Table 14a–1
Ranking of Possible Carcinogenic Hazards*

Possible Hazard: HERP (%)	Daily Human Exposure	Carcinogen Dose per 70-kg Person	Potency of Carcinogen: TD$_{50}$ (mg/kg)	
			Rats	Mice
Environmental Pollution				
0.001†	Tap water 1 L	Chloroform, 83 µg (US average)	(119)	90
0.004†	Well water, 1 L contaminated (worst well in Silicon Valley)	Trichloroethylene, 2800 µg	(−)	941
0.0004†	Well water, 1 L contaminated, Woburn	Trichloroethylene, 267 µg	(−)	941
0.0002†		Chloroform, 12 µg	(119)	90
0.0003†		Tetrachloroethylene, 21 µg	101	(126)
0.008†	Swimming pool, 1 h (for child)	Chloroform, 250 µg (average pool)	(119)	90
0.6	Conventional home air (14 h/d)	Formaldehyde, 598 µg	1.5	(44)
0.004		Benzene, 155 µg	(157)	53
2.1	Mobile home air (14 h/d)	Formaldehyde, 2.2 mg	1.5	(44)
Pesticide and Other Residues				
0.0002†	PCBs: daily dietary intake	PCBs, 0.2 µg (US average)	1.7	(9.6)
0.0003†	DDE/DDT: daily dietary intake	DDE, 2.2 µg (US average)	(−)	13
0.0004	EDB: daily dietary intake (from grains and grain products)	Ethylene dibromide, 0.42 µg (US average)	1.5	(5.1)
Natural Pesticides and Dietary Toxins				
0.003	Bacon, cooked (100 g)	Dimethylnitrosamine, 0.3 µg	(0.2)	0.2
0.006		Diethylnitrosamine, 0.1 µg	0.02	(+)
0.003	Sake (250 ml)	Urethane, 43 µg	(41)	22
0.03	Comfrey herb tea (1 cup)	Symphytine, 38 µg (750 µg of pyrrolizidine alkaloids)	1.9	(?)
0.03	Peanut butter (32 g; one sandwich)	Aflatoxin, 64 ng (US average, 2 ppb)	0.003	(+)
0.06	Dried squid, broiled in gas oven (54 g)	Dimethylnitrosamine, 7.9 µg	(0.2)	0.2
0.07	Brown mustard (5 g)	Allyl isothiocyanate, 4.6 mg	96	(−)
0.1	Basil (1 g of dried leaf)	Estragole, 3.8 mg	(?)	52
0.1	Mushroom, one raw (*Agaricus bisporus;* 15 g)	Mixture of hydrazines, etc.	(?)	20,300
0.2	Natural root beer (12 ounces; 354 ml; now banned)	Safrole, 6.6 mg	(436)	56
0.008	Beer, before 1979 (12 ounces; 354 ml)	Dimethylnitrosamine, 1 µg	(0.2)	0.2
2.8†	Beer (12 ounces; 354 ml)	Ethyl alcohol, 18 ml	9110	(?)
4.7†	Wine (250 ml)	Ethyl alcohol, 30 ml	9110	(?)
6.2†	Comfrey–pepsin tablets (nine daily)	Comfrey root, 2700 mg	626	(?)
1.3	Comfrey–pepsin tablets (nine daily)	Symphytine, 1.8 mg	1.9	(?)
Food Additives				
0.0002	AF-2: daily dietary intake before banning	AF-2 (furylfuramide), 4.8 µg	29	(131)
0.06†	Diet cola (12 ounces; 354 ml)	Saccharin, 95 mg	2143	(−)
Drugs				
[0.3]	Phenacetin pill (average dose)	Phenacetin, 300 mg	1246	(2137)
[5.6]	Metronidazole (therapeutic dose)	Metronidazole, 2000 mg	(542)	506
[14]	Isoniazid pill (prophylactic dose)	Isoniazid, 300 mg	(150)	30
16†	Phenobarbital, one sleeping pill	Phenobarbital, 60 mg	(+)	5.5
17†	Clofibrate (average daily dose)	Clofibrate, 2000 mg	169	(?)
Occupational Exposure				
5.8	Formaldehyde: workers' average daily intake	Formaldehyde, 6.1 mg	1.5	(44)
140	EDB: workers' daily intake (high exposure)	Ethylene dibromide, 150 mg	1.5	(5.1)

Reprinted with permission from Ames BN, Magaw R, Gold LS: Ranking possible carcinogenic hazards. Science 236: 271–280, 1987.

* *Potency of carcinogens:* A number in parentheses indicates a TD$_{50}$ value not used in HERP calculation because it is the less sensitive species; (−) = negative in cancer test; (+) = positive for carcinogenicity in tests not suitable for calculating a TD$_{50}$; (?) = not adequately tested for carcinogenicity. TD$_{50}$ values shown are averages calculated by taking the harmonic mean of the TD$_{50}$ of the positive tests in that species from the Carcinogenic Potency Database. Results are similar if the lowest TD$_{50}$ value (most potent) is used instead. For each test the target site with the lowest TD$_{50}$ value has been used. The average TD$_{50}$ has been calculated separately for rats and mice, and the more sensitive species is used for calculating the possible hazard. The database, with references to the source of the cancer tests, is complete for tests published through 1984 and for the National Toxicology Program bioassays through June 1986. We have not indicated the route of exposure or target sites or other particulars of each test, although these are reported in the database. *Daily human exposure:* We have tried to use average or reasonable daily intakes to facilitate comparisons. In several cases, such as contaminated well water or factory exposure to EDB, this is difficult to determine; these are assigned the value for the worst levels found. The calculations assume a daily dose for a lifetime; where drugs are normally taken only for a short period, we have bracketed the HERP value. For inhalation exposures, we assume an inhalation of 9600 L per 8 h for the workplace and 10,800 L per 14 h for indoor air at home. *Possible hazard:* The amount of rodent carcinogen indicated under carcinogen dose is divided by 70 kg to give a milligram per kilogram of human exposure, and this human dose is given as the percentage of the TD$_{50}$ dose in the rodent (mg/kg) to calculate the HERP.

† HERP from carcinogens thought to be nongenotoxic.

expressed, although the human exposure is likely to be less than daily for a lifetime. The HERP values are not risk assessments, because it is impossible to extrapolate to low doses (see "Error 4"), but provide a way to compare possible hazards of exposures so as to put them in perspective and set priorities (see Table 14a–1).

This analysis suggests that the amounts of pollution humans ingest from pesticide residues or water pollution appear to be trivial relative to the background of natural or traditional (*e.g.,* from cooking food) carcinogens.[3,26]

Nature's Pesticides ■

Americans ingest in their diet at least 10,000 times more natural pesticides (by weight) than man-made pesticide residues.[26] These natural "toxic chemicals" have an enormous variety of chemical structures, appear to be present in all plants, and serve as protection against fungi, insects, and animal predators.[8,26] Although only a few dozen are found in each plant species, they commonly make up 5% to 10% of the plant's dry weight.[26] There has been relatively little interest in the toxicology or carcinogenicity of these compounds until quite recently, although they are by far the main source of "toxic chemicals" ingested by humans.

Although most chemicals tested for carcinogenicity in rodent bioassays are synthetic compounds, the proportion of positive tests is about as high for natural pesticides as for synthetic chemicals. Because more than 99.99% of the pesticides we ingest are "nature's pesticides,"[3,8,26] our diet is likely to be very high in natural carcinogens. Their concentration is usually in parts per thousand or more, rather than parts per billion, as is usual for synthetic pesticide residues or water pollution.[3] The known natural carcinogens in mushrooms, parsley, basil, parsnips, fennel, pepper, celery, figs, mustard, and citrus oil are no doubt just the beginning of the list because so few of nature's pesticides have been tested.[3,8,26] For example, a recent analysis[27] of lima beans showed an array of 23 natural alkaloids (those tested have biocidal activity) that ranged in concentration in stressed plants from 0.2 to 33 parts per thousand fresh weight. None appears to have been tested for carcinogenicity or teratogenicity.

Man-made Pesticide Residues ■

The intake of man-made pesticide residues from food in the United States, including residues of industrial chemicals such as polychlorinated biphenyls (PCBs),

has been estimated by the Food and Drug Administration (FDA). They assayed food for residues of the 70 compounds thought to be of greatest importance.[28] The human intake averages about 150 μg/day. Most of this intake (105 μg) is composed of three chemicals (ethylhexyl diphenyl phosphate, malathion, and chlorpropham), shown to be noncarcinogenic in tests in rodents.[3] Thus, the intake of carcinogens from residues (45 μg/day if all the other residues are carcinogenic, which is unlikely) is extremely small relative to the background of natural substances.[3,26]

The latest figures from the FDA about actual exposures do not include every known man-made pesticide, but represent a reasonable attempt to do so. In a recent National Research Council/National Academy of Sciences (NRC/NAS) report, *Regulating Pesticides in Food,*[29] it is suggested that some of the pesticides not covered by the FDA sampling, particularly those used on tomatoes, should have their allowable limits lowered and presumably should be added to the FDA sampling program. Nevertheless, the estimate of 45 μg of possibly carcinogenic pesticide residues consumed in a day is likely to be a reasonable one, as is our conclusion that the possible hazards from these residues are minimal compared to the background of nature's pesticides. For comparison,[3] there are about 500 μg of carcinogens in a cup of coffee (hydrogen peroxide and methylglyoxal), 185 μg of carcinogenic formaldehyde in a slice of bread, about 2000 μg of formaldehyde in a cola, 760 μg of carcinogenic estragole in a basil leaf, a gram of burnt material from cooking our food, plus nitrosamines formed in gas ovens.

An alternative to synthetic pesticides is to raise the level of natural plant toxins by breeding. However, it is not clear that this approach, even where feasible, is preferable. One consequence of disproportionate concern about tiny traces of synthetic pesticide residues, such as ethylene dibromide,[3] is that plant breeders are developing highly insect-resistant plants, thus creating other risks. Two recent cases are instructive. A major grower introduced a new variety of highly insect-resistant celery into commerce. There was soon a flurry of complaints to the Centers for Disease Control (CDC) from all over the country, because people who handled the celery developed a severe rash when they were subsequently exposed to sunlight. Some detective work revealed that the pest-resistant celery contained 9000 parts per billion (ppb) psoralens (light-activated mutagenic carcinogens) instead of the level of 900 ppb psoralens in normal celery.[30,31] It is unclear whether other natural pesticides in the celery were increased as well.

Solanine and chaconine (the main natural alkaloids in potatoes) are cholinesterase inhibitors that were widely introduced into the human diet about 400 years ago with the dissemination of the potato from the Andes. They can be detected in the blood of all potato eaters. Total alkaloids are present in potatoes at a level of 15,000 μg per 200 g potato, which is only about a sixfold safety margin from the toxic level for humans.[3] Neither alkaloid has been tested for carcinogenicity. By contrast, the pesticide malathion, the main synthetic organophosphate cholinesterase inhibitor present in our diet (17 μg/day), has been thoroughly tested and is not a carcinogen in rodents. Plant breeders produced an insect-resistant potato that had to be withdrawn from the market because of its acute toxicity to humans, a consequence of higher levels of solanine and chaconine.

There is a tendency for laymen to think of chemicals as being only man-made, and to characterize them as toxic, as if every natural chemical were not also toxic at some dose. Even a recent NRC/NAS report states that "Advances in classical plant breeding . . . offer some promise for nonchemical pest control in the future. Nonchemical approaches will be encouraged by tolerance revocations if more profitable chemical controls are not available. . . ."[29] The report was particularly concerned with some pesticides used on tomatoes. Of course, tomatine, one of the alkaloids in tomatoes, is a chemical too, and was introduced from the New World 400 years ago. It has not been tested in rodent cancer bioassays, is present at 36,000 μg/100 g tomato, and is orders of magnitude closer to the toxic level than are man-made pesticide residues.

The Idea That Nature Is Benign ■

The notion that evolution has allowed us to cope with the toxic chemicals in the natural world[32] is not compelling[7] for several reasons: First, there is no reason to think that natural selection should eliminate the carcinogenic hazard of a plant toxin that causes cancer past the reproductive age, although there could be selection for resistance to the acute effects of particular carcinogens. For example, aflatoxin, a mold toxin that presumably arose early in evolution, causes cancer in trout, rats, mice, monkeys, and probably people, although the species are not equally sensitive.[5,33] Many of the common metal salts are carcinogens (*e.g.*, lead, cadmium, beryllium, nickel, chromium, selenium, and arsenic) despite their presence during all of evolution. Second, it is argued by some that humans, as opposed to rats or mice, may have developed resistance to each specific plant toxin or chemical in cooked food.[32] This is unlikely, because both rodents and humans have developed many types of general defenses against the large amounts and enormous variety of nature's pesticides.[3,8,26] These defenses include the constant shedding of the surface layer of cells of the digestive system, the detoxification of alkylating agents by glutathione transferases, the active excretion of hydrophobic toxins out of liver or intestinal cells, numerous defenses against oxygen radicals, and DNA excision repair. The fact that defenses usually are general, rather than specific for each chemical, makes good evolutionary sense and is supported by various studies. Experimental evidence indicates that these general defenses are effective against both natural and synthetic compounds,[34] since basic mechanisms of carcinogenesis are not unique to either. Third, the human diet has changed drastically in the last few thousand years, and most of us are eating recently introduced plants (coffee, potatoes, tomatoes, and kiwi fruit) that our ancestors did not eat. Fourth, the argument that plants contain anticarcinogens which protect us against plant carcinogens is irrelevant: plant antioxidants, the major known type of ingested anticarcinogens, do not distinguish whether oxidant carcinogens are synthetic or natural in origin, and thus help to protect us against both. Fifth, it has been argued that synthetic carcinogens can be synergistic. However, this is also true of natural chemicals and is irrelevant to the argument that synthetic pesticide residues in food or water pollution appear to be a trivial increment over the background of natural carcinogens.

Dioxin Compared to Alcohol and Broccoli ■

Common sense suggests that a chemical pollutant should not be treated as a significant hazard if its possible hazard level is far below that of common food items. Dioxin (TCDD) is a substance of great public concern, because it is an extremely potent carcinogen and teratogen in rodents, yet the doses humans are exposed to are very low relative to the effective level in rodents. TCDD can be compared to alcohol, as an example. Alcohol is an extremely weak carcinogen and teratogen, yet the doses humans are exposed to are very high relative to the effective dose in rodents (or humans). Indeed, alcoholic beverages are the most important known human teratogen, and the effective dose level of alcohol in humans (in milligrams per kilogram) is similar to the level that causes birth defects in mice. By contrast, there is no convincing evidence that TCDD is carcinogenic or teratogenic in man, although it is in rodents. If one compares the teratogenic potential of TCDD to that of alcohol for causing birth defects, after adjusting for their potency in rodents,[3] then a daily consumption of the Environmental Protection Agency (EPA) "reference dose" (formerly "acceptable dose limit") of TCDD, 6 pg/kg per day, is equivalent in teratogenic potential to the amount of alcohol ingested daily from 1/3000 of a beer, the equivalent of drinking one beer (15 g ethyl alcohol) over a period of 8 years. A daily slice of bread or glass of orange juice contains much more natural alcohol than this.

Alcoholic beverages are clearly carcinogenic in man (at a daily dose of about 5 drinks), although only one of several tests on ethyl alcohol in rats was positive.[22,23] This test should be replicated as confirmation that ethyl alcohol is the active ingredient, although the evidence for that is fairly strong.[22] A comparison of the carcinogenic potential of TCDD with that of alcohol, adjusting for potency in rodents, shows that the equivalence for the TCDD reference dose of 6 pg/kg per day is 1 beer every 5 months. Since the average *per capita* consumption of alcohol in the United States is equivalent to more than one beer per day, the great concern over TCDD at levels in the range of the reference dose seems unreasonable.

The assumption of a worst-case linear dose–response, often used for carcinogens, is not plausible for TCDD, yet extrapolations to man using such assumptions have generated great concern. TCDD binds to a receptor in mammalian cells, the Ah receptor, and the evidence suggests strongly that all of TCDD's effects are mediated through this binding.[35] Moreover, a wide variety of natural substances bind to the Ah receptor, and, as far as they have been examined, they have all of the properties of TCDD. A cooked steak contains polycyclic hydrocarbons, which bind to the Ah receptor and mimic TCDD. In addition, our diet contains a variety of flavones and other substances from plants, which bind to the Ah receptor. The most interesting of such substances is indole carbinol (IC), which is present in large amounts in broccoli (500 mg/kg), cabbage, cauliflower, and other members of the *Brassica* family.[36] The two substances induce the same set of enzymes.[37] When given before aflatoxin or other carcinogens, IC protects against carcinogenesis, as does TCDD.[38] However, when it is given after aflatoxin or other carcinogens, IC is a strong promoter of carcinogenesis, as is TCDD.[39] This stimulation of carcinogenesis has also been shown for cabbage itself.[40] When IC is exposed to acid pH (equivalent to that of the stomach), it is converted to a series of dimers and trimers that are similar to TCDD in size and shape, bind to the Ah receptor, and induce the set of TCDD-inducible enzymes, thus mimicking TCDD.[37,41] The 360 pg/day TCDD EPA reference dose should be compared with 50 million pg of IC per 100 g of broccoli (one portion); the affinity of the indole derivatives in binding to the Ah receptor is less by a factor of about 8000, suggesting that the broccoli portion might be roughly 20 times the possible hazard. Although these IC derivatives appear to be much more of a possible hazard than TCDD, it is not clear whether, at these low doses, either represents any danger.

Another study[42] also shows that when sunlight oxidizes tryptophan, a normal amino acid, it converts it to a variety of indoles (similar to the broccoli IC dimers), which bind to the Ah receptor and mimic the action of TCDD. It seems likely that many more of these "natural dioxins" will be discovered in the future.

Water Pollution ■

The possible hazards from carcinogens in contaminated well water (*e.g.,* the Santa Clara, or "Silicon," Valley, in California, and Woburn, Massachusetts) should be compared to the possible hazards of ordinary tap water (see Table 14a–1).[3] Of the 35 wells shut down in Santa Clara Valley because of a supposed carcinogenic hazard—low traces of trichloroethylene—only two were of a possible hazard greater than ordinary tap water. Well water is not usually chlorinated and therefore lacks the 83 ppb chloroform present in average chlorinated tap water.[3] Water from the most polluted well had a relative hazard that was orders of magnitude less than that for the carcinogens in an equal volume of cola, beer, or wine, or many natural carcinogens in our daily diet. The consumption of tap water is only about 1 or 2 liters/day, and the animal evidence cited[3] provides no good reason to expect that chloroform in water or current levels of man-made pollution of water would pose a significant carcinogenic hazard.

The trace amounts of chemicals found in polluted wells should be a negligible cause of birth defects, when compared to the background level of known teratogens such as alcohol. Most agents causing birth defects would also be expected to be harmless at low doses. Important risk factors for birth defects in humans include age of mother, alcohol ingestion, smoking, and rubella virus.

Air Pollution ■

A person inhales about 20,000 liters of air in a day. Thus, even modest contamination of the atmosphere results in inhalation of appreciable doses of a pollutant. Indoor air pollution is, in general, considerably more of a health hazard than outdoor air pollution, partly because of cigarette smoke, formaldehyde, benzene, and radon.[3,43] The most important indoor air pollutant is radon gas.[43] Radon is a natural radioactive gas that is present in the soil, gets trapped in houses, and gives rise to radioactive decay products that are known to be carcinogenic in humans.[43] It has been estimated that one million homes in the United States have a level of exposure to products of radon decay higher than that received by today's uranium miners. Two particularly contaminated houses had a risk estimated to be equivalent to receiving about 1200 chest x-rays a day. Approximately 10% of the lung cancer in the United States has been tentatively attributed to radon pollution in houses.[43] Many of these cancers may be preventable, because the most hazardous houses can be identified and modified to minimize radon contamination.[43]

General outdoor air pollution is a small risk relative to indoor air pollution or to the pollution inhaled by a smoker: a person breathing Los Angeles smog for a year inhales the same amount of burnt material that a smoker does in one day (two packs).[3,26] It is difficult for epidemiologists to determine cancer risk from outdoor air pollution because smoking and radon exposure must be accurately controlled.

Cooking Food ■

The cooking of food generates a variety of mutagens and carcinogens. The total amount of browned and burnt material eaten in a typical day is at least several hundred times more than that inhaled from severe outdoor air pollution.[26] Nine heterocyclic amines, isolated on the basis of their mutagenicity from proteins or amino acids that were heated in ways that reproduce cooking methods, have now been tested; all have been shown to be potent carcinogens in rodents.[44,45] Many others are still being isolated and characterized.[44,45] Three mutagenic nitropyrenes present in diesel exhaust have been shown to be carcinogens,[46] but the intake of these carcinogenic nitropyrenes from grilled chicken is estimated to be much higher than that from air pollution.[44,45–47]

Gas flames generate NO_2, which can form both the carcinogenic nitropyrenes[23,24] and the potently carcinogenic nitrosamines in food, such as fish, cooked in gas ovens. It seems likely that food cooked in gas ovens may be a major source of dietary nitrosamines and nitropyrenes.

Occupational Exposures ■

Occupational exposures to chemicals are often significant.[3,48] The potential carcinogenic hazards to US workers has been ranked using the PERP index (analogous to the HERP index,[3] except that the Oc-

cupational Safety and Health Administration permitted exposure levels replace actual exposures).[48] The PERP values differ by more than 100,000-fold. For 12 substances, the permitted levels for workers are greater than 10% of the rodent TD_{50} dose. Priority attention should be given to reduction of the allowable worker exposures that appear most hazardous in the PERP ranking.

Error 4: Extrapolating Risks Without Understanding Mechanisms of Carcinogenesis ■

Rodent Carcinogenesis Tests ■

It is prudent to assume that if a chemical is a carcinogen in rats and mice at the MTD, it is also likely to be a carcinogen in humans at the MTD. However, until we understand more about mechanisms of carcinogenesis, we cannot reliably predict risk to humans at low doses, often hundreds of thousands of times below the dose where an effect is observed in rodents. Thus, quantitative risk assessment currently is not scientifically possible.[3,4,7]

Carcinogenesis Mechanisms and the Dose–Response Curve ■

The study of mechanisms of carcinogenesis is a rapidly developing field and is essential for rational risk assessment. Both mutations and cell proliferation (*i.e.,* promotion) are required in carcinogenesis.[3,49,50] There is an enormous spontaneous rate of damage to DNA from endogenous oxidants, which we have discussed in relation to cancer and aging.[51,52] There is also a basal spontaneous rate for cell proliferation in some organs, e.g., colon, but not others, e.g., liver.[10,11] Thus, increasing either mutation or cell proliferation should be carcinogenic. Additional complications are that several mutations appear necessary for carcinogenesis, and there are many layers of defense against carcinogens. These considerations suggest a sublinear dose–response relationship, which is consistent with both the animal and human data,[3–7] and indicate that multiplicative interactions will be common in human cancer causation. Administering chemicals in cancer tests at the MTD commonly causes cell proliferation and inflammatory reactions.[3,49,50,53] Inflammatory reactions with release of oxygen radicals from phagocytic cells are equivalent to irradiating the tissue. If a chemical is nonmutagenic and its carcinogenicity is due to cell proliferation resulting from near-toxic doses, one might commonly expect a threshold.[3,49,50]

The fact that high doses of a chemical cause tumors does not necessarily mean that small doses will. Most chemicals may, in fact, be harmless at low levels. A list of carcinogens is not enough. The main rule in toxicology is that the "dose makes the poison:" at some level, every chemical becomes toxic, but there are safe levels below that. A scientific consensus evolved in the 1970s that we should treat carcinogens differently—that we should assume that even low doses could possibly cause some harm, even though we do not have the methods to measure effects at low levels. This idea evolved because most carcinogens appeared to be mutagens (agents that damage the DNA). The precedent of radiation, which is both a mutagen and carcinogen, gave credence to the idea that there could be effects of chemicals even at low doses. Some recent work on radiation, however, suggests that low doses may be of no harm or even protective.[54,54a,55,55a]

The idea that most of the classical carcinogens were mutagens that damaged DNA (about 90% in our studies),[56,57] along with work on oncogenes,[58] reinforced the mutagen–carcinogen connection. However, in recent years there has been a change in the picture. About half of all chemicals tested in animals are carcinogens, but only about half of these appear to be mutagenic. It is now standard in cancer tests to be rigorous about giving the MTD of the chemical for the lifetime of the animal, and this may be a factor. It seems quite reasonable that nonmutagens cause cancer, and mutagens in part cause cancer, because dosing at the MTD accelerates the promotional step of carcinogenesis.[59,60]

Promotion, or cell proliferation, can also be accelerated by viruses, such as the human carcinogenic hepatitis B viruses, a major cause of liver cancer around the world,[25] or human papilloma virus 16 (HPV-16), a contributor to cancer of the cervix.[24] Both cause chronic cell killing and consequent cell proliferation. Promotion can also be induced by hormones, which cause cell proliferation. Hormones appear to be major risk factors for certain human cancers, such as breast cancer, and appear to only increase cell proliferation.[10] The promotional step of cancer causation can also be accelerated by chemicals. Alcohol, for example, causes cirrhosis of the liver, leading to cancer. The classical chemical promoters, such as phenobarbital and tetradecanoyl phorbol acetate, would be expected to be, and are, carcinogens when tested in thorough animal tests at the MTD.[60] There is increasing evidence to show that low doses of promoters are not active.[49,50] It seems likely, therefore, that a high percentage of all chemicals, both man-made and natural, will cause cell proliferation at the MTD and be classified as carcinogens, but most of these may be acting as promoters and therefore may not be of interest at doses much below the toxic dose.[3]

Thus, the common water pollutants, such as trichloroethylene (TCE) and perchloroethylene (PCE), are unlikely to be of public health significance because [a] the amounts we are exposed to in pollution are trivial relative to the background of natural carcinogens, and [b] the evidence is that they are likely to be acting as promoters, not as DNA-damaging carcinogens, and therefore should be ignored at low concentrations.

Error 5: Storks Bring Babies, and Pollution Causes Cancer and Birth Defects ■

The number of storks in Europe has been decreasing for decades. At the same time, the European birth rate has also been decreasing. We would be foolish to accept this high correlation[61] as evidence that storks bring babies. The science of epidemiology tries to sort out from the myriad chance correlations those that are meaningful and involve cause and effect. However, it is not easy to obtain convincing evidence by epidemiologic methods because of inherent methodologic difficulties.[9] There are many sources of bias in observational data, and chance variation is also an important factor. For example, because there are so many different types of cancer or birth defects, by chance alone one might expect some of them to occur at a high frequency in a small community. Toxicology provides evidence to help decide whether an observed correlation might be causal or accidental.

There is no convincing evidence from epidemiology or toxicology that pollution is a significant source of birth defects and cancer. For example, the epidemiologic studies of Love Canal, dioxin in Agent Orange,[62,63] Contra Costa County refineries,[64,65] Silicon Valley,[66] Woburn,[3,8] and the use of DDT provide no convincing evidence that pollution was the cause of human harm in any of these well-publicized exposures. Even in Love Canal, where people were living next to a toxic waste dump, the epidemiologic evidence for an effect on public health is equivocal. Analysis of the toxicology data on many of these cases suggests that the amounts of the chemicals involved were much too low relative to the background of natural and traditional carcinogens to be credible sources of increased cancer risk to humans.[3] A comparative analysis of teratogens using a HERP-type index expressing the human exposure level as a percentage of the dose level effective in rodents would be of interest (see Error 3), but this has not been done in a systematic way.

Environmental exposure to TCE, PCE, trichloroethane, ethylene dibromide (EDB), and other pollutants is thousands of times lower than the exposure to these same agents in the workplace.[3,48] Thus, if parts per billion of these pollutants were causing cancer or birth defects, one might expect to see an effect in the workplace. The studies on these chemicals to date do not provide any evidence for a causal association,[33] although epidemiologic studies are inherently insensitive. Historically, cases of cancer due to workplace exposure resulted mainly from exposures to chemicals at very high levels. For example, the permissible and actual EDB levels for workers were shockingly high (see Table 14a–1). (I testified in California in 1981 that our calculations showed that the workers were allowed to breathe in a dose higher than the TD_{50} in rats.) California lowered the permissible worker exposure by more than 100-fold. Despite the fact that the epidemiology of EDB in highly exposed workers does not show any significant effect, the uncertainties in our knowledge make it important to have strict rules because workers can be exposed to extremely high doses.

Error 6: Technology Is Doing Us In ■

Modern technologies are almost always replacing older, more hazardous technologies. The reason that billions of pounds of TCE (one of the most important industrial nonflammable solvents) and PCE (the main dry-cleaning solvent in the United States) are used is that they have low toxicity and are not flammable. Is it advisable to go back to the age when industry and dry cleaners used flammable solvents and fires were frequent? Eliminating a carcinogen may not always be a good idea. For example, EDB, the main fumigant in the United States before it was banned, was present in trivial amounts in our food: the average daily intake was about one-tenth of the possible carcinogenic hazard of the aflatoxin in the average peanut butter sandwich, a trivial risk in itself (see Table 14a–1).[3] Elimination of fumigation results in insect infestation and subsequent contamination of grain by carcinogen-producing molds. This might result in a regression in public health, not an advance, and would also greatly increase costs. The proposed alternatives, such as irradiating food, could possibly be more hazardous than EDB, as well as more expensive. Similarly, modern pesticides replaced more hazardous substances such as lead arsenate, one of the major pesticides before the modern era. Lead and arsenic are both natural, highly toxic, and carcinogenic. Pesticides have increased crop yields and brought down the price of foods, a major public health advance.

Every living thing and every industry "pollutes" to some extent. How much does society wish to spend to get the last part per billion of TCE out of the wells in Silicon Valley, or to remove PCE from dry-cleaning plants? We are currently spending enormous amounts of money trying to eliminate lower and lower levels of pollution; one estimate is about $80 billion annually.[7] The fact that scientists have developed methods to measure parts per billion (one part per billion is equivalent to one person in all of China) of carcinogens and are developing methods to measure parts per trillion does not mean that significant pollution is increasing, or that the pollution found is a cause of human harm.

Conclusion ■

Everyone knows that spending all of one's effort on trivia without focusing on important problems is counterproductive. If we divert too much of our attention to traces of pollution and away from important public health concerns such as smoking (400,000 deaths per year), alcohol (100,000 deaths per year), unbalanced diets (e.g., too much saturated fat and cholesterol), acquired immunodeficiency syndrome, radioactive radon in our homes, and high-dose occupational exposure, we do not improve public health, and the important hazards are lost in the confusion. It is the inexorable progress of modern technology and scientific research that will continue to provide the knowledge resulting in steady progress to decrease cancer and birth defects and lengthen life span.

The author thanks Lois Gold and David Freedman for helpful discussion and criticisms. This work was supported by Outstanding Investigator Grant CA-39910 from the National Cancer Institute and by National Institute of Environmental Health Sciences Center Grant ES-01896.

References ■

1. National Cancer Institute: 1987 Annual Cancer Statistics Review Including Cancer Trends: 1950–1985. NIH Publication No. 88-2789 Bethesda, MD, National Institutes of Health, 1988
2. Doll R, Peto R: The Causes of Cancer. Oxford, England, Oxford University Press, 1981
3. Ames BN, Magaw R, Gold LS: Ranking possible carcinogenic hazards. Science 236:271–280, 1987
4. Ames BN, Magaw R, Gold LS: Response to letter: Risk assessment. Science 237:235, 1987
5. Ames BN, Magaw R, Gold LS: Response to letter: Carcinogenicity of aflatoxins. Science 237:1283–1284, 1987

6. Ames BN, Gold LS, Magaw R: Response to letter: Risk assessment. Science 237:1399–1400, 1987

7. Ames BN, Gold LS: Response to letter: Paleolithic diet, evolution, and carcinogens. Science 238:1634, 1987

8. Ames BN, Gold LS: Response to technical comment: Carcinogenic risk estimation. Science 240:1045–1047, 1988

9. Higginson J: Changing concepts in cancer prevention: Limitations and implications for future research in environmental carcinogenesis. Cancer Res 48:1381–1389, 1988

10. Henderson BE, Ross R, Bernstein L: Estrogens as a cause of human cancer: The Richard and Hinda Rosenthal Foundation Award Lecture. Cancer Res 48:246–253, 1988

11. Lipkin M: Biomarkers of increased susceptibility to gastrointestinal cancer: New application to studies of cancer prevention in human subjects. Cancer Res 48:235–245, 1988

12. Peto R: Epidemiological reservations about risk assessment. In Woodhead AD, Shellabarger CJ, Pond V, Hollaender A (eds): Assessment of Risk from Low-Level Exposure to Radiation and Chemicals, pp 3–16. New York, Plenum, 1985

13. Yang CS, Newmark HL: The role of micronutrient deficiency in carcinogenesis, CRC Crit Rev Oncol Hematol 7:267–287, 1987

14. Pence BC, Buddingh F: Inhibition of dietary fat-promoted colon carcinogenesis in rats by supplemental calcium or vitamin D_3. Carcinogenesis 9:187–190, 1988

15. Gold LS, Bernstein L, Magaw R, Slone TH: Interspecies extrapolation in carcinogenesis: Prediction between rats and mice. Environ Health Perspect (in press)

16. Gold LS, Sawyer CB, Magaw R, Backman GM, de Veciana M, Levinson R, Hooper K, Havender WR, Bernstein L, Peto R, Pike MC, Ames BN: A carcinogenic potency database of the standardized results of animal bioassays. Environ Health Perspect 58:9–319, 1984

17. Gold LS, Slone TH, Backman G, Magaw R, Da Costa M, Ames BN: Second chronological supplement to the carcinogenic potency database: Standardized results of animal bioassays published through December 1984 and by the National Toxicology Program through May 1986. Environ Health Perspect 74:237–329, 1987

18. Innes JRM, Ulland BM, Valerio MG, Petrucelli L, Fishbein L, Hart ER, Pallotta AJ, Bates RR, Falk HL, Gart JJ, Klein M, Mitchell I, Peters J: Bioassay of pesticides and industrial chemicals for tumorigenicity in mice: A preliminary note. JNCI 42:1101–1114, 1969

19. Schardein JL, Schwetz BA, Kenal MF: Species sensitivities and prediction of teratogenic potential. Environ Health Perspect 61:55–67, 1985

20. Reddy BS, Cohen LA (eds): Diet, Nutrition, and Cancer: A Critical Evaluation, Vols I and II. Boca Raton, FL, CRC Press 1986

21. Joossens JV, Hill MJ, Geboers J (eds): Diet and Human Carcinogenesis. Amsterdam, Elsevier Science Publishers, 1986

22. Ames BN: Review of evidence for alcohol-related carcinogenesis. Report for Proposition 65 Meeting, Sacramento, CA, December 11, 1987

23. IARC Monographs on the Evaluation of Carcinogenic Risks to Humans: Alcohol Drinking. Lyon, France, International Agency for Research on Cancer (in press)

24. Peto R, zur Hausen H (eds): Banbury Report 21. Viral Etiology of Cervical Cancer. Cold Spring Harbor, NY, Cold Spring Harbor Laboratory, 1986

25. Yeh F-S, Mo C-C, Luo S, Henderson BE, Tong MJ, Yu MC: A seriological case-control study of primary hepatocellular carcinoma in Guangxi, China. Cancer Res 45:872–873, 1985

26. Ames BN: Dietary carcinogens and anticarcinogens: Oxygen radicals and degenerative diseases. Science 221:1256–1264, 1983

27. Harborne JB: The role of phytoalexins in natural plant resistance. In Green MB, Hedin PA (eds): Natural Resistance of Plants to Pests. Roles of Allelochemicals. ACS Symposium 296, pp 23–35. Washington DC, American Chemical Society, 1986

28. Gartrell MJ, Craun JC, Podrebarac DS, Gunderson EL: Pesticides, selected elements, and other chemicals in adult total diet samples, October 1980–March 1982. J Assoc Off Anal Chem 69:146, 1986

29. National Research Council, Board on Agriculture: Regulating Pesticides in Food. Washington, DC, National Academy Press, 1987

30. Berkley SF, Hightower AW, Beier RC, Fleming DW, Brokopp CD, Ivie GW, Broome CV: Dermatitis in grocery workers associated with high natural concentrations of furanocoumarins in celery. Ann Intern Med 105:351–355, 1986

31. Seligman PJ, Mathias CGT, O'Malley MA, Beier RC, Fehrs LJ, Serrill WS, Halperin WE: Phytophotodermatitis from celery among grocery store workers. Arch Dermatol 123:1478–1482, 1987

32. Davis DL: Paleolithic diet, evolution, and carcinogens. Science 238:1633–1634, 1987

33. IARC Monographs on the Evaluation of Carcinogenic Risks to Humans: Overall Evaluations of Carcinogenicity: An Updating of IARC Monographs Volumes 1–42, Supplement 7. Lyon, France, International Agency for Research on Cancer

34. Jakoby WB (ed): Enzymatic Basis of Detoxification, Vols 1 and 2. New York, Academic Press, 1980

35. Knutson JC, Poland A: Response of murine epidermis to 2,3,7,8-tetrachlorodibenzo-p-dioxin: Interaction of the *Ah* and *hr* loci. Cell 30:225–234, 1982

36. Bradfield CA, Bjeldanes LF: High-performance liquid chromatographic analysis of anticarcinogenic indoles in Brassica oleracea. J Agric Food Chem 35:46–49, 1987

37. Bradfield CA, Bjeldanes LF: Structure-activity relationships of dietary indoles: A proposed mechanism of action as modifiers of xenobiotic metabolism. J Toxicol Environ Health 21:311–323, 1987

38. Dashwood RH, Arbogast DN, Fong AT, Hendricks JD, Bailey GS: Mechanisms of anti-carcinogenesis by indole-3-carbinol: Detailed *in vivo* DNA binding dose-response studies after dietary administration with aflatoxin B1. Carcinogenesis 9:427–432, 1988

39. Bailey GS, Hendricks JD, Shelton DW, Nixon JE, Pawlowski NE: Enhancement of carcinogenesis by the natural anticarcinogen indole-3-carbinol. JNCI 78:931–934, 1987

40. Birt DF, Pelling JC, Pour PM, Tibbels MG, Schweickert L, Bresnick E: Enhanced pancreatic and skin tumorigenesis in cabbage-fed hamsters and mice. Carcinogenesis 8:913–917, 1987

41. Bradfield C, Bjeldanes L: Personal communication, 1988

42. Rannug A, Rannug U, Rosenkranz HS, Winqvist L, Westerholm R, Agurell E, Grafstrom A-K: Certain photooxidized derivatives of tryptophan bind with very high affinity to the Ah receptor and are likely to be endogenous signal substances. J Biol Chem 262:15422–15427, 1987

43. Nero AV Jr: Controlling indoor air pollution. Scientific American 258:42–48, 1988

44. Sugimura T, Sato S, Ohgaki H, Takayama S, Nagao M, Wakabayashi K: Overview: Mutagens and carcinogens in cooked food. In Knudsen I (ed): Genetic Toxicology of the Diet, pp 85–107. New York, Alan R Liss, 1986

45. Sugimura T: Studies on environmental chemical carcinogenesis in Japan. Science 233:312–318, 1986

46. Ohgaki H, Hasegawa H, Kato T, Negishi C, Sato S, Sugimura T: Absence of carcinogenicity of 1-nitropyrene, correction of previous results, and new demonstration of carcinogenicity of 1,6-dinitropyrene in rats. Cancer Lett 25:239–245, 1985

47. Kinouchi T, Tsutsui H, Ohnishi Y: Detection of 1-nitropyrene in yakitori (grilled chicken). Mutation Res 171:105–113, 1986

48. Gold LS, Backman GM, Hooper NK, Peto R: Ranking the potential carcinogenic hazards to workers from exposures to chemicals that are tumorigenic in rodents. Environ Health Perspect 76:211–219, 1987

49. Pitot HC, Goldsworthy TL, Moran S, Kennan W, Glauert HP, Maronpot RR, Campbell HA: A method to quantitate the relative initiating and promoting potencies of hepatocarcinogenic agents in their dose-response relationships to altered hepatic foci. Carcinogenesis 8:1491–1499, 1987

50. Farber E: Possible etiologic mechanisms in chemical carcinogenesis. Environ Health Perspect 75:65–70, 1987

51. Adelman R, Saul RL, Ames BN: Oxidative damage to DNA: Relation to species metabolic rate and life span. Proc Natl Acad Sci USA 85:2706–2708, 1988

52. Richter C, Park J-W, Ames BN: Normal oxidative damage to mitochondrial and nuclear DNA is extensive. Proc Natl Acad Sci USA 85:6465–6467, 1988

53. Swenberg JA, Richardson FC, Boucheron JA, Deal FH, Belinsky SA, Charbonneau M, Short BG: High- to low-dose extrapolation: Critical determinants involved in the dose response of carcinogenic substances. Environ Health Perspect 76:57–63, 1987

54. Wolff S, Afzal V, Wiencke JK, Olivieri G, Michaeli A: Human lymphocytes exposed to low doses of ionizing radiations become refractory to high doses of radiation as well as to chemical mutagens that induce double-strand breaks in DNA. Int J Radiat Biol 53:39–48, 1988

54a. Yalow RS: Biologic effects of low-level radiation. In Burns ME (ed): Low-Level Radioactive Waste Regulation: Science, Politics, and Fear, pp 239–259. Chelsea, MI, Lewis Publishers, Inc, 1988

55. Ootsuyama A, Tanooka H: One hundred percent tumor induction in mouse skin after repeated β irradiation in a limited dose range. Radiation Res 115:488–494, 1988

55a. Kondo S: Mutation and cancer in relation to the atomic-bomb radiation effects. Jpn J Cancer Res (Gann) 79:785–799, 1988

56. McCann J, Choi E, Yamasaki E, Ames BN: Detection of carcinogens as mutagens in the Salmonella/microsome test: Assay of 300 chemicals. Proc Natl Acad Sci USA 72:5135–5139, 1975

57. McCann J, Ames BN: The detection of carcinogens as mutagens in the Salmonella/microsome test: Assay of 300 chemicals: Discussion. Proc Natl Acad Sci USA 73:950–954, 1976

58. Stowers SJ, Maronpot RR, Reynolds SH, Anderson MW: The role of oncogenes in chemical carcinogenesis. Environ Health Perspect 75:81–86, 1987

59. Butterworth BE, Slaga TJ (eds): Banbury Report 25. Nongenotoxic Mechanisms in Carcinogenesis. Cold Spring Harbor, NY, Cold Spring Harbor Laboratory, 1987

60. Iversen OH (ed): Theories of Carcinogenesis. Washington, DC, Hemisphere, 1988

61. Sies H: A new parameter for sex education. Nature 332:495, 1988

62. Lathrop GD, Machado SG, Karrison PG, Grubbs WD, Thomas WF, Wolfe WH, Michalek JE, Miner JC, Peterson MR, Ogerskok RW: Air Force Health Study: Epidemiologic Investigation of Health Effects in Air Force Personnel Following Exposure to Herbicides. First Follow-Up Examination Results. Brooks Air Force Base, TX, US Air Force, 1987

63. Gough M: Dioxin, Agent Orange: The Facts. New York, Plenum Press, 1986

64. Austin DF, Nelson V, Swain B, Johnson L, Lum S, Flessel P: Epidemiological Study of the Incidence of Cancer as Related to Industrial Emissions in Contra Costa County, California, NTIS Publication No. PB84-199785. Washington, DC, US Government Printing Office, 1984

65. Smith AH, Waller K: Air Pollution and Cancer Incidence in Contra Costa County: Review and Recommendations. Report Prepared for the Contra Costa County Department of Health Services, 1985

66. California Department of Health Services, Epidemiological Studies and Services Section: Pregnancy Outcome in Santa Clara County, 1980–1985. Berkeley, CA, California Department of Health Services, 1988

Frederica P. Perera

Paolo Boffetta

Ian C. T. Nisbet

What Are the Major Carcinogens in the Etiology of Human Cancer?

Industrial Carcinogens 14b

Introduction ■

The vast majority of human cancer can be attributed to a broad category of environmental factors and is thus potentially preventable. Although there is general agreement that occupational exposures and certain life-style factors, such as cigarette smoking and diet, contribute significantly to the human cancer burden, the contribution of nonoccupational exposures to industrial or man-made carcinogens is much more controversial. We define man-made or industrial carcinogens occurring outside of the workplace to include pesticides, synthetic chemicals, metals, and fibers that are present in drinking water, in ambient and indoor air, and in food and beverages as a result of human activities. (Naturally occurring carcinogens, strictly speaking, are those present in the diet, air, and water in the absence of human activities, and should be distinguished from dietary carcinogens resulting from certain avoidable food preparation and storage techniques.)

Nonoccupational exposure to man-made carcinogens has been variously described as "trivial" and "important," depending on the data and assumptions invoked. Here we hope to shed light on the debate by critically reviewing the various tools and strategies that have been deployed to identify and quantify the role of environmental carcinogens. Using particular examples, we illustrate the methodologic strengths and limitations of each approach: environmental monitoring, epidemiology, molecular epidemiology, quantitative risk assessment, and carcinogen ranking using a recently proposed human exposure/rodent potency (HERP) system. Finally, we briefly discuss nonscientific considerations, such as preventability of risk and equity, that help shape the debate, whether or not they are openly acknowledged.

Our conclusion is that there is a high degree of uncertainty in estimates of attributable and comparative risk. Nonetheless, available data suggest that industrial and man-made carcinogens in the air, water, and food supply are important because of their pervasiveness, their widespread human exposure, and their ability to interact with life-style factors such as cigarette smoking and diet. In addition, ethical considerations argue against allowing individuals to be involuntarily exposed to carcinogens, especially as the scientific data base does not allow precise calculation of risk. On both counts, therefore, it is prudent to control involuntary exposures to carcinogenic industrial chemicals and pesticides as part of an overall strategy to prevent human cancer.

Major Tools in Risk Identification and Quantification ■

Environmental Monitoring ■

The lack of adequate data on human exposure to specific chemicals or mixtures is often referred to as the "Achilles heel" of epidemiology and risk assessment. For example, the Clean Air Act requires surveillance only of six ambient airborne pollutants. With respect to drinking water, up until the present time only 22 pollutants have been periodically monitored under the Safe Drinking Water Act, and it has been estimated that less than 1% of the food supply is monitored for pesticide residues.[1] Thus, only a small available fraction of chemical pollutants have been subject to routine data collection.

Even for this limited number of chemicals, the resultant data constitute only a crude estimate of actual exposure. For example, during the past several decades, the only ambient air carcinogen that has been routinely monitored is benzopyrene (BP). Unfortunately, the conventional method used for monitoring this carcinogen (extraction from noncontinuous samples of total particulate matter collected from a limited number of sites) provided only a crude estimate of the amount of deeply respirable fine particulate BP to which persons were exposed. In addition, BP could be lost by evaporation and photodegradation, while analytic methods were subject to inaccuracy. Wide seasonal and geographic variations in BP concentrations were masked by the annual average values generally used as pollution indices. Nonetheless, investigators have, by default, often relied on these data to approximate individual exposure.

Despite these limitations, the available federal, state, and local environmental monitoring data show that there is widespread contamination of the ambient and indoor air, the drinking water, and the food supply. Data accumulated since the 1940s demonstrate that ambient air has been polluted by a substantial number of mutagenic and carcinogenic substances, including synthetic organic chemicals released during their manufacture, use, and disposal, as well as products of fossil fuel combustion.[2-5] Carcinogenic trace metals, polycyclic aromatic hydrocarbons (PAHs), and volatile organic chemicals have been widely detected in ambient air.[6] Over 700 organic chemicals have been measured in the US drinking water supply, including 40 known or suspected carcinogens.[7] These include dozens of pesticides and industrial chemical carcinogens frequently found in surface water, ground water, and drinking water.[8-12]

The National Academy of Sciences (NAS) has recently evaluated the potential risk of a number of carcinogenic pesticide residues present in the food supply.[13] The NAS report notes that approximately 480 million pounds of herbicides are used each year in the United States, of which about 300 million pounds, or 63%, are agents known or presumed by the US Environmental Protection Agency (EPA) to be oncogenic. It states that the presumed oncogens account for 35% to 50% of all insecticide acre treatments and expenditures and that about 90% of all agricultural fungicides are positive in oncogenicity

bioassays. However, despite the importance of the problem, the NAS committee found "very little actual data" on pesticide residues in food upon which to base risk estimates, and it was forced to rely on a surrogate measure.

Another difficulty is that environmental monitoring data are frequently presented as average exposure estimates that do not reflect the wide variation resulting from geographic, economic, and host factors in the human population. For example, in most cases, the distribution of exactly measured exposures is right-skewed (*i.e.,* whereas half of the population is exposed to concentrations between zero and the median, some people have exposure many times higher than the median), so that the use of any average exposure is likely to significantly underestimate the risk to that subset of the population.[14] As another example, children have a higher exposure (on a kilogram per body weight basis) to pollutants in drinking water and food than adults.[11,15,16] This is illustrated in Table 14b–1, which shows a 5–15-fold variation between child and adult in dietary intake of daminozide from three common foods containing residues of this chemical. For all these reasons, estimates of human exposure are highly uncertain. Yet, as will be discussed, they are used to provide the cornerstone both for conclusions about the etiology of cancer and for quantitative risk assessment.

Finally, with respect to exposure, humans are frequently exposed to the same carcinogen in many different media (workplace air, drinking water, ambient and indoor air, food and beverages). This is true for BP and other PAHs, benzene, vinyl chloride, trichloroethylene, polychlorinated biphenyls (PCBs), asbestos, arsenic, lead, and other substances. Yet risk assessments rarely factor in cumulative exposure from multiple sources.

Table 14b–2 provides some representative data for common environmental pollutants in the United States to illustrate the average carcinogen dose resulting from exposure in multiple media and to show the significant reductions in exposure that have occurred as a result of regulation. For several drinking

Table 14b–1
Variation in Dietary Intake of Daminozide*

Source	Daily Dose		
	Child (1–6 yr)	Adult (>20 yr)	Ratio
Apples	1.2	0.26	4.6
Apple juice	0.38	0.025	15.2
Peanuts	0.19	0.034	5.6

* Data are from the Environmental Protection Agency.[15,16] Doses are given in micrograms per kilogram of body weight per day.

water pollutants, worst-case estimates are provided to illustrate the extent to which use of average values will underestimate risk to the most highly exposed individuals by as much as 1 to 2 orders of magnitude. All values are in terms of daily dose per 70 kg adult to facilitate comparisons.

Epidemiology ■

CANCER TRENDS □

The analysis of trends in cancer incidence and mortality to bolster arguments about the importance of specific etiologic agents is problematic for the following reasons. First, overall trends in a particular type of cancer are the net result of a decrease following reduction in some risk factors and an increase attributable to new, unidentified risk factors. They may therefore mask important changes caused by specific etiologic agents. Second, artifactual changes in cancer rates may result from changes in diagnosis or coding. Third, cancer may be more common as a cause of death because of reduction in other diseases. Fourth, as discussed below, cancers are generally due to multiple factors, but are often inappropriately attributed to single causes.

Some investigators have concluded that lung cancer is the only cancer that is increasing, and that the increase is totally due to cigarette smoking (and possibly to asbestos).[45] Yet, mortality from other cigarette-related cancers, such as bladder cancer, has declined

Table 14b–2
Exposure Estimates for Selected Carcinogens (per 70 kg Adult)*

Carcinogenic Exposure	Average Daily Carcinogen Dose	Worst-Case Carcinogen Dose	Refs.
Man-made Chemicals in Foods and Beverages			
DDT, DDD, and DDE in food (preregulatory, 1968–1969)	29.0 μg		17–19
DDT, DDD, and DDE in food (postregulatory, 1980–1982)	2.3 μg		17–19
Dieldrin in food (preregulatory, 1968–1969)	1.5 μg		17, 19
Dieldrin in food (postregulatory, 1980–1982)	1.1 μg		17, 19
PCBs in food (preregulatory, 1971)	15 μg		19, 20
PCBs in food (postregulatory, 1980–1982)	0.2 μg		19, 20
Ambient Air Pollutants			
Benzene (Los Angeles, preregulatory, 1968)	1.0 mg		6, 21
Benzene (Los Angeles, postregulatory, 1984)	0.32 mg		6, 21
DDT (US rural areas preregulatory, 1972)	2.0 μg		22
DDT (US rural areas, postregulatory, 1974)	.24 μg		22
Formaldehyde (Los Angeles, 1966)	1.9 mg		23, 24
Formaldehyde (Los Angeles, 1979)	370 μg		23, 24
PCBs (US suburban areas, preregulatory, 1975)	2 μg		25, 26
PCBs (US urban areas, postregulatory, 1979)	150 ng		25, 26
Indoor Air Pollutants			
Benzene (personal average, NJ, 1981)	173 μg		12
Formaldehyde in conventional homes (average of all reported US data)	600 μg		27, 28
Formaldehyde in mobile homes (US average, 1984)	2.2 mg		27, 28
Tetrachloroethylene (personal average, NJ, 1981)	80 μg		12
Water Pollutants			
EDB (Florida, ground water, 1983)	7.8 μg	200 μg	29
PCBs (US surface water, preregulatory, 1971–1974	0.4 μg		30
Tetrachloroethylene (NJ water supplies, 1985)	12 μg	3000 μg	9, 31
Trichloroethylene (TCE) (US water supplies, 1985)	14 μg	70 mg	31, 32
Vinylidene chloride (NJ water supplies, 1985)	4 μg	18 μg	31
Occupational Exposures			
Benzene (rubber industry preregulatory, 1942)	1.2 g		33–35
Benzene (rubber industry, postregulatory, 1980s)	2.4 mg		33–35
Formaldehyde (resin and paper manufacture, 1961)	110 mg		36–40
Formaldehyde (resin and plastic manufacture, 1980s)	3.2 mg		36–40
TCE (small factories, preregulatory, 1940s)	4.1 g		41, 42
TCE (postregulatory, 1980s)	0.1 g		41, 42

* To calculate average daily dose over an individual lifetime, we assumed: [a] food consumption according to nationwide surveys; [b] water consumption-2 L/day; [c] ambient air-inhalation of 20,000 L/day; [d] indoor air-inhalation of 10,800 L/14 h day; [e] workplace air-inhalation of 9600 L/day, 5 days/wk, 50 wk/yr, 40 out of 70 yr (*i.e.*, 3768 L/day over an average lifetime).[43] We also calculated exposure for a 70 kg male adult, although a 60 kg adult is more reasonable.[44] When only a range of values was reported in the literature, their geometric mean was used as the average exposure.

between 1968 and 1983, suggesting that factors other than smoking may be important in changes in lung cancer rates.[46] Moreover, according to a recent report, brain cancer mortality rose by 8% annually and multiple myeloma by 2.75% from 1968 to 1983 in the 75–84 age group (US white males and females).[46] The authors believe that it is unlikely that these changes are artifactual and speculate that one possible cause may be exposure to carcinogenic substances in the workplace and general environment, since this cohort has been more highly exposed to carcinogens than younger age groups.[46] They note that further research is needed to pursue these clues. In addition, according to the most recent report on cancer statistics (1950–1985) in the United States cancer mortality rates for all sites except lung have declined for whites. However, there has been a 37% overall increase in cancer *incidence* for whites, and a 23% increase when lung cancer is excluded. Recent data also indicate that incidence rates have been rising, slightly more for blacks than for whites.[47] Further research is needed to pursue these clues. Certainly, the above discussion suggests that a simplistic interpretation of cancer trends to set public policy should be avoided.

EPIDEMIOLOGIC DATA ON ETIOLOGIC FACTORS □

The following discussion is not intended to provide an encyclopedic review of data on human carcinogens but to illustrate the methodologic strengths and limitations of this discipline in elucidating the role of environmental pollutants. The focus is on epidemiology pertaining to occupation and air pollution because these areas are the best developed. For an in-depth discussion of epidemiologic methods, the reader is referred elsewhere.[48–50]

Cancer epidemiologic studies include case reports based on data from individual cancer patients who were exposed to a specific agent; descriptive epidemiologic comparing the incidence of cancer among human populations having different levels of exposure to the agents under study, and analytic epidemiology studies (case-control and cohort studies) that investigate the association between exposure and increased risk of cancer at the individual level. The latter type of study is the most powerful but the most difficult and expensive to carry out.

Clearly, the advantage of epidemiology is the opportunity to study the real-life human situation in all its complexity. When a causal relationship is clearly demonstrated, there is no debate over its relevance. On the other hand, epidemiology is subject to confounding and to errors of data collection. It is also insensitive to modest increases in common cancers.[50] Epidemiology is also constrained by cost, feasibility,

and problems in identifying suitable study and comparison populations. There are difficulties in attributing increases to specific agents and in understanding dose–response relationships, in part because of the lack of adequate exposure data discussed above. As a result, conclusive epidemiologic data exist only for certain occupational cancers, drugs, cigarette smoking, and rare cancers in children. We discuss these methodologic problems with respect to the various known or suspected etiologic agents; exposure to occupational, ambient air, or drinking water carcinogens; passive smoking; diet; and radon.

Occupation □ The International Agency for Research on Cancer (IARC) series, *Monographs on the Evaluation of the Carcinogenic Risk to Humans,* is one of the most respected sources of judgment on the carcinogenicity of chemical substances. To date, 19 chemicals or groups of chemicals that occur in occupational settings and 11 industrial processes have been recognized by the IARC as being carcinogenic on the basis of evidence from human studies.[51] An additional 24 occupational exposures have been classified, on the basis of sufficient evidence from animal tests, as "probably carcinogenic" in humans. The IARC states that "chemicals for which there is sufficient evidence of carcinogenicity in experimental animals [should] be regarded as if they presented a carcinogenic risk to humans." Thus, other similar compilations of known or suspected carcinogens have included sufficient animal carcinogens.[52,53]

Table 14b–3 illustrates the large variability in estimates of the cancer risk attributable to occupations, which arises from differences in data sets and assumptions.* (See, for example, discussion by Davis and colleagues.[61]) Most of the published estimates of the fraction of cancers attributed to occupations are not based on accurate measures of the proportions of exposed subjects, the levels of exposure, or the carcinogenic risk. Therefore, it is preferable to estimate the proportion of organ-specific cancers attributable to occupations for defined populations, time periods, and geographical areas.[62] Table 14b–4 shows the place- and time-specific estimates of the proportion of bladder cancer in males attributable to occupations, as calculated by the authors of selected studies, and

---

* The attributable risk (AR) is the total disease experience in a population that would not have occurred if the effect associated with the risk factor of interest were absent.[59,60] It may be estimated for the exposed population, as well as for a broader population (population attributable risk, or PAR). AR is derived from the relative risk of disease among exposed in comparison with unexposed individuals, according to the formula $AR = (RR - 1)/RR$, where RR is the relative risk. PAR depends on the proportion of exposed subjects in the population (P): $P(RR - 1)/[P(RR - 1) + 1]$.[59]

Table 14b–3
Estimated Proportions of Cancer (PAR) Attributable to Occupations

Study	Population	PAR	Comments
Higginson[54]	Not stated	1% oral cancer 1%–2% lung cancer 10% bladder 2% skin cancer	No detailed presentation of exposure levels and other assumptions
Higginson and Muir[55]	Not stated	1%–3% total cancer	No detailed presentation of assumptions
Wynder and Gori[56]	Not stated	4% total cancer in men, 2% for women	Based on one PAR for bladder cancer and two personal communications
Bridbord et al[57]	United States	23%–38% total cancer (13%–18% for asbestos alone)	PAR to exposure to asbestos, arsenic, benzene, chromium, nickel and petroleum products; based on worst-case scenario both in terms of levels of exposure and proportion of exposed subjects (subsequently revised; see Davis et al[61])
Higginson and Muir[58]	West Midland, United Kingdom	6% total cancer in men, 2% total cancer in women	Based on 10% of non-tobacco-related lung cancer, mesothelioma, bladder cancer (30%), and leukemia (30%)
Doll and Peto[45]	United States	4% (range, 2%–8%) total cancer	Based on all studied cancer sites; reported as "tentative" estimate

as estimated by Vineis and Simonato,[72] using standardized criteria in order to obtain comparable estimations. The 20-fold variation between estimates results largely from differences in proportions of study populations that were occupationally exposed.

Workers are often among the first subjects to be exposed to industrial chemicals that eventually reach the remaining population and the environment. They are exposed to higher concentrations than other people, and suffer more severe consequences. It is noteworthy that a large amount of today's knowledge on human carcinogenesis derives from studies on occupationally exposed groups. Furthermore, a small attributable risk in the population at large may correspond to a very high risk within smaller groups of highly exposed workers. For example, it has been estimated that an attributable risk of 3% in the overall population, comparable to that estimated by most of the analyses reported above, corresponds to 25% of all those cancers among blue collar male workers that have known etiologic factors and are thus theoretically preventable.[73,74]

Air Pollution □ Cigarette smoking is the major cause of lung cancer, alone or in combination with other environmental agents. Epidemiologic data suggest

Table 14b–4
Proportion of Bladder Cancers Attributable to Occupations Among Men: Comparison of Selected Case-Control Studies

Study	Geographic Area	Time Period	Attributable % Risk According to:	
			Study Authors	Vineis and Simonato[72a]*
Wynder et al[63]	New York City	Late 1950s	NA†	1
Anthony and Thomas[64]	Leeds, United Kingdom	Late 1960s	>20	4
Cole et al[65]	Boston	Early 1970s	18	16
Davies et al[66]	London, United Kingdom	Mid 1970s	5	NA
Howe et al[67]	3 Canadian Provinces	Mid 1970s	8‡	3
Tola et al[68]	Finland, industrial areas	Mid 1970s	NA	5
Cartwright[69]	Leeds, United Kingdom	Late 1970s	20	19
Silverman et al[70]	Detroit	Late 1970s	NA	7
Schoenberg et al[71]	New Jersey	Late 1970s	20–22	2
Vineis and Magnani[72]	Torino, Italy	Early 1980s	10	7

* On the basis of standard criteria.

† NA = not available.

‡ Proportion attributed to occupational exposure to dust or fumes = 19%.

that industrial air pollutants are also important. However, the difficulty in characterizing human exposure to ambient air pollutants poses an almost insurmountable challenge to the epidemiologist, for several reasons. First, air pollution itself is a highly complex mixture. Many different carcinogenic substances have been identified in extracts of polluted air. These include carcinogenic metals (*e.g.,* arsenic, beryllium, cadmium, chromium, and nickel), PAH, asbestos, radionuclides, benzene, vinyl chloride, chlorinated solvents (*e.g.,* carbon tetrachloride, chloroform, and trichloroethylene), formaldehyde, pesticides (*e.g.,* chlordane, dieldrin, and DDT), PCBs, polychlorinated dibenzodioxins and dibenzofurans, and nitrosamines.[12,75–82] Other carcinogenic compounds have been reported in emissions from vehicles, combustion sources, industrial facilities, and waste disposal sites. Polluted air also contains substances such as mineral dusts, sulfur dioxide, and ozone, which may act as cofactors or promoters of carcinogenesis.

Second, reported concentrations of carcinogenic substances in ambient air vary widely according to location and time of sampling. For most pollutants, reported concentrations are several times higher in urban air than in rural air; concentrations near industrial sources may be 1 to 3 orders of magnitudes higher than those in the general environment.[82] The composition, distribution, and levels of carcinogenic components of air pollution have also changed over the past several decades. Historical data on levels of carcinogenic air pollutants are virtually nonexistent, but there is evidence that airborne concentrations of BP in the United States and other industrialized countries declined by at least a factor of 10 between the 1930s and the mid-1970s.[83–85] These declines were presumably offset by a rise in emissions of other carcinogenic substances, including metals, asbestos, pesticides, and volatile organic compounds resulting from increased industrial activity, greater use of motor vehicles, and the growth of the organic chemical industry during the 1950s and 1960s. More recently, emissions of some carcinogens, such as asbestos, vinyl chloride, benzene, and dieldrin, have been lowered in the United States by specific health-based regulations. It is likely that emissions of many carcinogens have been reduced as a result of emission controls on vehicles, power plants, and industrial facilities; improved industrial and waste disposal practices; and the decline in primary metals processing. Thus, although overall human exposure to airborne carcinogens in the United States now appears to be decreasing, systematic data to document such a trend are lacking.

Haemisegger and colleagues[82] estimated the magnitude of cancer risks to the human population of the United States by combining survey data on concentrations of various carcinogenic pollutants in urban and rural air with estimates of cancer potency factors. These factors were calculated by the EPA from dose–response data derived from epidemiologic studies or experimental studies on animals. The analysis by Haemisegger and co-workers[82] suggested that the substances posing the greatest risks to the general US population were cadmium, arsenic, and benzene. The excess lifetime cancer risks posed to individuals exposed to average urban concentrations of these substances were roughly estimated to be in the range of 10^{-5} to 10^{-3}, increasing to 10^{-2} (1 cancer per 100 persons exposed) or even higher for people living near major industrial emission sources.

Direct investigations of the relationship between cancer incidence (or mortality) and air pollution by means of epidemiologic studies in the general population have been limited by the inadequacy of data on levels of carcinogenic air pollutants in past decades, and the total lack of exposure data for individuals. Most epidemiologic studies that have been reported to date involved geographic comparisons, in which location of residence was used as a surrogate measure of likely past exposure to air pollution. In some studies, data on levels of noncarcinogenic air pollutants (*e.g.,* particulates, dustfall, or sulfur dioxide) were used as surrogate measures of likely past exposure to carcinogenic pollutants. In all such studies, effects of air pollution are subject to confounding with other factors (*e.g.,* smoking habits or occupational exposures) that may be correlated with location of residence.

For example, ecologic studies have shown that lung cancer rates are increased in heavily industrialized counties of the United States[86,87] and in the vicinity of coke oven and solvent refinery plants and iron foundries.[88,89] In addition, cancers at many sites are consistently more frequent in urban populations than in rural populations;[90] this difference is correlated not only with an urban–rural gradient in air pollution but with urban–rural gradients in smoking habits and in occupational exposures to many potential carcinogens.[45] The issue addressed in many reported studies is whether an urban–rural differential in cancer frequency remains after controlling for the urban–rural differentials in smoking, occupational exposures, and other confounding factors.

Nisbet and colleagues[81] reviewed 48 epidemiologic studies of cancer (mostly lung cancer) in human populations. In 28 of these studies, a statistical association was reported between cancer rates and one or more measures of air pollution; most of the rest reported an urban–rural differential in cancer rates. Only 7 or 8 studies reported no association between cancer rates and either urban location or measures of air pollution.

A number of the studies included attempts to control for smoking habits. However, strict control for the effects of smoking is difficult, because these effects are large and depend on several different aspects of smoking behavior.[45] An unpublished study by Dean and co-workers[91] controlled for a number of these aspects of smoking behavior and still found a strong urban–rural differential in lung cancer rates. Among seven studies limited to nonsmokers, five showed a strong urban–rural differential in lung cancer mortality rates.[81,85] Data from one study (Hammond and Garfinkel;[92] reanalyzed by Nisbet and co-workers[81]) show a strong urban–rural differential in lung cancer mortality rates after controlling for both occupational exposure and smoking. Overall, therefore, there is substantial evidence for an urban–rural gradient in lung cancer rates after controlling for the major known confounding factors.[93]

A number of reviewers[75,94,95] have attempted to define dose–response relationships for lung cancer mortality, using airborne levels of BP as a surrogate measure of air pollution. Nisbet and colleagues[81] reviewed 13 such studies, and concluded that the data were consistent with the hypothesis that about 19% (range of estimates, 11%–33%) of lung cancer deaths in the United States were associated with urban factors, including air pollution. Most of the studies were conducted between the late 1950s and the early 1970s, so that the estimate of 19% refers specifically to cancer deaths in that period, which would have been attributable to exposures starting in the 1930s or 1940s. There is insufficient information to estimate the proportion of current cancer deaths attributable to exposures in the 1950s or 1960s, or the proportion of future deaths that can be expected to result from current exposures.

Drinking Water □ Concern about carcinogenic risk from drinking water is based on the fact that known or suspected carcinogens have been found in drinking water, and several ecologic studies have reported a positive correlation between certain inorganic and organic contaminants and mortality from cancer at various sites.[9,11,85,97] Specifically, contamination of water from carcinogenic inorganic chemicals, such as arsenic, chromium, and nitrates, has been associated with increased risk of specific cancers at the ecologic level: the only published case-control study on nitrates in drinking water showed an association with stomach cancer.[98] There are conflicting data regarding the carcinogenicity of water hardness and fluoride.[85]

The role of organic chemicals has been more widely studied because of their large number and widespread occurrence: out of 309 volatile organic contaminants studied by the Safe Drinking Water Committee of the National Academy of Sciences, 22 are known or suspected carcinogens, and 60 have insufficient data on chronic toxicity.[11] Chloroform and other trihalomethanes, which result from disinfection of water with chlorine,[99] form the most important group of organic carcinogens found in drinking water. However, for reasons discussed below, results from both ecologic and case-control studies of the carcinogenic role of organic contaminants have not been conclusive.[97,100]

These studies exemplify the difficulties faced by epidemiologists when studying environmental exposures. For example, sources of bias in assessing exposure to water contaminants include the use of proxy variables, such as surface or ground water, when estimates of contaminant concentration or chlorination are not available; the use of state, county, or city data when estimates of individual exposure are not available; the lack of data on contaminant concentrations or chlorination in the past; the failure to account for use of water from different sources in the same area and time period (home versus work) or the use of bottled water; possible errors in recall of quantitative water intake; and the mobility of the population.[97] By contrast to most prior investigations, a recent study on bladder cancer in 10 areas of the United States was able to obtain a lifetime residential history of enrolled cases and controls with detailed data on chlorination of drinking water by utilities that provided water to subjects' residences. Results from this study support an increase in risk of bladder cancer with total intake of tap water for users of a chlorinated surface water supply for at least 40 years. The authors estimated the risk for bladder cancer attributable to ingestion of tap water from chlorinated surface sources at 12% (27% among nonsmokers) of all bladder cancers.[101] This estimate needs to be confirmed by other studies, and the potential risk from chloroform and other chlorination by-products must be compared with the benefits derived from water disinfection. This research illustrates the need to study the most heavily exposed subgroups in a population to avoid dilution of the effect in a population in which most people have low exposure.

Pesticides, Chemical Preservatives and Additives in the Diet □ No epidemiologic data are available concerning the carcinogenic risk of pesticide residues in the diet. Nor are there conclusive epidemiologic data showing that dietary nitrosamines (resulting in part from the addition of nitrite preservatives) are carcinogenic.[102] Some epidemiologic investigations of saccharin (a bladder carcinogen in rodents) have been of such low power as to be of little value. Among studies of adequate power, the results have been inconsistent.[103] Thus, it is not possible to estimate the percentage of cancer attributable to these sources based on epidemiologic data. Estimates such as that by Doll and Peto[45] that food contaminants, together with air and water pollutants, are responsible for 2% of cancer risk (range, <1%–5%) are highly arbitrary. Epidemiologists have, however, attributed the observed drop in stomach cancer rates in the United States to changes in food preservation and storage, specifically the replacement of salting, smoking, and pickling by refrigeration.[104]

Active and Passive Cigarette Smoking □ Probably the most exhaustively studied exposure to human carcinogens is cigarette smoke. Epidemiology has demonstrated a direct causal relationship between lung cancer and the number of cigarettes smoked, with no apparent threshold for the effect. Cancer at other sites, including mouth, pharynx, larynx and esophagus, bladder and pancreas, is also causally related to cigarette smoking.[100]

The contribution of environmental tobacco smoke (ETS), or passive smoking, to human cancer has recently been reviewed.[100,105] The NRC estimated that, based on results of no less than 13 case-control studies, the overall summary relative risk of lung cancer among nonsmokers from ETS exposure was 1.34. This means that the estimated increased risk in nonsmokers married to smokers compared with nonsmokers is about 35%, with a best estimate of about 24% after adjusting for reasonable exposure misclassification.[100] Doll and Peto[45] have estimated that active cigarette smoking was responsible in 1978 for about 30% of all US cancer deaths. This estimate will be discussed below.

Natural Constituents in the Diet □ As noted by Doll and Peto,[45] "diet is a chronic source of both frustration and excitement to epidemiologists" in that the potential reduction in cancer risk from modification of national dietary practices is great; yet the most important dietary factors have still not been definitively and reliably identified. Here we will discuss only natural constituents of food and those produced during the normal storage and preparation of food; chemical preservatives and additives have been mentioned above. We note, however, that the concentrations of microorganisms or their carcinogenic products, such

as aflatoxin B_1, are largely determined by the storage techniques used and are, therefore, in part man-made. Of the specific dietary carcinogens identified as such in laboratory animals (cycasin, safrole, pyrrolizidene alkaloids, PAHs, and other pyrolysis products) only aflatoxin B_1 has been related to cancer in humans. There is, for example, as yet no conclusive human evidence that endogenous (or exogenous) dietary N-nitroso compounds contribute to gastric cancer. A number of dietary factors are being actively studied as either "enhancers" or "protectors," including fat and fiber, certain vitamins and minerals (such as vitamin E, selenium, β-carotene and other carotenoids, and vitamin A or retinol) and overnutrition. However, it may not be possible to obtain clear-cut human evidence for the role of single dietary factors, given the difficulty in finding appropriate comparison populations.[45] Despite the paucity of data, Doll and Peto have "guesstimated" that 35% is a "plausible total" for the contribution of diet to US cancer death rates, emphasizing that the figure is based on parts that are "uncertain in the extreme" and that they "make no pretense of its reliability."[45]

More recent reviews[102,104,106] have also concluded that the role of specific dietary constituents such as fat and fiber, vitamins, and minerals in various human cancers has proved elusive, with epidemiologic studies frequently showing weak or inconsistent associations. The association between dietary fat and breast cancer, although limited, appears strongest, followed by that between fat intake and colon cancer.[104] Therefore, while recognizing the influence of diet, we concur with the NRC[102] that it is impossible, given the available data, to estimate its precise contribution to overall cancer risk.

Among the few dietary factors that have been shown to be carcinogenic to humans are alcoholic beverages. They have usually been related to cancer of the oral cavity, pharynx, larynx, esophagus, and liver[107] alone and in interaction with smoking. It is still not clear whether the effect of alcoholic beverages depends on alcohol itself or on other compounds found in wines, spirits, and beer, such as nitrosamines.[108] Cancer of the breast has recently been associated with alcohol; however, the evidence is, as yet, not conclusive.[109] According to an early estimate, 3% of all cancers in the United States are attributable to alcohol.[45]

Indoor Radon □ Levels of gaseous radon, a decay product of uranium, vary widely in US homes according to geographic and geologic area and season.[110] Indoor levels of radon tend to be highest in areas with permeable soil over granite and shales with high concentrations of uranium. They are also elevated during the winter months. There are few epidemiologic studies of the general population concerning the risk of indoor radon. However, the epidemiologic studies of uranium and other minerals have clearly demonstrated an increased frequency of lung cancer deaths resulting from radon exposure, with a multiplicative effect of cigarette smoking and uranium.[111] These data have provided the basis for the estimate that exposure to indoor radon results in 6,000–25,000 excess lung cancer deaths per year, with a best estimate of 13,000, or about 10% of total lung cancer deaths.[110,112,113] Based on the observed synergism between cigarette smoking and radon in the occupational setting, the great majority of these projected radon-related deaths are also smoking-related.

Remediation strategies include monitoring to identify "hot spots" and alert homeowners, the use of engineering techniques to ventilate existing structures, and standards for new construction.[110] It also appears that reduction of cigarette smoking would be the most direct approach to lowering the lung cancer risk of radon.[110]

Interactions Between Exposures and Life-style Factors □ In the epidemiologic literature, there are several other examples of interactions between cigarette smoking and other environmental exposures. The classic example is asbestos and cigarette smoking;[114] however, nickel has also been shown to interact synergistically with smoking. There is also some evidence of synergism between cigarette smoking, industrial pollutants, and ambient air pollution in the causation of lung cancer.[95,115–119]

Interactions have not been elaborated between viruses and industrial or man-made chemicals. However, there is evidence of interactions between dietary factors and viruses as in the case of aflatoxin B_1 and hepatitis B and liver cancer.[120]

Cancer is a multistage, multicausal process,[121–123] in which external exposures and internal factors act before the disease is detected clinically. It is likely that most cancers depend on two or more etiologic factors acting sequentially or simultaneously. Thus, smokers exposed to asbestos have a relative risk of developing lung cancer, in comparison with nonsmokers unexposed to asbestos, that is close to the product of the risks for the two risk factors (*i.e.,* the risk of smoking among subjects unexposed to asbestos and the risk for asbestos exposure among nonsmokers).[84,114] Similarly, alcohol per se appears to be a minor cause of cancer, but the risks of cancer in sites such as the oral cavity[125] for smokers who drink are much higher than the risk for those exposed to either factor alone. If two carcinogens interact, that is, if they affect two different stages of the carcinogenic process, cancers occurring in subjects exposed to both risk factors can be attributed to either factor.[57] The sum of the proportions of cancers attributable to known and unknown risk factors will therefore exceed 100%. In the hypothetic case where a risk factor accounts for 75% of all cancer, this does not imply that all remaining etiologic factors cause 25% of cancers, but that 75% of all cancers would be avoided if that exposure were eliminated. Figure 14b–1 shows the hypothetic example of a disease with two-stage etiology, in whose causation two factors interact. This important aspect of cancer prevention must be borne in mind when looking at the overall quantification

FIG. 14b–1   Hypothetical example of multiple causation and interaction. Two factors are needed to cause the disease: one "early" factor and one "late" factor. X is the only known early factor and Y is the only known late factor: 75% of disease is attributable to X (35% in interaction with Y, 40% with unknown late factors), and 50% is attributable to Y (35% with X, 15% with unknown early factors). Yet 10% of disease is attributable to neither X nor Y.

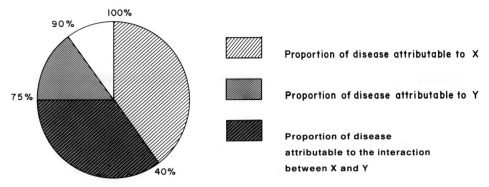

of cancer attributable to difference causes, such as that by Doll and Peto.[45]

Molecular Cancer Epidemiology ■

A relatively new approach in the study of environmental carcinogenesis and prevention has been the use of biologic markers to elucidate exposure dose–response relationships of carcinogens.[126-129] In particular, markers of dose and early response to carcinogens such as those shown in Table 14b–5 can improve human risk assessment by permitting early identification of carcinogenic hazards and estimates of potential risk on the group level. They can also improve extrapolation from quantitative cancer risks in high-dose laboratory experiments or high-exposure epidemiologic studies to lower exposure situations in humans. In quantitative risk assessment (QRA), population variability in response to exposure is a key consideration, but one that is usually not accounted for in the process. Biologic markers provide a means of assessing the extent of human variation in effective dose and early preclinical response. Biologic markers can not only allow epidemiology to become a more timely instrument in qualitative risk assessment but also significantly increase the power of epidemiologic studies to detect a true effect by allowing accurate classification of exposed versus unexposed individuals, where the former have received a significant, biologically effective dose. By providing an earlier and more commonly occurring endpoint than cancer incidence, markers of response that reflect early events in the pathogenic process can significantly increase the statistical power of an epidemiologic study to detect causal relationships. At present, available biologic markers can and do serve as indicators of carcinogenic hazard. In most cases, however, considerable work remains to validate them for use in QRA.

A consistent observation in molecular epidemiologic studies thus far has been the significant variability in markers of biologically effective dose and response between individuals with comparable environmental exposure to carcinogens. For example, the level of BP–DNA adduct formation in cultured human tissues and cells shows as much as a 350-fold variation.[131] Less than 30% of exposed coke oven workers tested for BP–DNA antibodies in sera had measurable adducts.[132] The extent of cis-platinum–DNA adduct formation in treated cancer patients also varies widely, with about 50% of subjects forming measurable adducts.[133] Studies on 1–2 pack/day smokers show considerable individual variation in formation of BP–DNA and 4-aminobiphenyl (4-ABP)–hemoglobin adducts, as well as in sister chromatid exchange frequencies.[134]

A second common finding, equally relevant to risk estimation, is that measurable levels of biologic markers have been seen in virtually all so-called "unexposed control" groups studied. For example, substantial "background" levels of various carcinogen–protein and carcinogen–DNA adducts have been

Table 14b–5
Examples of Human Studies

Endpoint	Sample*	Study Population	Exposure
Protein adducts	RBC	Sterilization plant workers, smokers, controls	Ethylene oxide
Protein adducts	RBC	Smokers, nonsmokers	4-APB
DNA adducts	WBC	Lung cancer patients, nonsmokers, roofers, foundry workers, coke oven workers, controls	BP in mixture
DNA adducts	WBC	Chemotherapy patients, controls	cis-platinum
Antibodies to DNA adducts	WBC	Coke oven workers	BP in mixture
DNA adducts (excised)	Urine	African outpatients	Aflatoxin B$_1$
DNA adducts	Placenta	Pregnant women, smokers, nonsmokers	Cigarette smoke
Unscheduled DNA synthesis	WBC	Workers, controls	Propylene oxide
DNA adducts	Buccal mucosa	Betel and tobacco chewers, controls	Betel nut, tobacco
Chromosomal aberrations	WBC	Workers, controls	Vinyl chloride
Sister chromatid exchange	WBC	Workers, controls	Ethylene oxide
Micronuclei	Lymphocytes	Tank cleaners, controls	Organic solvents, heavy metals
Somatic cell mutation	RBC	Cancer patients	Chemotherapy agents
Somatic cell mutation	Lymphocytes	Medical technicians	Radiotherapy

Reviewed in Perera.[130]

* RBC = red blood cells; WBC = white blood cells.

seen in nonsmokers and worker controls.[134,135] Both of these findings support the concept of low-dose linearity in human cancer risk estimation (discussed below).

Quantitative Risk Assessment Based on Animal Data ■

Because of the limitations of epidemiology, described above, chronic bioassays in rodents are currently the most reliable and widely used basis for predicting carcinogenic effects in humans and for estimating the magnitude of human risk. Historical data demonstrate an excellent correlation between human and experimental carcinogenicity for those substances and agents that have been adequately tested. According to the IARC, of the agents for which there is sufficient or limited evidence of carcinogenicity in humans, all 37 that have been tested adequately produce cancer in at least one animal species.[51] Although this association cannot establish that all agents that cause cancer in experimental animals also do so in humans, the IARC considers that it is both biologically plausible and prudent to regard agents with sufficient animal evidence as being carcinogenic in humans.[51] The IARC has listed 37 chemicals, agents, or industrial processes as probably carcinogenic in humans, mostly on the basis of sufficient evidence of carcinogenicity in laboratory animals and limited evidence in humans.[51]

The process of extrapolating human risk from animal data involves a number of important assumptions about interspecies relationships and the nature of the carcinogenic process itself. These assumptions guide the selection of the data set (most sensitive or less sensitive species), the dose conversion factor (surface area or body weight) and, very importantly, the mathematical model to use in predicting low-dose carcinogenic risk to humans. A variety of mathematic models have been developed that are based on assumptions or information about population tolerance and mechanisms or stages involved in carcinogenesis, or tumor latency. Unfortunately, in most cases the observed data do not provide a guide to model selection, since many models fit the high-dose data equally well. However, the resultant estimates of low-dose risk can vary by many orders of magnitude. The EPA and other federal and state agencies have, as a general rule, used the linearized multistage model, which incorporates the plausible concept that the carcinogenic process usually involves multiple stages, at least one of which can be affected by ex-

posure to the carcinogen of concern. It also assumes that the chemical of interest is capable of adding to the effect of background exposures and processes.[136,137] Epidemiologic data regarding radiation, arsenic, aflatoxin, and cigarette smoking do not indicate that human thresholds or safe levels of exposure exist for these agents,[138] and thus support the linearized model.

Although it is generally conservative, the linearized multistage model does not account for possible interactions between chemicals or between a chemical and a life-style or host factor. Nor does it explicitly account for the significant variability that has been demonstrated for metabolism, cellular and tissue susceptibility, and genetic predisposition in the human population.[128,139] Thus in certain instances, the model may underestimate human risk.

An advantage of QRA based on animal data is that risk estimates generated for a series of chemicals or agents using consistent assumptions and procedures can provide a means of setting priorities for regulation. On the other hand, the major disadvantage of QRA is that, because of the numerous uncertainties inherent in the process, the estimates really represent "guesstimates" of low-dose risk, which may overestimate or (with more serious consequences for public health) underestimate the true risk by several orders of magnitude. This fact is often ignored—in part because the actual uncertainty is belied by the apparent precision of the numbers.

In a few instances, it is possible to compare human cancer risk estimates for the same carcinogen based on experimental and human data (see Table 14b–6). The two appear to be generally consistent when procedures and models are used that incorporate low-dose linearity using either direct proportionality or a fitted model (Refs. 96, 140–143, plus Hertz-Picciotto, personal communication). Although these data are limited, they support the reliance on animal data as a basis for QRA in the usual case where epidemiologic data are not available.

Table 14b–6
Comparisons of Human and Animal-based Lifetime Risk Estimates*

Carcinogen	Animal Data	Human Data
Asbestos	0.009–0.021	0.001–0.165
Benzene	0.000078–0.000170	0.000048–0.000120
Gasoline	0.0035	0.0011
Cadmium	0.000110–0.000180	0.000002–0.000012

Data are from Hertz-Picciotto; Personal communication.

* Human and animal exposures were equivalent for each substance.

Table 14b–7
HERP Indices for Natural and Man-made Carcinogens

	HERP (%)	
Carcinogenic Exposure*	Ames et al[23]	Perera and Boffetta
Man-made Chemicals in Food and Beverages		
DDE/DDT in food		
Preregulatory	—	0.003
Postregulatory	0.0003	0.0002
EDB in grains	0.0004	0.0004
PCBs in food		
Preregulatory	—	0.01
Postregulatory	0.0002	0.0002
Sodium saccharin in diet sodas	.06†	0.003
Natural Carcinogens in Foods and Beverages		
Aflatoxins in peanuts and peanut butter	0.03†	0.003
DMN in cured meat and bacon	0.003†	0.001
DEN in cured meat	0.006†	0.002
Estragole in basil	0.1†	<0.0001
Ethyl alcohol in beer	2.8†	1.6
Ethyl alcohol in wine	4.7†	0.4
Hydrazines in mushrooms	0.1†	0.01
Ambient Air Pollutants		
Formaldehyde in conventional home air	0.6	0.6
Formaldehyde in mobile home air	2.1	2.1
Water Pollutants		
Chloroform in water	0.001	0.003
Tetrachlorethylene in water	0.0003†	0.0002‡
TCE in water	0.004†	0.00002§
Occupational Exposures		
Formaldehyde in workplace air	5.8	3.0

From: Perera and Boffetta.[149]

* EDB, ethylene dibromide; PCBs, polychlorinated biphenyls; DMN, N-nitrosodimethylamine; DEN, N-nitrosodiethylamine; TCE, trichloroethylene.

† Worst-case exposure.

‡ Worst-case assumption: HERP% = 0.007.

§ Worst-case assumption: HERP% = 0.1.

For ethylene oxide, 9.2 total leukemia deaths were predicted extrapolating from animal data using the multistage model. Eight leukemia deaths were observed.[143]

The Human Exposure Rodent Potency (HERP) Index ■

Ames and colleagues[27] have suggested a novel approach to ranking possible carcinogenic hazards and have applied it to a selection of man-made and naturally occurring carcinogens, with resultant controversy.[144] Their possible hazard index is determined by expressing the human exposure (in milligrams per kilogram) as a percentage of the rodent TD_{50} dose (milligrams per kilogram).* They compared HERP indices for five pollutants in drinking water and indoor air, five man-made chemicals in foods and beverages, ten naturally occurring dietary toxins, five drugs, and two occupational carcinogens. Their conclusion: viewed against the background of natural carcinogens (largely in the diet), the carcinogenic hazard of man-made environmental pollutants, such as pesticide residues and drinking water contami-

* The TD_{50} is the average daily dose rate to halve the percentage of tumor-free animals by the end of a standard lifetime.[145] The average TD_{50} is the harmonic mean of the TD_{50}s of the positive tests in the most sensitive species. For each test, the target site with the lowest TD_{50} value was used. The source of TD_{50} values is the Carcinogenic Potency Database.[145–148]

nants, is minimal, and their control should not be a priority for public health policy.

Although the HERP system is attractive in its simplicity, it is highly susceptible to the effects of chemical selection and assumptions about human exposure. The reader is referred to a detailed critique of the HERP approach.[149] It therefore cannot provide a sound basis for public health policy concerning environmental carcinogens. However, we note that when estimates of average exposure are consistently used in these comparisons, and when the comparison is based on a more representative sample of chemical pollutants to which the US population is commonly exposed, the HERP indices are fairly comparable for "natural" and man-made carcinogens (see Table 14b-7). Furthermore, the postregulatory HERPs are generally at least one order of magnitude lower than preregulatory HERPs, illustrating the efficacy of regulation.

Nonscientific Considerations ■

The moral and ethical questions involved in the regulation of carcinogens are numerous and thorny.[150-152] Should involuntary exposures to carcinogens over which the person has no feasible control and of which he or she is often ignorant be emphasized by regulators in contrast to voluntary exposures to cigarette smoke and dietary constituents that can be addressed primarily by educational programs to guide the public in their choices? If the answer is yes, to what extent should we as a society be concerned about protecting the most heavily exposed individuals (those in the right-hand tail of the exposure frequency distribution) and the most sensitive segments of the population (children, the elderly, those with impaired health)? How should we address the basic inequity that in most cases the individuals who bear the risks of environmental pollution are not the same people who benefit from production?

A second set of "nonscientific" considerations includes the economic and technical feasibility of controlling exposures by regulatory means. In virtually all cases where man-made carcinogens in the workplace, air, water, and food supply have been identified as candidates for regulation, technical means have readily been found to substantially reduce those exposures. Indeed, in contrast to voluntary exposures (such as smoking and diet) which are not so amenable to regulation, environmental pollution is highly tractable to regulations requiring technical and engineering controls.

Conclusion ■

A major purpose of this review has been to illustrate the pitfalls of using oversimplified "accounting systems" to dictate priorities in cancer prevention. Rather, given both the available data and the gaps in our knowledge about cancer risks, our conclusion is that prevention of this complex, multifactorial disease requires action on many fronts: educational programs regarding life-style choices (*i.e.*, smoking, diet, sexual behavior) that subject people to carcinogenic hazards, as well as control of involuntary exposures to toxic chemicals generated by human activities. The latter requires an active program of environmental monitoring and testing to identify chemicals with the potential to cause cancer in humans. Because of the limitations of epidemiology, for most environmental exposures to carcinogens, conclusive epidemiologic data do not exist, nor are they likely to be developed. However, their absence does not mean that action should not be taken. Rather, on the basis of positive experimental data, efforts should be made to minimize or eliminate environmental exposures to carcinogens. Our present review of a subset of these carcinogens, certain industrial chemicals and pesticides, suggests that their contribution to the burden of human cancer is significant, particularly to certain segments of the population. On the basis of scientific and nonscientific considerations, therefore, public health and environmental policy should be preventive in orientation and should include the control of involuntary exposures to these chemicals.

References ■

1. US General Accounting Office: Pesticides: Need to Enhance FDA's Ability to Protect the Public From Illegal Residues (RCEC-87-7). Washington, DC, GAO, 1987
2. Sawicki E: Chemical composition and potential genotoxic aspects of polluted atmospheres. In Mohr U, Schmal D, Tomatis W, Davis W (eds): Air Pollution and Cancer in Man, pp 127–157. IARC S Publ No. 16. Lyon, France, International Agency for Research on Cancer, 1977
3. US Environmental Protection Agency: Human Exposure to Atmospheric Concentrations of Selected Chemicals. EPA 68-02-3066. Washington, DC, EPA, 1980
4. Hunt WF Jr, Raoro RB, Curran TC, Muntz J: Estimated cancer incidence rates for selected toxic air pollutants using ambient air pollution data. Research Triangle Park, NC, US Environmental Protection Agency, Office of Air and Radiation, 1984
5. Nriagu JO, Pacyna JM: Quantitative assessment of worldwide contamination of air, water and soils by trace metals. Nature 333:134–139, 1988

6. Hunt WF Jr, Faoro RB, Freas W: Report on the Interim Data Base for State and Local Air Toxic Volatile Organic Chemical Measurements. (EPA-450/4-86-012). Washington, DC, US Environmental Protection Agency, 1986

7. Harris RH, Page T, Reiches NA: Carcinogenic hazards of organic chemicals in drinking water. In Hiatt HH, Watson JD, Winsten JA (eds). Book A. Incidence of Cancer in Humans. Cold Spring Harbor, NY, Cold Spring Harbor Laboratory, 1977

8. Council on Environmental Quality: Contamination of Groundwater by Toxic Organic Chemicals. Washington, DC, US Government Printing Office, 1981

9. Crump KS, Guess HA: Drinking water and cancer: Review of recent epidemiological findings and assessment of risks. Annu Rev Publ Health 3:339–357, 1982

10. US Congress Office of Technology Assessment: Protecting the Nation's Groundwater from Contamination. OTA-0-233. Washington, DC, OTA, 1984

11. National Research Council: Drinking Water and Health. Washington, DC, National Academy Press, 1977–1987

12. Wallace LA, Pellizzari ED, Hartwell TD, Sparacino C, Whitmore R, Sheldon L, Zelon H, Perrit R: The TEAM study: Personal exposures to toxic substances in air, drinking water, and breath of 400 residents of New Jersey, North Carolina and North Dakota. Environ Res 43:290–307, 1987

13. National Academy of Sciences: Regulating Pesticides in Food: The Delaney Paradox. Washington, DC, National Academy Press, 1987

14. Schneiderman MA: Expectation and limitation of human studies and risk assessment. In Andelman JB, Underhill DW (eds): Health Effects from Hazardous Waste Sites. Chelsea, MI, Lewis Publishing, 1987

15. US Environmental Protection Agency: Daminozide Special Review. Phase III Market Basket Survey. Uniroyal's Submissions Dated February 13 and 20, 1987 and April 13, 1987. Memo from L Cheng to W Waldrop, May 18, 1987

16. US Environmental Protection Agency: Tolerance Assessment System. Annualized Chronic Consumption Data, Based Upon the United States Department of Agriculture 1977 Nationwide Food Consumption Survey. Washington, DC, EPA, Office of Pesticide Programs, 1987

17. Duggan RE, Corneliussen PE: Dietary intake of pesticide chemicals in the United States (III), June 1968–April 1970. Pesticide Monitoring Journal 5:331–341, 1972

18. US Environmental Protection Agency: DDT: A review of scientific and economic aspects of the decision to ban its use as a pesticide: EPA-540/1-75-022. Washington, DC, EPA, 1975

19. Gartell MJ, Craun JD, Podrebarac DS, Gunderson EL: Pesticides, selected elements and other chemicals in adult total diet samples, October 1980–March 1982. J Assoc Off Anal Chem 69:146–161, 1986

20. Jelinek CF, Corneliussen PE: Levels of PCBs in the U.S. food supply. In Proceedings of the National Conference on Polychlorinated Biphenyls, Chicago, 1975. EPA-560/6-75-004. Washington, DC, US Environmental Protection Agency, 1976

21. Lonneman WA, Bellar TA, Altshuller AP: Aromatic hydrocarbons in the atmosphere of the Los Angeles basin. Environ Sci Toxicol 2:1017–1020, 1968

22. Arthur RD, Cain JD, Barrentine BF: Atmospheric levels of pesticides in the Mississippi Delta. Bull Environ Contamin Toxicol 15:129–134, 1976

23. Patterson RM, Bornstein MI, Garshick E: Assessment of Formaldehyde as a Potential Air Pollution Problem, Vol 8. Bedford, MA, US Environmental Protection Agency, GCA, 1976

24. Versar Inc: Human Exposure to Formaldehyde: Draft Report. Contract No. 68-01-5791, Office of Pesticides and Toxic Substances, US Environmental Protection Agency. Springfield, VA, Versar Inc, 1980

25. Kutz FW, Yang HSC: A note on polychlorinated biphenyls in air. In Proceedings of the National Conference on Polychlorinated Biphenyls, Chicago, 1975. EPA-560/6-75-004. Washington, DC, US Environmental Protection Agency, 1976

26. Eisenreich SJ, Looney BB, Thornton JD: Airborne organic contaminants in the Great Lakes ecosystem. Environ Sci Technol 15:30–38, 1981

27. Ames BN, Magaw R, Gold LS: Ranking possible carcinogenic hazards. Science 236:271–280, 1987

28. Connor TH, Theiss JC, Hanna HA, Montkeith DK, Matney TS: Genotoxicity of organic chemicals frequently found in the air of mobile homes. Toxicol Lett 25:33–40, 1985

29. US Environmental Protection Agency: Ethylene Dibromide (EDB). Position Document 4. Washington, DC, EPA, September 27, 1983

30. Dennis DS: Polychlorinated biphenyls in the surface waters and bottom sediments of the major drainage basins of the United States. In Proceedings of the National Conference on Polychlorinated Biphenyls, Chicago, 1975, pp 183–194. EPA Publication 560/6-75-004, Washington, DC, 1975

31. New Jersey Department of Environmental Protection: Results of Testing for Hazardous Contaminants in Public Water Supplies under Assembly Bill A-280. Final Report. Trenton, NJ, NJDEP, 1987

32. AWWA: Materials for Research Workshop on Volatile Organic Chemicals. Denver, CO, 1972 American Water Works Association

33. International Agency for Research on Cancer: IARC Monograph on the Evaluation of the Carcinogenic Risk of Chemicals to Humans, Vol 29. Some Industrial Chemicals and Dyestuffs. Lyon, France, IARC, 1982

34. US Environmental Protection Agency: SAI-Human Exposure to Atmospheric Concentrations of Selected Chemicals, Vols, 1 and 2. Research Triangle Park, NC, Office of Air Quality Planning and Standards, 1980

35. Runion HE, Scott LM: Benzene exposure in the United States 1978–1983: An overview. Am J Ind Med 7:385–393, 1985

36. National Institute for Occupational Safety and Health: Criteria for a Recommended Standard. Occupational Exposure to Formaldehyde. DHEW (NIOSH) Publ. No. 77-125. Washington, DC, NIOSH, 1976

37. National Research Council: Formaldehyde—An Assessment of its Health Effects. Washington, DC, National Academy Press, 1980

38. Siegel DM, Frankos VH, Schneiderman MA: Formaldehyde risk assessment for occupationally exposed workers. Reg Toxicol Pharmacol 3:355–371, 1983

39. Bernstein RS, Stayner LT, Elliott LJ, Kimbrough R, Falk H, Blader L: Inhalation exposure to formaldehyde: An overview of its toxicology, epidemiology, monitoring and control. Am Ind Hyg Assoc J 45:778–785, 1984

40. US Environmental Protection Agency: Technical Document. Formaldehyde. Washington, DC, Office of Pesticides and Toxic Substances, November 16, 1981

41. Flinn FB: Industrial exposures to chlorinated hydrocarbons. Am J Med 1:388–394, 1946

42. Kimbrough RD, Mitchell FL, Houk VN: Trichloroethylene: An update. J Toxicol Environ Health 15:369–383, 1985

43. Gold LS, Backman GM, Hooper NK, Peto R: Ranking the potential carcinogenic hazards to workers from exposures to chemicals that are tumorigenic in rodents. Environ Health Perspect (in press)

44. US Environmental Protection Agency: Captan Special Review Position Document 2/3. Washington, DC, EPA, Office of Pesticides and Toxic Substances, 1985

45. Doll R, Peto R: The Causes of Cancer: Quantitative Estimates of Avoidable Risk of Cancer in the United States Today. New York, Oxford University Press, 1981
46. Davis DL, Schwartz J: Trends in cancer mortality: U.S. white males and females, 1968–83. Lancet 1:633–636, 1988
47. National Cancer Institute: New Cancer Statistics Released. JNCI Vol 8:8, 1988
48. Hutchinson GB: The epidemiologic method. In Schottenfeld D, Fraumeni JF Jr (eds): Cancer Epidemiology and Prevention. Philadelphia, WB Saunders, 1982
49. Berg MT: Occupational cancer epidemiology. In Brandt-Rauf P (ed): Occupational Medicine: Occupational Cancer and Carcinogenesis. Philadelphia, Hanley and Belfus, 1987
50. Day NE: Statistical considerations. In Wald NJ, Doll R (eds): Interpretation of Negative Epidemiologic Evidence of Carcinogenicity. Lyon, France, International pp 13–27
51. International Agency for Research on Cancer: Overall Evaluations of Carcinogenicity: An Updating of IARC Monographs, Vols 1–42, Suppl 7. Lyon, France, IARC, 1987
52. Simonato I, Saracci R: Cancer, occupational. In Parmeggiaini L (ed): Encyclopedia of Occupational Health and Safety, 3rd ed, pp 369–375. Geneva, International Labour Office, 1983
53. Decouflé P: Occupation. In Schottenfeld D, and Fraumeni JF Jr (eds): Cancer Epidemiology and Prevention, pp 318–335. Philadelphia, WB Saunders Company, 1982
54. Higginson J: Present trends in cancer epidemiology. Proc Canadian Cancer Res Conf 8:40–75, 1969
55. Higginson J, Muir CS: The role of epidemiology in elucidating the importance of environmental factors in human cancer. Cancer Detect Prev 1:79–105, 1976
56. Wynder EL, Gori GB: Contribution of the environment to cancer incidence: An epidemiologic exercise. JNCI 58:825–832, 1977
57. Bridbord K, Decouflé P, Fraumeni JF, Hoel DG, Hoover RN, Rall DP, Saffiotti U, Schneiderman MA, Upton AC, Day N: Estimates of the fraction of Cancer in the United States Related to Occupational Factors. Reproduced in Peto R, Schneiderman M (eds): Quantification of Occupational Cancer. Banbury Report 9, pp 701–726. Cold Spring Harbor, NY, Cold Spring Harbor Laboratory, 1981
58. Higginson J, Muir CS: Environmental carcinogenesis: Misconceptions and limitations to cancer control. JNCI 63:1291–1298, 1979
59. Cole P, MacMahon B: Attributable risk percent in case-control studies. Br J Prev Soc Med 25:242–244, 1971
60. Miettinen OS: Proportion of disease caused or prevented by a given exposure, trait or intervention. Am J Epidemiol 99:325–332, 1974
61. Davis DL, Bridbord K, Schneiderman M: Estimating cancer causes: Problems in methodology, production and trends. In Peto R, Schneiderman M (eds): Quantification of Occupational Cancer. Banbury Report 9, pp 285–316, Cold Spring Harbor, NY, Cold Spring Harbor Laboratory, 1981
62. Cole P, Merletti F: Chemical agents and occupational cancer. J Environ Path Toxicol 3:399–417, 1980
63. Wynder EL, Onderdonk J, Mantel N: An epidemiological investigation of cancer of the bladder. Cancer 16:1388–1407, 1963
64. Anthony HM, Thomas GM: Tumors of the urinary bladder: An analysis of the occupations of 1,030 patients in Leeds, England. JNCI 45:879–895, 1970
65. Cole P, Hoover R, Friedell GH: Occupation and cancer of the lower urinary tract. Cancer 29:1250–1260, 1972
66. Davies JM, Somerville SM, Wallace DM: Occupational bladder tumor cases identified during ten years' interviewing patients. Br J Urol 48:561–566, 1976
67. Howe GR, Burch JD, Miller AB, Cook GM, Esteve J, Morrison B, Gordon P, Chambers LW, Fodor G, Winsor GM: Tobacco use, occupation, coffee, various nutrients, and bladder cancer. JNCI 64:701–713, 1980
68. Tola S, Tenho M, Korkala ML, Jarvinen E: Cancer of the urinary bladder in Finland. Int Arch Occup Environ Health 46:43–51, 1980
69. Cartwright R: Occupational bladder cancer and cigarette smoking in West Yorkshire. Scand J Work Environ Health 8(Suppl 1):79–82, 1982
70. Silverman DT, Hoover RN, Albert S, Graff KM: Occupation and cancer of the lower urinary tract in Detroit. JNCI 70:237–245, 1983
71. Schoenberg JB, Stemhagen A, Mogielnicki AP, Altma R, Toshi A, Mason TJ: Case-control study of bladder cancer in New Jersey: I. Occupational exposures in white males. JNCI 72:973–981, 1984
72. Vineis P, Magnani C: Occupation and bladder cancer in males: A case-control study. Int J Cancer 35:599–606, 1985
72a. Vineis P, Simonato L: Estimates of the proportion of bladder cancers attributable to occupation. Scand J Work Environ Health 12:55–60, 1986
73. Nicholson WJ: Quantitative estimates of cancer in the workplace. Am J Indust Med 5:341–342, 1984
74. Nicholson WJ: Research issues in occupational and environmental cancer. Arch Environ Health 39:190–202, 1984
75. National Academy of Sciences: Particulate Polycyclic Organic Matter. Washington, DC, National Research Council, NAS, 1972
76. National Academy of Sciences: Vapor Phase Organic Pollutants. Washington, DC, National Research Council, NAS, 1976
77. National Academy of Sciences: Polychlorinated Biphenyls. Washington, DC, National Research Council, NAS, 1979
78. US Environmental Protection Agency: Ambient Water Quality Criteria for Benzene. EPA 440/5-80/018. Washington, DC, EPA, 1980
79. Santodonato J, Howard P, Basu D: Health and ecological assessment of polynuclear hydrocarbons: 5.5. Human exposure from various media. J Environ Pathol Toxicol 5:162–171, 1981
80. Singh HB, Salas LJ, Stiles RE, Shigeishi H: Measurements of hazardous organic chemicals in the ambient atmosphere. Research Triangle Park, NC, Environmental Science Research Laboratory, Office of Research and Development, US Environmental Protection Agency, 1982
81. Nisbet ICT, Schneiderman MA, Karch NJ, Siegel DM: Review and Evaluation of Evidence for Cancer Associated with Air Pollution. EPA 450/5-83-006R. Research Triangle Park, NC, EPA, Office of Air Quality Planning and Standards, 1984
82. Haemisegger E, Jones A, Steigerwald B, Thompson V: The Toxics Air Problem in the United States: An Analysis of Cancer Risks for Selected Pollutants. U.S. Environmental Protection Agency, Office of Air and Radiation, May 1985
83. Wilson R, Colome SD, Spengler JD, Wilson DG: Health Effects of Fossil Fuel Burning: Assessment and Mitigation. Cambridge, MA, Ballinger, 1980
84. Council on Environmental Quality: Eleventh Annual Report of the Council on Environmental Quality. Washington, DC, US Government Printing Office, 1980
85. Shy CM, Struba RJ: Air and water pollution. In Schottenfeld D, Fraumeni JF (eds): Cancer Epidemiology and Prevention, pp 336–363. Philadelphia, WB Saunders
86. Blot WJ: Clues to environmental determinants of cancer from its geographic patterns: In Breslow NE, Whittemore AS (eds): Energy and Health, 1979. Proceedings of a SIMS Conference, Philadelphia, Society for Industrial and Applied Mathematics, pp 151–167, 1979

87. Blot WJ, Fraumeni JF Jr: Arsenical air pollution and lung cancer. Lancet 2:142–144, 1976

88. Maclure KM, MacMahon B: An epidemiologic perspective of environmental carcinogenesis. Epidemiol Rev 2:19–48, 1980

89. Smith GH, Williams FLR, Lloyd OLL: Respiratory cancer and air pollution from iron foundries in a Scottish town: An epidemiological and environmental study. Br J Industr Med 44:795–802, 1987

90. Goldsmith J: The "urban factor" in cancer: Smoking, industrial exposures, and air pollution as possible explanations. J Environ Pathol Toxicol 3:205–217, 1980

91. Dean G, Lee PN, Todd GF, Wicken AJ: Report on a second retrospective mortality study in North East England. Tobacco Research Council Research Paper 14, Pt. II. London, Tobacco Research Council, 1978

92. Hammond EC, Garfinkel L: General air pollution and cancer in the United States. Prev Med 9:206–211, 1980

93. Oleske DM: The epidemiology of lung cancer: An overview. Sem in Oncol Nursing 3:165–173, 1987

94. Pike MC, Gordon RJ, Henderson BE, Menck HR, Soohoo J: Air Pollution. In Fraumeni JF (ed): Persons at High Risk of Cancer, pp 225–239. An Approach to Cancer Etiology and Control. New York, Academic Press, 1975

95. Cederlof R, Doll R, Fowler B, et al: Air pollution and cancer: Risk assessment methodology and epidemiological evidence. Environ Health Perspect 22:1–12, 1978

96. California Department of Health Services: Health Effects of Benzene: Report to the Scientific Review Panel, Part B. Sacramento, CA, CDHS, 1984

97. Wilkins JR, Reiches NA, Kruse CW: Organic chemical contaminants in drinking water and cancer. Am J Epidemiol 110:420–448, 1979

98. Cuello C, Correa P, Haenszel W, Gordillo G, Brown C, Archer M, Tannenbaum S: Gastric cancer in Colombia. I. Cancer risk and suspect environmental agents. JNCI 57:1015–1020, 1976

99. Rook JJ: Formation of haloforms during chlorination of natural waters. Water Treat Exam 23:234–243, 1974

100. National Research Council: Environmental Tobacco Smoke: Measuring Exposures and Assessing Health Effects. Washington, DC, National Academy Press, 1986

101. Cantor KP, Hoover R, Hartge P, Mason TJ, Silverman DT, Altman R, Austin DF, Child MA, Key CR, Marrett LD, Myers MH, Narayana AS, Levin LI, Sullivan JW, Swanson GM, Thomas DB, West DW: Bladder cancer, drinking water source, and tap water consumption: A case-control study. JNCI 79:1269–1279, 1987

102. National Research Council: Diet, Nutrition and Cancer. Washington, DC, National Academy Press, 1982

103. Stellman S: Review of Saccharin. Workshop on Guidelines to the Epidemiology of Weak Associations. American Health Foundation. Dec 4–5, 1985. Publ Prevent Med 16:165–182, 1987

104. Cohen L: Diet and cancer. Sci Am 257:42–48, 1987

105. International Agency for Research on Cancer: Tobacco Smoking. Monograph on the Evaluation of Carcinogenic Risk of Chemicals to Humans, Vol 38. Lyon, France, 1986

106. Higginson J: Changing concepts in cancer prevention: Limitations and implications for future research in environmental carcinogenesis. Cancer Res 48:1381–1389, 1988

107. Tuyns AJ: Alcohol. In Schottenfeld D, Fraumeni JF (eds): Cancer Epidemiology and Prevention, pp 293–303. Philadelphia, WB Saunders, 1982

108. Preussman R: Occurrence and exposure to N-nitroso compounds and precursors. In O'Neill IK, Von Borstel RC, Miller CT, Long J, Bartsch H (eds): N-Nitroso Compounds: Occur-

rence, Biological Effects and Relevance to Human Cancer, pp 3–15. IARC Scientific Publ No 57. Lyon, France, International Agency for Research on Cancer, 1984

109. Graham S: Alcohol and breast cancer. N Engl J Med 316:1211–1213, 1987

110. Kerr RA: Indoor radon: The deadliest pollutant. Science 240:606–608, 1988

111. Archer VE: Enhancement of lung cancer by cigarette smoking in uranium and other miners. Carcinog Compr Serv 8:23–37, 1985

112. Committee on the Biological Effects of Ionizing Radiations, National Research Council: Health Risks of Radon and Other Internally Deposited Alpha-Emitters. Washington, DC, National Academy of Sciences Press, 1988

113. American Cancer Society: Cancer Facts and Figures—1987. New York, ACS, 1987

114. Hammond EC, Selikoff IJ, Seidman H: Asbestos exposure, cigarette smoking and death rates. Ann NY Acad Sci 330:473–490, 1979

115. Bingham E, Niemeier RW, Reid JB: Multiple factors in carcinogenesis. In Saffiotti U, Wagoner JK (eds): Occupational Carcinogenesis. Ann NY Acad Sci 271:14–21, 1976

116. Doll R: Atmospheric pollution and lung cancer. Environ Health Perspect 22:23–31, 1978

117. Menck HR, Casagrande JT, Henderson BE: Industrial air pollution: Possible effect on lung cancer. Science 183:210–212, 1974

118. Stocks P: Cancer in North Wales and Liverpool Regions. British Empire Cancer Campaign Annual Report (Supplement). London, 1957

119. Vena JE: Air pollution as a risk factor in lung cancer. Am J Epidemiol 116:42–56, 1982

120. Armstrong BK, McMichael AJ, MacLennan R: Diet. In Schottenfeld D, Fraumeni JF Jr (eds): Cancer Epidemiology and Prevention. Philadelphia, WB Saunders, 1982

121. Peto R: Epidemiology, multistage models and short term mutagenicity tests. In Hiatt HH, Watson JD, Winstein JA (eds): Origins of Human Cancer, pp 1403–1428. Cold Spring Harbor, NY, Cold Spring Harbor Laboratory, 1977

122. Weinstein IB, Gattoni-Celli S, Kirschmeier P, Lambert M, Hsiao W, Backer J, Jeffrey A: Multistage carcinogenesis involves multiple gene and multiple mechanisms. In Cancer Cells 1: The Transformed Phenotype, pp 229–237. Cold Spring Harbor, NY, Cold Spring Harbor Laboratory, 1984

123. Yuspa SH, Harris CC: Molecular and cellular basis of chemical carcinogenesis. In Schottenfeld D, Fraumeni JF Jr (eds): Cancer Epidemiology and Prevention. Philadelphia, WB Saunders, 1982

124. Saracci R: The interactions of tobacco smoking and other agents in cancer etiology. Epidemiol Rev 9:175–193, 1987

125. Blot WJ, McLaughlin JK, Winn DM, Austin DF, Greenberg RS, Preston-Martin S, Bernstein L, Schoenberg JB, Stemhagen A, Fraumeni JF: Smoking and drinking in relation to oral and pharyngeal cancer. Cancer Res 48:3282–3287, 1988

126. Perera FP: Molecular cancer epidemiology: A new tool in cancer prevention. JNCI 78:887–898, 1987

127. Committee on Biological Markers, National Research Council: Biological Markers in Environmental Health Research. Environ Health Perspect 74:3–9, 1987

128. Harris CC: Future directions in the use of DNA adducts as internal dosimeters for monitoring human exposure to environmental mutagens and carcinogens. Environ Health Perspect 62:185–191, 1985

129. Schulte PA: Methodologic issues in the use of biologic markers in epidemiologic research. Am J Epidemiol 126:1006–1015, 1987

130. Perera F: The significance of DNA and protein adducts in human biomonitoring studies. Mutat Res 205:255–269, 1988

131. Vahakangas K, Autrup H, Harris CC: Interindividual variation in carcinogen metabolism, DNA damage and repair. In Berlin A et al (eds): IARC International Seminar on Methods of Monitoring Human Exposure to Carcinogenic and Mutagenic Agents, pp 85–98. IARC Scientific Publ No 59. Lyon, France, International Agency for Research on Cancer, 1984

132. Shamsuddin AKM, Sinopoli NT, Hemminki K, Boesch RR, Harris CC: Detection of benzo[a]pyrene-DNA adducts in human white blood cells. Cancer Res 45:66–68, 1985

133. Reed E, Yuspa S, Zelling LA, Ozols RF, Poirier MC: Quantitation of cis-diamminedichloro-platinum II (cis-platin)-DNA-intrastrand adducts in testicular and ovarian cancer patients receiving cisplatin chemotherapy. J Clin Invest 77:545–550, 1986

134. Perera FP, Santella RM, Brenner D, Poirier MC, Munshi AA, Fischman HK, Van Ryzin J: DNA adducts, protein adducts and sister chromatid exchange in cigarette smokers and nonsmokers. JNCI 79:449–456, 1987

135. Perera F: Biological markers in risk assessment. In Travis C (ed): Carcinogen Risk Assessment. New York, Plenum Press, 1988

136. California Department of Health Services: Guidelines for Chemical Carcinogen Risk Assessments and Their Scientific Rationale. Sacramento, CA, CDHS, November, 1985

137. US Environmental Protection Agency: Guidelines for carcinogen risk assessment. Federal Register 51:33992-34003, 1986

138. Anderson E: Quantitative approaches in use to assess cancer risk. Risk Anal 3:277–295, 1983

139. Setlow RB: Variations in DNA repair among humans. In Harris CC, Autrup H (eds): Human Carcinogenesis, pp 231–254. New York, Academic Press, 1983

140. Hertz-Picciotto I, Gravitz N, Neutra RR: How do cancer risks predicted from animal bioassays compare with the epidemiologic evidence? The case of ethylene dibromide. Risk Anal (in press)

141. Rowe JN, Springer JA: Asbestos lung cancer risks: Comparison of animal and human extrapolation. Risk Anal 6:171–180, 1986

142. Hertz-Picciotto I, Neutra RR, Collins JF: Ethylene oxide and leukemia. JAMA 257:2290, 1987

143. Enterline PE: A method for estimating lifetime cancer risks from limited epidemiologic data. Risk Anal 7:91–96, 1987

144. Epstein SS, Schwartz JB: Carcinogenic risk estimation. Science 240:1043–1047, 1988

145. Peto R, Pike MC, Bernstein L, Gold LS, Ames BN: The TD_{50}: A proposed general convention for the numerical description of the carcinogenic potency of chemicals in chronic-exposure animal experiments. Environ Health Perspect 58:1–8, 1984

146. Gold LS, Sawyer CB, Magaw R, Backman GM, de Veciana M, Levinson R, Hooper NK, Havender WR, Bernstein L, Peto R, Pike MC, Ames BN: A carcinogenic potency data base of the standardized results of animal bioassays. Environ Health Perspect 58:9–13, 1984

147. Gold LS, de Veciana M, Backman GM, Magaw R, Lopipero P, Smith M, Blumenthal M, Levinson R, Bernstein L, Ames BN: Chronological supplement to the carcinogenic potency data base: Standardized results of animal bioassays published through December 1982. Environ Health Perspect 67:161–200, 1986

148. Gold LS, Slone TH, Backman GM, Magaw R, DaCosta M, Lopipero P, Blumenthal M, Ames BN: Second chronological supplement to the carcinogenic potency data base: Standardized results of animal bioassays published through December 1984. Environ Health Perspect 74:237–329, 1987

149. Perera F, Boffetta P: Perspectives in comparing the risks of environmental carcinogens. JNCI 80:1282–1293

150. Ashford NA: Alternatives to cost-benefit analysis in regulatory decisions. Ann NY Acad Sci 129–137, 1980

151. Bogen K: Quantitative risk-benefit analysis in regulatory decision-making: A fundamental problem and an alternative proposal. Journal of Health Politics, Policy, Law 8:121–141, 1983

152. Conservation Foundation: Cost-Benefit Analysis: A Tricky Game. The Conservation Foundation, Washington, DC, Conservation Foundation, 1980

Walter C. Willett

Meir J. Stampfer

Graham A. Colditz

Does Alcohol Consumption Influence the Risk of Developing Breast Cancer? Two Views

15a

Introduction ■

In recent years, evidence from a number of epidemiologic studies has suggested that alcohol intake may increase the risk of breast cancer in women. In this chapter, we examine studies addressing this topic and discuss the possibility that observed associations are due to chance, bias, or confounding variables. Secondary issues critical to both individual decision making and public health policy are also considered. These include the association of breast cancer risk with specific beverage type, the details of the dose–response relationship, data regarding temporal aspects of exposure, including the effect of stopping alcohol use and modification of the association by other variables.

Case-Control Studies of Alcohol and Breast Cancer ■

Case-control studies of alcohol and breast cancer are summarized in Table 15a–1. Of 14 case-control studies, 11 were published as full papers; of these, a positive association was observed in 8. The first study addressing the relationship of alcoholic beverage to breast cancer, reported by Williams and Horm in

1977, was based on an exploratory analysis of cancer cases ascertained by the US Third National Cancer Survey.[1] Approximately 600 breast cancer patients were included in the analysis; control subjects were patients with other forms of cancer deemed to be unrelated to alcohol intake. Analyses were controlled for age, smoking, and race; data on other risk factors for breast cancer were not available. Alcohol intake was calculated as ounces per week multiplied by years of consumption (ounce-years), which makes interpretation and comparison with other studies difficult. Compared with nondrinkers, the relative risk for women consuming less than 51 ounce-years was 1.28, and for women consuming 51 or more ounce-years the relative risk was 1.55. For women consuming 51 or more ounce-years of specific beverages, the relative risks compared with nondrinkers were 1.08 for wine, 1.35 for beer, and 1.44 for liquor. However, these relationships with specific beverages were not controlled for the use of other alcoholic beverages, with which they tend to be highly correlated.

Rosenberg and associates used data from a large drug surveillance program conducted in the United States, Canada, and Israel to examine the relationship of alcohol intake with breast cancer risk.[2] They identified 1152 breast cancer patients and compared their

Table 15a–1
Case-Control Studies of Alcohol and Breast Cancer*

Study	Population	No. of Cases	Controls	Amounts	Relative Risk Total	Wine	Beer	Liquor	Comment
Williams and Horm (1977)[1]	US Third National Cancer Survey	≈650	Large number, patients with other cancers	<51 oz-year	1.28	1.67	1.18	1.43	Controlled for smoking, age, race
				≥51 oz-year	1.55	1.08	1.35	1.44	
Rosenberg et al (1982)[2]	US, Canada, Israel	1152	Endometrial or ovarian cancer, N = 519	<4 d/wk	1.5	1.8	2.0	1.2	Control for SES and reproductive factors had minimal effect on RR
				≥4 d/wk	2.0	2.3	2.2	2.1	
				Ex-drinker	1.3	—	—	—	
			Nonmalignant disorders, N = 2702	<4 d/wk	1.9	2.2	1.2	1.2	
				≥4 d/wk	2.5	1.9	2.1	2.5	
				Ex-drinker	1.6				
Byers et al (1982)[3]	Roswell Park, NY	1314	Nonneoplastic conditions, N = 770	0 (Never)	1.0				No relation with beer, wine, liquor
				0 (Ex)	0.59				
				<1 drink/mo	1.11				
				1–8 drink/mo	1.02				
				9–25 drink/mo	1.09				
				26+ drink/mo	1.13				
Paganini-Hill et al (1983)[4]	US retirement community	239 (prevalent cases)	Matched community controls, N = 239	Never drink	1.0				No effect for beer, wine, liquor
				≤1 drink/d	1.0				
				1+ drink/d	1.0				
Begg et al (1983)[5]	US Eastern Oncology Group	997	Other cancers, N = 730	0 drinks/wk	1.0				Adjusted for age and smoking
				1–7 drink/wk	0.9 (0.9, 1.1)†				
				7+ drink/wk	1.4 (0.9, 2.0)				
Webster et al (1983)[6]	US multicenter study, based on tumor registries	1226 <55 yr	Random-digit dialing, 85% participation = 1279	0 g/wk	1.0				Alcohol questions not clearly directed to period before diagnosis; no effect of beer or wine
				<50 g/wk	0.9 (0.7–1.2)				
				50–149 g/wk	0.9 (0.7–1.2)				
				150–199 g/wk	1.1 (0.7–1.7)				
				200–249 g/wk	1.1 (0.7–1.9)				
Le et al (1984, 1986)[7,8]	France, private clinics	Total = 1010; 500 with detailed data	Surgical clinic patients, 945/1950 with detailed data	Alcohol with meals (vs none)	1.48 ($p = 10^{-4}$)	1.48	2.18	1.21‡	Unknown participation rates
				0 g/wk	1.0				Significantly increased risks for beer and wine use; cider and liquor use uncommon; control for reproductive factors and dairy products did not affect risk
				1–79 g/wk	1.0 (0.7–1.4)				
				80–159 g/wk	1.4 (1.0–2.0)				
				160–239 g/wk	1.5 (1.0–2.0)				
				240+ g/wk	1.2 (0.7–2.0)				

Reference	Location	Cases	Controls/Cohort	Exposure	RR	CI[†]	Comments
Talamini et al (1984)[9]	Northern Italy	368	Acute conditions, N = 373	Ever vs never Wine: not used ≤0.5 l/d >0.5 l/d	2.5 1.0 2.4 16.7	(1.7–3.7) (1.6–3.5) (3.1–89.7)	High participation rates, controlled for SES and reproductive factors
LeVecchia et al (1985)[10]	Milan, Italy	437	Acute conditions, N = 437	0 drinks/d ≤3 drinks/d >3 drinks/d	1.0 1.25 2.10	 (0.91–1.75) (1.2–3.95)	High participation: any use of beer, RR = 1.32 (NS) or liquor RR = 1.44 (NS); adjusted for SES and reproductive factors and limited dietary variables; effect strongest among youngest
O'Connell et al (1987)[11]	North Carolina	276	Community residents, N = 1519	0, <1 drink/wk ≥1 drink/wk	1.0 1.45	 (0.97–2.12)	Adjusted for race, estrogen or oral contraceptive use, cigarette smoking; effect limited to premenopausal women (RR = 1.92); for postmenopausal group RR = 1.17; no specific beverage data
Harvey et al (1987)[12]	Participants in a US national cancer screening	Diagnosed 3+ yrs after entry, N = 1524	Program participants, N = 1896	Never 0.1–13 g/wk 14–91 g/wk 92–182 g/wk 183+ g/wk	1.0 1.12 1.06 1.31 1.66	 (0.9–1.3) (0.9–1.3) (1.0–1.7) (1.2–2.4)	Controlled for SES and reproductive factors; effect almost entirely attributable to alcohol before age 30; independent effects for beer and liquor
Katsouyanni et al (1986)[13]	Greece, hospitalized cases	120	Orthopedic patients, N = 120	Nonsignificant inverse trend. Alcohol intake levels not specified			Low statistical power; alcohol consumption not provided, probably low
Harris et al (1988)[14]	New York	1467	Hospitalized patients, N = 10,178	No alcohol <5 g/d 5–15 g/d 15+ g/d	1.0 1.0 0.9 0.9	 (0.8–1.2) (0.7–1.0) (0.8–1.1)	No data on most known risk factors
Rohan and McMichael (1988)[15]	Australia	451	Population controls, N = 451	No alcohol <3 g/d 3–9 g/d 9+ g/d	1.0 0.8 1.2 1.6	 (0.5–1.3) (0.7–1.9) (1.0–2.5)	Adjustment for known risk factors did not alter findings

* RR = relative risk, NS = not significant; oz-year = (ounce/week) × (years); SES = socioeconomic status.

† 95% Confidence intervals.

‡ Relative risk for cider consumption.

alcohol use with that of two control series: 519 women with endometrial or ovarian cancer and 2702 women hospitalized for nonmalignant diseases. The measure of alcohol intake was crude; drinkers of each specific beverage were asked whether they consumed that beverage on fewer than 4 or on 4 or more days per week. Using the cancer series as a control group, women who drank on fewer than 4 days/week experienced a relative risk of 1.5 compared with nondrinkers; the corresponding relative risk for those drinking ≥4 days/week was 2.0. With the nonmalignant series as the control group, the relative risk was 1.9 for <4 days/week and 2.5 for ≥4 days/week. Control for socioeconomic and reproductive variables in multiple logistic regression analysis did not appreciably alter the relationship of alcohol use with breast cancer. When examined by specific beverage type, similar relative risks were observed for beer, wine, and liquor, although these analyses were not controlled for correlated use.

Byers and co-workers, responding in a letter to the report of Rosenberg and associates, provided data from a large case-control study conducted at Roswell Park Memorial Hospital in the United States.[3] The drinking habits of 1314 breast cancer patients were compared with those of 770 patients with nonneoplastic conditions from the same institution. These investigators found no relationship of breast cancer risk with alcohol use at any level, nor with consumption of beer, wine, or liquor, specifically. However, the authors noted their subjects were raised in a rural area during the Prohibition era, which may have resulted in a low overall level of alcohol consumption.

Paganini-Hill and colleagues, also in a letter responding to the report of Rosenberg and associates, examined the relationship of alcohol intake and breast cancer in a US retirement community.[4] These authors identified 239 prevalent cases and compared their current alcohol intake with that of 239 matched community controls of similar social class. No elevation in risk was found for those consuming ≥1 drinks/day. Among a subsample of 25 cases, women denied reducing alcohol intake after the diagnosis of cancer.

In another letter following the report of Rosenberg, Begg and associates compared the alcohol use among 997 breast cancer cases from the US Eastern Oncology Group with that among 730 patients with other malignancies not thought to be related to alcohol use.[5] After adjustment for age and smoking, the relative risks were 0.9 for the use of 1–7 drinks/week, and 1.4 (95% confidence interval [CI], 0.9–2.0) for >7 drinks/week.

Webster and co-workers examined the relation of alcohol use with breast cancer in a large, multicentered US case-control study primarily designed to address the effect of steroid hormone use on risk of this disease.[6] Cases consisted of 1226 women younger than 55 years who were compared with 1279 controls identified by random-digit telephone dialing. No relation of alcohol use with breast cancer risk was observed; even for the use of more than 300 g/week, the relative risk was 1.1. The participation rates, although less than desirable, were good for contemporary US studies: 82% for cases and 85% for those identified as potential controls. However, the number of controls not contacted at all is never known when the random-digit dialing procedure is used.

In a study from France, Le and associates reported on the association of alcohol use with breast cancer risk among patients attending a group of private surgical clinics.[7,8] A simple measure of alcohol intake (i.e., whether or not it was usually consumed with meals) was available for the entire group of 1010 cases and 1950 clinic controls. After a positive relationship with breast cancer risk was observed during the study, additional detailed questions on alcohol use were posed to the remaining 500 cases and 945 controls. Among the total group, a highly significant ($p = 0.0004$) relative risk of 1.48 was found. Among the women for whom detailed data were available, the relative risks were 1.0 for 1–79 g/week, 1.4 for 80–159 g/week, 1.5 for 160–239 g/week, and 1.2 for 240 or more g/week. Statistical control for the effects of reproductive factors and a limited set of dietary questions (mainly regarding dairy products) did not appreciably alter the relative risks. In this population, the preponderance of alcohol intake was in the form of wine. In addition to wine, a significant elevation in risk was associated with beer consumption; no significant association was found for alcohol in the form of cider, but the use of this beverage was relatively low.

Talamini and associates conducted a case-control study in a Northern Italian population that included information on the use of wine, the primary form of alcohol in that area.[9] They identified 368 cases; controls consisted of 373 women hospitalized with acute conditions. Participation rates were remarkably high for both cases and controls. Multivariate analyses were used to control for the effects of socioeconomic and reproductive variables; these analyses did not appreciably alter the crude relationships. Compared with nondrinkers, the relative risk for the use of less than 0.5 liters of wine per day was 2.4 (95% CI, 1.6–3.5); for the use of 0.5 or more liters/day, the relative risk was 16.7 (95% CI, 3.1–89.7).

In another study from northern Italy, LaVecchia and colleagues obtained information on the number of drinks per day of specific alcoholic beverages from 437 patients with breast cancer and 437 patients hospitalized with acute conditions.[10] Analyses were conducted adjusting for socioeconomic and reproductive variables; these adjustments did not materially alter results of observations that accounted for age alone. For women consuming ≤3 drinks/day, the relative risk was 1.25, and for those drinking >3 drinks/day the relative risk was 2.10 (95% CI, 1.12–3.95). For >3 drinks/day of wine, the relative risk was 2.24.

In a study from North Carolina, O'Connell and colleagues examined alcohol intake among 276 cases and 1519 community controls.[11] Analyses were adjusted for race, estrogen and oral contraceptive use, and cigarette smoking. For women consuming ≥1 drink of any alcoholic beverage per week compared with those consuming no alcohol or <1 drink/week, the relative risk was 1.45 (95% CI, 0.99–2.12). No specific beverage data were available. In this study, the effect of alcohol was limited to premenopausal women, among whom the relative risk was 1.92 as compared with 1.17 among postmenopausal women.

Harvey and associates conducted a nested case-control study within a cohort of women participating in a national US cancer screening program.[12] Cancer cases (1524) were identified who were diagnosed at least 3 years after entry in the screening program. Control subjects (1896) were identified from participants who did not develop cancer. In contrast with other case-control studies, this design provided a clearly identified base population from which to sample controls. Compared with women who never consumed alcohol, relative risks were 1.12 for 0.1–13 g/week, 1.06 for 14–91 g/week, 1.31 for 92–182 g/week, and 1.66 for ≥183 g/week. Control for socioeconomic and reproductive factors did not appreciably affect these relative risks. Independent associations were observed for beer (relative risk = 1.71 for ≥92 g/week) and liquor (relative risk = 2.05 for the same level of alcohol intake), but no independent effect for wine was observed (relative risk = 0.77 for ≥92 g/week); however, because the use of wine alone was limited to only a few women, the confidence limits around the point estimate of 0.77 must have been wide. The influence of alcohol use at different ages was also examined; the positive association with breast cancer was entirely attributable to alcohol use before the age of 30. For women who consumed 92 g/day of alcohol before age 30, the risk of breast cancer was elevated whether or not they drank at later ages. However, the number of women who drank before age 30 and later stopped was small (15 cases); consequently, the comparison between those who continued and those who stopped is statistically unstable. For alcohol consumption at age 30, the association with risk of breast cancer did not vary by age at diagnosis, suggesting that a latent period effect was not present.

In a small Greek case-control study, Katsouyanni and associates observed a nonsignificant inverse relationship between alcohol intake and risk of breast cancer.[13] Alcohol intake was not a focus of this study and few details are provided; levels of alcohol intake were not described but are likely to have been low.

Harris and co-workers used data from a multipurpose study in which information was collected from unselected hospitalized patients in New York to compare the reported alcohol consumption of 1467 women with breast cancer with that of 10,178 women having other diagnoses, presumably unrelated to smoking or alcohol intake.[14] Overall, no association was observed, although a marginally significant positive relationship was seen among the leanest women. The diagnoses of the control subjects are only broadly defined and the appropriateness of the comparison series is difficult to evaluate. In addition, information on other risk factors for breast cancer was not obtained, precluding an evaluation of potentially confounding effects.

In a case-control study from southern Australia, Rohan and McMichael compared reports of previous alcohol consumption by 451 women with breast cancer with intake reported by 451 matched population controls.[15] A statistically significant positive dose–response relationship was observed; for women consuming >9 g/day of alcohol, the relative risk was 1.6 (95% CI, 1.0–2.5) compared with nondrinkers.

Cohort Studies of Alcohol and Breast Cancer ■

Five general-population cohort studies that examine the association of alcohol intake and breast cancer have been published (Table 15a–2). A positive association has been observed in all five.

The largest cohort study of alcohol and breast cancer was published in a non-peer-reviewed journal by Seidman and associates, based on data from the American Cancer Society study.[16] These data represented 365,812 women aged 30 to 84 years without previous diagnosis of cancer who were followed for 6 years, during which time 3130 cases of breast cancer were diagnosed. Data were very incompletely analyzed; information can only be interpolated from a figure and is interpretable only among women with no other risk factors for breast cancer. Alcohol intake was dichotomized as less than daily versus daily drinking. Among women drinking daily, the relative risk was approximately 1.2 for both those aged 30 to 54 years and those aged 55 to 84 years.

Hiatt and Bawol followed approximately 95,000 female members of a US health care plan who were

Table 15a-2
Prospective Studies of Alcohol and Breast Cancer*

Study	Population	Cases		Relative Risks			Comment
				Ages 30–54	*Ages 55–84*		
Seidman et al (1982)[16**]	American Cancer Society; 365,812 ages 30–84 yr; followed 6 yr	3130	<Daily alcohol	1.0	1.0		Incompletely analyzed
			Daily alcohol	1.2	1.2		
Hiatt and Bawol (1984)[17]	~95,000 US health plan members; up to 13 yr of follow-up; ages > 15 yr	1169	0 drinks/d	1.0			Could not divide group with <3 drinks/d; no data on specific beverages; controlled for race, education, smoking, BMI, reproductive factors
			<3 drinks/d	0.98			
			≥3 drinks/d	1.40†			
Hiatt et al (1987, 1988)[18,19]	US health plan members, N = 69,000, follow-up = 5 yr	303	Nondrinkers	1.0			Controlled for age, race, BMI, smoking; effect not limited to any specific beverage; RR strongest among white or Hispanic and postmenopausal women
			Past drinkers	2.2 (1.2–3.9)†			
			1–2 drinks/d	1.5 (1.0–2.3)			
			3–5 drinks/d	1.5 (0.8–2.8)			
			6+ drinks/d	3.3 (1.2–9.3)			
Schatzkin et al (1987)[20]	US, First National Health and Nutrition Examination Survey 7188 women aged 25 to 74 yr, median follow-up = 10 yr	121	No drinks in last year	1.0			Adjusted for education, BMI, dietary fat, and reproductive factors; no data on specific beverage use; highest RR among youngest and thinnest women
			>0–1.2 g/d	1.4 (0.8–2.5)			
			1.3–4.9 g/d	1.6 (0.9–3.1)			
			≥5 g/d	2.0 (1.1–3.7)			
Willett et al (1987)[21]	US, 89,538 registered nurses aged 34 to 59 yr; follow-up = 4 yr	601	0 g/d	1.1			Significantly increased RR independently for 5+ g/d of beer (1.4; 1.1–1.8) and liquor (1.4; 1.2–1.7), but not wine (1.1; 0.9–1.4); RR strongest among younger and thinner women and those without other risk factors for breast cancer (2.5; 1.5–4.2)
			<1.5 g/d	1.0 (0.8–1.3)			
			1.5–4.9 g/d	0.9 (0.7–1.2)			
			5.0–14.9 g/d	1.3 (1.0–1.6)			
			≥15 g/d	1.6 (1.3–2.0)			

* RR = relative risk; BMI = body mass index; **rates for Seidman et al study are interpolated from figure, among women with no other risk factors.

† $p = 0.03$.

‡ Confidence intervals.

older than 15 years at enrollment.[17] In up to 13 years of follow-up, 1169 cases of breast cancer occurred. After controlling for race, education, smoking, body mass index, and reproductive factors (all of which made only small differences), relative risks were 0.98 for <3 drinks/day and 1.40 for ≥3 drinks/day ($p = 0.03$). The wording of the alcohol use questions did not allow the authors to subdivide the group consuming <3 drinks/day or to examine the effects of specific beverages.

Hiatt and co-workers have presented data based on a separate cohort of 69,000 women who belonged to the same health care plan.[18,19] During 5 years of follow-up, 303 cases of breast cancer occurred among these women. After controlling for age, race, body mass index, and cigarette smoking, the relative risks were 1.5 for those consuming 1–2 drinks/day, 1.5 for 3–5 drinks/day, and 3.3 for ≥6 drinks/day. Relative risks were highest among white or Hispanic women and among those who were postmenopausal.

Schatzkin and associates analyzed data on alcohol intake and breast cancer from the US First National Health and Nutrition Examination Survey.[20] At enrollment, 7188 women 25 to 74 years of age were available for analysis. During follow-up (median = 10 years), 121 cases of breast cancer were diagnosed. After controlling for the effects of education, body mass index, dietary fat (based on a single 24-hour recall), and reproductive factors, the adjusted relative risks were similar to or slightly higher than the crude relationships. Compared with women reporting no alcohol use during the previous year, the relative risks were 1.4 (95% CI, 0.8–2.5) for 0.1–1.2 g/day, 1.6 (95% CI, 0.9–3.1) for 1.3–4.9 g/day, and 2.0 (95% CI, 1.1–3.7) for ≥5 g/day. No data were available for the use of specific beverages. The authors speculated that the elevated risk seen even in the lowest consumption group might be due to underreporting of alcohol intake by some women. Highest relative risks were seen among the youngest and thinnest women.

Willett and co-workers examined the risk of breast cancer in relation to alcohol intake among the US-based Nurses' Health Study cohort.[21] Among 89,538 women aged 34 to 59 years who were followed for 4 years, 601 incident cases of breast cancer were ascertained. Compared with women reporting no alcohol intake during the year before the baseline questionnaire, the relative risks were 1.0 (95% CI, 0.8–1.3) for <1.5 g/day of alcohol, 0.9 (95% CI, 0.7–1.2) for 1.5–4.9 g/day, and 1.3 (95% CI, 1.0–1.6) for 5.0–14.9 g/day. Fairly comprehensive data on other dietary factors were collected. Controlling for these nutritional factors, family history of breast cancer, and reproductive variables had no influence on the association

of alcohol with risk of breast cancer. When the use of ≥5 g/day of specific alcoholic beverages was examined, controlling for the use of other specific alcoholic beverages simultaneously in a multivariate model, significant associations were found for beer (relative risk = 1.4; 95% CI, 1.1–1.8) and liquor (relative risk = 1.4; 95% CI, 1.2–1.7), but not for wine (relative risk = 1.1; 95% CI, 0.9–1.4). The confidence interval for wine includes the estimates for the other beverages, indicating that a similar association with wine is not excluded. The association with breast cancer risk was strongest among the women who were younger and thinner. A particularly strong association was observed among those who had no other risk factors for breast cancer (relative risk = 2.5; 95% CI, 1.5–4.2). Information on remote alcohol intake was not collected; however, no elevation in risk of breast cancer was seen among women who were currently nondrinkers but reported that their alcohol intake had greatly decreased during the previous 10 years.

The association of alcohol intake with breast cancer mortality was examined among the 2641 women participating in the Framingham Heart Study.[22] Only 28 fatal cases were ascertained. A small and statistically nonsignificant negative logistic regression coefficient was noted for alcohol intake in one table. Because of the small number of cases and incomplete analysis, this report will not be considered further.

Cohort Studies of Breast Cancer in Alcoholics ■

Because of their extreme level of exposure, the breast cancer experience of alcoholic women is of some interest. Several such studies have been reported and will be noted here (Table 15a–3). These are based on the follow-up of women who were institutionalized for treatment of their alcoholism. Typically, little is known about potentially confounding variables for these individuals: only mortality rather than incidence data are available, and the number of breast cancer cases is very small.

Schmidt and de Lint followed 1119 Canadian women treated for alcoholism for a period of up to 14 years.[23] Two cases of breast cancer were observed; this was said to be not significantly different from an unstated number of expected cases.

Nicholls and associates identified 275 British women discharged from a hospital with a diagnosis of abnormal drinking and followed them for a period of 10 to 15 years.[24] Three cases of breast cancer were

Table 15a–3
Cohort Studies of Breast Cancer in Alcoholic Women*

Study	Population	Cases†	Association	Comments
Schmidt and deLint (1972)[23]	1119 Canadian women treated for alcoholism followed 1–14 yr	2	Not significant	Minimal information, no control of confounding variables
Nicholls et al (1974)[24]	275 UK women discharged with diagnosis of abnormal drinking, followed 10–15 yr	3	Elevated risk, p = 0.05	Minimal information, no control of confounding variables
Monson and Lyons (1975)[25]	243 chronic US alcoholic women	3	PCMR = 0.7	Low follow-up rate; PCMR probably needs to be multiplied by 2 or 3 to estimate excess rate in alcoholics; no control of potential confounding factors
Adelstein and White (1976)[26]	475 UK hospitalized alcoholic women followed 10–15 yr	10	Two-fold elevation	No control of confounding variables

* PCMR = proportional cancer mortality rate.

† In the Adelstein and White study, the expected number of cases was 4.5; number of expected cases is not known for the other studies.

observed; this was said to be a statistically significant excess above the expected number.

Monson and Lyons identified 243 US women who were hospitalized for chronic alcoholism between 1930 and 1940 and attempted to trace them for up to 40 years.[25] Since follow-up proved difficult and was incomplete, the proportion of breast cancers in total cancer mortality was compared with the general US population to estimate the association of alcoholism with risk of breast cancer. This proportional rate, which was 0.7 (based on only 3 observed cases), should be multiplied by a factor of 2 or 3 to estimate the relationship with rates in the general population because the overall risk of cancer in alcoholics is elevated by a factor of 2 or 3.

Adelstein and White identified 475 alcoholic women hospitalized in the United Kingdom and ascertained deaths for a period up to 21 years.[26] Ten deaths due to breast cancer occurred, compared with an expected number of 4.5, yielding a relative risk of approximately 2.0. No control for confounding effects was possible.

Summary of Published Studies of Alcohol and Breast Cancer ■

Can the Association Be Explained by Chance? ■

The first consideration in reviewing the studies described above is whether an overall association with alcohol intake exists beyond that expected by chance.

A positive association between alcohol intake and breast cancer incidence was seen in 9 of 14 case-control and all of 5 large prospective studies in general populations. Thus, it is clear, even discounting the Williams and Horm study (which can be considered hypothesis-generating) and possible publication biases, that an association exists between alcohol intake and breast cancer incidence that is extremely unlikely to be the result of chance. Longnecker and co-workers have conducted a formal meta-analysis of these studies and found statistically significant dose–response relationships among both case-control studies and cohort studies.[27] Weighting by study quality and the inclusion of several unpublished studies did not alter these findings. Given the substantial possibility for biases to obscure a weak or modest association in the context of a case-control study, the overall consistency, even in the case-control studies, is remarkable. Nevertheless, it may prove instructive to examine the inconsistent case-control studies to consider whether the failure to observe an association is the result of a biologic factor (such as the age structure of the study population or the type of alcoholic beverage used in that group) or a methodologic difference.

Does Bias Explain Differences in the Findings of Case-Control Studies? ■

In case-control studies, the true relation between alcohol intake and breast cancer could be distorted by selective exclusion or inclusion of study subjects with respect to their alcohol intake. It has been suggested that hospital patient controls may consume less alcohol than members of the community at large, perhaps because of a reduction of intake secondary to their illness.[28] Although the majority of positive case-control studies did use hospital or clinic patient controls, three recent studies did not.[11,12,15] Thus, it seems unlikely that the positive associations in the earlier studies are due to the use of ill subjects as controls. Conversely, the lower participation rates in the positive studies using community-based controls raise concern that women with higher alcohol intake selectively refused to participate. It remains a concern that the control group in the null study reported by Webster and associates[6] selectively included women in both groups with higher than typical alcohol intake.

Differential errors in recall of alcohol intake between cases and controls could also distort the relation with breast cancer risk. Since alcohol consumption is a very value-laden behavior in many cultures, it would not be surprising if the occurrence of a grave illness colored recall. Since even a slight difference in recall could obscure the moderate associations observed in the positive studies, the degree of consistency among studies is remarkable. In several studies of dietary recall, it has been noted that current dietary intake has a major influence on the reporting of remote diet. It is thus likely that the use of prevalent cases of breast cancer[4,5,12] will be less reliable than newly diagnosed cases, even if alcohol intake does not influence prognosis. However, the studies that included prevalent cases are not themselves consistent in their findings.

Selection and recall bias are not issues in prospective cohort studies, which makes them much more likely to be valid. Bias could occur in a cohort study if the detection of breast cancer were related to alcohol intake. However, the follow-up rates in the prospective studies were sufficiently high to ensure that the observed associations were not simply due to differential tracing of subjects. Differential detection of breast cancer among alcohol users is unlikely to explain the positive associations because, even with the use of mammography or physician examination, the lead time for this disease gained by early diagnosis is only 1 or 2 years. In the study of Willett and co-workers, the percentage of cases with positive nodes was similar among the users and nonusers of alcohol.[21] Similarly, the percentage of women with tumors smaller than 2 cm among nondrinkers (59%) was similar to that (65%) among those drinking >15 g/day of alcohol (unpublished data). It thus seems clear that the findings of the prospective studies cannot be explained on the basis of methodologic bias.

Can the Association Be Explained by Confounding Variables? ■

It will probably never be feasible to exclude, with complete certainty, the possibility that the association between alcoholic beverage intake and breast cancer is due to confounding by another determinant of breast cancer. The classic breast cancer risk factors (including age at first birth, menopausal status, age at menarche, parity, and family history of breast cancer), as well as other factors that are not established determinants of breast cancer (including relative weight and cigarette smoking) were controlled in the prospective studies of Hiatt and co-workers,[13,18] Schatzkin and co-workers,[20] and Willett and co-workers,[21] and most of the case-control studies. Adjusting for these factors did not perceptibly alter the association of alcohol intake with breast cancer. Because the earlier studies did not include an assessment of dietary intake, concern exists that the positive associations found might be secondary to an association of alcohol intake with a dietary factor that causes breast cancer. Two conditions must exist for this to occur: alcohol must be associated with the dietary factor, and the dietary factor must be associated with breast cancer. With additional evidence it now seems that neither of these associations exist with sufficient strength to account for the effect of alcohol. In the study reported by Willett and associates, moderate alcohol intake was minimally associated with dietary fat, protein, fiber, vitamin A and a variety of other nutrients.[21] Moreover, within this cohort, dietary fat intake was not associated with breast cancer risk;[29] this lack of association is consistent with most epidemiologic evidence based on studies of individuals. Thus, in those studies in which data were collected on a few specific foods,[7-10] or a more comprehensive assessment of diet was done,[20,21] adjustment for diet did not reduce the association of alcohol intake with breast cancer whatsoever. Because dietary intake will always be measured imperfectly in epidemiologic studies, it is not possible to completely control for confounding by this variable. If adjustment for dietary factors had partially explained the association with alcohol, one would be concerned that a more perfect measure of diet would fully explain the association. Thus, the lack of any appreciable effect of adjusting for dietary factors is notable. It could be postulated that the relevant confounding dietary factor has not been identified or examined. Although this is quite possible, it is unlikely that such a factor would be strongly associated with alcoholic beverage use because the dietary factors already examined were only minimally associated with moderate alcohol intake, and dietary factors tend to be intercorrelated.

Another set of potentially confounding variables includes factors related to income, education, and psychosocial status. It is less tenable to consider these as true potential confounding variables because they are not likely to be, or have not been shown to be, direct causes of breast cancer. Nevertheless, the case for causality would be strengthened if the association with alcohol intake could be shown to be independent of these factors. Therefore, the fact that positive findings have been reported from multiple countries with different social contexts of alcohol use reduces the likelihood that the association with alcohol intake is secondary to socioeconomic factors. In a number of studies, socioeconomic factors (usually income and education) were controlled in the design or analysis.[2,9,10,12,17,20] In the study by Willett and associates, socioeconomic status was largely controlled by restriction of the study group to a single occupational group, registered nurses.[21]

Because the established risk factors for breast cancer are generally associated with modest relative risks of a magnitude similar to the effect of alcohol (*i.e.,* relative risks of 1.5 or 2.0), an unmeasured confounding variable would need to be stronger than known risk factors and strongly associated with alcohol intake to explain the effect of alcohol seen in the majority of studies. This remains possible but seems unlikely. The potential for an unmeasured confounding variable to explain an association is generally reduced with increasing magnitude of the observed relative risk; thus, it may be helpful to examine subgroups where the relative risk would be expected to be large. Such subgroups include women with high alcohol intake and those with low baseline risk. Thus, the findings of a relative risk of 3.3 among women consuming ≥6 drinks/day in the study of Hiatt and colleagues[17] and the relative risk of 2.5 among low-baseline-risk women in the study of Willett and associates[21] enhance the likelihood that the more modest increases in risk observed overall are not due to confounding variables.

What Are the Effects of Potential Errors in Measuring Alcohol Intake? ∎

Errors in the measurement of alcohol intake, if unbiased with respect to disease status, would generally reduce the strength of associations with breast cancer. The published studies reviewed above have each used different questions to assess alcohol intake. Some have been extremely crude—asking about alcohol intake only as a dichotomy—whereas others have asked separate questions regarding the use of each alcoholic beverage and have allowed for a continuum of frequency responses. In only one study was the validity of the alcohol measurement evaluated.[21] In that study, alcohol intake, assessed by a standardized questionnaire, was compared with intake measured by a detailed day-by-day recording of all foods and beverages among a subgroup of 173 participants. The mean intake assessed by the two methods was virtually identical; the correlation between methods was 0.86 for the questionnaire completed before the detailed recording and 0.90 for the questionnaire completed after the recording. Further, highly significant correlations ($r = 0.33$–0.44) were observed between the questionnaire measure of alcohol intake and plasma high-density lipoprotein levels (known to be sensitive to alcohol ingestion), thus providing qualitative physiologic evidence of the alcohol intake measured by questionnaire.

With a correlation as high as 0.9 between questionnaire measurement of alcohol intake and an independent assessment, it is unlikely that the relative risks for current intake observed by Willett and associates[21] were attenuated by measurement error to any substantial degree. However, if current alcohol intake only acts as a surrogate measure for alcohol intake at a more biologically relevant time (*e.g.,* before age 30, as suggested by the data of Harvey and colleagues[12]), the impact of alcohol may have been substantially underestimated. Even if it is the cumulative effect of alcohol over the 10- or 15-year period preceding diagnosis that is biologically relevant, individual changes in consumption during that period will cause some misclassification, resulting in some unknown attenuation of associations. Although current alcohol intake may be measurable with a high degree of accuracy and precision, it will be necessary to conduct studies that assess consumption at different points in life, and to investigate the validity of these measurements over longer periods, to improve our quantitative interpretation of observed relative risks.

Is There an Association with Specific Types of Alcoholic Beverages? ∎

Whether breast cancer risk is related to specific types of alcoholic beverages is of considerable interest because this would address the possibility that some chemical other that ethanol is responsible for an observed association with overall alcohol intake. Data on intake of specific alcoholic beverages were collected in only seven of the published studies. Wine,[2,7,9,10] beer,[2,7,12,21] and liquor[2,12,15,21] were each significantly associated with breast cancer in four studies.

The examination of specific beverage effects is complicated by the tendency of women who drink one alcoholic beverage to also consume other types of alcohol. The effects of specific beverages are thus best studied with multivariate analyses that control the use of each beverage for the use of the others. This form of analysis was used only in the studies of Harvey and associates,[12] Willett and associates,[21] and Rohan and McMichael:[15] the first two studies found independent effects of beer and liquor but not of wine, whereas the third found an independent effect for liquor. The number of wine drinkers who did not regularly consume other beverages was small; consequently, a similar positive association of wine could not be excluded with reasonable confidence. This issue again illustrates the usefulness of studies in multiple cultures where the patterns of alcoholic beverage consumption are distinct (*e.g.,* in France and Italy, where wine is the dominant beverage).

Given the data noted above, it is clear that the association of alcohol intake and breast cancer cannot be attributed to a single beverage. Although further data on this issue would be very useful, evidence exists from multiple studies that beer, wine, and liquor all contribute to increased risk. This increases the likelihood that alcohol *per se* is the responsible factor. However, the lower risk associated with wine in several studies should not be dismissed entirely; Herbert and associates have suggested that this may be due to a protective effect of sulfites added during the preparation of wine.[30]

What Are the Dose–Response Relationships? ■

Appropriate individual and public responses to evidence of an overall association of alcohol intake and breast cancer risk depend on knowledge of the dose–response relationship. However, information on this relationship is generally rather crude and inconsistent. In the earlier studies, only simple questions were posed, and this did not allow a quantitative estimate of alcohol intake. The studies with more quantitative data have all used different units and categories to describe the relationship of alcohol intake to breast cancer risk. For purposes of summarizing the data, we assumed three rough categories of alcohol use among those who reported any use: <1 drink/day, 1–2 drinks/day, and ≥3 drinks/day. For this purpose, it will be assumed that one drink contains approximately 12 g of alcohol.

Of the studies that found any association with alcohol intake, 11 provided data on the use of <1 drink/day. Of these, four observed an elevated risk.[2,15,20,21] In the study of Willett and associates, no increase was found below 0.5 drink/day,[21] whereas in the report of Schatzkin and co-workers, an elevated risk was seen even below that level.[20] Of the same 11 studies, 10 found an elevated risk at the level of about 1 or 2 drinks/day.[2,3,7,9,11,12,15,19,20,21] (In some instances, this was not strictly clear since the highest category was "one or more drinks per day.") The magnitude of relative risk for this level of intake has ranged from 1.3 to 2.4. In 2 of the 11 positive studies with relevant data, an increased risk was only found with ≥3 drinks/day.[10,12] Relative risks have varied considerably for ≥3 drinks/day in the 5 positive studies that have examined this group separately.[7,9,10,17,19] The extremely high relative risk (16.7) found in the study of Talamini and associates is an outlier value based on only a small number of controls.[9] If this value is excluded, the relative risks range from 1.2 to 3.3 for ≥6 drinks/day.

It could be argued that quantitative estimates are best obtained from the prospective studies with substantial numbers of breast cancer cases because there is less potential for methodologic bias. If this is done, the relative risk estimates are more—although not completely—consistent. For very light drinking (<5 g/day, *i.e.,* about half a drink), a positive association was seen only in the study of Schatzkin and associates.[20] In the study by Willett and co-workers, a significantly elevated risk (1.3) was found in the range of 5–14.9 g/day.[21] The other studies did not examine this group separately because they were included with all women drinking <3 drinks/day in the study of Hiatt and Bawol (among whom the relative risk was 1.0),[17] with all women drinking >5 g/day in the study of Schatzkin and associates (relative risk, 2.0),[20] and with women who drank 1 or 2 drinks/day in the study of Hiatt and associates (relative risk, 1.5).[19] For women drinking more than 15 g/day (>1 drink), the relative risk estimates fall within a fairly narrow range: 1.4 for ≥3 drinks/day in the study of Hiatt and Bawol,[17] 1.5 for 3–5 drinks/day and 3.3 for ≥6 drinks/day in the study of Hiatt et al.,[19] and 1.6 for ≥15 g/day in the study of Willett and co-workers.[21] The effect of heavier alcohol intake is more difficult to define. Few studies had sufficient participants with very heavy alcohol intake; the study of Hiatt suggests that some additional increase in risk may be observed among these women.[19] Although the studies of alcoholic women tend to support the hypothesis that alcohol increases risk of breast cancer, they also suggest that the increase in risk is not extreme with heavy intake.

Taken together, these data quite consistently indicate that there is a 50% to 100% increase in risk for consuming 1 or 2 drinks/day and suggest that a smaller increment in risk may exist for the use of <1 drink/day.

In the meta-analysis reported by Longnecker and associates, the relative risk based on the analysis of case-control studies was estimated to 1.4 (95% CI, 1.0–1.8) for 24 g/day of alcohol.[27] The data based on cohort studies were most compatible with a nonlinear relationship, with the risk gradient being the steepest at higher intake. For these cohort studies, the summary relative risk for women drinking 12 g/day of alcohol was 1.4 (95% CI, 1.1–1.7) and for 24 g/day was 1.7 (95% CI, 1.4–2.2).

Attributable Risk ■

The population attributable risk percentage—the proportion of cases of breast cancer in the study population that would be prevented if no woman consumed alcohol—provides information on the overall impact of this behavior, assuming that the relationship represents cause and effect. Using data (see Table 15a–2) from the study of Willett and associates, this attributable risk can be calculated as being 14%.[21] However, because of the relatively young age of women in this study, it is difficult to generalize this percentage to all women. This estimate, however, is very close to that of 13% obtained by Longnecker and co-workers using all available studies on this relationship.[27]

Temporal Aspects of Exposure ■

In addition to the overall relationship between alcoholic beverage intake and risk of breast cancer, the temporal aspects of exposure and risk are of major practical importance. These include whether the breast is particularly sensitive to alcohol intake at any specific age, whether a latent period exists between exposure and onset of breast cancer, and whether (and how soon) reducing alcohol intake reduces the risk of breast cancer.

Few investigators have collected data that even begin to address these issues. The only reported study that assessed alcohol intake at different ages was that by Harvey and colleagues.[12] In their investigation, alcohol intake before the age of 30 years accounted for the entire positive association. Although the number of women who drank before age 30 and later stopped was small, their elevation in risk was similar to that for women who continued to drink. This relationship with drinking at younger ages is consistent with other data indicating that the breast is particularly susceptible to cancer risk factors during early adult life. In this same study, the relative risk did not appear to vary according to age at diagnosis among women who drank before age 30; thus, an effect of latency was not observed.

In several studies, information has been obtained on the risk associated with past alcohol intake. However, it is generally not known for how long alcohol use had ceased or what the prior level of intake was. Hiatt and associates found an increased risk among past drinkers compared with women who never drank (relative risk = 2.2; 95% CI, 1.3–3.9),[19] as did Rosenberg and colleagues (relative risks of 1.3 compared with the cancer control group and 1.6 compared with the no-malignancy control group).[2] Willett and associates did not find evidence of an increased risk among the small number of women who currently drank no alcohol but who reported that their alcohol intake had greatly decreased during the previous 10 years; however, nothing is known about their drinking more than 10 years before.[21] It is clear that additional data on these important issues are needed.

Modification of the Association by Other Variables ■

The possibility that the effect of alcohol intake may vary among subgroups of women with different levels of underlying risk for breast cancer has potential practical importance. Whereas effect modification (interaction) can be examined either in the scale of attributable risk (rate difference) or relative risk (rate ratio), only the latter has been used in published studies. Most reports have not included data on effect modification, and those that have vary in the subgroups analyzed. In general, such analyses require substantially more data to identify significant variation in effects among subgroups than to examine the effect of alcohol in the total group.

The potential effect modifiers that have been examined most frequently are age and menopausal status; because of their high correlation, these variables can be considered synonymous for this purpose. Of the seven studies that examined this interaction, five observed a higher relative risk among younger or premenopausal women,[10,11,15,20,21] one reported no evidence for an interaction,[12] and one found a higher relative risk among postmenopausal women.[18] Although this is insufficient information from which to derive conclusions, it is tempting to speculate that a higher relative risk among younger women might be related to the finding of Harvey and associates that the effect of alcohol was entirely attributable to use before age 30.[12] If this is indeed the relevant exposure, the use of current or recent alcohol intake as a measure of exposure would lead to increasing misclassification with advancing age, and a reduction in relative risk. A different relative risk at various ages could conceivably explain discrepant findings between studies. However, it does not explain the major inconsistent study because the participants in that case-control study were all younger than 55 years.[6]

The only other interaction suggested in more than one study is the observation of a higher relative risk among thin women.[14,20,21] It is possible that this simply represents a higher dose per kilogram of body mass; however, expressing alcohol intake in this way did not appreciably alter the relationship of alcohol intake to risk of breast cancer in the study by Willett and associates.[21] The relative risks among women without other risk factors for breast cancer tended to be slightly higher in that study; as noted previously, the relative risk was 2.5 for ≥15 g/day of alcohol among women without other risk factors compared with 1.5 among women not in the low risk group. It is possible that this difference is simply a statistical expression of the fact that the effect of alcohol more closely approximates a constant attributable risk than a factor that is multiplicative with respect to other risk factors. However, it is clear that the issues of interaction will not be resolved without substantially larger data sets.

Ecologic Studies ■

Breslow and Enstrom examined the association between *per capita* alcoholic beverage consumption and age-adjusted breast cancer mortality rates in 41 states; a positive association was observed for beer but not wine or liquor.[31] Similarly, among 46 prefectures in Japan, positive associations were reported for beer and whiskey consumption, but not for sake or wine.[32] In a comparison of data from 14 countries, no association was observed between *per capita* intake of alcohol and breast cancer mortality.[33]

Geographic comparisons are generally considered to be among the weakest form of epidemiologic data; in the case of alcohol and breast cancer, their limitations are particularly serious. Most importantly, the data on alcohol intake are typically compiled on a *per capita* basis that includes men, women, and children, whereas breast cancer occurs virtually only among women. Because alcohol intake varies markedly according to gender in many cultures, these methods of estimating intake will result in serious

misclassification. Further, even if the observed association of alcohol consumption and breast cancer is causal, alcohol would be only part of the etiology of a disease that is clearly multifactorial, and one should not expect that alcohol would explain a major part of the large international difference in rates. For example, because the population attributable risk of alcohol can be estimated to be approximately 10% to 15%, an otherwise similar population that consumed no alcohol, such as Seventh Day Adventists, would be expected to experience a breast cancer rate only 10% to 15% lower. Indeed, Seventh Day Adventist women have breast cancer mortality rates that are 11% lower (p = NS) than the general US rates;[44] however, a difference this small could easily be due to other life-style factors or differences in detection and treatment of breast cancer. At the other extreme, French women do appear to drink more alcohol than US women. If the data from the control series in the study by Le and associates[7] are considered representative, it can be estimated that approximately one-third of French women drink ≥15 g/day of alcohol as compared with about one-sixth of the women in the US study by Willett and associates.[21] (About one-third of the women in both studies reported no alcohol intake.) If the relative risk of 1.6 for ≥15 g/day of alcohol reported by Willett and colleagues also applied to the one-sixth greater proportion of French women consuming this amount, then the French population would be expected to have a breast cancer rate only about 10% higher than the US population. Clearly, a difference of this magnitude could easily be obscured by the numerous other potentially relevant factors that differ among countries.

Attempts to evaluate the hypothesis that alcohol intake increases the risk of breast cancer by using geographic correlation are obviously futile intellectual exercises. Fortunately, alcohol consumption varies much more among women within most countries than does average intake between countries. Thus, case-control and cohort studies provide not only a much greater contrast in exposures but also the possibility of controlling for potential confounding variables at the individual level.

Animal Studies ■

The effects of alcohol and alcoholic beverages on the occurrence of mammary tumors in animals have been minimally examined. Schrauzer and co-workers found that long-term alcohol administration markedly depressed prolactin levels in C3H mice, while causing a strikingly earlier appearance of mammary tumors.[34] Red wine administration had a generalized growth-depressing effect and did not increase tumor incidence. Further animal studies could be useful; however, the relevance of these models to human breast cancer will always be uncertain.

Mechanisms by Which Alcohol May Lead to Breast Cancer ■

Because the pathologic events leading to breast cancer are so poorly understood, any discussion of mechanisms by which alcohol (or any other) exposure may lead to breast cancer is purely speculative. Alcohol is clearly implicated as a cause of upper gastrointestinal cancer[35] and readily reaches the breast tissue,[36] where it may alter membrane permeability[37] or have direct toxic effects. The primary metabolite of alcohol, acetaldehyde, is highly reactive and a known carcinogen under some circumstances.[38] Alcohol can increase lipid peroxidation[39] and may therefore lead to DNA damage by free radicals.[40]

Herbert and associates have noted that superoxide, which has been implicated in carcinogenesis, can be formed in alcohol metabolism, and that sulfite, which is added to wine during processing, can inhibit the formation of superoxide.[30] Williams has hypothesized that alcohol might increase the risk of breast cancer by stimulating prolactin release;[41] however, the effect of moderate alcohol intake on prolactin levels has not been defined. Stevens and Hiatt have suggested that alcohol may increase breast cancer risk by suppressing the diurnal variation in melatonin secretion.[42] The same moderate levels of alcohol consumption associated with elevated breast cancer risk have a major effect on liver metabolism,[21] and could thereby influence sex hormone levels and the activation or deactivation of exogenous carcinogens. Some have commented that the amounts of alcohol reported to be associated with elevated breast cancer risk are implausibly low. However, similar amounts are strongly associated with elevated HDL levels[21] and, in other studies, with substantially reduced risk of coronary heart disease,[43] thus indicating that these are potent pharmacologic doses.

Speculation regarding possible mechanisms for effect of alcohol on breast cancer risk may be useful in generating new and testable hypotheses that could ultimately enhance our basic understanding of this disease. However, lack of an established mechanism cannot be considered as evidence against the existence of a causal relationship because our basic understanding of the etiology of breast cancer is so limited.

Conclusion ■

Current epidemiologic data are reasonably consistent in demonstrating an association between alcohol intake and risk of breast cancer. The association appears to be present for all forms of alcoholic beverages and is very unlikely to be the result of chance. There seems to be a dose–response effect, but the shape of the curve is not well delineated. The present evidence is insufficient to conclude that the association is one of cause and effect, but no more plausible explanation has been proposed. The most definitive proof, a randomized trial, is not possible for ethical and feasibility reasons. Although the magnitude of the observed effect is relatively modest, the potential public health impact is large because moderate alcohol intake is so common and because there are few known ways to reduce risk of breast cancer. Moderate alcohol intake may confer a reduced risk of heart disease,[43] and this should also be considered in weighing risks and benefits.

References ■

1. Williams RR, Horm JW: Association of cancer sites with tobacco and alcohol consumption and socioeconomic status of patients. Interview study from the Third National Cancer Survey. JNCI 58:525–547, 1977
2. Rosenberg L, Slone D, Shapiro S, et al: Breast cancer and alcoholic beverage consumption. Lancet 1:267–271, 1982
3. Byers T, Funch DF: Letter: Alcohol and breast cancer. Lancet 1:799–801, 1982
4. Paganini-Hill A, Ross RK: Breast cancer and alcohol consumption (letter). Lancet 2:826–827, 1983
5. Begg CB, Walker AM, Wessen B, Zelen M: Letter: Alcohol consumption and breast cancer. Lancet 1:293–294, 1983
6. Webster LA, Layde PM, Wingo PH, Dry HW: Alcohol consumption and risk of breast cancer. Lancet 2:724–726, 1983
7. Le MG, Hill C, Kramar A, Flamant R: Alcohol beverage consumption and breast cancer in a French case-control study. Am J Epidemiol 120:350–357, 1984
8. Le MG, Moulton LH, Hill C, Kramar A: Consumption of dairy produce and alcohol in a case-control study of breast cancer. JNCI 77:633–636, 1986
9. Talamini R, La Vecchia C, Decarli A, et al: Social factors, diet and breast cancer in a northern Italian population. Br J Cancer 49:723–729, 1984
10. La Vecchia C, Decarli A, Francesci S, Pampallona S, Tognoi G: Alcohol consumption and the risk of breast cancer in women. JNCI 75:61–65, 1985
11. O'Connell OL, Hulka BS, Chambless LE, Wilkinson WE, Deubner DC: Cigarette smoking, alcohol consumption and breast cancer risk. JNCI 78:229–234, 1987
12. Harvey E, Schairer C, Brinton LA, Hoover RN, Fraumeni JF: Alcohol consumption and breast cancer. JNCI 78:657–661, 1987
13. Katsouyanni K, Trichopoulos D, Boyle P, Xirouchaki E, Trichopoulou A, Lisseas B, Vasilaros S, MacMahon B: Diet and

breast cancer: A case-control study in Greece. Int J Cancer 38: 815–820, 1986

14. Harris RE, Wynder EL: Breast cancer and alcohol consumption: a study in weak association. JAMA (in press)

15. Rohan TE, McMichael AJ: Alcohol consumption and risk of breast cancer. Int J Cancer: (in press)

16. Seidman H, Stellman SD, Muchinshi MH: A different perspective on breast cancer risk factors: Some implications of nonattributable risk. CA 32:3–15, 1982

17. Hiatt RA, Bawol RD: Alcoholic beverage consumption and breast cancer incidence. Am J Epidemiol 120:676–683, 1984

18. Hiatt RA, Klatsky A, Armstrong MA: Heavy alcohol consumption may increase the risk of breast cancer (abstr). Fed Proc 46:883, 1987

19. Hiatt RA, Klatsky AL, Armstrong MA: Alcohol consumption and the risk of breast cancer in a pre-paid health plan. Cancer Res 48:2284–2287, 1988

20. Schatzkin A, et al: Alcohol consumption and breast cancer in the epidemiologic follow-up study of the First National Health and Nutritional Examination Study. N Engl J Med 316:1169–1173, 1987

21. Willett WC, Stampfer MJ, Colditz GA, Rosner BA, Hennekens CH, Speizer FE: Moderate alcohol consumption and the risk of breast cancer. N Engl J Med 316:1174–1179, 1987

22. Gordon T, Kannel WB: Drinking and mortality: The Framingham study. Am J Epidemiol 126:97–107, 1984

23. Schmidt W, de Lint J: Causes of death of alcoholics. Q J Stud Alcohol 33:171–185, 1972

24. Nicholls P, Edwards G, Kyle E: Alcoholics admitted to four hospitals in England. Q J Stud Alcohol 35:841–855, 1974

25. Monson R, Lyons L: Proportional mortality among alcoholics. Cancer 36:1077–1079, 1975

26. Adelstein A, White G: Alcoholism and mortality. Population Trends 6:7–13, 1976

27. Longnecker P, Berlin JA, Orz MJ, Chalmers TC: A meta-analysis of alcohol consumption in relation to breast cancer risk. JAMA (in press)

28. Editorial: Does alcohol cause breast cancer? Lancet 1:1311–1312, 1985

29. Willett WC, Stampfer MJ, Colditz GA, Rosner BA, Hennekens CH, Speizer FE: Dietary fat and risk of breast cancer. N Engl J Med 316:22–28, 1987

30. Herbert V, Jayatilleke E, Shaw S: Letter: Alcohol and breast cancer. N Engl J Med 317:1287–1288, 1987

31. Breslow N, Enstrom J: Geographic correlation between cancer mortality rates and alcohol-tobacco consumption in the United States. JNCI 53:631–639, 1974

32. Kono S, Ikeda M: Correlation between cancer mortality and alcoholic beverage in Japan. Br J Cancer 40:449–455, 1979

33. La Vecchia C, Franceschi S, Cuzick J: Alcohol and breast cancer. Lancet 1:621, 1982

34. Schrauzer GN, McGinness JE, Ishmael D, Bell LJ: Alcoholism and cancer. I. Effects of long-term exposure to alcohol on spontaneous mammary adeno-carcinoma and prolactin levels in C3H/St mice. J Stud Alcohol 40:240–246, 1979

35. Tuyns AJ: Epidemiology of alcohol and cancer. Cancer Res 39:2840–2843, 1979

36. Lawton ME: Alcohol in breast milk. Aust NZ J Obstet Gynaecol 25:71–73, 1985

37. Freund G: Possible relationships of alcohol in membranes to cancer. Cancer Res 39:2899–2902, 1979

38. Ames BN, Magaw R, Gold LS: Ranking possible carcinogenic hazards. Science 236:271–280, 1987

39. Videla LA, Valenzuela Z: Alcohol ingestion, liver glutathione and lipoperoxidation: Metabolic interrelations and pathological implications. Life Sci 3:2395–2407, 1982

40. Ames BN: Dietary carcinogens and anticarcinogens: Oxygen radicals and degenerative diseases. Science 221:1256–1264, 1983

41. Williams RR: Breast and thyroid cancer and malignant melanoma promoted by alcohol-induced pituitary secretion of prolactin, T.S.H., and M.S.H. Lancet 1:996–999, 1976

42. Stevens RG, Hiatt RA: Letter: Alcohol and breast cancer. N Engl J Med 317:1287, 1987

43. Moore RD, Pearson TA: Moderate alcohol consumption and coronary artery disease: A review. Medicine 65:242–267, 1986

44. Phillips RL, Snowdon DA: Association of meat and coffee use with cancers of the large bowel, breast, and prostate among Seventh Day Adventists: Preliminary results. Cancer Res 43 (Suppl 5):2403s–2408s, 1983

Ernst L. Wynder
Randall E. Harris

Does Alcohol Consumption Influence the Risk of Developing Breast Cancer? Two Views

15b

Introduction ■

Epidemiologists find themselves embroiled in yet another controversy involving a cancer risk factor. The issue at hand is whether alcohol consumption increases the risk of breast cancer. The stakes are high. On the one hand, if breast cancer is indeed preventable by reduction in alcohol consumption, the public needs to be so informed. On the other hand, if the breast cancer–alcohol link is merely a red herring, or if definitive conclusions regarding the issue are premature, then notifying the public is of no benefit and, in fact, may do harm by creating alarm and confusion.

Epidemiologists have made key contributions to our understanding of factors influencing human cancer risk. In earlier years, epidemiology dealt with associations of relatively large magnitude, such as those linking smoking with lung cancer or alcohol abuse with cancer of the oral cavity. These associations were so sizable that even if a methodologic error had occurred, it would have been unlikely to seriously affect the conclusions reached. Now that the more obvious associations have been identified, we are left with associations of smaller magnitude (generally yielding relative risks of less than 3) that are more susceptible to errors in method or (what is particularly worrisome) questions of bias.

The proceedings of two workshops on the "Epidemiology of Weak Associations" have recently been published.[1,2] In both workshops, considerable concern

was expressed that such factors as case-control selection, confounding variables, bias (both in replies of interviewees and on the part of the investigators), and problems of subgroup analyses could lead to spurious "weak associations."

Weak associations between diseases and potential risk factors have often led to controversy and debate among epidemiologists and public health officials. Typically, an investigator first reports an association based on preliminary data and suggests hypothetic (unconfirmed) mechanisms of causality. The association, which may in fact be artifactual, indirect (noncausal), or direct (causal), then becomes the subject of intense independent investigation and debate. The possibility of an artifactual or spurious result can be eliminated only if the studies are adequately designed and conducted, and if research conducted in different geographic areas by independent investigators produces the same or similar statistical associations. Numerous examples of weak associations exist that apparently have not withstood the scrutiny of subsequent independent investigation (*viz.,* saccharin and bladder cancer, hair dye and breast cancer, coffee and cancer of the pancreas).[1] Even if an artifactual association can be ruled out, it is still necessary to determine whether the association is direct (causal) or indirect (noncausal) and merely due to confounding factors.

The relationship between moderate drinking and cancer of the breast, the subject of this chapter, has

283

received widespread public attention and has been the focus of many independent studies. Here, we summarize the various studies currently in the literature and interpret the available data, with particular emphasis on consistency with what is known in general about breast cancer epidemiology. As a basis for our evaluation, we have used the "criteria of judgment" so eloquently described in the Surgeon General's 1964 report on smoking and health.[3] We teach our students about these criteria of causality, yet we tend to overlook them when presenting our own data on the association between a risk factor and a serious disease, particularly when their application does not fit our hypothesis. Notable among these criteria are internal and external consistency and biologic plausibility. Clearly, if different investigators produce different results, we must question the reasons for such divergence, and if biologic mechanisms are postulated, they should be examined by metabolic studies to confirm causality.

It is our hope that an epidemiologic debate on the subject of alcohol and breast cancer will prove helpful in drawing appropriate conclusions from the available data that will benefit the scientific community and the public, and will also aid in crystallizing problems inherent in the epidemiology of weak associations.

Method ■

In evaluating the causal significance of the reported association between alcohol consumption and breast cancer, five criteria were utilized. These criteria, as specified by the 1964 report of the Surgeon General,[3]

comprise [a] consistency of the association; [b] strength of the association; [c] specificity of the association; [d] temporal relationship of the association; and [e] coherence of the association.

When considered together, these five criteria allow one to make a judgment about the weight of evidence supporting a causal interpretation of an association. In essence, the stronger the evidence for each criterion, the greater the likelihood that a given association has biologic relevance.

Results ■

Consistency of the Association ■

As defined in the Surgeon General's 1964 report,[3]

"This criterion implies that diverse methods of approach in the study of an association will provide similar conclusions. Consistency requires that the association be repeatedly observed by multiple investigators, in different locations and situations, at different times, using different methods of study. Such replication insures that the association is not likely to be an artifact due to bias and study methodology or subject selection, and that it is not indirect due to confounding variables such as diet, occupation, or genetics."

Basic results of the published studies of alcohol consumption and breast cancer are summarized in Figures 15b–1 and 15b–2. As of this writing, 5 prospective studies[4–8] and 12 case-control studies[9–21] have been reported. Of these 17 studies, 10 found a significant elevation in the relative risk (or odds ratio)

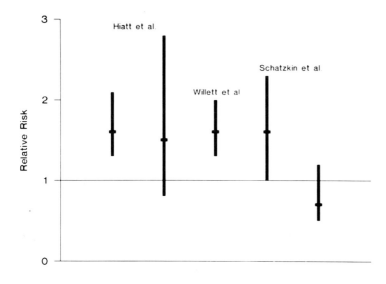

FIG. 15b–1 Prospective studies of alcohol and breast cancer. Studies are current to April 1988. Relative risks are estimated for moderate versus no consumption of alcohol, with 95% confidence intervals.

of breast cancer for moderate versus no alcohol consumption, where "moderate" refers to at least one drink of any alcoholic beverage per day (one shot of whiskey, one 4 oz glass of wine, or one 12 oz bottle of beer). However, among the positive studies, only a weak association is suggested, with reported odds ratios generally less than 2.0 for women who drink versus those who abstain.

Five cohort studies have now been published in which the incidence of breast cancer was prospectively determined and compared for women reporting different levels of alcohol consumption at baseline.[4-8] The four positive prospective studies[4-7] show remarkable consistency among the estimates of relative risk (see Fig. 15b–1), and suggest that women who report moderate levels of alcohol consumption are about 1.6 times more likely to develop breast cancer than those who report no consumption of alcohol. In marked contrast, the prospective study by Schatzkin and colleagues,[8] which is based on a recent analysis of the Framingham data, yielded a relative risk of 0.7, indicating just the opposite relationship—that women who abstain are about 1.4 times more likely to develop breast cancer than women who drink. Since the average relative risk value among the positive studies differs significantly from the single value of the negative study (1.6 versus 0.7, $p < 0.01$), these results do not appear to be consistent; that is, there is no indication that these relative risks scatter about some underlying true positive value.

A total of 12 case-control investigations have focused on the breast cancer and alcohol issue (see Fig. 15b–2).[9-21] Six of these studies show significant elevations in the odds ratios relating breast cancer and alcohol consumption,[9-15] whereas the remaining six do not.[16-21] The results of these studies also cluster into two distinct groups. Among the six positive studies, the average odds ratio is 1.62, with 95% confidence intervals (CI) of 1.46 to 1.80. Among the six negative studies, the average odds ratio is 0.98, with a 95% CI of 0.96 to 1.04. These average values differ from one another by more than 8 standard deviations ($p < 0.001$), indicating the presence of marked bimodal heterogeneity among the existing case-control investigations.

To assess the likelihood of publication bias, it is often useful to plot the logarithm of the relative risk (which is on a uniform scale) against the standard error of the logarithm of the relative risk and to then inspect this scatter plot for various patterns.[22] If the error among studies behaves like a random event, this procedure should yield a "funnel," wherein the point of the funnel points to the underlying true value. On the other hand, if there is publication bias, no such pattern should be visible, and the data would cluster in different quadrants. In Figure 15b–3, we have plotted results of the 17 studies of breast cancer and alcohol. Obviously, the data tend to cluster into two groups. The 11 positive studies have a mean relative risk of 1.60, with a 95% CI of 1.51 to 1.70, and the 7 negative studies have a mean relative risk of 0.94, with a 95% CI of 0.90 to 0.97. Mean values of these two clusters differ markedly, and the difference is highly significant ($p < 0.001$).

FIG. 15b–2 Case-control studies of breast cancer and alcohol consumption.

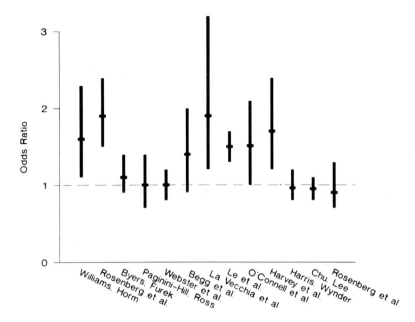

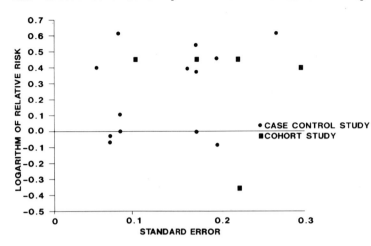

FIG. 15b–3 Plot of relative risk (on logarithmic scale) versus its standard error among studies of breast cancer and alcohol.

In summary, our evaluation indicates a marked lack of consistency in the magnitude of the reported odds ratios. The studies cluster into two groups, positive and negative, with little in between. We find no evidence to support the idea that the relative risk estimates that have been reported scatter around some true underlying value that is on the positive side of 1. This pattern of results argues against consistency of the alleged association between breast cancer and moderate alcohol consumption.

CONFOUNDING VARIABLES □

A major issue in all studies of any socioeconomic variable is the adjustment for potentially confounding variables. In our recent large case-control investigation of alcohol consumption and breast cancer,[21] several factors were found to influence alcohol consumption, including age, religion, education, occupation, marital status, body mass, and cigarette smoking. Specifically, women who drink are more frequently found among younger age groups, whites versus blacks or hispanics, divorcees versus other marital subgroups, highly educated women versus others, women in career-oriented professions versus others, and lean women. In addition, cigarette smoking generally shows a positive association with drinking; that is, the tendency to smoke cigarettes decreases with increasing age and body mass.

In our study,[21] we compared alcohol consumption patterns among 1467 patients with newly diagnosed and histologically confirmed breast cancer and 10,178 age-matched controls. As shown in Figure 15b–4, there were no significant differences in the frequency of drinking between cases and controls in any of the age groups examined. Further, in subsequent com-

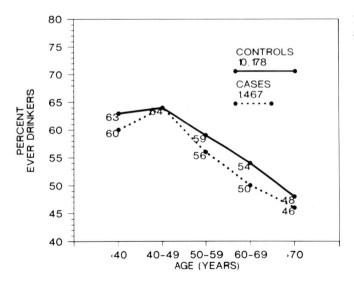

FIG. 15b–4 Alcohol consumption in breast cancer cases and hospital controls.

parisons of cases and controls for over 30 different subgroups of the data, the resultant odds ratios adjusted for pertinent confounders and interactions fluctuated randomly about 0.94 (SD = 0.12) and showed no consistent trend with increasing alcohol consumption. Nevertheless, one small subgroup of lean women (Quetelet Index <22) had elevated unadjusted odds ratios for breast cancer of 2.1, 1.7, and 1.4 associated with consuming <5, 5–15, and >15 g/day of alcohol, respectively. However, adjustment for a risk profile of confounding factors, including education and occupation (which are strong correlates of age at first pregnancy and parity) reduced these estimates to 1.4, 1.2, and 0.9, none of which differed significantly from 1.0 (Fig. 15b–5). The implication is that the observed elevations in the unadjusted odds ratios in the lean subgroup could merely have been the result of confounding by the other factors. Our interpretation is that social factors, including social drinking, have an impact on, or are confounded with, reproductive history, which in turn is the true risk factor associated with breast cancer.

Strength of the Association ■

Interpretation of the strength of an observed association is based on the following guidelines:[3]

> A relative risk ratio measures the strength of an association and provides an evaluation of the importance of that factor in the production of a disease. The greater the relative risk ratio . . . , the stronger the relationship between the etiologic agent and the disease. Important to the strength, as well as to the coherence of the association, is the presence of a dose–response phenomenon in which

a positive gradient between degree of exposure to the agent and incidence or mortality rates of the disease can be demonstrated.

A recent workshop on the epidemiology of weak associations focused on such problems as case-control selection, confounding variables, biases, subgroup analysis, criteria of judgment, and biologic plausibility.[20] Clearly, when it comes to alcohol consumption and breast cancer, we are dealing with a weak association. The reported odds ratios, even in positive studies, are less than 2.0 for women who drink versus those who abstain, and the weakness of the association is not further enhanced by clear dose–response relationships.

In the two positive cohort studies by Willett and colleagues[5] and Schatzkin and associates,[6] the increase in risk appears to reach an early plateau at <1 drink/day, as opposed to rising substantially with increasing dose. If alcohol were indeed a factor in breast cancer, one would expect that the relationship would be stronger in heavier drinkers (≥3 drinks/day). Hiatt and colleagues[7] recently reported relative risks for various levels of alcohol consumption among breast cancer patients and a random 10% sample of noncases in 58,347 women being followed prospectively. These relative risks also show an unusual dose–response pattern, ranging from nonsignificant values of 1.17 for <1 drink/day to 1.37 for 3–5 drinks/day, but then abruptly increasing to a significantly elevated value of 3.18 for ≥6 drinks/day. However, the estimate for the heavy-drinking category is based on only four breast cancer patients.

In the lean subgroup of females examined in our negative case-control investigation,[21] the unadjusted

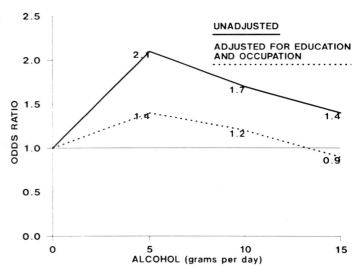

FIG. 15b–5 Odds ratios of breast cancer by increasing alcohol consumption in the lean subgroup of females.

estimates of risk also reached a plateau at <1 drink/day and then declined with increasing dose; more importantly, adjustments for confounding socioeconomic factors, themselves correlates of established breast cancer risk factors (late reproduction and nulliparity), reduced the estimates to near unity (see Fig. 15b–5). Moreover, the other positive studies do not reflect clear dose–response patterns, nor do they show that the risk increases with increasing duration of drinking,[9–14] and there is no evidence of any dose–response in the remaining negative studies.[8,16–20]

The absence of strength in this association, along with the "early plateau" dose–response patterns observed in positive studies, the disappearance of risk with adjustment for important confounding variables in one study, and a complete lack of dose–response relationships in the negative studies, provides little support for the thesis that alcohol has an etiologic role in breast cancer.

Specificity of the Association ■

Our evaluation of the specificity of the alcohol–breast cancer relationship is based on the following principles:[3]

> Specificity implies that a causal agent invariably leads to a single specific disease, an event rarely observed. A one to one relationship between the presence of an etiologic agent and disease would reflect a causal relationship. However, several points must be kept in mind in interpreting specificity in biological systems. First, an agent may be associated with multiple diseases. Second, many responses considered to be disease states have multiple causes. Third, a single pure substance in the environment may produce a number of different diseases. Fourth, a single factor may be the vehicle for several different substances. And fifth, there is no reason to assume that the relationships between one factor and different diseases have similar explanations. In summary, despite the fact that the demonstration of specificity in an association makes a causal hypothesis more acceptable, lack of specificity does not negate such an hypothesis, since many biological and epidemiologic aspects of the association must be considered.

Alcoholic beverages are somewhat complex mixtures consisting of many chemical substances[23] capable of producing more than a single biologic response. The three basic categories of alcoholic beverages are spirits, wine, and beer. The concentration of alcohol is in an approximate ratio of 8:2:1 for spirits, wine, and beer, which have alcohol concentrations of 40%, 10%, and 5%, respectively.

Only a few of the published studies have examined the question of specificity with respect to the type of alcohol consumed. In the study by Willett and colleagues,[5] statistically significant relative risks of about 1.5 were obtained for each type of beverage for women consuming at least 5 g/day of alcohol versus those who abstained. In that study, adjustment of the effect of each category attributable to the remaining two categories reduced the effect of wine to a nonsignificant level, whereas the effects of beer and spirits retained statistical significance even after adjustment. Similarly, the investigation by Harvey and coworkers[15] suggested the presence of independent effects of liquor and beer (odds ratios = 2.05 and 1.71 for at least 92 g/week of alcohol derived from liquor and beer, respectively) but not of wine (odds ratio = 0.77). In the latter study, the effects were confined to reported alcohol consumption before age 30. Finally, in the recent study by Hiatt and colleagues,[7] regular users of wine, liquor, and beer had similar but nonsignificantly higher risks of breast cancer compared to infrequent users of the corresponding type of alcohol relative to lifelong abstainers, and preference for specific beverage types had no independent effects on breast cancer risk.

We also examined type of alcohol in the case-control study described above.[21] As shown in Table 15b–1, the examination of total alcohol, as well as of alcohol from beer, wine, and spirits, provided no evidence of a positive relationship with breast cancer.

Thus, of the few results pertaining to specificity, three studies indicate weak specific effects of alcohol irrespective of the type of alcoholic beverage consumed, whereas one study indicates no effect of any specific type of alcoholic beverage on breast cancer risk. Again, there is inconsistency among studies in the specificity of the estimated effects, and these inconsistencies argue against alcohol as being etiologically important in breast cancer.

Temporal Relationship of the Association ■

The issue of temporality in reported risk associations is straightforward:[3]

> In any evaluation of the significance of an association, exposure to an agent presumed to be causal must precede, temporally, the onset of the disease which it is purported to produce.

Obviously, the criterion of temporality requires that alcohol consumption antedate the onset of disease,

Table 15b–1
Odds Ratios of Breast Cancer for Levels of Alcohol Consumption by Type of Alcohol, with 95% Confidence Levels (in Parentheses)*

Type of Beverage	Alcohol Consumption, g/day		
	<5	5–15	>15
Beer	0.9 (0.7–1.3)	1.0 (0.7–1.6)	1.0 (0.8–1.2)
Wine	1.3 (1.0–1.7)	1.4 (1.1–1.9)	0.9 (0.8–1.1)
Spirits	1.3 (1.0–1.7)	1.0 (0.9–1.2)	1.1 (0.9–1.4)
All types	1.0 (0.8–1.3)	1.1 (0.8–1.3)	1.0 (0.9–1.1)

* Estimates were adjusted for age and year at diagnosis in a multiple logistic regression model.

but temporality is more difficult to establish for diseases with long latency periods, such as breast cancer. Prospective studies minimize this difficulty, although they do not exclude the possibility that the disease was present in an undetected form before exposure to the specific agent.

In the case of strong causal associations between a risk factor and a cancer, *per capita* consumption or use of the specific factor can sometimes be shown to correlate with subsequent mortality rates of the resultant malignancy. For example, the antecedent pattern of *per capita* cigarette use in the United States strikingly parallels the rates of lung cancer following an approximate 20-year latency.[24] With respect to breast cancer mortality, however, the rates over time are remarkably constant and reflect no obvious secular trend,[25] whereas *per capita* alcohol consumption has nearly doubled in the United States since about 1935[26] and, as expected, has resulted in rising mortality due to cirrhosis of the liver (Fig. 15b–6). The

constancy of annual breast cancer mortality rates argues against the existence of a temporal relationship between breast cancer and antecedent alcohol consumption.

Indirect support for an association between a risk factor and disease can sometimes be obtained by examining ecologic correlations. Table 15b–2 presents a set of such ecologic correlations between 1975 age-adjusted breast cancer mortality and selected measures of alcohol consumption in women in 22 Western industrialized countries. Correlations are given for mortality rates due to cirrhosis of the liver, laryngeal cancer, and breast cancer in women[27] and the apparent alcohol consumption *per capita* in 1960 in these 22 nations.[28,29] The correlations involving cirrhosis of the liver, laryngeal cancer, and the crude measures of alcohol consumption utilized are positive and statistically significant. In contrast, breast cancer mortality is negatively correlated with mortality due to cirrhosis of the liver (r = −0.47, $p < 0.05$) and

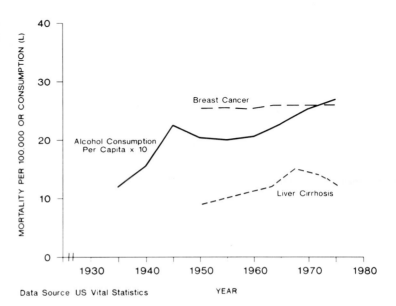

FIG. 15b–6 Trend data on breast cancer mortality, apparent alcohol consumption, and mortality due to cirrhosis of the liver in the United States.

Table 15b–2
Ecologic Correlations Between 1975 Age-Adjusted Breast Cancer Mortality and Measures of Alcohol Consumption in 22 Western Industrialized Countries

1975 Female Mortality	Cirrhosis of Liver	1960 Apparent Alcohol Consumption *per Capita**	
		Total	Women
Cirrhosis of liver	1.00	0.73†	0.81†
Laryngeal cancer	0.52†	0.57†	0.59†
Breast cancer	−0.41‡	−0.06	0.11

* Apparent alcohol consumption in liters *per capita,* was derived from data in Brenner[28] for each country (except Japan) by weighting the amounts of spirits, wine, and beer by factors of 0.40, 0.10, and 0.06, respectively, and then summing over the three beverage sources. Data for Japan were obtained from the Japanese Bureau of Tax.[29] Apparent alcohol consumption levels for women were estimated by weighting the total *per capita* levels by the ratio of female cirrhosis mortality to total cirrhosis mortality in each country.

† Statistically significant, $p < 0.01$.

‡ Statistically significant, $p < 0.05$.

shows no relationship to the 1960 *per capita* levels of alcohol consumption. The absence of an ecologic correlation between breast cancer mortality and antecedent alcohol consumption can be visualized in the scatter plot shown in Figure 15b–7. Further, other reported geographic and secular correlations between breast cancer incidence and alcohol consumption are nonsignificant or only weakly positive,[30,31] and significant effects of duration of drinking on breast cancer risk apparently have not been found either in cohort or case-control studies.[4–21] The existing evidence therefore does not support a temporal relationship between alcohol consumption and breast cancer.

Coherence of the Association ■

An important criterion in evaluating the causal significance of an association is its coherence with knowledge of the natural history and biology of the disease. As stated in the Surgeon General's 1964 report,[3]

Coherence requires that descriptive epidemiologic results on disease occurrence correlate with measures of exposure to the suspected agent. Perhaps the most important consideration here is the observation of a dose–response relationship between agent and disease, that is, the progressively increasing occurrence of disease in increasingly heavily exposed groups. [Inconsistencies in observed dose–responses are discussed in the section on strength of the association.] In order to establish the coherence of a specific association, other possible explanations for the association must be systematically considered and excluded or taken into account. Coherence is clearly established when the actual (physiologic) mechanism of disease production is defined.

Biologic plausibility is a key element in establishing coherence. At least four physiologic mechanisms have been proposed to explain the effect of alcohol on the development of breast cancer. It is important to stress that none of these mechanisms has been proved. The proposed mechanisms are induction of estrogens with stronger mitogenic and mutagenic activity, stimulation of prolactin release, increasing membrane permeability to carcinogens, and direct damage to the DNA.[4,6,7]

The potential role of estrogens (in particular, free estradiol) in breast cancer etiology has been extensively studied and reviewed,[32,33] and firm associations exist between breast cancer risk and early menarche,

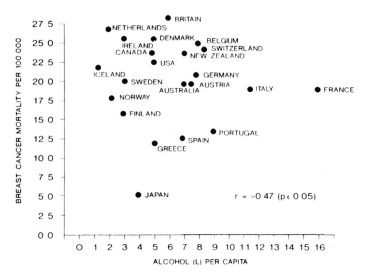

FIG. 15b–7 Plot of breast cancer mortality and 1960 alcohol consumption per capita.

late age at first pregnancy or nulliparity, and late menopause.[34] Although there is no general agreement on the role of estrogens in breast cancer, one view is that the crucial factor is the cumulative number of menstrual cycle-associated hormonal fluctuations to which the breast is exposed.[35]

There are few data on the effect of alcohol on female reproductive physiology and endocrine function. It is known, however, that women who are heavy drinkers tend to be infertile, have irregular menstrual cycles, and are more prone to amenorrhea.[36] Because these conditions generally are associated with low levels of estrogens, and amenorrhea may be protective with respect to breast cancer risk, these results appear incompatible with a role for alcohol-induced changes in endocrine function in elevating breast cancer risk.

Studies have also shown that alcohol consumption is associated with increased levels of sex-hormone-binding globulin (SHBG), which binds estradiol with high affinity.[37] Consequently, alcohol would be expected to increase plasma levels of SHBG, thereby reducing circulating levels of free estradiol, which is the biologically active fraction of the estrogen profile. This chain of events would therefore be expected to reduce rather than increase breast cancer risk by diminishing proliferation of breast ductal epithelium by free estradiol.

With respect to other postulated mechanisms unrelated to estrogens, there is no evidence regarding potentially carcinogenic membrane changes, toxicity, or DNA damage from alcohol in the ductal epithelium of breast tissue. Further, studies of the hypothalamic–pituitary axis indicate that high alcohol intake tends to suppress rather than increase circulating levels of prolactin.[38] Biologic plausibility, therefore, remains to be confirmed in this association.

STUDIES OF HEAVY DRINKERS □

Inhibition of estrogen metabolism by alcohol-induced damage to the liver has been suggested as an indirect mechanism by which alcohol might be involved in the etiology of breast cancer.[7] However, if this were true, then heavy-drinking subgroups should manifest high breast cancer rates, and known alcohol-related conditions such as alcoholism, cirrhosis of the liver, and pancreatitis should occur concomitantly with breast neoplasms more often than would be expected by chance. Contrary to these expectations, Monson and Lyon[39] found no increase in the proportionate rate of breast cancer among female alcoholics in the United States, and Lindegard[40] found no association of breast cancer with alcoholism, liver cirrhosis, or pancreatitis in a cohort of Swedish women. In the latter study, although alcohol-related conditions varied significantly with marital status, breast cancer did not. Nevertheless, Garfinkel and co-workers[41] observed increased standardized breast cancer mortality rates of 1.65 and 1.89 among heavy drinkers (5 or 6 drinks/day, respectively) in a cohort of 581,321 US women, but the numbers of cases in the heavy-drinking classes were relatively small, and rates for regular drinkers of 1–4 drinks/day were not significantly elevated.

Recently, we examined proportionate morbidity rates of breast cancer and other neoplasms in women veterans diagnosed in Veterans Administration (VA) hospitals.[42] In this cohort, which had an approximate twofold higher prevalence of alcohol abuse and chronic cigarette smoking than expected, the proportionate rates of neoplasms known to be related to alcohol and tobacco (cancers of the oral cavity, larynx, esophagus, and lung) were significantly elevated, but the rates of breast cancer were not. The standardized proportionate morbidity rates of breast cancer for white, black, and all women veterans were 0.92, 0.85, and 0.91, respectively. Based on these results, chronic alcohol abuse and its consequent medical conditions do not appear to be consistently associated with heightened breast cancer risk.

Conclusion ■

In this chapter, we have evaluated the association between alcohol consumption and breast cancer using the criteria of judgment specified in the 1964 Surgeon General's report.[3] The results can be summarized as follows:

1. There is a marked lack of consistency in the magnitude of relative risk estimates reported among studies, which cluster about a positive value of 1.60 and a null value of 0.96.
2. The strength of the association is weak, even in positive studies, with reported relative risk estimates generally being less than 2.0. Further, dose–response patterns are not consistent from study to study and, in positive studies, exhibit an early plateau that is not compatible with known mechanisms of carcinogenesis.
3. There is a paucity of information on the effects of specific types of alcohol, but again inconsistencies exist among different studies regarding the effects of wine, beer, and liquor.
4. Trend data do not support a temporal relationship between apparent *per capita* consumption of alcohol and breast cancer mortality either within the United States or internationally.

5. Although several biologic mechanisms have been postulated, none has been proven and, in fact, current results tend to argue against the biologic plausibility of an alcohol-induced endocrine effect that would result in heightened breast cancer risk. Studies of proportionate breast cancer rates in heavy-drinking populations do not indicate elevated rates of the disease, nor do they show an association with known alcohol-related diseases such as cirrhosis of the liver.

In conclusion, our evaluation of the existing experimental evidence does not support moderate alcohol consumption as an etiologically important factor in the development of breast cancer. However, we are *not* advocating the consumption of alcoholic beverages at any level. Prior investigations clearly indicate that heavy alcohol consumption is linked to cancers of the oral cavity, larynx, esophagus, and liver.[43–47] Moreover, the combined social costs of problem drinking in the United States, measured in terms of accidents, lost productivity, crime, other diseases, and death, amount to tens of billions of dollars annually, and the cost in broken homes, wasted lives, loss to society, and human misery is beyond calculation.[48] Nevertheless, as pointed out by Andrianopoulos and Nelson,[49] alcohol consumption is associated with many behavioral and psychosocial factors, and it is important that the data on breast cancer and alcohol be interpreted within the framework of the myriad of confounding variables that may accompany or be triggered by moderate or social drinking. Indeed, additional epidemiologic and metabolic studies will be required to determine definitively whether the association between moderate alcohol intake and breast cancer is real, or whether we are dealing with a web of confounding variables with social status at its center.

Epilogue ■

There have been a number of weak epidemiologic associations that have not withstood the scrutiny of independent investigation over time. One lesson to be learned from these examples is that epidemiologists should present exploratory data conservatively so that they will not be exploited by the media and cause unnecessary concern to society.

As epidemiologists, we need to be particularly aware of problem areas, such as case-control selection bias, confounding variables, and subgroup analysis, that may affect our findings either by yielding elevated relative risks that could be artifactual or indicating no risk when indeed a real risk may exist. Caution is

the order of the day. Data should be carefully interpreted by distinct guidelines such as the "criteria of judgment." Where a fit exists between rigid criteria and existing data, we should emphasize this, but at the same time we should not ignore those data that do not fit. Selective reporting and interpretation are not helpful.

Independent study with the passage of time tends to resolve epidemiologic controversy. On the basis of scientific discussions and the further exploration of existing or new data, we will eventually reach a consensus as to whether a particular epidemiologic association (in this case, social drinking and breast cancer) is causative or not. We are convinced that while the study of weak associations at times strains the epidemiologic tools available to us, in the long run, we have the capacity to determine the true nature of an observed association.

References ■

1. Wynder EL: Workshop on guidelines to the epidemiology of weak associations. Prev Med 16:139–141, 1987
2. Wynder EL: Workshop on the epidemiology of breast cancer and alcohol. Prev Med (in press)
3. US Public Health Service: Smoking and Health, Report of the Advisory Committee to the Surgeon General of the Public Health Service. US PHS Publ. No. 1103. Washington, DC, Department of Health, Education, and Welfare, Public Health Service, Centers for Disease Control, 1964
4. Hiatt RA, Bawol RD: Alcoholic beverage consumption and breast cancer incidence. Am J Epidemiol 120:676–683, 1984
5. Willett WC, Stamfer GA et al: Moderate alcohol consumption and the risk of breast cancer. N Engl J Med 316:1174–1180, 1987
6. Schatzkin A, Jones Y et al: Alcohol consumption and breast cancer in the epidemiologic follow-up study of the first national health and nutrition examination survey. N Engl J Med 316: 1169–1173, 1984
7. Hiatt RA, Klatsky AL, Armstrong MA: Alcohol consumption and the risk of breast cancer in a prepaid health plan. Cancer Res 48:2284–2887, 1988
8. Schatzkin A et al: Alcohol consumption and breast cancer in the NHANES I epidemiologic follow-up study and the Framingham heart study. Abstract in "Workshop on Breast Cancer and Alcohol." Prev Med (in press)
9. Williams RR, Horm JM: Association of cancer sites with tobacco and alcohol consumption and socioeconomic status of patients: Interview study from the Third National Cancer Survey. JNCI 58:525–547, 1977
10. Rosenberg L, Stone D, Shapiro S et al: Breast cancer and alcoholic-beverage consumption. Lancet 1:267–271, 1982
11. Begg CB, Walker AM, Wessen B et al: Alcohol consumption and breast cancer. Lancet 1:293–294, 1983
12. Le MG, Hill C, Kramar A et al: Alcoholic beverage consumption and breast cancer in a French case-control study. Am J Epidemiol 120:350–357, 1984
13. La Vecchia C, Decarli A, Franceschi S et al: Alcohol consumption and the risk of breast cancer in women. JNCI 75: 61–65, 1985

14. O'Connell DL, Hulka BS et al: Cigarette smoking, alcohol consumption, and breast cancer risk. JNCI 78:229–234, 1987

15. Harvey EB, Schairer C et al: Alcohol consumption and breast cancer. JNCI 78:657–661, 1987

16. Byers T, Funch DP: Alcohol and breast cancer. Lancet 1:799–800, 1982

17. Paganini-Hill A, Ross RK: Breast cancer and alcohol consumption. Lancet 2:626–627, 1983

18. Webster LA, Layde PM, Wingo PA et al: Alcohol consumption and risk of breast cancer. Lancet 2:724–726, 1983

19. Chu S, Lee N: Alcohol consumption and breast cancer: (case-control study of CDC. Abstract in "Workshop on Breast Cancer and Alcohol." Prev Med (in press)

20. Rosenberg L, Palmer JR, Moller DR, Clark A, Shapiro S: Alcohol and Breast Cancer: A case-control study. Abstract in "Workshop on Breast Cancer and Alcohol." Prev Med (in press)

21. Harris RE, Wynder EL: Breast cancer and alcohol: A study in weak associations. JAMA 259:2867–2871, 1988

22. Vandenbroucke JP: Passive smoking and lung cancer: A publication bias? Br Med J 296:391–392, 1988

23. Tuyns AJ: Alcohol. In Schottenfeld D, Fraumini JF Jr (eds): Cancer Epidemiology and Prevention, pp 293–303. Philadelphia, WB Saunders, 1982

24. Peto R, Doll R: Keynote address: The control of lung cancer. In Mizell M, Correa P (eds): Lung Cancer: Causes and Prevention, pp 1–19. Deerfield Beach, Verlag Chemie International, 1984

25. National Cancer Institute; Annual Cancer Statistics Review Including Cancer Trends: 1950–1985. NIH Publ. No. 88-2789. Bethesda, MD, US Department of Health and Human Services, 1988

26. Malin H, Coakley J, Kaelber C: An epidemiologic perspective on alcohol use and abuse in the United States. In Alcohol and Health Monograph No. 1, Alcohol Consumption and Related Problems, pp 99–153. Washington DC, US Government Printing Office, 1982

27. Cancer mortality and morbidity statistics, Japan and World. In Segi M, Tominago S, Aoki K, Fujimoto I (eds): GANN Monograph on Cancer Research No. 26. Tokyo, Japan, Japan Scientific Societies Press, 1981

28. Brenner MH: International trends in alcohol consumption and related pathologies. In Alcohol and Health Monograph No. 1, Alcohol Consumption and Related Problems, p 953. Washington, DC, US Government Printing Office, 1982

29. The Annual Report of Statistics. Tokyo, Japan, Japan National Bureau of Tax, 1980

30. Breslow NE, Enstrom JE: Geographic correlations between cancer mortality rates and alcohol-tobacco consumption in the United States. JNCI 53:631–639, 1974

31. Kono S, Ikeda M: Correlation between cancer mortality and alcohol beverage in Japan. Br J Cancer 40:440–449, 1979

32. Petrakis NL, Wrensch MR, Ernster VL et al: Influence of pregnancy and lactation on serum and breast fluid estrogen levels: Implications for breast cancer risk. Int J Cancer 40:587–591, 1987

33. Ernster VL, Wrensch MR, Petrakis NL et al: Benign and malignant breast disease: Initial study results of serum and breast fluid analyses of endogenous estrogens. JNCI 79:949–960, 1987

34. Kelsey JL: A review of the epidemiology of human breast cancer. Epidemiol Rev 1:47, 1979

35. Vorherr H: Breast Cancer: Epidemiology, Endocrinology, Biochemistry, and Pathology, p 487. Baltimore, Urban and Schwarzenberg

36. Blume SB: Women and alcohol. JAMA 256:1467–1470, 1986

37. Rose D: Effects of alcohol consumption on the endocrine system. In "Workshop on Alcohol and Breast Cancer." Prev Med (in press)

38. Witorsch RJ: Letter to the editor. N Engl J Med 317:1288, 1987

39. Monson RR, Lyon JL: Proportional mortality among alcoholics. Cancer 36:1077–1079, 1975

40. Lindegard B: Letter to the Editor. N Engl J Med 317:1285, 1987

41. Garfinkel L, Boffetta P, Stellman SD: Alcohol and breast cancer: a cohort study. In "Workshop on Breast Cancer and Alcohol." Prev Med (in press)

42. Harris RE, Spritz NE, Wynder EL: Studies of breast cancer alcohol. In "Workshop on Breast Cancer and Alcohol." Prev Med (in press)

43. Wynder EL, Bross IJ, Hirayama T: A study of the epidemiology of cancer of the breast. Cancer 13:559–601, 1960

44. Wynder EL, Bross IJ, Day EA: A study of environmental factors in cancer of the larynx. Cancer 9:86–110, 1957

45. Wynder EL, Hultberg S, Jacobsson F, Bross IJ: Environmental factors in cancer of the upper alimentary tract: A Swedish study with special reference to Plummer-Vincent (Patterson-Kelly) syndrome. Cancer 10:470–487, 1957

46. Harris RE, Hebert JR, Spritz NE, Wynder EL: Cancer risk in male veterans utilizing the Veterans Administration Medical System. Cancer (submitted for publication)

47. Yu H, Harris RE, Kabat GC, Wynder EL: Cigarette smoking, alcohol consumption, and primary liver cancer, a case-control study in the USA. Int J Cancer 42:325–328, 1988

48. Jaffe JH: Drug addiction and drug abuse. In Gilman AG, Goodman LS, Gilman A (eds): The Pharmacological Basis of Therapeutics, pp 535–584. New York, Macmillan, 1980

49. Andrianopoulos G, Nelson RL: Letter to the Editor. N Engl J Med 317:1286, 1987

Index

Page numbers followed by *f* indicate figures; numbers followed by *t* indicate tabular material.

A

abl oncogene, 11–12
Air pollution
    as carcinogen, 242–243
    epidemiologic studies of, 253–255
Alcohol
    breast cancer and, 267–292. *See also* Breast cancer
    as carcinogen and teratogen, 241–242
Anal cancer, 161–176
    at anal margin, 175
    anatomy in, 161–162, 162f
    etiology of, 163
    histology in, 162, 162f
    historical treatment of, 161
    incidence of, 162–163
    inguinal lymph node metastasis in, 174
    pathology in, 163–164, 164f
    patterns of treatment failure in, 165–166
    routes of spread of, 164
    staging of, 164–165, 165t
    symptoms and diagnosis of, 166–167
    therapy in, 167–174
        chemotherapy, 169
        combined, 169–172
        current, 172–174, 173f–174f
            chemoradiation schema in, 174f
            cisplatin in, 173
            mitomycin C in, 173
            radiation field in, 173, 173f
        radiation, 167–169
        surgical, 167
    treatment prospects in, 174–175

Anorectal fistula, malignant, 175
Antibody, monoclonal, with recombinant interleukin–2, 100–104, 103t, 104f
Antigens, major histocompatibility, recombinant cytokine effects on, 115–117, 116t–117t
Antisense compounds, 79–96. *See also* Oligos
Azidothymidine (AZT), 30

B

BKV early region genes, in transgenic mice, 66
BPV–1 early region genes, in transgenic mice, 67
Breast cancer
    inflammatory, 129–148
        axillary nodal involvement in, 132–133
        classification of, 132, 132t
        clinical signs and symptoms of, 130–131, 130f
        combination chemotherapy in, 138t–139t, 139–141
        differential diagnosis of, 131
        distant metastatic disease in, 133
        estrogen and progesterone receptors in tumor in, 133
        historical, 129
        hormonal manipulation in, 137–139
        incidence of, 129
        National Cancer Institute experience with, 142–147
            BMT and melphalan vs maintenance chemotherapy in, 146–147
            bone marrow transplant and melphalan in, 143
            disease-free and overall survival in, 145–146, 145f–147f

Breast cancer, inflammatory, National Cancer Institute experience with (*continued*)
    future directions of, 147–148
    growth factor therapy in, 148
    induction and maintenance chemotherapy in, 142–143
    initial and follow-up evaluation in, 142
    patient selection for, 142
    radiotherapy and mastectomy in, 143
    response to induction chemotherapy in, 144, 144f
    response to local therapy in, 144
    results of, 143–144, 144t
    statistical analysis of, 143
    toxicities in, 144–145, 145t
  natural history of, 133–134
  pathology in, 131–132
  patient characteristics with, 129–130
  prognostic factors in, 132–133
  radiation therapy in, 134–136, 135t
  surgery in, 134, 134t
  surgery plus radiation therapy in, 136–137, 137t
  Tunisian experience with, 133
  negative alcohol correlations in, 283–291
    causal significance of associations in, 284
    coherence of association in, 290–291
    confounding variables in, 286–287, 286f–287f
    consistency of association in, 284–287, 284f–287f
    heavy drinkers and, 291
    specificity of association in, 288, 289t
    strength of association in, 287–288, 287f
    temporal relationship of association in, 288–290, 289f–290f, 290t
    weak associations and, 283–284
  positive alcohol correlations in, 267–280
    alcohol intake measurement in, 276
    in alcoholics, 273–274, 274t
    animal studies of, 279–280
    attributable risk in, 278
    beverage type in, 276–277
    bias in case control studies of, 274–275
    case control studies of, 267–271, 268t–269t
    chance associations in, 274
    cohort studies of, 271–273, 272t
    confounding variables in, 275–276
    dose-response relationships in, 277–278
    ecologic studies of, 279
    effect modifiers in, 278–279
    mechanisms of, 280
    temporal aspects of exposure in, 278
  stage I (node-negative), 151–158
    Cardiff trial in, 157
    Eastern Cooperative and Southwest Oncology group trial in, 157
    future directions for adjuvant therapy in, 157–158
    Mainz adjuvant trial in, 155
    Milan adjuvant trial in, 156, 156f
    natural history of, 151–154
    NSABP adjuvant trial in,
      past, 154

    recent, 156–157
    oncogene amplification in, 153
    OSAKO adjuvant trial in, 155
    physical examination of axillary nodes in, 151, 152t
    relapse rate by estrogen receptor status in, 152, 153t
    relapse rate by tumor cell kinetic studies in, 152–153, 154f
    relapse rate by tumor size in, 151, 152t, 153t
    Scandinavian adjuvant trial in, 154–155
    tumor grading in, 152
    Wein adjuvant trial in, 156
    West Midlands adjuvant trial in, 155
  tamoxifen in, 179–189
    as adjuvant monotherapy in postmenopausal patients, 181–182, 182t
    chemotherapy plus, 182–184, 183f–184f
    extended monotherapy with, 184–185
    improving effectiveness of, 185–186, 185t, 186f
    long-term toxicology of, 186–188, 187f–188f
    in premenopausal patients, 185
Broccoli, as carcinogen, 242
Burkitt's lymphoma
  myc oncogene in, 16–17
  sis oncogene and, 8

C
Cancer, two-mutation theory of, 52–53
Cancer cell
  genetic changes in, 3–4
  propagation of, normal cellular propagation vs, 3
Cancer rates, 237
Carcinogens, 237–261
  animal models for predictions about, 259–260, 259f
  cancer trends and, 251–252
  cooking food and, 243
  dioxin vs alcohol and broccoli as, 241–242
  dose-response curve and, 243–244
  epidemiologic studies of, 252–258
    active and passive cigarette smoking in, 256
    air pollution in, 253–255
    dietary factors in, 256
    drinking water in, 255
    indoor radon in, 256–257
    interactions between life-styles and exposure in, 257–258, 257f
    molecular, 258–259, 258t
    occupation in, 252–253, 253t
    pesticides and chemical preservatives in, 255–256
  exposure estimates for, 251t
  human exposure rodent potency (HERP) index of, 238, 239t, 260–261, 260t
  industrial, 249–261
    environmental monitoring of, 249–251, 250t–251t
  man-made pesticides as, 240–241
  natural, 237–245
    evolution and, 241

natural pesticides as, 240
nonscientific considerations in, 261
occupational, 243
pollution as, epidemiologic studies of, 244–245
rodent tests of, 243
technologic advances and, 245
Carcinoma
anal. *See* Anal cancer
breast. *See* Breast cancer
extrapulmonary small cell, chromosomal heterozygosity in, 57, 57t
hepatocellular, *myc* oncogene in, 17
non-small cell lung, chromosome 3p in, 57
renal cell, chromosomal deletions in, 48–54. *See also* Renal cell carcinoma
small cell lung
chromosome 3p polymorphisms in, 46–47, 54–57, 54t, 55f–56f
*erb*A oncogene in, 17
squamous cell, epidermal growth factor receptor in, 10
Chemicals, carcinogenic and teratogenic, 237–238
Chondrosarcoma, neutron irradiation in, 231–232, 232t
Chordoma, neutron irradiation in, 230
Choroid plexus tumors, in transgenic mice, harboring SV40 early region genes, 63–64
Chromosome
DNA polymorphism in, 41–42
Philadelphia, in chronic myelogenous leukemia, 11–12
Chromosome 3
banding pattern of, 44f, 45
linkage maps for, 48, 48f
Chromosome 3p
linkage maps for, 48, 48f
in non-small cell lung carcinoma, 57
polymorphic probes for, 47–48, 47t
in renal cell carcinoma, 45–46, 45f–46f, 49–52, 49f–51f, 52t
in small cell lung carcinoma, 46–47, 54–57, 54t, 55f–56f
Chromosome 11p, in renal cell carcinoma, 52
Chromosome 13, in small cell lung carcinoma, 56–57
Chromosome 17, in small cell lung carcinoma, 56–57
Cigarette smoking, active and passive, 256
Cisplatin, side effects of, renal, 217, 217t
Condyloma acuminatum, squamous cell carcinoma with, 175
crk oncogene, 13
Cyclophosphamide
host component in effectiveness of, 119–120
with recombinant interleukin–2, 99–121, 100–102, 100f–101f, 102t
with recombinant tumor necrosis factor, 111, 112f, 113t

D
Daminozide, dietary intake of, 250, 250t
Diabetes mellitus, transgenic mouse model and, 73

Diet, carcinogenesis and, 256
Dioxin, as carcinogen, 241–242
DNA polymorphism
chromosomal, 41–42
in linkage analysis, 44–45
in solid tumors, detection of, 43–44, 43f–44f
Down's syndrome
ets–2 oncogene in, 19
transgenic mouse model and, 73
Doxorubicin, with recombinant tumor necrosis factor, 111

E
Environmental monitoring, of industrial pollutants, 249–251, 250t–251t
*erb*A oncogene, 17
*erb*B oncogene, epidermal growth factor receptor and, 9
Ethyl phosphotriesters, new chemotherapy with, 94
ets–2 oncogene, 18–19
Ewing's sarcoma, *sis* oncogene and, 8

F
5-Fluorouracil, with recombinant tumor necrosis factor, 111
fms oncogene, 8–9
fos oncogene, 14–16

G
Gallium, 205–218
bone cell function effects of, 209–210, 209f–210f
bone mineral effects of, 208–209, 208f
bone protein effects of, 210–211
in cancer-related hypercalcemia, 211–213, 211f–213f, 212t
historical development of, 205–206
as anticancer agent, 205–206
as medical radionuclide, 205
hypocalcemic effects of, 206
incorporation and anatomic localization in bone of, 206–208, 207f
laboratory studies of, 206–211
in malignant osteolysis, 215–217, 216f–217f
in parathyroid carcinoma, 213–214, 214f
pharmacology of, 206
side effects of, 217–218, 217t
hematologic, 218
metabolic, 218
renal, 217, 217t
Genes, retroviral, malignant transformation by, 4
G-proteins, 13
Growth factor
defective, oncogene proteins and, 8–9
in inflammatory breast cancer therapy, 148
in mitogenesis, 6–7
GTP-binding regulatory proteins, 13

H

Head and neck cancer, neutron irradiation in, 227, 228f
Heart disease, transgenic mouse model and, 73
Hematopoietic disease, transgenic mouse model in, 68–69
Hemophilia B, transgenic mouse model and, 73
Hepatitis B, transgenic mouse model and, 73
Hepatocellular carcinoma, *myc* oncogene in, 17
HTLV–1/*tat* fusion genes, in transgenic mice, 70–71
Human exposure rodent potency (HERP) index, 238, 239t, 260–261, 260t
Human immunodeficiency virus (HIV)
  life cycle of, 29
  oligos in genetic inhibition of, 86–89, 88f–89f
Hypercalcemia, cancer-related, gallium in, 211–213, 211f–213f, 212t

I

Impotence, 193–202
  in cancer patients, 198–202
    arterial revascularization for, 200
    hormonal therapy for, 199
    intracavernous injection of vasoactive agents in, 199–200, 199t–200t
    penile prosthesis for, 201–202, 201f–202f
    penile vein excision and ligation for, 200
    psychotherapy for, 198–199
    vacuum suction devices for, 200–201
  cavernous artery evaluation in, 198
  etiology of, 195–196
    associated conditions in, 196
    neurovascular injury in, 195
    radiation therapy in, 195
  evaluation of, 196–198
  laboratory examination in, 197
  medical and sexual history in, 196
  penile vein evaluation in, 198
  pharmacologic evaluation of, 197–198
  physical and neurologic examination in, 196–197
Interferon
  recombinant
    host component in effectiveness of, 117–119, 119t
    MHC antigen effects of, 115–116
    with tumor necrosis factor, 109–110
    with recombinant interleukin–2, 104–108, 105t–107t
    with recombinant interleukin–2 and tumor-infiltrating lymphocytes, 108–109, 108t
Interleukin–2, recombinant
  with chemotherapeutic agents, 99–121, 100–102, 100f–101f, 102t
  host component in effectiveness of, 117–119, 119t
  with interferons, 104–108, 105t–107t
  with interferons and tumor-infiltrating lymphocytes, 108–109, 108t
  MHC antigen effects of, 115, 116t–117t
  with monoclonal antibody, 100–104, 103t, 104f
  with tumor necrosis factor, 110–111, 110f, 111t
Interleukin–4, recombinant, 112–115, 113t–114t

J

JCV early region genes, in transgenic mice, 66
jun oncogene, 17–18

L

Leukemia
  acute lymphocytic, Philadelphia chromosome in, 12
  acute myelocytic, Philadelphia chromosome in, 12
  chronic myelogenous
    Philadelphia chromosome in, 11–12
    sis oncogene and, 8
Lung carcinoma
  non-small cell, chromosome 3p polymorphisms in, 57
  small cell
    chromosome 3p polymorphisms in, 46–47, 54–57, 54t, 55f–56f
    chromosome 13 and 17 polymorphisms in, 56–57
    *erb*A oncogene in, 17
Lymphocytes, tumor infiltrating
  host component in effectiveness of, 120–121
  with interferons and recombinant interleukin–2, 108–109, 108t
Lymphokine combinations, immunotherapy with, 99–121. *See also* Interleukin–2, recombinant
Lymphoma, Burkitt's
  myc oncogene in, 16–17
  sis oncogene in, 8

M

Major histocompatibility antigens, recombinant cytokine effects on, 115–117, 116t–117t
Methotrexate (MTX), transgenic mouse model of resistance to, 71
met oncogene, 10
Methylphosphonates, new chemotherapy with, 94
Mitogenic signal pathway
  amplified gene expression in, 20
  components of, 5f, 6f
  insertional genetic activation in, 20
  intermediate steps in, 12–13
  oncogenes in, 3–27
  point mutations in, 21
  specific repression in, 20
MMTV/H*ras* fusion genes, in transgenic mice, 67t, 68
MMTV/*myc* fusion genes, in transgenic mice, 67–68, 67t
MMTV/*onc* fusion genes, in transgenic mice, 67–68, 67t
Mouse model, transgenic, 61–74
  chemotherapeutic resistance in, 71
  further applications of, 73
  harboring BKV early region genes, 66
  harboring BPV–1 early region genes, 67
  harboring HTLV–1/*tat* fusion genes, 70–71
  harboring JCV early region genes, 66
  harboring MMTV/H*ras* fusion genes, 67t, 68

harboring MMTV/*myc* fusion genes, 67–68, 67t
harboring MMTV/*onc* fusion genes, 67–68, 67t
harboring PyV early region genes, 66–67
harboring SV40 early region genes, 63–66
    choroid plexus tumors in, 63–64
    other tumors in, 63t, 65–66
    pancreatic tumors in, 64–65
in hematopoietic disease, 68–69
pleuripotential mouse embryonic stem cell lines in, 71–73, 72f
preimplantation infection with retroviral vectors in, 73
promiscuous oncogene expression in, 69–70
pronuclear injection for creation of, 61–62, 62f
proto-oncogene deregulated expression in, 70
tissue specificity of oncogene action in, 69
myc oncogene, 16–17
    oligos inhibition of, 93–94, 93f

N
neu oncogene, 10
Neutron irradiation, 221–232
    advantages of, 221
    in chondrosarcoma, 231–232, 232t
    in chordoma, 230
    in head and neck tumors, 227, 228f
    historical, 221–222
    in osteogenic sarcoma, 230–231, 231t
    in prostate tumors, 223–226, 224f–225f, 226t
    in salivary gland tumors, 222–223, 222f–223f, 223t–224t
    in soft tissue sarcoma, 227–230, 229t

O
Oligos
    automated synthesis of, 82f
    cancer and, 93–94, 93f
    cellular uptake of, 80–82, 84f–85f
    with covalently linked groups, 90–92, 91f–92f
    hybridization of, 82–83, 86f–88f
    in vivo stability of, 79–80
    as inhibitors of gene expression, 83–90
        HIV gene and, 86–89, 88f–89f
        viral genes and, 84–86
    as inhibitors of mRNA expression, in cell-free and bacterial systems, 89–90
    mechanisms of action of, 92–93, 92f
    new chemotherapy with, 94–95, 94f–95f
    normal and modified, structure of, 80
Oncogene
    abl, 11–12
    crk, 13
    definition of, 4, 37
    *erb*A, 17
    *erb*B, 9
    ets–2, 18–19
    fms, 8–9

fos, 14–16
jun, 17–18
met, 10
in mitogenic signal pathway, 3–27
myc, 16–17
    oligos inhibition of, 93–94, 93f
neu, 10
nuclear, 14–19
proteins encoded by, 4
ras, 13–14
recessive, criteria for, 53–54
sis, 7–8
src, 10–11
in stage I (node-negative) breast cancer, 153
in transgenic mouse model, 69–70
Osteogenesis imperfecta, transgenic mouse model and, 73
Osteogenic sarcoma, neutron irradiation in, 230–231, 231t
Osteolysis, malignant, gallium in, 215–217, 215f–216f

P
Pancreatic tumors, in transgenic mice, harboring SV40 early region genes, 64–65
Parathyroid carcinoma, gallium in, 213–214, 214f
Penis. *See also* Impotence
    erection of
        mechanism of, 194
        pharmacology of, 194–195, 194t
    functional anatomy of, 193, 194f
Pesticides
    as carcinogens, 255–256
    man-made, 240–241
    natural, 240
Philadelphia chromosome, in chronic myelogenous leukemia, 11–12
Phosphatidylinositol, in mitogenic signal pathway, 12
Phosphorothioates, new chemotherapy with, 94
Pollution
    air, 242–243
        epidemiologic studies of, 253–255
    as carcinogen, 244–245
    industrial, environmental monitoring of, 249–251, 250t–251t
    technologic advances and, 245
    water, 242
Preservatives, chemical, as carcinogens, 255–256
Prostate tumors, neutron irradiation in, 223–226, 224f–225f, 226t
Protein, encoded by oncogenes, 4
Protein kinase C, in mitogenic signal pathway, 12
Protein tyrosine kinase, in mitogenic signal pathway, 12
Proto-oncogene
    definition of, 4
    deregulated expression of, in transgenic mouse model, 70
PyV early region genes, in transgenic mice, 66–67

300 Index

R

Radiotherapy, neutron, 221–232. *See also* Neutron irradiation
Radon, carcinogenesis and, 256–257
Radon gas, 242–243
ras oncogene, 13–14
Receptor
  colony-stimulating factor–1, *fms* oncogene and, 8–9
  epidermal growth factor
    *erb*B oncogene and, 9
    platelet derived growth factor receptor vs, 10
    in squamous cell carcinoma, 10
  growth factor
    in mitogenesis, 6–7
    oncogene proteins and, 7–8
  platelet derived growth factor
    activation of, 10
    epidermal growth factor receptor vs, 10
    sis oncogene and, 7–8
Renal cell carcinoma, 48–54
  chromosome 3p in, 45–46, 45f–46f
  familial, 48–49
  onset of somatic mutations in, 54
  sporadic
    chromosome 3p polymorphism in, 45f–46f, 49–52, 49f–51f, 52t
    chromosome 11p polymorphism in, 52
Renal oncocytoma, 49
Retroviral genes, malignant transformation by, 4
Retrovirus, in mitosis and malignancy studies, 4
Reverse transcriptase, HIV, 29–38
  chemotherapy and, 37–38
  drug screening and drug design and, 35–36
  expression in *E. coli* of, 30–33, 31f–33f
  monoclonal antibodies and, 36–37, 36f
  mutagenic studies of, 33–35, 34t
  structural studies of, 33
Ribosomal protein S6 kinase, in mitogenic signal pathway, 12

S

Salivary gland tumors, neutron irradiation in, 222–223, 222f–223f, 223t–224t

Sarcoma, Ewing's, *sis* oncogene and, 8
sis oncogene, 7–8
Soft tissue sarcoma, neutron irradiation in, 227–230, 229t
Southern transfer analysis, 42
Squamous cell carcinoma, epidermal growth factor receptor in, 9
src oncogene, 10–11
SV40 early region genes, in transgenic mice, 63–66

T

Tamoxifen
  in breast cancer, 179–189. *See also* Breast cancer
  in dimethylbenzanthracene-induced rat mammary carcinoma, 179–180, 180f
  evidence of chemosuppression with, 181
  in heterotransplanted breast cancer in athymic mice, 181, 181f
  metabolism of, 179, 180f
  in n-nitrosomethylurea-induced rat mammary carcinoma, 180
  in spontaneous mouse mammary tumors, 180–181
Tumor inflitrating lymphocytes, host component in effectiveness of, 120–121
Tumor necrosis factor, recombinant
  with chemotherapeutic agents, 111, 112f, 113t
  host component in effectiveness of, 118–119, 119f
  with interleukin–2, 110–111, 110f, 111t
  with recombinant interferon, 109–110
Tumor promoters, cellular, 3

V

von Hippel-Lindau disease
  familial, 48
  genetic predisposition to, 54

W

Water, drinking, as carcinogen, 255
Water pollution, as carcinogen, 242

ISBN 0-397-51004-7